Lung Cancer Metastasis

Novel Biological Mechanisms and Impact on Clinical Practice

Venkateshwar Keshamouni · Douglas
Arenberg · Gregory Kalemkerian
Editors

Lung Cancer Metastasis

Novel Biological Mechanisms and Impact
on Clinical Practice

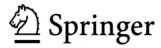 Springer

Editors

Venkateshwar G. Keshamouni
Division of Pulmonary and Critical
  Care Medicine
Department of Internal Medicine
University of Michigan Health System
109 Zina Pitcher Place
Ann Arbor MI 48109-2200
Biomedical Science Res. Bldg.
USA
vkeshamo@umich.edu

Douglas A. Arenberg
Division of Pulmonary and Critical
  Care Medicine
University of Michigan Medical Center
Department of Internal Medicine
1150 W. Medical Center Dr.
6301 MSRB III
Ann Arbor, MI 48109–5642
darenber@umich.edu

Gregory P. Kalemkerian
Division of Hematology/Oncology
Department of Internal Medicine
University of Michigan
C350 MIB - SPF 5848
1500 E. Medical Center Drive
Ann Arbor, MI 48109-5848
USA
kalemker@umich.edu

ISBN 978-1-4419-0771-4   e-ISBN 978-1-4419-0772-1
DOI 10.1007/978-1-4419-0772-1
Springer New York Dordrecht Heidelberg London

Library of Congress Control Number: 2009933691

Printed on acid-free paper

Springer is part of Springer Science+Business Media (www.springer.com)

Preface

Lung cancer is the leading cause of cancer-related mortality, killing more than the combined tolls of breast, prostate, and colorectal cancers. In spite of this, the number of investigators studying this disease and the volume of funding devoted to lung cancer lag far behind these common solid tumors and other less lethal diseases. Metastatic lung cancer is responsible for more than 90% of lung cancer-related deaths. However, relatively little progress has been made in understanding the process of metastasis. The two main aims of this book are (a) to introduce clinical concepts to basic scientists and basic molecular and cellular concepts to clinical investigators, in order to promote collaboration and foster much needed translational research and (b) to introduce new and emerging concepts and approaches in metastasis research to the lung cancer research community at large. To accomplish these goals, this book covers a broad spectrum of subjects ranging from current trends in the clinical management of metastatic disease to the systems biology approach for gaining insights into the mechanisms of metastasis. Some of the subjects covered include defining basic hallmarks of the metastatic process, the concept of tumor stem cells, epithelial–mesenchymal transitions, evasion of immune surveillance, tumor–stromal interactions, angiogenesis, molecular imaging, and biomarker discovery. Authors who are actively involved in lung cancer research or lung cancer patient care and have made original contributions in their area of expertise have written the chapters of this book. While seeking contributions, we realized how little we know about the various aspects that are covered, re-emphasizing the need for a book like this. We hope that this book will stimulate others to take up the investigation of lung cancer metastasis. In writing and editing the chapters, we have put forth our best effort to make the material accessible to graduate students, postdoctoral fellows, and clinical fellows who are at the beginning of their careers, while maintaining utility for the more seasoned investigator. We hope that this book will provide a stimulating overview for both clinical and basic science investigators in the field of lung cancer research. Finally, we thank all the authors for their outstanding contributions in preparing this book.

Ann Arbor, Michigan

Venkateshwar G. Keshamouni
Douglas A. Arenberg
Gregory P. Kalemkerian

Contents

Contributors

Steven M. Albelda, M.D. Thoracic Oncology Research Laboratory, Pulmonary and Critical Care Division, University of Pennsylvania Medical Center, Philadelphia, PA 19104-6160, USA, albelda@mail.med.upenn.edu

Angel Alvarez Department of Chemical Engineering, University of Michigan, Ann Arbor, MI 48109, USA, angelpr@umich.edu

Douglas A. Arenberg, M.D. Division of Pulmonary and Critical Care Medicine, Department of Internal Medicine, University of Michigan, Ann Arbor, MI 48109-5642, USA, darenber@umich.edu

Mahaveer Swaroop Bhojani, Ph.D. Center for Molecular Imaging, Department of Radiation Oncology, University of Michigan, Ann Arbor, MI 48109, USA, mahaveer@umich.edu

Bizhan Bandarchi, M.D. Ontario Cancer Institute and Princess Margaret Hospital, University Health Network and University of Toronto, Toronto, Ontario M5G 2M9, Canada, bbandarc@uhnres.utoronto.ca

M. Cecilia Crisanti, M.D. Thoracic Oncology Research Laboratory, Department of Surgery, University of Pennsylvania Medical Center, Philadelphia, PA 19104-6160, USA, ceciliacrisanti@yahoo.com

James D. Cavalcoli, Ph.D. Center for Computational Medicine & Biology, University of Michigan Medical School, Ann Arbor, MI 48109-2218, USA, cavalcol@umich.edu

Steven M. Dubinett, M.D. Division of Pulmonary and Critical Care Medicine and Hospitalists, Department of Medicine, UCLA Lung Cancer Research Program, Jonsson Comprehensive Cancer Center, David Geffen School of Medicine at UCLA, Los Angeles, CA 90095, USA, sdubinett@mednet.ucla.edu

Zvi G. Fridlender, M.D. Thoracic Oncology Research Laboratory, Pulmonary and Critical Care Division, University of Pennsylvania Medical Center, Philadelphia, PA 19104-6160, USA, gfrid@mail.med.upenn.edu

Mark M. Fuster, M.D. Division of Pulmonary and Critical Care, Department of Medicine, University of California San Diego and VA San Diego Healthcare System, San Diego, CA, USA, mfuster@ucsd.edu

Shirish M. Gadgeel, M.D. Wayne State University/Karmanos Cancer Institute, Detroit, MI 48201, USA, gadgeels@karmanos.org

Edward Garon, M.D. Division of Hematology and Oncology, Department of Medicine, UCLA Lung Cancer Research Program, Jonsson Comprehensive Cancer Center, David Geffen School of Medicine at UCLA, Los Angeles, CA 90095, USA, egaron@mednet.ucla.edu

Kaustabh Ghosh, Ph.D. Vascular Biology Program, Children's Hospital/ Harvard Medical School, Boston, MA 02115, USA, kaustabh.ghosh@childrens.harvard.edu

James Hayman, M.D., M.B.A. Department of Radiation Oncology, University of Michigan, Ann Arbor, MI 48109, USA, hayman@umich.edu

Saswati Hazra, Ph.D. Division of Pulmonary and Critical Care Medicine and Hospitalists, Department of Medicine, UCLA Lung Cancer Research Program, Jonsson Comprehensive Cancer Center, David Geffen School of Medicine at UCLA, Los Angeles, CA 90095, USA, shazra@mednet.ucla.edu

Jaclyn Y. Hung, Ph.D. Greehey Children's Cancer Research Institute and Department of Pediatrics, University of Texas Health Science Center, San Antonio, Texas 78229-3900, USA, hungj@uthscsa.edu

David M. Jablons, M.D. Thoracic Oncology Program, Comprehensive Cancer Center, University of California San Francisco, CA, USA, jablonsd@surgery.ucsf.edu

Michael R. Johnston, M.D. Division of Thoracic Surgery, Department of Surgery, Dalhousie University, Halifax, Nova Scotia, Canada, mrj2@mac.com

Gregory P. Kalemkerian, M.D. Division of Hematology/Oncology, Department of Internal Medicine, University of Michigan, Ann Arbor, MI 48109-5848, USA, kalemker@umich.edu

Ella A. Kazerooni, M.D., M.S. Department of Radiology, University of Michigan, Ann Arbor, MI 48109, USA, ellakaz@umich.edu

Ellen C. Keeley Division of Cardiovascular Medicine, Department of Medicine, University of Virginia, Charlottesville, VA 22908, USA, eck6v@virginia.edu

Venkateshwar G. Keshamouni, Ph.D. Division of Pulmonary and Critical Care Medicine, Department of Internal Medicine, University of Michigan, Ann Arbor, MI 48109-2200, USA, vkeshamo@umich.edu

Venkataramu Krishnamurthy, M.D. Department of Radiology, University of Michigan, Ann Arbor, MI 48109, USA, venkkris@umcih.edu

Jay M. Lee, M.D. Division of Cardiothoracic Surgery, Department of Surgery, UCLA Lung Cancer Research Program, Jonsson Comprehensive Cancer Center, David Geffen School of Medicine at UCLA, Los Angeles, CA 90095, USA, jaymoonlee@mednet.ucla.edu

Jiang Liu, M.D., PhD. Division of Applied Molecular Oncology, Princess Margaret Hospital, University Health Network, University of Toronto, Toronto, Ontario, M5G 2M9, Canada, jiang.liu@utoronto.ca

Borna Mehrad Division of Pulmonary and Critical Care Medicine, Department of Medicine, University of Virginia, Charlottesville, VA 22908, USA, mehrad@virginia.edu

Aristidis Moustakas Ludwig Institute for Cancer Research, Uppsala University, SE-751 24 Uppsala, Sweden, aris.moustakas@licr.uu.se

Roya Navab, Ph.D. Ontario Cancer Institute and Princess Margaret Hospital, University Health Network and University of Toronto, Toronto, Ontario M5G 2M9, Canada, rnavab@uhnres.utoronto.ca

Shyam Nyati, Ph.D. Center for Molecular Imaging, Department of Radiation Oncology, University of Michigan, Ann Arbor MI 48109 USA, shyamnya@umich.edu

Kevin S. Oh, M.D. Massachusetts General Hospital, Boston, MA, USA, koh2@partners.org

Gilbert S. Omenn, M.D. Center for Computational Medicine & Biology, University of Michigan Medical School, Ann Arbor, MI 48109-2218, USA, gomenn@umich.edu

Charlie Pan, M.D. Department of Radiation Oncology, University of Michigan, Ann Arbor, MI 48109, USA, cpan@umich.edu

Allan Pickens, M.D. Section of Thoracic Surgery, Department of Surgery, University of Michigan, Ann Arbor, MI 48109, USA, allanp@umich.edu

Suresh S. Ramalingam, M.D. Emory University School of Medicine, Emory Winship Cancer Institute, Atlanta, GA, USA, suresh.ramalingam@emoryhealthcare.org

Hyma R. Rao Center for Molecular Imaging, Department of Radiation Oncology, University of Michigan, Ann Arbor, MI 48109, USA, hrrao@umich.edu

Alnawaz Rehemtulla, Ph.D. Center for Molecular Imaging, Department of Radiation Oncology, University of Michigan, Ann Arbor, MI 48109, USA, alnawaz@umich.edu

M. Roshni Ray Thoracic Oncology Program, Comprehensive Cancer Center, University of California, San Francisco, CA, USA, roshni.ray@ucsf.edu

Brian D. Ross, Ph.D. Center for Molecular Imaging, Department of Radiology, University of Michigan, Ann Arbor, MI 48109, USA, bdross@umich.edu

Katia Savary Ludwig Institute for Cancer Research, Uppsala University, Biomedical Center, SE-751 24 Uppsala, Sweden, katia.savary@licr.uu.se

Bryan J. Schneider, M.D. Division of Hematology/Oncology, Department of Internal Medicine, Presbyterian-Weill Cornell Medical Center, Payson Pavilion, NY 10065, USA, bjs2004@med.cornell.edu

Sherven Sharma, Ph.D. Division of Pulmonary and Critical Care Medicine and Hospitalists, Department of Medicine, UCLA Lung Cancer Research Program, Jonsson Comprehensive Cancer Center, David Geffen School of Medicine at UCLA, Los Angeles, CA 90095, USA, ssharma@mednet.ucla.edu

Robert M. Strieter, M.D. Division of Pulmonary and Critical Care Medicine, Department of Medicine, University of Virginia, Charlottesville, VA 22908, USA, strieter@virginia.edu

Baskaran Sundaram, M.B.B.S., M.R.C.P., F.R.C.R. Department of Radiology, University of Michigan, Ann Arbor, MI 48109, USA, sundbask@umich.edu

Stefan Termén Ludwig Institute for Cancer Research, Uppsala University, Biomedical Center, SE-751 24 Uppsala, Sweden, stefan.termen@licr.uu.se

Charles Kumar Thodeti, Ph.D. Vascular Biology Program, Children's Hospital/Harvard Medical School, Boston, MA 02115, USA, charles.thodeti@childrens.harvard.edu

Sylvie Thuault Ludwig Institute for Cancer Research, Uppsala University, Biomedical Center, SE-751 24 Uppsala, Sweden, sylvie.thuault@licr.uu.se

Ming-Sound Tsao, M.D. Ontario Cancer Institute and Princess Margaret Hospital, University Health Network and University of Toronto, University Avenue, Toronto, Ontario M5G 2M9, Canada, ming.tsao@uhn.on.ca

Judith A. Varner Moores UCSD Cancer Center, University of California San Diego, La Jolla, CA, USA, jvarner@ucsd.edu

Malini Venkatram, M.D. Department of Internal Medicine, Sinai-Grace/ Wayne State University, Detroit, MI, USA, malinive@umich.edu

Tonya Walser, Ph.D. Division of Pulmonary and Critical Care Medicine and Hospitalists, Department of Medicine, UCLA Lung Cancer Research Program, Jonsson Comprehensive Cancer Center, David Geffen School of Medicine at UCLA, Los Angeles, CA 90095, USA, twalser@mednet.ucla.edu

Peter J. Woolf, Ph.D. Departments of Chemical Engineering and Biomedical Engineering, University of Michigan, Ann Arbor, MI 48109, USA, pwoolf@umich.edu

Jane Yanagawa, M.D. Division of Pulmonary and Critical Care Medicine and Hospitalists, Department of Medicine, UCLA Lung Cancer Research Program, Jonsson Comprehensive Cancer Center, David Geffen School of Medicine at UCLA, Los Angeles, CA 90095, USA, jyanagawa@mednet.ucla.edu

Lung Cancer: Overview

Shirish M. Gadgeel and Gregory P. Kalemkerian

Abstract Lung cancer is the leading cause of cancer-related death in the world and 90% of all cases are caused by tobacco smoking. Lung cancer is divided into two major histologic subtypes, non-small cell (NSCLC) and small cell (SCLC), with distinct biological behavior, genetic alterations, and therapy. Thus far, screening for lung cancer has not been proven effective since no modality has been shown to decrease mortality. Most patients with both SCLC and NSCLC present with symptoms of either locally advanced or metastatic disease, with only about 25% of patients with NSCLC having early-stage, resectable disease. For patients with stage I or II NSCLC, surgical resection is the treatment of choice and results in long-term survival in 60–80% or 40–50% of patients, respectively. For patients with stage III, locally advanced NSCLC or limited-stage SCLC, aggressive chemotherapy plus radiotherapy can offer a cure in 20–25% of patients. Stage IV, or metastatic, NSCLC and extensive-stage SCLC are incurable diseases in which chemotherapy can prolong survival and palliate symptoms. Recent advances in our understanding of the molecular biology of lung cancer have led to novel therapeutic strategies targeting relevant pathways that regulate the proliferation and/or progression of lung cancer. Several of these molecularly targeted therapies have now demonstrated significant clinical benefits in subsets of patients with lung cancer.

Introduction

Lung cancer is the most common cancer in the United States and the leading cause of cancer-related death in both men and women, accounting for more deaths annually than breast, colon, prostate, and pancreatic cancer *combined* [1]. By gender, lung cancer is the second most common cancer in both men (after prostate cancer) and women (after breast cancer). In 2009, there will be an

G.P. Kalemkerian (✉)
Division of Hematology/Oncology, Department of Internal Medicine, University of Michigan, Ann Arbor, MI 48109-5848, USA
e-mail: kalemker@umich.edu

V. Keshamouni et al. (eds.), *Lung Cancer Metastasis*,
DOI 10.1007/978-1-4419-0772-1_1, © Springer Science+Business Media, LLC 2009

estimated 219,440 new cases and 159,390 deaths due to lung cancer in the United States [1]. Worldwide, lung cancer is also the leading cause of cancer-related death, killing an estimated 1.5 million people annually [2].

Epidemiology

At the beginning of the 20th century, lung cancer was a relatively rare disease, but by the end of the century it had become the major cancer-related public health problem in the world [3, 4]. As early as the 1930s it was noted that the incidence of lung cancer was rising at an alarming rate, and astute clinicians suspected that the increasing prevalence of tobacco smoking was to blame. In the 1950s, case–control studies firmly established the association between smoking and lung cancer [5, 6]. Although tobacco had been widely smoked for several centuries, the rise of lung cancer over the past 100 years has been attributed to the introduction of mass-produced cigarettes with enhanced addictive potential and milder smoke, which resulted in lower cost, increased daily usage, and sustained exposure of the lungs to inhaled carcinogens [7]. The distribution of free, mass-produced cigarettes to millions of troops during World War I also led to a rapid rise in smoking prevalence.

The incidence of lung cancer began to rise in American men in the 1930s and peaked in the mid-1980s [3, 4, 8]. Since then, the incidence rate has declined in proportion to the decreasing prevalence of smoking. In women, the incidence of lung cancer began to rise sharply in the 1960s following the drastic increase in the prevalence of tobacco use by women during World War II. The peak incidence in women occurred in the early part of this decade with only a slight downward trend noted in more recent years (Fig. 1). From 2000 to 2004, the US Surveillance Epidemiology and End Results (SEER) database reported lung cancer incidence and mortality rates of 81.2/100,000 and 73.4/100,000 in men and 52.3/100,000 and 41.1/100,000 in women, respectively [8].

Lung cancer incidence rates in the United States vary based on race as well as gender [9, 10]. Interestingly, racial differences are gender specific, with a greater incidence in black men than white men, but no significant difference between black women and white women. From 2000 to 2004, the SEER database reported that the incidence rates of lung cancer in black and white men were 109.2/100,000 and 88.3/100,000, respectively [8]. Though the precise reasons for this racial disparity are unclear, differences in lifestyle, smoking habits, and socioeconomic class, as well as potential genetic influences, have all been implicated in various epidemiological studies.

Socioeconomic status, as measured by income and level of education, is inversely correlated with the risk of lung cancer, even after adjustment for the prevalence of smoking [11–14]. Socioeconomic status is closely associated with several other determinants of lung cancer, including the prevalence of tobacco use, diet, and exposure to carcinogens in the home and workplace. Lower

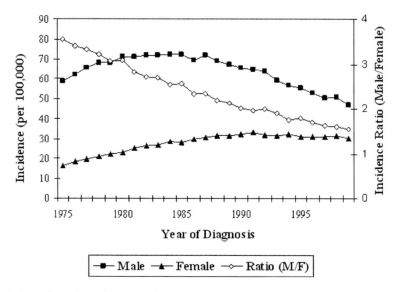

Fig. 1 Age-adjusted, gender-specific incidence rates of lung cancer, 1975–1999 (adapted from [117])

socioeconomic status is also associated with the diagnosis of lung cancer at a more advanced stage of disease.

The median age of patients with lung cancer in the United States is now 70 years and is expected to continue to rise with aging of the population [15]. Elderly patients often have comorbidities and age-related changes in organ function that can confound efforts to provide optimal anticancer therapy. In addition, elderly patients are significantly underrepresented in clinical trials, limiting the applicability of study data to their clinical care.

Survival after the diagnosis of lung cancer has changed little over the past 20 years, with overall 5-year survival rates increasing from 12.7% in 1975–1977 to 15.1% in 1996–2003 (http://seer.cancer.gov/csr/1975_2004). Survival also varies based on gender and race. The 5-year survival rates are 13.2% for white men, 10.3% for black men, 17.8% for white women, and 14.7% for black women. Regardless of race or gender, the primary reason for these dismal overall survival rates is that 75% of patients with lung cancer already have locally advanced or metastatic disease at the time of initial diagnosis.

Etiologic Factors

Smoking

Nearly 90% of all cases of lung cancer are caused by chronic exposure of the bronchial mucosa to carcinogens found in cigarette smoke. Case–control studies published in the 1950s by Wynder and Graham in the United States and Doll and Hill in England provided the first strong scientific link between lung cancer and tobacco use [5, 6]. Subsequently, many other prospective epidemiologic studies have confirmed this causal, dose–response relationship. In 2004, the prevalence of smoking among adults in the United States was 20.9% (23.2% in men, 19.2% in women) [16]. Cigarette smoking is directly responsible for 85–90% of lung cancers [17]. The strongest determinants of lung cancer in smokers are the duration of tobacco use and the number of cigarettes smoked. Thus, the risk of lung cancer is 60- to 70-fold higher in a person who smoked 2 packs (40 cigarettes) a day for 20 years (40 pack-years) than in a lifelong never-smoker. Lung cancer risk is increased to a lesser degree in cigar and pipe smokers. Further support for the causal role of smoking comes from data demonstrating that the risk of lung cancer decreases steadily over time in those who quit smoking [17]. While early epidemiologic studies focused on male smokers, similar risks of lung cancer have been reported in females [18]. Passive, or secondhand, exposure to cigarette smoke can increase the risk of lung cancer by up to 25% [19].

Lifelong non-smokers account for 10–15% of patients with lung cancer [20]. Some have had exposure to secondhand cigarette smoke or another known carcinogen, but in many, no specific carcinogen exposure can be identified [21–24]. The incidence of lung cancer is higher in female than male never-smokers. However, it is unclear if this gender disparity is due to increased susceptibility to lung cancer in women or to a greater likelihood of exposure to secondhand cigarette smoke.

The biology of lung cancer differs between smokers and never-smokers. Nearly all lung cancers occurring in non-smokers are adenocarcinomas, frequently well-differentiated tumors with bronchioloalveolar features, and they have an improved survival compared to smokers [20, 25, 26]. Recent data have shown that lung cancers in never-smokers are much more responsive to epidermal growth factor receptor tyrosine kinase inhibitors (EGFR-TKIs) and that this tumor susceptibility is due to a greater likelihood of somatic mutation in the kinase domain of the *EGFR* gene [27–29]. In addition, K-ras mutations, which predict a poor response to therapy and shorter survival, are found frequently in smokers, but less so in non-smokers [30, 31].

Other Causes

Numerous environmental exposures, both occupational and non-occupational, have been associated with an increased risk of lung cancer, including radon, asbestos, air pollution, chromium, nickel, polycyclic aromatic hydrocarbons, and arsenic [17]. Each of these may account for a percentage of lung cancers in non-smokers, but more commonly, exposure to these agents appears to act synergistically with tobacco carcinogens to increase the risk of lung cancer in smokers.

Asbestos is an independent lung carcinogen. In a retrospective cohort study published in 1955, Doll noted a 10-fold increased risk of lung cancer in asbestos textile workers [32]. Radon exposure in underground miners was connected to lung cancer risk in the early 1900s. More recently, residential, indoor radon exposure has been implicated as a risk factor for lung cancer, though the relative risk is much lower than that noted for miners [33]. However, it is estimated that indoor radon exposure may account for up to 15,000 lung cancer deaths per year in the United States.

Certain lung diseases are associated with an increased risk of lung cancer even after adjustment for tobacco use. The clearest association is with chronic obstructive pulmonary disease (COPD) [34, 35]. Both COPD and lung cancer are so highly related to cigarette use that statistical adjustments may not completely eliminate the confounding effect of smoking on the causal link between COPD and lung cancer. Interstitial lung disease and systemic sclerosis have also been reported as risk factors for lung cancer, possibly due to the presence of chronic lung inflammation which may lead to genetic changes in bronchial epithelial and stromal cells [36].

Epidemiologic studies have implicated various dietary factors in the risk of lung cancer. Diets rich in fruits and vegetables are associated with a lower incidence of lung cancer, and higher dietary intake and blood levels of β-carotene and total carotenoids correlate with a 30–80% lower risk of lung cancer, even after adjusting for smoking, age, and gender [37, 38]. However, two large, randomized, interventional trials demonstrated that β-carotene supplementation actually resulted in a significant increase in lung cancer risk in active smokers [39, 40]. One possible explanation for this finding is that β-carotene has an oxidative, mitogenic effect in the high oxygen tension environment present in the lungs of smokers [41–43]. These results do not contradict the protective effect of diets rich in fruits and vegetables since such diets contain many other micronutrients, such as folic acid, flavones, and isoflavonoids, which may reduce the risk of lung cancer.

Although the vast majority of lung cancer is caused by tobacco use, only 10–15% of all smokers develop lung cancer. This raises the question of individual susceptibility, possibly due to genetic variations that affect carcinogen activation or catabolism. Familial aggregation of lung cancer was first reported over 40 years ago [44]. Since then, studies have demonstrated a familial aggregation of lung cancer even after adjustment for exposure to tobacco smoke [45–47]. Some of these studies suggest that the pattern is consistent with Mendelian inheritance of a rare major gene, particularly when there is early onset of disease [48]. However, a study in twins did not support a genetic basis for lung cancer [49]. Despite reports of lung cancer in some patients with Li–Fraumeni syndrome, which is due to inherited mutations in *p53*, few known cancer susceptibility syndromes have been linked to lung cancer [50].

A specific "lung cancer gene" has not been identified. Candidate suscept-ibility genes include those associated with carcinogen metabolism and DNA repair. *CYP1A1* is a P450 enzyme involved in metabolizing several potential carcinogens, and two specific polymorphisms of the *CYP1A1* gene have been linked to increased lung cancer risk, although other studies have found no such association [51]. Similarly, relative deficiency of *GSTM1*, an enzyme involved in detoxifying metabolites of constituents in cigarette smoke, has been associated with lung cancer risk [52]. Inherited variability in DNA repair capacity may also contribute to inherited susceptibility to lung cancer by allowing the accumula-tion of genetic changes [53]. Additional large-scale studies are needed to better define the gene–gene and gene–environment interactions that drive susceptibil-ity to lung cancer in an effort to identify those at highest risk.

Pathology

The term lung cancer comprises all malignant neoplasms arising from the bronchial, bronchiolar, or alveolar epithelium. Lung cancers are categorized by histologic characteristics defined by light microscopy with four major histo-logic types: adenocarcinoma, squamous cell carcinoma, large cell carcinoma, and small cell carcinoma (Table 1) [54]. Lung cancers are commonly divided into non-small cell lung cancer (NSCLC) and small cell lung cancer (SCLC). NSCLC includes adenocarcinoma, squamous cell carcinoma, and large cell carcinoma. These tumors are grouped due to similarities in their prognosis and management. Clear definition of the specific histologic subtype of

Table 1 WHO classification of malignant epithelial lung tumors

Squamous cell carcinoma
    Variants: papillary, clear cell, small cell, basaloid
Small cell carcinoma
    Variants: combined small cell lung carcinoma
Adenocarcinoma
    Variants: acinar, papillary, bronchioloalveolar, solid adenocarcinoma with mucin,
    adenocarcinoma with mixed subtypes, fetal, mucinous, signet ring, clear cell
Large cell carcinoma
    Variants: large cell neuroendocrine carcinoma, basaloid, lymphoepithelioma-like,
    clear cell, rhabdoid phenotype
Adenosquamous carcinoma
Sarcomatoid carcinoma
    Variants: pleomorphic, spindle cell, giant cell, carcinosarcoma, pulmonary blastoma
Carcinoid tumors
    Variants: typical, atypical
Carcinomas of the salivary gland type
    Variants: mucoepidermoid, adenoid cystic, epithelial–myothelial

Adapted from Beasley MB et al. [54].

NSCLC can be difficult in patients who are diagnosed by cytology or in those with very poorly differentiated tumors, leading to the designation of "non-small cell lung cancer, not otherwise specified (NOS)." SCLC is a poorly differentiated neuroendocrine tumor characterized by aggressive tumor growth and early lymphatic and hematogenous metastases. The clinical course and management of patients with SCLC differ in several important ways from those with NSCLC.

Bronchioloalveolar carcinoma (BAC) is a subtype of adenocarcinoma. According to the World Health Organization, BAC is characterized by "growth of neoplastic cells along pre-existing alveolar structures, without evidence of stromal, vascular or pleural invasion" [54]. Patients with tumors that have focal areas of BAC but evidence of invasion or metastasis are considered to have "adenocarcinoma with BAC features."

Over the past 25 years, notable shifts have occurred in the incidence rates of the various histologic subtypes of lung cancer [55, 56]. Prior to the mid-1980s, squamous cell carcinoma was the most common histologic type of lung cancer in the United States and SCLC accounted for 20% of all lung cancers. Since then, adenocarcinoma has become the most common histologic type, while the incidences of squamous cell carcinoma and SCLC have declined. The precise reasons for these histologic shifts remain unclear, although it has been proposed that changes in cigarettes, such as the introduction of filters, may have resulted in the decreased inhalation of particulate matter which deposits in the proximal airway where squamous cell carcinoma and SCLC primarily form and the increased carcinogen exposure in the distal airway where adenocarcinoma predominates [57]. Currently, in the United States, adenocarcinoma accounts for 40% of lung cancers, squamous cell carcinoma 30%, large cell carcinoma 15%, and SCLC 15%.

Pathogenesis

The specific events that trigger the malignant transformation of bronchial epithelial cells are not well defined [58]. The genetic theory of carcinogenesis assumes that exposure to carcinogens induces genetic alterations that result in the malignant phenotype. These carcinogens or their metabolites may directly cause genetic damage in epithelial cells or they may induce an inflammatory response that ultimately leads to epigenetic or genetic alterations in epithelial and stromal cells. Some individuals appear to have an increased susceptibility to acquire these genetic mutations, perhaps due to inherited genetic variations in metabolic enzymes.

The accumulation of genetic mutations by bronchial epithelial cells results in the activation of protooncogenes and the inactivation of tumor suppressor genes. Loss of specific regions of chromosomes 9p (involving *p16*) and 3p has been recognized as an early event in premalignant lung lesions and normal appearing bronchial epithelial cells in smokers [59, 60]. Inactivating point mutations of the *p53* tumor suppressor gene have also been noted in normal appearing epithelial cells in smokers [61]. However, 17p deletions involving the p53 locus have only been observed in carcinoma in situ. Other common genetic and epigenetic changes observed in lung cancer cells include overexpression of Notch-3 due to a translocation of chromosomes 15 and 19, K-ras mutation, and promoter methylation which inhibits the expression of tumor suppressor genes [62]. It is clear that lung cancers display an astonishing range of molecular heterogeneity, both between and within individual patients. Chronic exposure to tobacco carcinogens results in a multitude of genetic derangements in each individual patient, leading to a level of molecular complexity that is likely responsible for the severe limitation in our ability to treat advanced disease. Some of these molecular changes reverse after smoking cessation, but others have been found to persist in the bronchial epithelial cells in former smokers for decades after their last cigarette. Lung cancers that arise in never-smokers tend to have fewer accumulated molecular abnormalities, a finding that probably explains the improved survival and response to targeted therapy in this patient population [63, 64].

The histologic progression of premalignant lesions appears to differ for each histologic subtype of lung cancer, and this process has been presumptively delineated for adenocarcinoma and squamous cell carcinoma [65, 66]. Premalignant events have been better defined in squamous cell carcinoma since these cancers tend to occur in the central airways where they are more amenable to bronchoscopic evaluation. The pathogenesis of squamous cell carcinoma proceeds from basal cell hyperplasia to squamous metaplasia to dysplasia to carcinoma in situ to invasive carcinoma. The precursor lesions of adenocarcinoma remain more elusive due to the primarily peripheral site of origin of these tumors. However, atypical adenomatous hyperplasia (AAH), a focal proliferation of alveolar cells, is often found in association with adenocarcinoma and bronchioloalveolar carcinoma, suggesting that AAH may be a precursor lesion. Although diffuse idiopathic neuroendocrine cell hyperplasia (DIPNECH), which occurs in response to lung injury and impaired gas exchange, has been associated with the development of bronchial carcinoid, it does not appear to be associated with SCLC [67].

Chemoprevention

Chemoprevention is based on the concept that carcinogenesis is a multistep process that can be reversed through clinical intervention prior to the development of the full malignant phenotype. Smoking cessation is the most important step that a smoker can take to reduce their risk of lung cancer. The normalization of histologic and molecular precancerous defects has been well documented after sustained smoking cessation [68]. Although the risk of lung cancer in a former smoker will never return to that of a never-smoker, after 10 years of smoking cessation, lung cancer incidence is reduced by about 50% [69].

A major focus of chemoprevention for lung cancer has been the evaluation of various nutritional supplements. This approach is primarily based on observations that populations and individuals with high intake of fruits and vegetables have a lower risk of lung cancer. Based on such epidemiologic data, two large studies evaluated the role of β-carotene in lung cancer prevention, but both trials reported a higher incidence of lung cancer in active smokers who took supplemental β-carotene [39, 40]. Studies of vitamin E and vitamin A (retinol) have also failed to demonstrate a reduction in lung cancer risk [70]. A large US trial evaluated the potential for isotretinoin (13-cis-retinoic acid) to reduce the risk of second primary lung cancers in patients who had undergone resection of stage I NSCLC [71]. As was noted in the β-carotene trials, isotretinoin increased mortality in current smokers and failed to reduce the incidence of second primary lung cancer.

Chronic inflammation is believed to play a crucial role in the formation of many cancers, including lung cancer [72]. Arachidonic acid metabolites are major mediators of inflammation and are known to induce procarcinogenic effects, such as cellular proliferation, inhibition of apoptosis, and angiogenesis. Aspirin inhibits the activity of COX-2, an inducible cyclooxygenase enzyme that metabolizes arachidonic acid into prostaglandins and is overexpressed in many premalignant and malignant lesions. In two studies, aspirin resulted in a non-significant reduction in the risk of lung cancer [73, 74]. The chemopreventive potential of selective COX-2 inhibitors, such as celecoxib, is currently being evaluated in clinical trials [75].

Epidemiological studies have noted an inverse association between serum selenium levels and lung cancer risk, possibly due to alterations of gene expression, modification of oxidative stress pathways, or inhibition of cyclooxygenase and lipooxygenase pathways. In a trial evaluating the potential role of selenium in skin cancer prevention, a secondary analysis revealed a 26% reduction in the risk of lung cancer [76]. A large US intergroup trial is currently underway to evaluate the role of selenium in reducing the risk of second primary lung cancers in patients who have undergone surgery for stage I NSCLC.

Chemopreventive trials traditionally require the accrual of a large number of subjects who need to be followed for long periods of time. The great expense and logistical challenges of such studies have resulted in a recent focus on the development of surrogate biological endpoints that will facilitate the assessment of many agents over a shorter time period. Examples of such surrogate endpoints that may be useful in lung cancer chemoprevention studies include bronchial dysplasia, expression of proteins such as Ki-67 and p53, and genomic or proteomic assays. Although promising, none of these markers has been prospectively validated in clinical trials.

Screening

The goal of cancer screening is to detect disease at an early stage when curative interventions can improve the overall mortality of the disease. The potential impact of screening is greater if a high-risk population can be identified. This is clearly the case in lung cancer where tobacco use accounts for the vast majority of cases. In addition, the poor overall survival in lung cancer is primarily due to the fact that 75% of patients present with either locally advanced disease, in which the potential for cure is relatively low, or metastatic disease, in which cure is virtually non-existent. Prognosis is much better in patients with earlier stages of disease in which complete surgical resection is possible. Therefore, the early detection of disease through screening offers the best, and most realistic, opportunity to significantly improve the overall outcome of people with lung cancer.

In the 1970s and 1980s, several randomized studies evaluated the utility of chest X-ray and sputum cytology for lung cancer screening in high-risk populations of smokers [77–79]. These studies found that even though these techniques could detect lung cancer at an earlier stage, they did not improve lung cancer-specific or overall mortality. One explanation for this apparent paradox is that screening may detect small, slow-growing, non-aggressive cancers that may have a similar outcome even if they are detected when they become symptomatic, while aggressive cancers that cause the majority of deaths develop and progress beyond curability during the interval between screening exams.

Recently, a great deal of interest has been focused on computed tomography (CT) as a screening tool for the early detection of lung cancer. Uncontrolled studies have shown that CT can detect four times as many cancers as plain chest X-rays and that most screen-detected cancers are found at an early stage. One of the largest uncontrolled studies of screening CT is the International Early Lung Cancer Action Program (I-ELCAP), which screened 31,567 individuals at high-risk for lung cancer due to a history of smoking, secondhand smoke exposure, or occupational carcinogen exposure [80]. Lung cancer was diagnosed in 484 subjects and 85% of them had stage I disease with an estimated 10-year survival rate of 80–88%. However, the lack of a control group makes it impossible to determine if CT improved lung cancer mortality. Two large, randomized trials of CT screening are on-going in order to address this important question. Thus far, the potential benefits and risks of CT for lung cancer screening have not been adequately defined and, thus, CT screening is not recommended.

A wide variety of blood and sputum biomarkers have been identified in patients with lung cancer. However, their utility as screening tools has yet to be validated in prospective cohorts of high-risk individuals. Nevertheless, the use of high-yield imaging modalities in a high-risk population that has been enriched through the use of blood or sputum biomarkers holds great promise for the early detection of lung cancer.

Clinical Presentation

The primary reason that most patients with lung cancer present with advanced stage disease is that early-stage disease does not usually cause significant symptoms, especially when arising in the periphery of the lung. Overall, only 5–10% of lung cancer patients are asymptomatic at the time of diagnosis [81, 82]. Most of these asymptomatic cancers are detected during the evaluation of an unrelated medical problem. The absence of symptoms, physical signs, and abnormal laboratory tests in these patients is associated with a lower incidence of metastatic disease, and patients who are asymptomatic have a much better prognosis than those who are symptomatic. Most of the presenting symptoms of lung cancer are due to the direct effects of locally advanced or metastatic disease. In addition, constitutional symptoms, such as anorexia, fatigue, and weight loss, are very common in patients with lung cancer [83].

Symptoms of Local Disease

Cough is the most common symptom in patients with lung cancer, occurring in at least 50% of patients at presentation and eventually developing in most who are not cured of the disease [84]. Cough may be due to airway obstruction, postobstructive pneumonia, excessive mucus production, parenchymal metastases, or pleural effusion and can lead to significant functional debility and impairment of quality of life. Many patients have a chronic "smokers' cough," leading them to ignore the gradual change brought on by a developing lung tumor. Tumor-directed therapy and opiates are the most successful approaches for relieving lung cancer-related cough, but in many cases, cough persists despite appropriate therapy [85].

Hemoptysis due to a friable endobronchial tumor frequently results in the production of blood-streaked sputum. As with cough, many patients presenting with hemoptysis are initially treated with antibiotics, delaying the diagnosis of lung cancer. Massive hemoptysis, most commonly due to a tumor-induced fistula between a pulmonary artery and the airway, is a relatively uncommon, but usually fatal, complication of lung cancer. The management of hemoptysis depends on its severity. Mild to moderate hemoptysis requires only cancer-directed therapy, such as radiation, and antitussive medications. Severe hemoptysis may call for emergent lung resection, selective arterial embolization, endobronchial vasoconstrictors, or balloon tamponade [86, 87].

Dyspnea occurs in most patients with lung cancer during the course of their disease due to a wide variety of causes, including direct impingement of the airway, underlying chronic lung disease, radiation- or chemotherapy-induced pneumonitis, infection, pleural effusion, or pulmonary embolism. Management of dyspnea requires treatment of the underlying etiology, with recognition that the tumor is not always the primary cause. Symptomatic therapy includes supplemental oxygen, opioids, anxiolytics, and sedatives [88, 89]. Dyspnea is an extremely distressing symptom for both patients and their families, so optimal and aggressive management of dyspnea must be a primary goal of lung cancer therapy.

Chest pain is a common symptom that may occur even in early-stage lung cancer without frank evidence of invasion of the pleura, chest wall, or mediastinum. The origin of such pain is unclear since the lung parenchyma is not supplied with pain receptors. Retrosternal pain may arise from hilar or mediastinal lymphadenopathy, direct invasion of the mediastinum, or involvement of the pericardium. Chest wall pain is typically due to invasion of the parietal pleura or ribs or to rib metastases. Analgesics, including narcotics, should be used to optimally control pain along with appropriate anticancer therapy.

Symptoms of Locally Advanced Disease

Superior vena cava (SVC) syndrome is characterized by cough, dyspnea, and facial, neck, and upper extremity edema and venous distention. It is usually due to obstruction of the SVC by massive right paratracheal lymphadenopathy or by direct extension of a primary right upper lobe tumor into the mediastinum. The severity of symptoms depends on how rapidly the obstruction progresses and on the development of collateral circulation. Rarely, SVC obstruction can result in potentially fatal cerebral or laryngeal edema. In the United States, 80% of patients with SVC syndrome have an underlying lung cancer. Once considered a medical emergency, current practice is to ensure that a tissue diagnosis is obtained expeditiously prior to the initiation of therapy [90]. Due to relative chemoresistance, radiotherapy is the preferred treatment for patients with NSCLC. Stenting of the SVC can be useful as part of the initial therapy or in patients who have not responded to other treatments.

Approximately 15% of lung cancer patients present with pleural effusion. Although most effusions are ultimately found to be malignant, about half are cytologically negative on initial thoracentesis. It is important to determine if an effusion is due to pleural involvement since this finding indicates incurable disease. In patients with a good performance status and reasonable life expectancy, aggressive interventions such as thoracoscopic talc pleurodesis can usually relieve symptoms by preventing the reaccumulation of fluid [83]. Patients with more advanced disease may be better served by placement of a flexible, indwelling, small-bore catheter. However, patients whose lung cannot re-expand due to extensive parenchymal or pleural disease will not benefit from drainage of pleural fluid.

Pancoast tumors are lung cancers that involve the apex of the lung and invade into adjacent structures, such as the upper ribs and lower brachial plexus, causing pain, Horner's syndrome, brachial plexopathy, and reflex sympathetic dystrophy. Unfortunately, diagnosis is frequently delayed in such patients by evaluation of musculoskeletal causes of pain. For patients without mediastinal lymph node involvement, treatment consists of chemotherapy and radiation followed by surgical resection, while those with mediastinal lymph node involvement are treated with definitive chemoradiotherapy [91]. Pain can be difficult to control, often requiring large doses of narcotics and neurolytic medications as well as nerve blocks.

Symptoms of Metastatic Disease

Both NSCLC and SCLC are highly invasive diseases with high metastatic potential. The commonest sites of hematogenous metastases are contralateral lung, brain, liver, bone, adrenal gland, and extrathoracic lymph nodes. However, lung cancer can spread to any site in the body, including skin, soft tissues, pancreas, bowel, ovary, and thyroid.

Lung cancer is the most common cause of brain metastases [92]. Up to 60% of patients with SCLC and 33% with NSCLC develop symptomatic brain metastases during the course of their disease [92, 93]. Improved control of intrathoracic disease in patients with locally advanced NSCLC has led to an increase in the incidence of brain metastases in these patients [94]. The symptoms of brain metastases vary depending on the location of the lesion and the degree of associated edema or hemorrhage and include headache, nausea, vomiting, focal weakness, seizures, confusion, ataxia, and visual disturbances. Leptomeningeal carcinomatosis may present as headache and cranial nerve palsies without structural abnormalities on brain imaging. On initial lumbar puncture, cytology is positive in only 50–70% of patients with leptomeningeal disease, requiring repeated evaluation for diagnosis [95]. Magnetic resonance imaging (MRI) is more sensitive than CT for the identification of parenchymal and leptomeningeal metastases [96]. The initial management of brain metastases consists of corticosteroids to control edema followed by whole brain radiation, stereotactic radiosurgery, or surgical resection depending on the size, number, and location of the lesions as well as the extent of extracranial disease and the general condition of the patient. Leptomeningeal carcinomatosis is poorly responsive to therapy, particularly in patients with NSCLC, and is usually associated with progressive systemic disease and very short survival. In patients with SCLC, intrathecal chemotherapy can be beneficial, but prognosis remains extremely poor.

Although lung cancer can metastasize to any bone, the axial skeleton and proximal long bones are most commonly involved. Pain due to bone metastases is present in up to 25% of patients at initial diagnosis. Radiation can relieve pain in 60–70% of patients with symptomatic bone metastases. In selected patients with lytic metastases in weight-bearing bones, surgery should be considered to minimize fracture potential and optimize function. Non-steroidal anti-inflammatory drugs can be useful adjuncts to narcotics in patients with painful bone metastases. Zoledronic acid, a bisphosphonate, can significantly decrease the incidence of skeletal-related adverse events in lung cancer patients with bone metastases.

Liver metastases are common in patients with lung cancer, resulting in fatigue, weight loss, abdominal pain, and refractory nausea, which can lead to significant debility and a poor prognosis. Adrenal metastases are usually asymptomatic and are frequently detected on staging CT scans. Large adrenal metastases can cause abdominal or back pain, but adrenal insufficiency is rare. Surgical resection of solitary adrenal metastases has been associated with long-term survival in small series and case reports, but this approach remains controversial [97].

Constitutional Symptoms

Constitutional symptoms, such as depression, fatigue, anxiety, insomnia, anorexia, and cachexia, cause significant debility in patients with lung cancer. Depression and psychological distress are very common, but are infrequently recognized and treated [98]. Fatigue, which is the commonest symptom in patients with lung cancer, is usually due to multiple factors, including anemia, dyspnea, anorexia, cachexia, pain, and therapy. Appropriate assessment and management of these symptoms can substantially improve quality of life, particularly in patients with advanced disease where the benefits of anticancer therapy are limited.

Paraneoplastic Syndromes

Paraneoplastic syndromes are effects of cancer that occur systemically or at sites distant from tumor and, as such, are not related to direct anatomic involvement by tumor. They are usually caused by either an aberrant autoimmune response to tumor antigens or an ectopic cytokine or hormone production by tumor cells. Paraneoplastic syndromes are most commonly seen in patients with SCLC due to the neuroendocrine nature of these cells. Syndromes associated with SCLC include subacute cerebellar degeneration, Lambert–Eaton myasthenia, inappropriate secretion of antidiuretic hormone, and Cushing's syndrome. Paraneoplastic syndromes more commonly seen in patients with NSCLC include clubbing, hypertrophic pulmonary osteoarthropathy, humoral hypercalcemia, and migratory thrombosis (Trousseau's syndrome).

Staging

Stage is the most important prognostic factor in patients with lung cancer. After a diagnosis of lung cancer is made, a variety of examinations and tests are performed to delineate the anatomic extent, or stage, of disease. For most cancers, including NSCLC, the TNM system is used for staging based on the evaluation of three factors: tumor (T), lymph nodes (N), and metastases (M). From the scoring of these three factors, the numerical stage of disease (stage I through stage IV) can be determined. The current TNM staging criteria for lung cancer are presented in Table 2; however, a newly revised system has been proposed and is likely to be adopted in 2009 (Table 3) [99, 100]. Although the TNM system can be used for SCLC, the two-stage Veterans Administration system is usually used: limited-stage, disease confined to one hemithorax that

Table 2 Current AJCC TNM staging system for lung cancer

Primary tumor (T)

T1 – Tumor ≤3 cm diameter without invasion more proximal than lobar bronchus

T2 – Tumor >3 cm diameter *or* tumor of any size with any of the following:
  Invades visceral pleura
  Atelectasis or obstructive pneumonitis involving less than the entire lung
  Proximal extent ≥2 cm from carina

T3 – Tumor of any size with any of the following:
  Invasion of chest wall, diaphragm, mediastinal pleura, or parietal pericardium
  Atelectasis or obstructive pneumonitis involving the entire lung
  Proximal extent <2 cm of carina

T4 – Tumor of any size with any of the following:
  Invasion of mediastinum, heart, great vessels, trachea, esophagus, vertebral body, or
    carina
  Malignant pleural or pericardial effusion
  Satellite tumor nodule(s) within same lobe as primary tumor

Nodal involvement (N)

N0 – No regional node involvement

N1 – Metastasis to ipsilateral peribronchial and/or ipsilateral hilar lymph nodes

N2 – Metastasis to ipsilateral mediastinal and/or subcarinal nodes

N3 – Metastasis to contralateral mediastinal, contralateral hilar nodes, ipsilateral or
    contralateral scalene, or supraclavicular nodes

Metastasis (M)

M0 – No distant metastasis

M1 – Distant metastasis (includes tumor nodules in a different lobe from the primary tumor)

Stage groupings of TNM subsets

Stage IA	T1	N0	M0
Stage IB	T2	N0	M0
Stage IIA	T1	N1	M0
Stage IIB	T2	N1	M0
	T3	N0	M0
Stage IIIA	T3	N1	M0
	T1-3	N2	M0
Stage IIIB	Any T	N3	M0
	T4	Any N	M0
Stage IV	Any T	Any N	M1

Adapted from Mountain CF [99].

Table 3 Proposed revised TNM staging system for lung cancer

Primary tumor (T)

T1 – Tumor ≤3 cm diameter without invasion more proximal than the lobar bronchus

T1a – Tumor ≤2 cm diameter

T1b – Tumor >2 cm but ≤3 cm diameter

T2 – Tumor >3 cm but ≤7 cm diameter *or* tumor with any of the following:
   Invasion of visceral pleura
   Atelectasis or obstructive pneumonitis involving less than the entire lung
   Proximal extent ≥2 cm from carina

T2a – Tumor >3 cm but ≤5 cm diameter

T2b – Tumor >5 cm but ≤7 cm diameter

T3 – Tumor >7 cm diameter or tumor with any of the following:
   Invasion of chest wall, diaphragm, phrenic nerve, mediastinal pleura, or parietal
     pericardium
   Atelectasis or obstructive pneumonitis involving the entire lung
   Proximal extent <2 cm of carina
   Separate tumor nodule(s) in the same lobe

T4 – Tumor of any size with any of the following:
   Invasion of mediastinum, heart, great vessels, trachea, esophagus, recurrent laryngeal
     nerve, vertebral body, or carina
   Separate tumor nodule(s) in a different ipsilateral lobe

Nodal involvement (N)

N0 – No regional node involvement

N1 – Metastasis in ipsilateral peribronchial and/or ipsilateral hilar lymph nodes

N2 – Metastasis in ipsilateral mediastinal and/or subcarinal lymph nodes

N3 – Metastasis in contralateral mediastinal, contralateral hilar, ipsilateral or contralateral
     scalene, or supraclavicular nodes

Metastasis (M)

M0 – No distant metastasis

M1 – Distant metastasis

M1a – Separate tumor nodule(s) in a contralateral lobe; pleural nodules or malignant
     pleural or pericardial effusion

M1b – Distant metastasis

Stage groupings of TNM subsets

Stage IA	T1a–T1b	N0	M0
Stage IB	T2a	N0	M0
Stage IIA	T2b	N0	M0
	T1a–T2a	N1	M0
Stage IIB	T2b	N1	M0
	T3	N0	M0
Stage IIIA	T1a–T3	N2	M0
	T3	N1	M0
	T4	N0-1	M0
Stage IIIB	T4	N2	M0
	Any T	N3	M0
Stage IV	Any T	Any N	M1a–M1b

Adapted from Goldstraw P et al. [100].

can be safely encompassed in one radiation field; and extensive-stage, anything beyond limited-stage, including contralateral lung lesions, malignant pleural effusion, or hematogenous metastases [101]. Staging not only defines the extent of disease but also serves as the basis for treatment decision making and prognostication.

Staging Procedures

A detailed history and physical examination is the most important first step in planning appropriate management. The presence of specific symptoms or physical findings may help direct further staging studies. The presence of constitutional symptoms, such as weight loss, fatigue, or poor performance status, greatly increases the likelihood of metastatic disease. The primary purpose of laboratory tests is to detect abnormalities in organ function, particularly of the liver and kidneys, which may affect tolerance to various therapeutic interventions.

CT scan of the chest, preferably with intravenous contrast to delineate mediastinal structures, is performed in all patients with lung cancer unless they are so debilitated that no specific therapy is being considered. CT scans should extend into the upper abdomen to include the liver and adrenal glands, which are common sites of metastatic spread. CT provides initial information on the potential involvement of mediastinal lymph nodes based on size criteria, while also assessing for hematogenous metastases. The accuracy of CT for mediastinal lymph node involvement is limited, with sensitivity of 50–60% and specificity of 85% [102].

Positron emission tomography (PET) is based on the concept that the uptake of glucose and the rate of glycolysis are greater in cancer cells than in normal cells. During PET, patients receive an intravenous injection of radiolabeled ^{18}F-2-deoxy-D-glucose (FDG), which is taken up by cancers at an increased rate relative to normal tissues. The anatomic accumulation of FDG is then detected by a positron-sensitive camera. PET provides information on the differential metabolic function of tissues, while CT provides high-resolution anatomic details. In patients with lung cancer, PET can be helpful in detecting mediastinal lymph node involvement and distant metastases. However, FDG avidity on PET is not a definitive sign of malignancy since benign inflammatory lesions may also yield an FDG-avid signal. Conversely, small or indolent tumors, such as well-differentiated adenocarcinoma or bronchioloalveolar carcinoma, may not be FDG avid. The sensitivity and the specificity of PET for the detection of mediastinal lymph node involvement are 74% and 85%, respectively [102]. PET scans can also detect distant metastases in 10% of patients with presumed early-stage disease based on traditional staging modalities. As a general rule, FDG-avid mediastinal lymph nodes or distant foci that will alter treatment if they truly reflect metastatic disease need to be biopsied to confirm or refute involvement with tumor.

The brain is an important metastatic site in patients with both NSCLC and SCLC. In patients with early-stage NSCLC who do not have neurologic symptoms, the utility of routine brain imaging has a relatively low yield and is not recommended. However, once mediastinal lymph node involvement has been documented, the risk of brain metastasis rises, particularly in patients with adenocarcinoma, increasing the utility of brain imaging. In patients with SCLC, brain imaging is recommended for all patients due to the high incidence of brain metastases.

Prognostic Factors

Prognostic factors are patient- and tumor-related characteristics that impact on outcome independent of therapy [99, 103, 104]. Stage at diagnosis is the most important determinant of an individual patient's prognosis. For example, the 5-year survival rate of patients with stage I NSCLC is 70%, while that of patients with stage IV disease is 1%. Performance status (PS), a physician's assessment of a patient's ability to perform routine physical activity, is the second most important clinical prognostic factor. PS represents the impact of tumor-related symptoms, comorbidities, and complications of medical interventions on the patient. Other important clinical and pathologic prognostic factors include age, gender (women have a better prognosis than men), and histologic subtype.

The expression or mutation status of numerous tumor-associated gene products has also been found to have varying degrees of prognostic significance. Such biomarkers include bcl-2, p53, Ki-67, COX-2, vascular endothelial growth factor (VEGF), and K-ras. Genomic analyses of lung cancers have been conducted to define genetic profiles that can identify good or poor prognostic groups of patients. None of these biomarkers are currently being utilized for routine clinical assessment due to the retrospective and univariate nature of most analyses and the need for prospective validation in larger cohorts of patients. It is likely that some of these biomarkers will complement known clinical prognostic factors and will be of significant utility in the not-too-distant future. In addition, early studies have begun to identify molecular factors that appear to be predictive for response or resistance to specific therapeutic agents, such as ERCC1 expression for platinum sensitivity and *EGFR* mutation for sensitivity to EGFR tyrosine kinase inhibitors. Such predictive factors hold great promise for achieving individualized therapy tailored to each patient's own host- or tumor-associated characteristics.

Management of Lung Cancer

The primary objectives of lung cancer management are to maximize patient survival while optimizing quality of life. Many clinical factors need to be considered in determining a rational care plan for an individual patient, including the stage and histology of the disease and the symptoms, performance status, and comorbid conditions of the patient. In general, all of the subtypes of NSCLC are managed in a similar manner, but there are significant differences in the management of NSCLC and SCLC.

Management of NSCLC

The ultimate goal of therapy for patients with NSCLC is dependent on stage: cure for patients with stage I–III disease and palliation for those with stage IV disease. Basically, three questions regarding the extent of disease drive therapeutic decision making: (1) Is the primary tumor confined to the lung? (stage I/II); (2) Has the cancer metastasized to the mediastinal lymph nodes? (stage III); and (3) Are there distant metastases? (stage IV).

NSCLC Confined to the Lung

In 25% of patients, NSCLC is confined to the lung (T1-2) with or without metastases to hilar or peribronchial (N1) lymph nodes (stages I/II). The goal of therapy in these patients is cure, which is achievable in 60–80% of patients with stage I disease and 40–50% of patients with stage II disease. The primary, curative modality is surgical resection by lobectomy or pneumonectomy [105]. Although lesser resections (wedge resection or segmentectomy) have been associated with increased recurrence rates and decreased survival in prior studies, these lung-sparing procedures are being re-evaluated in light of the recent trend toward presentation with smaller, more peripheral tumors due to the increased use of lung imaging and the rising incidence of adenocarcinoma. Distant relapse is the primary cause of death in patients who die within 5 years of a complete surgical resection. Thus, even when the cancer appears to be limited to the lung, undetected micrometastases remain a common problem. Recently, randomized clinical trials have demonstrated a 5–15% improvement in the 5-year survival rate for patients with stage II and III NSCLC who receive adjuvant chemotherapy after complete surgical resection. However, there is no clear benefit for adjuvant chemotherapy in patients with stage I disease [106]. Due to the high rate of cigarette use in patients with lung cancer, many patients are unable to tolerate adequate lung resections because of coexisting chronic lung or cardiovascular disease. In such patients, alternative therapies, such as external beam radiation, stereotactic body radiotherapy, and radiofrequency ablation, are available, although the long-term disease-control rates and survivals associated with these modalities appear substantially lower than those with surgical resection.

Mediastinal Involvement Without Distant Metastases

In 35% of patients with NSCLC, the primary tumor has directly invaded local structures or the cancer has spread to the mediastinal lymph nodes (stage III). These locally advanced tumors are generally not amenable to primary surgical resection, though advances in surgical techniques and the increasing use of combined modality therapy have led to a re-examination of the role of surgery in stage III disease. Patients with mediastinal involvement have a high incidence of hematogenous micrometastatic disease that frequently results in distant relapse and a relatively high mortality rate. Nevertheless, the goal of therapy remains cure, with about 20% of patients with stage III disease remaining disease-free 5 or more years after initial definitive therapy. Historically, radiotherapy and surgical resection were the primary treatments for locally advanced NSCLC, yielding 5-year survival rates of 5% or less. Subsequently, the use of systemic chemotherapy along with thoracic radiotherapy has led to significant improvements in survival by increasing local control and decreasing distant relapse [107, 108]. Sequential chemotherapy followed by radiotherapy initially raised 5-year survival rates to 10–15%. Concurrent chemotherapy and radiotherapy have now further improved long-term survival rates to 20–25%, although median survival remains only 18–21 months. Standard chemotherapy regimens used in this setting incorporate cisplatin or carboplatin along with a second agent, usually etoposide, a taxane, or a vinca alkaloid, while definitive radiotherapy is given over 6–7 weeks to a total dose of 60–70 Gy [107, 108]. As is usually the case in oncology, increases in survival are mirrored by increases in toxicity, in this case, primarily esophagitis and pneumonitis. Many patients with locally advanced NSCLC are not able to tolerate concurrent chemotherapy and radiation due to poor performance status or comorbid conditions. In such patients, the treatment plan needs to be individualized to allow control of symptoms and disease without inducing excessive treatment-related complications.

Several studies have evaluated "trimodality" therapy, utilizing induction chemotherapy or chemoradiotherapy prior to surgical resection with further chemotherapy or radiotherapy after surgery, in patients who are relatively fit and who have relatively low-bulk mediastinal disease. Thus far, these studies have failed to demonstrate a clear survival benefit of this approach over standard, definitive chemoradiotherapy for patients with stage III NSCLC [109].

Distant Metastases

Approximately 40% of patients with NSCLC already have distant, hematogenous metastases (stage IV) or a malignant pleural effusion at the time of diagnosis. Patients with such advanced disease are incurable and almost all will die from the disease. The objectives of therapy in such patients are to control the cancer, prolong survival, palliate symptoms, and optimize quality of life. The primary initial treatment for patients with advanced NSCLC is chemotherapy, usually with one of several "standard" two-drug combinations of cytotoxic agents. The expected outcomes from any of these regimens are similar, with 20–25% of patients exhibiting an objective response (significant tumor shrinkage) and another 30–40% having stability or control of disease [109, 110]. However, each of the available treatment regimens induces its own particular set of toxicities which usually influence the choice of a particular regimen in each individual patient. Recently, a large clinical trial has demonstrated that the addition of the antiangiogenic, anti-VEGF (vascular endothelial growth factor) antibody, bevacizumab, to standard chemotherapy can improve survival in some patients with advanced NSCLC [111]. Unfortunately, the benefits of chemotherapy have been demonstrated only in patients with good performance status. Therefore, supportive care with attention to symptom relief is the most reasonable management option for those with significant physical debility.

Treatment options for patients who progress on first-line chemotherapy or experience tumor regrowth after initial response include single-agent cytotoxic chemotherapy or molecularly targeted therapy with an epidermal growth factor receptor (EGFR) inhibitor, such as erlotinib [27, 112]. These treatments carry the potential for tumor control in approximately half of patients. Even with state-of-the-art therapy, the overall prognosis of patients with advanced NSCLC remains poor, with median survival of 8–10 months, 1-year survival of 30–40%, and 2-year survival of 10–20%. In light of these dire statistics, enrollment on investigational clinical trials remains an excellent option for patients with this disease. A more detailed discussion of the management of advanced NSCLC is provided in Chapter 20 (Ramalingam and Schneider).

Management of SCLC

The principles of management of patients with SCLC are predicated upon two observations: (1) SCLC is a highly aggressive disease that leads to early hematogenous metastases and (2) SCLC is highly sensitive to initial chemotherapy and radiotherapy. For these reasons, systemic chemotherapy is always included in the management of SCLC, regardless of the stage of disease. Surgery is rarely used for treatment of SCLC since over 95% of patients have mediastinal lymph node involvement at diagnosis. If surgery is performed for early-stage SCLC, it should be followed by adjuvant cisplatin-based chemotherapy. For the one-third of patients with limited-stage disease, standard treatment consists of concurrent chemotherapy plus thoracic radiotherapy delivered with curative intent [113]. Four cycles of cisplatin plus etoposide remain the optimal chemotherapy regimen. Radiotherapy can be delivered once a day to a total dose of 60–70 Gy or twice a day to a total dose of 45 Gy, although the twice-a-day regimen given early during the course of chemotherapy in appropriate patients significantly improves overall survival, albeit with increased acute toxicity [114]. With concurrent chemoradiotherapy, nearly 90% of patients with limited-stage SCLC will have an objective response and 20–40% will have a complete response, resulting in a median survival of 18 months and a 5-year survival rate of 20–25%.

Unfortunately, 70% of patients with SCLC have distant metastases at the time of diagnosis. Despite high initial response rates to standard chemotherapy, extensive-stage SCLC is an incurable disease with a median survival of 9 months and a 2-year survival rate of <5%. Up to 60% of patients with SCLC will develop brain metastases during the course of their disease. Recent clinical trials have demonstrated that prophylactic brain radiation provides a significant improvement in survival for patients with both limited- and extensive-stage disease who have responded favorably to initial therapy [115, 116]. Further information on the management of patients with extensive-stage SCLC is provided in Chapter 20 (Ramalingam and Schneider).

References

1. Jemal A, Siegel R, Ward E, et al. Cancer statistics. CA Cancer J Clin 2009; 59:225–249.
2. Youlden DR, Cramb SM, Baade PD. The international epidemiology of lung cancer: geographical distribution and secular trends. J Thorac Oncol 2008; 3:819–831.
3. Weiss W. Cigarette smoking and lung cancer trends. A light at the end of the tunnel? Chest 1997; 111:1414–1416.
4. Wingo PA, Cardinez CJ, Landis SH, et al. Long-term trends in cancer mortality in the United States, 1930–1998. Cancer 2003; 97:3133–3275.
5. Wynder EL, Graham EA. Tobacco smoking as a possible etiologic factor in bronchiogenic carcinoma; a study of 684 proved cases. J Am Med Assoc 1950; 143:329–336.
6. Doll R, Hill AB. Smoking and carcinoma of the lung; preliminary report. Br Med J 1950; 2:739–748.
7. Giovino GA. The tobacco epidemic in the United States. Am J Prev Med 2007; 33:S318–S326.
8. Espey DK, Wu XC, Swan J, et al. Annual report to the nation on the status of cancer, 1975–2004, featuring cancer in American Indians and Alaska natives. Cancer 2007; 110:2119–2152.
9. Abidoye O, Ferguson MK, Salgia R. Lung carcinoma in African Americans. Nat Clin Pract Oncol 2007; 4:118–129.
10. Gadgeel SM, Kalemkerian GP. Racial differences in lung cancer. Cancer Metastasis Rev 2003; 22:39–46.
11. Albano JD, Ward E, Jemal A, et al. Cancer mortality in the United States by education level and race. J Natl Cancer Inst 2007; 99:1384–1394.

12. Devesa SS, Diamond EL. Socioeconomic and racial differences in lung cancer incidence. Am J Epidemiol 1983; 118:818–831.
13. Krieger N, Quesenberry C, Jr., Peng T, et al. Social class, race/ethnicity, and incidence of breast, cervix, colon, lung, and prostate cancer among Asian, Black, Hispanic, and White residents of the San Francisco Bay Area, 1988–92 (United States). Cancer Causes Control 1999; 10:525–537.
14. Baquet CR, Horm JW, Gibbs T, et al. Socioeconomic factors and cancer incidence among blacks and whites. J Natl Cancer Inst 1991; 83:551–557.
15. Gridelli C, Langer C, Maione P, et al. Lung cancer in the elderly. J Clin Oncol 2007; 25:1898–1907.
16. State-specific prevalence of cigarette smoking and quitting among adults–United States, 2004. MMWR Morb Mortal Wkly Rep 2005; 54:1124–1127.
17. Alberg AJ, Ford JG, Samet JM. Epidemiology of lung cancer: ACCP evidence-based clinical practice guidelines (2nd edition). Chest 2007; 132:29S–55S.
18. Patel JD. Lung cancer in women. J Clin Oncol 2005; 23:3212–3218.
19. Taylor R, Najafi F, Dobson A. Meta-analysis of studies of passive smoking and lung cancer: effects of study type and continent. Int J Epidemiol 2007; 36:1048–1059.
20. Wakelee HA, Chang ET, Gomez SL, et al. Lung cancer incidence in never smokers. J Clin Oncol 2007; 25:472–478.
21. Gorlova OY, Zhang Y, Schabath MB, et al. Never smokers and lung cancer risk: a case-control study of epidemiological factors. Int J Cancer 2006; 118:1798–1804.
22. Neuberger JS, Field RW. Occupation and lung cancer in nonsmokers. Rev Environ Health 2003; 18:251–267.
23. Mayne ST, Buenconsejo J, Janerich DT. Previous lung disease and risk of lung cancer among men and women nonsmokers. Am J Epidemiol 1999; 149:13–20.
24. Wu AH, Fontham ET, Reynolds P, et al. Family history of cancer and risk of lung cancer among lifetime nonsmoking women in the United States. Am J Epidemiol 1996; 143:535–542.
25. Nordquist LT, Simon GR, Cantor A, et al. Improved survival in never-smokers vs current smokers with primary adenocarcinoma of the lung. Chest 2004; 126:347–351.
26. Brownson RC, Loy TS, Ingram E, et al. Lung cancer in nonsmoking women. Histology and survival patterns. Cancer 1995; 75:29–33.
27. Shepherd FA, Rodrigues PJ, Ciuleanu T, et al. Erlotinib in previously treated non-small-cell lung cancer. N Engl J Med 2005; 353:123–132.
28. Lynch TJ, Bell DW, Sordella R, et al. Activating mutations in the epidermal growth factor receptor underlying responsiveness of non-small-cell lung cancer to gefitinib. N Engl J Med 2004; 350:2129–2139.
29. Paez JG, Janne PA, Lee JC, et al. EGFR mutations in lung cancer: correlation with clinical response to gefitinib therapy. Science 2004; 304:1497–1500.
30. Tam IY, Chung LP, Suen WS, et al. Distinct epidermal growth factor receptor and KRAS mutation patterns in non-small cell lung cancer patients with different tobacco exposure and clinicopathologic features. Clin Cancer Res 2006; 12:1647–1653.
31. Le CF, Mukeria A, Hunt JD, et al. TP53 and KRAS mutation load and types in lung cancers in relation to tobacco smoke: distinct patterns in never, former, and current smokers. Cancer Res 2005; 65:5076–5083.
32. Doll R. Mortality from lung cancer in asbestos workers. Br J Ind Med 1955; 12:81–86.
33. Lubin JH, Boice JD, Jr., Edling C, et al. Lung cancer in radon-exposed miners and estimation of risk from indoor exposure. J Natl Cancer Inst 1995; 87:817–827.
34. Tockman MS, Anthonisen NR, Wright EC, et al. Airways obstruction and the risk for lung cancer. Ann Intern Med 1987; 106:512–518.
35. de Torres JP, Bastarrika G, Wisnivesky JP, et al. Assessing the relationship between lung cancer risk and emphysema detected on low-dose CT of the chest. Chest 2007; 132:1932–1938.

36. Daniels CE, Jett JR. Does interstitial lung disease predispose to lung cancer? Curr Opin Pulm Med 2005; 11:431–437.
37. Skuladottir H, Tjoenneland A, Overvad K, et al. Does insufficient adjustment for smoking explain the preventive effects of fruit and vegetables on lung cancer? Lung Cancer 2004; 45:1–10.
38. Holick CN, Michaud DS, Stolzenberg-Solomon R, et al. Dietary carotenoids, serum beta-carotene, and retinol and risk of lung cancer in the alpha-tocopherol, beta-carotene cohort study. Am J Epidemiol 2002; 156:536–547.
39. The effect of vitamin E and beta carotene on the incidence of lung cancer and other cancers in male smokers. The Alpha-Tocopherol, Beta Carotene Cancer Prevention Study Group. N Engl J Med 1994; 330:1029–1035.
40. Omenn GS, Goodman GE, Thornquist MD, et al. Effects of a combination of beta carotene and vitamin A on lung cancer and cardiovascular disease. N Engl J Med 1996; 334:1150–1155.
41. Paolini M, Cantelli-Forti G, Perocco P, et al. Co-carcinogenic effect of beta-carotene. Nature 1999; 398:760–761.
42. Paolini M, Antelli A, Pozzetti L, et al. Induction of cytochrome P450 enzymes and over-generation of oxygen radicals in beta-carotene supplemented rats. Carcinogenesis 2001; 22:1483–1495.
43. Arora A, Willhite CA, Liebler DC. Interactions of beta-carotene and cigarette smoke in human bronchial epithelial cells. Carcinogenesis 2001; 22:1173–1178.
44. Tokuhata GK, Lilienfeld AM. Familial aggregation of lung cancer in humans. J Natl Cancer Inst 1963; 30:289–312.
45. Schwartz AG, Yang P, Swanson GM. Familial risk of lung cancer among nonsmokers and their relatives. Am J Epidemiol 1996; 144:554–562.
46. Cote ML, Kardia SL, Wenzlaff AS, et al. Risk of lung cancer among white and black relatives of individuals with early-onset lung cancer. JAMA 2005; 293:3036–3042.
47. Etzel CJ, Amos CI, Spitz MR. Risk for smoking-related cancer among relatives of lung cancer patients. Cancer Res 2003; 63:8531–8535.
48. Sellers TA, Bailey-Wilson JE, Elston RC, et al. Evidence for mendelian inheritance in the pathogenesis of lung cancer. J Natl Cancer Inst 1990; 82:1272–1279.
49. Braun MM, Caporaso NE, Page WF, et al. Genetic component of lung cancer: cohort study of twins. Lancet 1994; 344:440–443.
50. Malkin D, Li FP, Strong LC, et al. Germ line p53 mutations in a familial syndrome of breast cancer, sarcomas, and other neoplasms. Science 1990; 250:1233–1238.
51. Vineis P, Veglia F, Benhamou S, et al. CYP1A1 T3801 C polymorphism and lung cancer: a pooled analysis of 2451 cases and 3358 controls. Int J Cancer 2003; 104:650–657.
52. Vineis P, Veglia F, Anttila S, et al. CYP1A1, GSTM1 and GSTT1 polymorphisms and lung cancer: a pooled analysis of gene–gene interactions. Biomarkers 2004; 9:298–305.
53. Yu D, Zhang X, Liu J, et al. Characterization of functional excision repair cross-complementation group 1 variants and their association with lung cancer risk and prognosis. Clin Cancer Res 2008; 14:2878–2886.
54. Beasley MB, Brambilla E, Travis WD. The 2004 World Health Organization classification of lung tumors. Seminars in Roentgenology 2005; 40:90–97.
55. Wingo PA, Ries LA, Giovino GA, et al. Annual report to the nation on the status of cancer, 1973–1996, with a special section on lung cancer and tobacco smoking. J Natl Cancer Inst 1999; 91:675–690.
56. Devesa SS, Shaw GL, Blot WJ. Changing patterns of lung cancer incidence by histological type. Cancer Epidemiol Biomarkers Prev 1991; 1:29–34.
57. Brooks DR, Austin JH, Heelan RT, et al. Influence of type of cigarette on peripheral versus central lung cancer. Cancer Epidemiol Biomarkers Prev 2005; 14:576–581.
58. Schuller HM. Mechanisms of smoking-related lung and pancreatic adenocarcinoma development. Nat Rev Cancer 2002; 2:455–463.

59. Pan H, Califano J, Ponte JF, et al. Loss of heterozygosity patterns provide fingerprints for genetic heterogeneity in multistep cancer progression of tobacco smoke-induced non-small cell lung cancer. Cancer Res 2005; 65:1664–1669.
60. Sundaresan V, Heppell-Parton A, Coleman N, et al. Somatic genetic changes in lung cancer and precancerous lesions. Ann Oncol 1995; 6:27–31.
61. Franklin WA, Gazdar AF, Haney J, et al. Widely dispersed p53 mutation in respiratory epithelium. A novel mechanism for field carcinogenesis. J Clin Invest 1997; 100:2133–2137.
62. Panani AD, Roussos C. Cytogenetic and molecular aspects of lung cancer. Cancer Lett 2006; 239:1–9.
63. Sanchez-Cespedes M, Ahrendt SA, Piantadosi S, et al. Chromosomal alterations in lung adenocarcinoma from smokers and nonsmokers. Cancer Res 2001; 61:1309–1313.
64. Sun S, Schiller JH, Gazdar AF. Lung cancer in never smokers – a different disease. Nat Rev Cancer 2007; 7:778–790.
65. Gradowski JF, Mantha GS, Hunt JL, et al. Molecular alterations in atypical adenomatous hyperplasia occurring in benign and cancer-bearing lungs. Diagn Mol Pathol 2007; 16:87–90.
66. Wistuba II, Behrens C, Milchgrub S, et al. Sequential molecular abnormalities are involved in the multistage development of squamous cell lung carcinoma. Oncogene 1999; 18:643–650.
67. Davies SJ, Gosney JR, Hansell DM, et al. Diffuse idiopathic pulmonary neuroendocrine cell hyperplasia: an under-recognised spectrum of disease. Thorax 2007; 62:248–252.
68. The Surgeon General's 1990 Report on The Health Benefits of Smoking Cessation. Executive Summary. MMWR Recomm Rep 1990; 39:i-12.
69. Kenfield SA, Stampfer MJ, Rosner BA, et al. Smoking and smoking cessation in relation to mortality in women. JAMA 2008; 299:2037–2047.
70. The HOPE and HOPE-TOO Trial Investigators. Effects of long-term Vitamin E supplementation on cardiovascular events and cancer: A randomized controlled trial. JAMA 2005; 293:1338–1347.
71. Lippman SM, Lee JJ, Karp DD, et al. Randomized phase III intergroup trial of isotretinoin to prevent second primary tumors in stage I non-small-cell lung cancer. J Natl Cancer Inst 2001; 93:605–618.
72. Balkwill F, Coussens LM. Cancer: an inflammatory link. Nature 2004; 431:405–406.
73. Peto R, Gray R, Collins R, et al. Randomised trial of prophylactic daily aspirin in British male doctors. Br Med J (Clin Res Ed) 1988; 296:313–316.
74. Cook NR, Lee IM, Gaziano JM, et al. Low-dose aspirin in the primary prevention of cancer: the Women's Health Study: a randomized controlled trial. JAMA 2005; 294:47–55.
75. Kim ES, Hong WK, Lee JJ, et al. A randomized double-blind study of the biological effects of celecoxib as a chemopreventive agent in current and former smokers. J Clin Oncol (Meeting Abstracts) 2008; 26:1501.
76. Clark LC, Combs GF, Jr., Turnbull BW, et al. Effects of selenium supplementation for cancer prevention in patients with carcinoma of the skin. A randomized controlled trial. Nutritional Prevention of Cancer Study Group. JAMA 1996; 276:1957–1963.
77. Frost JK, Ball WC, Jr., Levin ML, et al. Early lung cancer detection: results of the initial (prevalence) radiologic and cytologic screening in the Johns Hopkins study. Am Rev Respir Dis 1984; 130:549–554.
78. Marcus PM, Bergstralh EJ, Fagerstrom RM, et al. Lung cancer mortality in the Mayo Lung Project: impact of extended follow-up. J Natl Cancer Inst 2000; 92:1308–1316.
79. Melamed MR, Flehinger BJ, Zaman MB, et al. Screening for early lung cancer. Results of the Memorial Sloan-Kettering study in New York. Chest 1984; 86:44–53.
80. Henschke CI, Yankelevitz DF, Libby DM, et al. Survival of patients with stage I lung cancer detected on CT screening. N Engl J Med 2006; 355:1763–1771.

81. Carbone, PP, Frost, JK, Feinstein, AR, et al. Lung cancer: perspectives and prospects. Ann Intern Med 1970; 73:1003–1024.
82. Chute CG, Greenberg ER, Baron J, et al. Presenting conditions of 1539 population-based lung cancer patients by cell type and stage in New Hampshire and Vermont. Cancer 1985; 56:2107–2111.
83. Spiro SG, Gould MK, Colice GL. Initial evaluation of the patient with lung cancer: symptoms, signs, laboratory tests, and paraneoplastic syndromes: ACCP evidenced-based clinical practice guidelines (2nd edition). Chest 2007; 132:149S–160S.
84. Muers MF, Round CE. Palliation of symptoms in non-small cell lung cancer: a study by the Yorkshire Regional Cancer Organisation Thoracic Group. Thorax 1993; 48:339–343.
85. Fuller RW, Jackson DM. Physiology and treatment of cough. Thorax 1990; 45:425–430.
86. Gottlieb LS, Hillberg R. Endobronchial tamponade therapy for intractable hemoptysis. Chest 1975; 67:482–483.
87. Hsu AA. Thoracic embolotherapy for life-threatening haemoptysis: a pulmonologist's perspective. Respirology 2005; 10:138–143.
88. Jennings AL, Davies AN, Higgins JP, et al. A systematic review of the use of opioids in the management of dyspnoea. Thorax 2002; 57:939–944.
89. Bruera E, de SN, Velasco-Leiva A, et al. Effects of oxygen on dyspnoea in hypoxaemic terminal-cancer patients. Lancet 1993; 342:13–14.
90. Rice TW, Rodriguez RM, Light RW. The superior vena cava syndrome: clinical characteristics and evolving etiology. Medicine (Baltimore) 2006; 85:37–42.
91. Rusch VW. Management of Pancoast tumours. Lancet Oncol 2006; 7:997–1005.
92. Kelly K, Bunn PA, Jr. Is it time to reevaluate our approach to the treatment of brain metastases in patients with non-small cell lung cancer? Lung Cancer 1998; 20:85–91.
93. Hirsch FR, Paulson OB, Hansen HH, Vraa-Jensen J. Intracranial metastases in small cell carcinoma of the lung: correlation of clinical and autopsy findings. Cancer 1982; 50:2433–2437.
94. Carolan H, Sun AY, Bezjak A, et al. Does the incidence and outcome of brain metastases in locally advanced non-small cell lung cancer justify prophylactic cranial irradiation or early detection? Lung Cancer 2005; 49:109–115.
95. Chamberlain MC. Neoplastic meningitis. Oncologist 2008; 13:967–977.
96. Davis PC, Hudgins PA, Peterman SB, Hoffman JC, Jr. Diagnosis of cerebral metastases: double-dose delayed CT vs contrast-enhanced MR imaging. AJNR Am J Neuroradiol 1991; 12:293–300.
97. Tanvetyanon T, Robinson LA, Schell MJ, et al. Outcomes of adrenalectomy for isolated synchronous versus metachronous adrenal metastases in non-small-cell lung cancer: a systematic review and pooled analysis. J Clin Oncol 2008; 26:1142–1147.
98. Carlsen K, Jensen AB, Jacobsen E, et al. Psychosocial aspects of lung cancer. Lung Cancer 2005; 47:293–300.
99. Mountain CF. Revisions in the International System for Staging Lung Cancer. Chest 1997; 111:1710–1717.
100. Goldstraw P, Crowley J, Chansky K, et al. The IASLC Lung Cancer Staging Project: proposals for the revision of the TNM stage groupings in the forthcoming (seventh) edition of the TNM Classification of malignant tumours. J Thorac Oncol 2007; 2:706–714.
101. Argiris A, Murren JR. Staging and clinical prognostic factors for small-cell lung cancer. Cancer J 2001; 7:437–447.
102. Toloza EM, Harpole L, Detterbeck F, et al. Invasive staging of non-small cell lung cancer: a review of the current evidence. Chest 2003; 123:157S–166S.
103. Mandrekar SJ, Schild SE, Hillman SL, et al. A prognostic model for advanced stage nonsmall cell lung cancer. Pooled analysis of North Central Cancer Treatment Group trials. Cancer 2006; 107:781–792.

104. Ou SH, Zell JA, Ziogas A, et al. Prognostic factors for survival of stage I non-small cell lung cancer patients: a population-based analysis of 19,702 stage I patients in the California Cancer Registry from 1989 to 2003. Cancer 2007; 110:1532–1541.

105. Scott WJ, Howington J, Feigenberg S, et al. Treatment of non-small cell lung cancer stage I and stage II: ACCP evidence-based clinical practice guidelines (2nd edition). Chest 2007; 132:234S–242S.

106. Pignon JP, Tribodet H, Scagliotti GV, et al. Lung adjuvant cisplatin evaluation: a pooled analysis by the LACE Collaborative Group. J Clin Oncol 2008; 26:3552–3559.

107. Robinson LA, Ruckdeschel JC, Wagner H, Jr., et al. Treatment of Non-small Cell Lung Cancer-Stage IIIA: ACCP Evidence-Based Clinical Practice Guidelines (2nd Edition). Chest 2007; 132:243S–265.

108. Jett JR, Schild SE, Keith RL, et al. Treatment of Non-small Cell Lung Cancer, Stage IIIB: ACCP Evidence-Based Clinical Practice Guidelines (2nd Edition). Chest 2007; 132:266S–276.

109. Albain KS, Swann RS, Rusch VR, et al. Phase III study of concurrent chemotherapy and radiotherapy (CT/RT) vs CT/RT followed by surgical resection for stage IIIA(pN2) non-small cell lung cancer (NSCLC): Outcomes update of North American Intergroup 0139 (RTOG 9309). J Clin Oncol (Meeting Abstracts) 2005; 23:7014.

110. Schiller JH, Harrington D, Belani CP, et al. Comparison of four chemotherapy regimens for advanced non-small-cell lung cancer. N Engl J Med 2002; 346:92–98.

111. Sandler A, Gray R, Perry MC, et al. Paclitaxel-carboplatin alone or with bevacizumab for non-small-cell lung cancer. N Engl J Med 2006; 355:2542–2550.

112. Hanna N, Shepherd FA, Fossella FV, et al. Randomized phase III trial of pemetrexed versus docetaxel in patients with non-small-cell lung cancer previously treated with chemotherapy. J Clin Oncol 2004; 22:1589–1597.

113. Simon GR, Turrisi A. Management of small cell lung cancer: ACCP evidence-based clinical practice guidelines (2nd Edition). Chest 2007; 132:324S–3339.

114. Turrisi AT, III, Kim K, Blum R, et al. Twice-daily compared with once-daily thoracic radiotherapy in limited small-cell lung cancer treated concurrently with cisplatin and etoposide. N Engl J Med 1999; 340:265–271.

115. Auperin A, Arriagada R, Pignon JP, et al. Prophylactic cranial irradiation for patients with small-cell lung cancer in complete remission. N Engl J Med 1999; 341:476–484.

116. Slotman B, Faivre-Finn C, Kramer G, et al. Prophylactic cranial irradiation in extensive small-cell lung cancer. N Engl J Med 2007; 357:664–672.

117. Fu JB, Kau Y, Severson RK, et al. Lung cancer in women: analysis of the national surviellance, epidemiology, and end results database. Chest 2005; 127:768–777.

Hallmarks of Metastasis

M. Roshni Ray and David M. Jablons

Abstract Metastasis is rarely due to accidental sloughing off of cancerous cells from a nonmalignant tumor and colonizing elsewhere; on the contrary, it is an active process requiring genetic and/or epigenetic mechanisms leading to the formation of a cell capable of responding to certain chemotactic signals that direct motility, interacting with other cells to be co-translocated, implanting in foreign locations, avoiding immune response, being refractory to growth inhibitory signals, and proliferating independently of growth factors for sustained cell division. The complexity of these processes necessitates a detailed understanding of the molecular and cellular mechanisms behind each of these steps. In this chapter, we will discuss hallmarks of metastatic process, along with theories proposed, genes involved, techniques to monitor, and therapeutic implications.

Introduction

Cancer is a general term describing hundreds of diseases in which cells aggressively proliferate without regard for normal growth limits of the original tissue or organ site and then invade surrounding and adjoining tissues. Most cancers are diseases of the epithelial tissue [1], where in late stages the cancerous cells invade the mesoderm and the endodermal layers. Metastasis, the subsequent spread of these invasive cells throughout the body to other organs, accounts for 90% of human cancer deaths [2]. Interestingly, 5-year survival of stage IV patients is a dismal 3%. By contrast, 5-year survival of early-stage cancers is 49% [3]. Thus, in addition to early detection efforts, understanding the mechanisms of metastasis and halting its course are imperative to the treatment of cancer.

D.M. Jablons (✉)
Thoracic Oncology Program, Comprehensive Cancer Center, University of California,
San Francisco, CA, USA
e-mail: jablonsd@surgery.ucsf.edu

V. Keshamouni et al. (eds.), *Lung Cancer Metastasis*,
DOI 10.1007/978-1-4419-0772-1_2, © Springer Science+Business Media, LLC 2009

Traditionally, metastasis has been characterized as a late-stage phenomenon in cancer. Pathologic staging describes first the size and local invasion of a primary tumor, then metastasis to lymph nodes, and finally distal metastases. Gene expression profiling studies [4] suggest that metastatic potential is intrinsic to all tumor cells and that metastatic spread could be an early event in tumorigenesis. However, there is some evidence for the existence of a small population of cells within a tumor, which exclusively are capable of metastasis – the so-called cancer stem cells.

Regardless of which cells are capable of metastasizing, metastasis is an extremely complex process and, thankfully, highly inefficient as only a small fraction of tumor cells are actually able to fully metastasize. The process involves migration of a cancerous cell out of the original location, overcoming barriers to implantation in a foreign location, subsequently dividing uncontrolled, and/or metastasizing further. Whereas in most cancers the cell cycle checkpoint arrest is overcome by at least one transformative event early in cancer development in the traditional model of metastasis, a second genetic or epigenetic event is usually necessary for transition of a non-metastatic tumor to metastatic. Metastasis is rarely due to accidental sloughing off of cancerous cells from a nonmalignant tumor and colonizing elsewhere; on the contrary, it is an active process requiring genetic and/or epigenetic mechanisms leading to the formation of a cell capable of responding to certain chemotactic signals that direct motility, interacting with other cells to be co-translocated, implanting in foreign locations, avoiding immune response, being refractory to growth inhibitory signals, and proliferating independently of growth factors for sustained cell division. The complexity of these processes necessitates a detailed understanding of the molecular and cellular mechanisms behind each of these steps.

The Metastatic Process

Cancer metastasis involves several interrelated steps, each of which can be rate limiting in that failure to achieve any state can shut down the entire metastatic process. Moreover, only certain cells within a heterogeneous tumor population are capable of achieving these steps. Metastasis consists of (1) detachment of epithelial cells from the extracellular matrix (ECM), (2) survival within the bloodstream, and (3) growth at the metastatic site (Fig. 1).

As metastasis tends to be the lethal aspect of cancer, dissecting its biological basis is of utmost importance in pinpointing therapeutic targets to prevent and cure it. The existence of lymph node metastases in a cancer is a strong indicator of survival in patients as well as a prognosticator of whether other distal metastases will develop. In some cancers, lymph node metastases are better indicators of distant metastasis than in other cancers. In head and neck cancer, for example, the correlation is strong – the presence of lymph node metastases in the neck halves the survival rate in patients [5]. Moreover, only 7% of

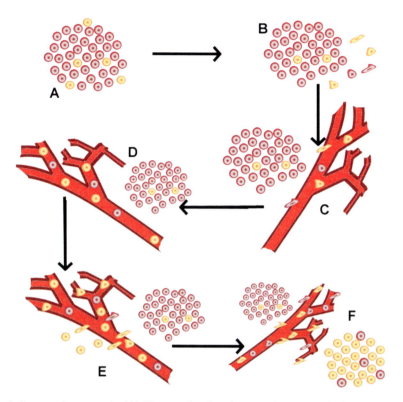

Fig. 1 Stages of metastasis. (**A**) Tumor; (**B**) detachment of tumor cells from the ECM; (**C**) intravasation of tumor cells into the bloodstream; (**D**) transport of tumor cells through the bloodstream; (**E**) extravasation of tumor cells at distal site; and (**F**) growth of metastatic lesion

patients whose necks are free of lymph node metastases develop distant metastases. This strong correlation seems to indicate that metastasis somehow involves infiltrating the lymphatic system and using it to migrate through the body. In other cancers such as breast cancer, however, 20–30% of patients whose axillary lymph nodes are free of disease still develop distant metastases. Thus, there seems to be another distinct pathway of metastatic cell dissemination that is independent of the lymphatic system. This second pathway has been shown to utilize hematogenous routes in the vascular system. Even so, the presence of axillary lymph node metastasis continues to serve as a good indicator of whether the disease will spread [6].

All cells have the default fate of apoptosis or programmed cell death. Most cells depend on extracellular signals to keep the trigger for apoptotic cascade of proteolysis at bay. Cancer cells, in general, are refractory to apoptotic signals, or their mitotic division is independent of stimulation by growth factors. As the potential for developing a tumor is directly correlated with resistance to apoptosis, so is resistance to apoptosis correlated with the metastatic potential of a tumor. The reason behind this correlation is somewhat unclear. It is possible that certain rare cells having the ability to undergo mitosis independently of growth factors preferentially become metastatic; alternatively, the same molecular events that give rise to metastatic transformation of a tumor cell cause it to be resistant to apoptosis. Therefore, anoikis (cell death by disruption of cell adhesion and cell–ECM interactions) and amorphosis (cell death by loss of cytoskeletal structure) are vital to preventing metastasis. Normally anoikis and amorphosis are triggered by detachment of usually adherent cells from the ECM and through disruption of the actin cytoskeleton [7], which is consistent with the general observation that specific cell–cell and/or cell–matrix contact and ligand-mediated signaling are necessary to keep the apoptotic cascade from being activated. Abrogation of the need for signaling through contact for suppressing apoptosis might, therefore, lead to both immortalization and cell detachment. Alternatively, the two processes might be unrelated.

Theories of Metastasis

It is currently unclear whether any given cell within a tumor once transformed into the metastatic stage can migrate and form a secondary tumor or whether a special group of cells within a solid tumor, cancer stem cells, a rare tumor cell type with indefinite self-renewal capability, is the only cell type capable of migrating and colonizing secondary tissues and organs. In the traditional model of cancer metastasis, every malignant tumor cell supposedly possesses metastatic potential. A normal cell accumulates random mutations eventually leading to cancer, and these neoplastic cells continue to accrue mutations until some become metastatic by chance. Nevertheless, small populations of cells in many malignant tumors, including acute myeloblastic leukemia (AML) [8], glioblastoma [9], small cell lung cancer [10], non-small cell lung cancer [11], malignant melanoma [12], and breast cancer [13], display properties reminiscent of stem cells, the cell group that indefinitely retains the property of self-renewal by mitosis [14]. It is conceivable that migration of these cells could in principle lead to metastasis and successful colonization at a distant site, and this may explain why successful primary metastasis is a relatively rare event. Strong evidence implicating these "cancer stem cells" (see Chapter 3) in metastasis is provided by the observation of overlap between the genes and signaling pathways necessary for normal stem cell motility and those for metastatic cancer cells [15]. Invasive metastasis appears, for a number of cancer types, to be a property of a subpopulation of tumor cells which appear to have stem cell-like properties. Since differentiated cells rarely reenter the somatic stem cell state, progeny of previously differentiated cells should rarely metastasize.

Dissemination from the Primary Tumor

The first stage of cancer metastasis is signaled by the detachment of cancer cells from the ECM before entering into the bloodstream. Changes in cell motility are major factors in enabling separation from the primary tumor, and changes in cell fate associated with cytoskeletal reorganization are needed for transition to the invading cell type. Cells display two major types of morphogenesis correlated with early metastatic ability. In the more common version – epithelial–mesenchymal transition (EMT) – the cell elongates, secretes extracellular enzymes to locally degrade the ECM, and migrates out (see Chapter 4 for discussion on EMT). While TGFβ in cooperation with the Ras-GTPase signaling pathways can induce EMT, it is unclear whether cells that are so transformed indeed constitute metastatic cells [16]. The other, more aggressive, type of motility is amoeboid transcription: the elongated cells take on a spherical morphology, and these spheroidal cells deform through pre-existing gaps in the ECM to disseminate into the bloodstream (Fig. 2). There is also a third, rarer, form of cellular motility called collective migration that involves simultaneous mesenchymal motion of a cluster of cells.

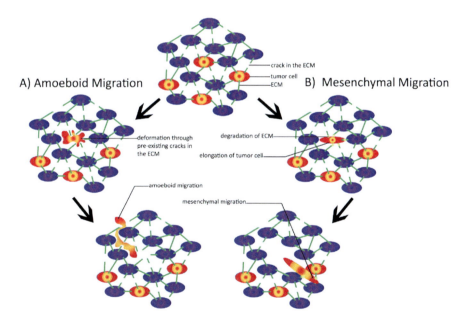

Fig. 2 (**A**) Amoeboid motility. (1) Epithelial tumor cells in the ECM. (2) Deformation through pre-existing gaps in the ECM. (3) Amoeboid migration through cracks in the ECM. (**B**) Mesenchymal motility. (1) Epithelial tumor cells in the ECM. (2) Elongation of tumor cell and degradation of ECM. (3) Degradation of ECM and mesenchymal migration

Intra- and intercellular signaling mechanisms enable these morphogenetic processes, and cell–cell cooperation is likely involved in controlling swarm-like behavior of rare metastasizing cells. Cells, however, appear to be capable of switching between different forms of motility, which renders therapeutics that target genes or proteins associated with distinct aspects of mobility somewhat refractory [17]. There is, nonetheless, evidence suggesting that certain transcriptional regulators may control entire sets of motility genes. For example, AP-1 transcription factor activity is correlated with expression of cell motility genes [18]. Twist, Six-1, and BRMS1, all transcriptional regulators, have also been implicated. Other genes involved in cell–cell signaling such as ErbB1, encoding epidermal growth factor receptor (EGFR), are implicated in cancer cell motility but not necessarily in growth of the primary tumor. Genes or proteins that are specifically implicated in cell motility in metastatic transformation are potential drug targets.

The significance of EMT lies in that disseminating metastatic cells must be able to survive without normal matrix components and evade anoikis. This survival is important in metastasis because intra/extravasating tumor cells either do not adhere to a matrix at all or encounter foreign matrices along the way [19]. Overexpression of BCL2 increases the metastatic potential of breast cancer epithelial cells by inhibiting matrix-degradation-induced apoptosis but does not affect primary tumor growth or cell motility [20, 21].

The developmental signaling pathways Wnt, Notch, and Hedgehog have also been linked to EMT [19]. Wnt signaling is of particular interest as it has been associated with collective migration and is aberrantly activated in lung cancers [22]. With regard to metastasis, loss of signaling by Wnt1, the first of the Wnt proteins to be discovered, has been shown to reduce the size of lung metastases in mice [23].

As stated earlier, most motile cells normally move mesenchymally (Fig. 2). After tumor cells undergo EMT, they migrate by polarizing and extending pseudopodia-like projections (lamellipods) on their anterior ends, binding specific cell surface or extracellular matrix ligands, pushing themselves forward through actin-based contractions of the cell body, and then releasing the adhesive bonds at the rear. Adhesion to the ECM substrate is mediated through interactions of beta-integrins, a major group of cell surface receptor ligands. Subsequently, signaling by the integrins, as well as integrins themselves, cooperate with and recruit cell surface proteases (such as matrix metalloproteinases, MMPs) to locally degrade the ECM. MMPs break down collagen in the ECM (collagenolysis). Mesenchymal motion is proteolytic and path generating: gaps in the ECM through which the cell ultimately passes are created by the cell itself [24]. Actin filaments are the dominant structural component of lamellipods [25]. H-, N-, and K-Ras are small GTPases that promote mesenchymal lamellipod extension by regulating $PtdIns(3,4,5)P3$ levels. Cdc42 and Rac1 are also small GTPases that promote formation of actin-rich protrusions. Unfortunately for patients, near-total inhibition of cell surface proteases by protease inhibitor treatment induces conversion of mesenchymal cells to spherical morphology and virtually no change in migration rates [24].

Amoeboid motion – where spherically shaped cells deform and slip through pre-existing cracks in the ECM – is protease independent and path finding (in contrast to the proteolytic path-generating nature of mesenchymal locomotion) (Fig. 2). RhoA (a small GTPase) activates the ROCK protein, which phosphorylates MLC2, a myosin light chain protein, which in turn activates a signaling cascade implicated in the development of spheroid structure and induction of cellular locomotion. The Smurf1 protein, an ubiquitin ligase, is responsible for targeting RhoA for degradation. When Smurf1 is activated, RhoA activity is depleted due to ubiquitin-mediated proteolysis, possibly involving the proteasome, and cells form lamellipods that aid in mesenchymal cell movement. On the other hand, when Smurf1 activity is downregulated, the RhoA cascade is activated and induces amoeboid cell invasion, which is actually more aggressive than mesenchymal motion [26].

The signaling cascades leading to different types of motion ultimately influence cytoskeletal elements to reorganize and the molecular motors to generate force that leads to cellular motion. Altered MLC organization is related to the amoeboid tumor cells' ability to generate sufficient mechanical force to deform the extracellular mesh of collagen fibers and to enable the cell to push through the ECM [27]. ROCK regulates MLC phosphorylation, and inhibition of ROCK (but not of MMPs) reduces in vivo cancer cell motility. The protein ezrin is localized in the direction of cell movement in amoeboid cells [28]. Ezrin provides a functional link between the plasma membrane and the cortical actin cytoskeleton of the cell. Forced ezrin expression induces a highly metastatic state in certain poorly metastatic tumor cell lines [27]. Combined blockade of extracellular proteases and ROCK prevents tumor cells from switching between types of motility and also blocks cell invasion.

In a study to identify a gene expression signature associated with the propensity for metastasis, invasive breast cancer tumor cells were collected in vitro by virtue of their chemotactic ability (migration toward a source of EGF), and their mRNA expression levels were assayed in relation to their less invasive counterparts [17]. Genes associated with motility were most strikingly differentially regulated in invasive cells compared to those in non-invasive cells. For example, cofilin, Arp2/3 complex, and capping protein, all involved in lamellipod protrusion, extension, and tail retraction, were coordinately upregulated in the invasive cells. Genes encoding Rho and ROCK were significantly upregulated. Upregulation of cofilin, Arp2/3, and capping protein results in increased protrusion velocities of up to 10-fold higher than those in cells with lower levels of expression of these proteins. By contrast, the ZBP1 gene is strongly downregulated in invasive breast carcinoma cells. ZBP1 binds to beta-actin mRNA and localizes the mRNA to the leading edge of cells. Beta-actin is the most common form of actin which is polymerized as filaments within the lamellipod and is acted on by cofilin, capping protein, and the Arp2/3 pathways. The site of sub-cellular localization of the ZBP1 protein likely determines, by controlling localization of the beta-actin mRNA (thus its site of translation), the site at which these pathways converge. Downregulation of ZBP1-mediated beta-actin mRNA targeting, which is associated with inhibition of lamellipod formation in mesenchymal cells, results in the formation of highly invasive amoeboid cells and increased chemotaxis [4].

Vascular Transport of Metastatic Cells

Even though both mesenchymal and amoeboid cells can migrate toward and intravasate into blood vessels, amoeboid cells are better suited to survive within the vascular system. A mesenchymal to amoeboid transformation is important during entry into blood vessels because elongated mesenchymal cells tend to shatter, or undergo amorphosis, in response to the force of blood flow (hemodynamic shearing). The spheroid morphology characteristic of amoeboid cells can better withstand high shear stress and hence these cells survive better in the bloodstream [29]. Thus, solitary cancer cells in circulation are sensitive to apoptosis, particularly to that induced by mechanical stress and immune-mediated destruction. Potentially metastatic cells that have entered the bloodstream are destroyed either by mechanical stress or, supposedly, by immune-directed cell death.

Once disseminated into the bloodstream, tumor cells are able to circulate throughout the body. Oftentimes cancer patients have significant quantities of these cells both in blood and in bone marrow long after removal of the primary tumor and before any sign of metastasis occurs [30]. Are each of these dormant cells capable of producing their own clonal metastases or do only a fraction possess the pluripotency to form the seed of metastatic malignancy? To answer this question, a distinction between the tumor cells circulating in peripheral blood (circulating tumor cells – CTCs) as opposed to those aggregated in the bone marrow (disseminated tumor cells – DTCs) must be established.

DTCs have been documented in the bone marrow for most types of epithelial cancers [30]. While a number of studies have revealed correlation between the presence of DTCs and postoperative metastatic relapse, viable use of DTCs as prognosticators of recurrence has yet to be unequivocally demonstrated. A point of interest is that presence of DTCs is associated not only with bone metastases but also with distal tumor development in lung, brain, and liver; thus, it is likely that DTCs accumulating in the bone marrow eventually reenter the vasculature to travel throughout the body [31]. Incidentally, the processes by which tumor cells disseminate appear to vary by cancer. In early-stage breast cancer, DTCs are heterogeneous and do not possess the same changes as the tumor; however, in late stages the DTC genotypes are largely homogeneous. This observation seems to indicate that dissemination of DTCs is an early event after which the cells accumulate other mutations, some of which eventually overwhelmingly favor metastasis. In prostate cancer, however, CTCs appear genotypically homogeneous and similar to cells in the primary tumor. This observation suggests that as the tumor develops, cells with metastatic potential eventually arise directly from the primary tumor and spread forth throughout the body [30].

At present, only limited data exist correlating DTCs with concurrent CTCs, and the significance of CTCs in peripheral blood is as yet unclear [30]. In most cancers, patients appear to present with a higher fraction of DTCs than CTCs, suggesting that bone marrow may provide better conditions for tumor cell homing and survival [30]. Another hypothesis of note is the speculation as to whether surgery itself can dislodge tumor cells from the primary malignancy, thereby allowing these cells to become CTCs. Bone marrow possibly forms a pre-metastatic niche and that it offers a site for dormancy is evidenced by the presence of DTCs in colorectal carcinomas, a cancer in which bone metastases are rare [31].

It is usually assumed that invasive tumor cells entering blood vessels and foreign tissues will be recognized and targeted by the immune system. Thomas and Burnet [32, 33] suggested that immunosurveillance was responsible for the targeted elimination of cancerous cells, particularly in that immune response is often associated with advanced carcinogenesis (for discussion on immunesurveilance and tumor progression see Chapter 6). Indeed, immune surveillance may contribute to dormancy in DTCs. The nature of dormancy is variable in that in some cases it is characterized by a balance between apoptosis and proliferation whereas in other cases it describes either non- or slowly proliferating cells. It has been shown in murine models that upon depletion of CD4 + and CD8 + leukocytes, progressive growth is initiated in previously dormant tumor cells [30]. In lung cancer, increased presence of CD8 + cytotoxic lymphocytes has been observed, but this escalation in immune response does not appear to correlate with outcome. Tumor cells appear to evade the immune system because, as native cells, they are poorly immunogenic. Moreover, tumor cells also downregulate antigens by interfering with antigen-presenting cells and secrete cytokines that may aid in both immune tolerance and suppression. Tumor cells are often also resistant to cytotoxic T-lymphocytes as evidenced by the cells' failure to undergo apoptosis upon attack. Nonetheless, reduction of malignant tumor has been observed alongside bacterial infection, leading to hope of an anti-tumor vaccine created from dead bacteria. Although no conclusively successful anti-tumor vaccines have yet been reported, a number of such vaccines have entered clinical trials [34].

All this being said, our understanding of the role immunosurveillance plays in maintaining dormancy is murky, at best. In most cases, tumor development appears to be similar in normal and in immunocompromised animal models, and any systematic correlation between immune deficiency and human cancer has yet to be demonstrated. Thus, it is unlikely that immune surveillance offers much protection against anything but pathogen-associated cancers [35].

What then of the heightened immune cell activity at primary tumor and metastatic sites? Macrophages have been observed to produce matrix metalloproteinases that promote tumor cell mobility by degrading the ECM. These tumor-associated macrophages (TAMs) express EGF and promote EGFR-dependent cell invasion (for more detailed discussion of TAMs and other immune cells see Chapter 11). TAMs tend to aggregate along blood vessels and tumor margins and create an EGF gradient responsible for directing chemotaxis. This gradient likely promotes intra- and extravasation. In fact, prior to extravasation, leukocytes are recruited when tumor cells attach to blood vessel walls, and the leukocytes are thought to extravasate ahead of the cancer cells, in essence by ushering them out [36].

Proliferative Ability at Site of Metastasis

Metastasis has been directly correlated, on a single animal basis, with the blood burden of tumor cells. A high concentration of CTCs in the bloodstream is related to a higher likelihood of metastasis [17]. Nevertheless, most cells die rapidly after extravasation [37, 38], which is likely why DTCs seem to correlate better with prognosis than CTCs. In as far back as 1889, Stephen Paget posited the "seed and soil" hypothesis [39] – that metastatic ability was dependent upon cross-communication between specific tumorigenic cells (seeds) and the distal organ microenvironment (soil). The more tumor "seeds" that are available in distal organs, the more likely it is that some will take root and metastasize. The actual site of metastasis is, incidentally, not directly linked to blood profusion through that specific organ. This is because certain markers at the secondary tumor site genetically predispose tumor cells to attach and develop into micro-metastases – the importance of "soil."

Organs with dense capillary beds (bone, liver, and lung) are common metastatic sites probably because CTCs are mechanically arrested in small vessels [7]. That being said, certain cancers are predisposed to metastasize to certain organs and there is no systematic correlation between blood burden and metastasis on an organ level. Instead, organs with high metastatic potential in a specific instance tend to exhibit predisposition toward angiogenesis. For example, cells of these tissues express high levels of growth factors such as VEGF, HGF, FGF, and EGF. These growth factors stimulate macrophages to produce MMPs that locally degrade the ECM and allow tumor cells to take root and proliferate. CD44 has been implicated in tumor cell adhesion and is important for endowing the expressing cells with the ability to form micrometastases at distal site. Disruption of the CD44–ECM interaction tends to induce apoptosis and prevent metastasis [40].

Without a blood supply, tumor cells adhered at a secondary site constitute foci of dormant micrometastases, and although they may remain dormant for years, they undergo rapid proliferation once angiogenesis occurs. While dormant, these cells are largely quiescent or, in some cases, proliferate at extremely slow rates. Once growth factor-induced angiogenesis takes place, however, the cells begin to rapidly divide. Blood supply provides oxygen, growth factors, and nutrients vital to the proliferation of metastatic cells. Angiogenesis is triggered when angiogenic inducers (mainly growth factors) are favored over inhibitors (for further discussion on angiogenic diversity see Chapters 7 and 8). The inhibitors tend to be ECM proteins or protein fragments such as thrombospondin and endostatin [31]. Inhibition of angiogenesis appears to stymie metastatic spread and has thus received much attention of late with regard to targeted therapeutics.

Genes Involved in Metastasis

Are metastatic cancer cells genetically different from non-metastatic cancer cells? The genetic variability usually associated with most solid tumor cells provides a window into the mechanism of metastatic spread. The spectrum of genetic variability among secondary tumors of diverse locations resembles more closely those present in cells of the primary tumors in the same individual than either is to the same cancer type from different individuals [41]. These results are consistent with the idea that metastatic cells are clonally derived from primary tumor cells but do not necessarily signify that metastatic tumors, or tumors in general from different individuals, are genetically heterogeneous. On the contrary, the question of whether the same or similar genetic or epigenetic changes are necessary for all metastatic cells remains open.

Given the complexity of the metastatic process, genetic mechanisms behind it are likely to be complex. The motivations for studying genes involved in metastasis are 2-fold: understanding the biological basis of the process and finding a molecular signature of metastasis for better diagnosis, prognosis, and therapeutic intervention to restrict it. Both motivations are well served by studies that aim to identify the predominant genetic factors correlated with metastasis. A groundbreaking step in understanding the genetic basis of metastasis was taken by Ramaswamy et al. [42] when the authors measured genome-wide gene expression profiles of 12 samples of confirmed metastatic adenocarcinomas of diverse origins (breast, lung, prostate, uterine, and ovarian cancers) and compared them with those obtained from 64 confirmed non-metastasizing cancers of the same types. The comparison yielded a best descriptor transcript set of 128 genes, of which 64 were overexpressed and 64 were underexpressed in the metastatic cancer samples. The descriptor gene set did not provide any obvious set of genes with related function. In fact, some genes that are underexpressed are unexpected (e.g., *MLC2*) and others that are overexpressed are of unknown significance for metastasis (e.g., glucose phosphate isomerase). From this larger gene set, the authors derived a core gene expression signature with a refined set of 17 metastasis markers (8 overexpressed and 9 underexpressed). These 17 genes performed well as predictors of metastasis on other unrelated tumors with or without metastasis. This refined core set of genes also included several genes whose expression signatures defy simple logical expectations: e.g., actin gamma 2, myosin heavy chain 11, and myosin light chain kinase genes are underexpressed, whereas lamin B and type 1 collagens $\alpha 1$ and $\alpha 2$ are overexpressed. Thus, despite the obvious utility of this core set of gene expression signature markers for more accurate prognosis, a biological understanding of their basis was not forthcoming.

The results of Ramaswamy et al. [42] can in principle be interpreted to mean that a majority of cells in solid tumors, which carry a signature set of gene expression values defining potential for metastasis, are able to metastasize. This conclusion could be drawn because a minority contribution of rare metastatic cells to the overall mRNA levels would have gone undetected in their experiments and could give credence to the traditional theory of metastatic progression. Alternatively, it might also mean that a small population of cancer stem cells in these tumors are actually capable of metastasis, yet by cell division, they give rise to two cell types: one along the linear stem cell line that maintains a constant cell number and the another that proliferates to differentiate into non-stem cell character but retains the epigenetic signature of the original metastatic stem cells. The reason for not detecting this core gene expression signature in non-metastatic tumors might just be that the stem cell populations in these tumors are below a critical number or that there is a reversal of epigenetic signatures among some of their progeny.

A biologically insightful understanding of metastasis has come from identifying genes that suppress tumor metastasis using several different in vivo metastasis assays [43]. Metastasis suppressor genes, or MSGs, are a special class of genes that are turned off in metastatic cells but, when re-expressed, inhibit metastasis without affecting tumorigenicity. At least 12 suppressor genes have been identified to date, beginning with the discovery of NM23 in 1988 [44]. Other MSGs include *NME1* – a member of the nucleoside diphosphate kinase family of proteins implicated in cell cycle regulation, *KISS1* – a regulator of metalloproteases and a ligand of a G-protein-coupled receptor [45], a mitogen-activated protein kinase gene (*MKK4*), and *BRMS1* which functions in gap junctions and reduces motility. Each of these genes provides interesting anchor to the spectrum of events thought to be responsible for distinct cellular stages of metastasis. In lung cancer, the invasion suppressor CRMP1 (collapsin response-mediator protein 1) has been identified as an invasion suppressor, but its efficacy as an MSG has only been demonstrated in vitro and thus has yet to be validated as a true MSG [44]. More work is needed in this direction to understand the detailed molecular pathways that integrate functions of MSGs in gene regulatory and signaling networks.

Techniques for Monitoring Metastasis

Because only a small fraction of malignant cells eventually metastasize, and these are difficult to identify early in a heterogeneous tumor cell population, studying metastasis has proven difficult until only recently. With the advent of refined optical imaging techniques, on both a whole-body and microscopic scale, and by the identification of cellular and molecular markers to define the metastatic stage, a better understanding of metastasis is now possible. Whole-body imaging allows non-invasive study of the tumorigenic and metastatic processes and their development within a single organism. Microscopic techniques allow morphological analysis on a cellular and sub-cellular level [46]. Currently, most in vivo techniques for studying metastasis are usable only in animal models.

Goodale et al. developed a flow cytometry method to quantify CTCs in mice and further adapted this technique along with laser scanning cytometry methods to study both bone marrow and lymph node dissemination of tumor cells [47]. Essentially, mice were injected with metastatic human breast cancer cells and at progressive time points, the animals were sacrificed for harvest of peripheral blood, lymph nodes, and bone marrow. These samples were then fluorescently labeled and studied using cytometric techniques. Unfortunately, since this method requires sacrifice of the animal model, it is not translatable to human research.

Multiphoton confocal microscopy has also been used to study metastatic cells in vivo by tagging these cells with green fluorescent protein and tracking their motion but again, this technology is not approved for use in clinic patients [46]. Sipkins and colleagues have used dynamic intravital confocal imaging to demonstrate unique regions within bone marrow to which metastatic leukemia cells may home [48]. A group at the University of Pennsylvania employed GFP tagging to study apoptosis in potentially metastatic melanomas and found that propensity to apoptose after arrest in pulmonary vasculature was a distinguishing factor between metastatic and non-metastatic cells [49].

Most human models of metastasis involve ex vivo analysis of cells purified from either blood or surgically resected samples [46]. Such methodology, however, limits the insight gained regarding the initial process of metastasis away from the original tumor. In terms of monitoring metastases in patients, PET and CT scans are used to regularly check cancer patients for new lesions and pathologists use traditional observation and staining methods to determine whether these lesions are new primary cancers or secondary or tertiary metastases.

Therapeutics and Future Directions

Since, as mentioned earlier, metastasis accounts for nearly 90% of cancer-related deaths, recognizing and preemptively treating carcinomas with high metastatic potential is vital to reducing disease mortality. Identifying and targeting the so-called cancer stem cells is a key step in such early treatment. However, to do so requires definite identification of such cancer stem cells as well as therapeutic regimens that demonstrably target only cancer stem cells but not normal stem cells [50].

Apoptosis resistance has been shown to be a key feature both in tumorigenesis and in metastatic spread but the direct correlation with metastasis has yet to be illuminated due to limited models [7]. Moreover, a cell's intrinsic survival properties likely play a role in its ability to survive in a distal microenvironment, and these properties must be elucidated to better target highly metastatic cells.

Total blood and bone marrow burdens of disseminated cells seem to play a role in the likelihood of cancer recurrence, so early detection of these disseminated tumor cells could perhaps determine whether patients should undergo systemic therapies adjuvant to surgical resection. Although all such therapies do target disease relapse, there is currently little selection in place to determine which patients are at greater statistical relapse than others, leading to toxic and unpleasant overtreatment of patients [51]. For example, currently less than 25% of breast cancer patients lacking overt lymph node metastases suffer from relapse within 10 years after operation, but greater than 90% receive chemotherapy [52]. In non-small cell lung cancer (NSCLC), patients presenting with early-stage disease generally forgo adjuvant therapy post-resection, but some of these patients, those who suffer relapse within 5 years of operation, need to be selectively identified for therapies complementing surgery [53].

Inhibition of cellular motility is also an important target, particularly in managing early-stage disease [17]. As early detection becomes more commonplace, targeted therapies limiting dissemination of cancers that have not yet undergone micrometastases become more important. Unfortunately, evaluating the effectiveness of therapies based on limiting invasiveness of tumor cells has proven difficult because cellular motility cannot be assessed in patients and histological analysis has thus far proven unreliable. In fact, this difficulty in assessing the efficacy of motility-targeting therapeutics was a likely cause for the failure of clinical trials using MMP inhibitors [54].

A major area of current study on therapeutic directions focuses upon the targeting of angiogenesis. Without its own blood supply, a distal micrometastasis is unable to continue proliferation. Angiogenesis appears to be closely linked to the presence of a variety of growth factors and their receptors, in particular basic fibroblast growth factor (bFGF), vascular endothelial growth factor (VEGF) [55], and epidermal growth factor receptor (EGFR) [56]. These factors have been shown to be of importance for tumor growth and invasiveness. A majority of lifetime non-smoking NSCLC patients, females of Caucasian and Asian descent in particular, present with an EGFR mutation treatable by the targeted small molecule EGFR inhibitor erlotinib (Tarceva) [57]. In recent years, various solid tumors have been treated with a reasonable degree of success by targeted monoclonal antibodies (MAbs) against EGFR and VEGF. Such therapies include cetuximab, panitumumab, and bevacizumab [56]. The two former antibodies target EGFR whereas bevacizumab is a humanized IgG1-type MAb directed against soluble VEGF. Bevacizumab, in particular, has become part of the standard first-line chemotherapy regimen for NSCLC patients [57].

In conclusion, the metastatic cascade is grossly implicated in the lethality of cancer, lung cancer included, and dissecting the process is essential to treating the disease. Medical scientists are faced with a number of key questions in metastasis to tackle: Is metastatic spread a capability intrinsic to all cells or to only a select few cancer stem cells? Which are the genes responsible for EMT? What genes control all subtypes of cellular locomotion? Are cell detachment from the ECM and the bypass of apoptosis separate or linked processes? How do DTCs and CTCs relate to each other, and what are their prognostic and mechanistic roles with regard to metastasis? What role does immunosurveillance play in the spread of cancer? What factors cause metastatic cells to "home" in on specific organs? How do dormant disseminated cancer cells begin to rapidly proliferate? By what biology do metastatic prognosticator genes actually aid and abet metastasis? How can MSGs be better characterized, and how can they be reactivated in later stage cancers? Although the processes leading up to cellular metastasis are still poorly understood, a great deal has been learned in recent years. As the chain of events leading to metastasis is better elucidated, our ability to medically target various parts of the process will in turn be enhanced.

Acknowledgments   The authors would like to thank Dr. Animesh Ray of the Keck Graduate Institute, Claremont, CA, for invaluable help and assistance in preparing this manuscript.

References

1. Cairns, J. Mutation selection and the natural history of cancer. Nature *255*: 187–200, 1975.
2. Weigelt, B., Peterse, J.L., and van 't Veer, L.J. Breast cancer metastasis: markers and models. Nature Rev Cancer *5*: 591–602, 2005.
3. Jemal, A., Siegel, R., Ward, E., Hao, Y., Xu, J., Murray, T., and Thun, M.J. Cancer statistics. Ca Cancer J Clin *58*: 71–96, 2008.
4. Wang, W., Goswami, S., Lapidus, K., Wells, A.L., Wyckoff, J.B., Sahai, E., Singer, R.H., Segall, J.E., and Condeelis, J.S. Identification and testing of gene expression signature of invasive carcinoma cells within primary mammary tumors. Cancer Res *64*: 8585–8594, 2004.
5. Leemans, C.R., Tiwari, R., Nauta, J.J., van der Waal, I., and Snow, G.B. Regional lymph node involvement and its significance in the development of distant metastases in head and neck carcinoma. Cancer Res *71*: 452–456, 1993.
6. Braun, S., Pantel, K., Mueller, P., Janni, W., Hepp, F., Kentenich, C.R.M., Gastroph, S., Wischnik, A., Dimpfl, T., Kindermann, G., Riethmueller, G., and Schlimok, G. Cytokeratin-positive bone marrow micrometastases an survival of breast cancer patients with stage I-III disease. N Engl J Med *342*: 525–533, 2000.
7. Mehlen, P. and Puisieux, A. Metastasis: a question of life or death. Nature Rev Cancer *6*: 449–458, 2006.
8. Lapidot, T., Sirard, C., Vormoor, J., Murdoch, B., Hoang, T., Caceres-Cortes, J., Minden, M., Paterson, B., Caligiuri, M.A., and Dick, J.E. A cell initiating human acute myeloid leukemia after transplantation into SCID mice. Nature *17*: 645–648, 1994.
9. Singh, S.K., Clarke, I.D., Terasaki, M., Bonn, V.E., Hawkins, C., Squire, J., and Dirks, P.B. Identification of a cancer stem cell in human brain tumours. Cancer Res *63*: 5821–5828, 2003.

10. Krystal, G.W., Hines, S.J., and Organ, C.P. Autocrine growth of small cell lung cancer mediated by coexpression of c-kit and stem cell factor. Cancer Res *56*: 370–376, 1996.

11. Kim, C.F., Jackson, E.L., Woolfenden, A.E., Lawrence, S., Babar, I., Vogel, S., Crowley, D., Bronson, R.T., and Jacks, T. Identification of bronchioalveolar stem cells in normal lung and lung cancer. Cell *121*: 823–835, 2005.

12. Klein, W.M., Wu, B.P., Zhao, S., Wu, H., Klein-Szanto, A.J.P., and Tahan, S.R. Increased expression of stem cell markers in malignant melanoma. Modern Pathol *20*: 102–107, 2007.

13. Al-Hajj, M., Wicha, M.S., Benito-Hernandez, A., Morrison, S.J., and Clarke, M.F. Prospective identification of tumorigenic breast cancer cells. Proc Natl Acad Sci USA *100*: 3983–3988, 2003.

14. Pardal, R., Clarke, M.F., and Morrison, S.J. Applying the principles of stem cell biology to cancer. Nature Rev Cancer *3*: 895–902, 2003.

15. Kucia, M., Reca, R., Miekus, K., Wanzeck, J., Wojakowski, W., Janowska-Wieczorek, A., Ratajczak, J., and Ratajczak, M.Z. Trafficking of normal stem cells and metastasis of cancer stem cells involve similar mechanisms: pivotal role of the SDF-1-CXCR4 axis. Stem Cells *23*: 879–894, 2005.

16. Oft, M., Akhurst, R.J., and Balmain, A. Metastasis is driven by sequential elevation of H-ras and Smad2 levels. Nature Cell Biol. *4*: 487–494, 2002.

17. Sahai, E. Mechanisms of cancer cell invasion. Curr Opin Gen Dev *15*: 87–96, 2005.

18. Ozanne, B.W., McGarry, L., Spence, H.J., Johnston, I., Winnie, J., Meagher, L., and Stapleton, G. Transcriptional regulation of cell invasion: AP-1 regulation of a multigenic invasion programme. Eur J Cancer *36*: 1640–1648, 2000.

19. Eccles, S.A. and Welch, D.R. Metastasis: recent discoveries and novel treatment strategies. Lancet *369*: 1742–1757, 2007.

20. Martin, S.S. and Leder, P. Human MCF10A mammary epithelial cells undergo apoptosis following actin depolymerization that is independent of attachment and rescued by Bcl-2. Mol. Cell Biol *21*: 6529–6536, 2001.

21. Pinkas, J., Martin, S. S., and Leder, P. Bcl-2-mediated cell survival promotes metastasis of EpH4 bMEKDD mammary epithelial cells. Mol Cancer Res *2*: 551–556, 2004.

22. Mazieres, J., He, B., You, L., Xu, Z., and Jablons, D.M. Wnt signaling in lung cancer. Cancer Lett *222*: 1–10, 2005.

23. You, L., Kim, J., He, B., Xu, Z., McCormick, F., and Jablons, D.M. Wnt-1 signal as a potential cancer therapeutic target. Drug News Perspectives *19*: 1–5, 2006.

24. Wolf, K., Mazo, I., Leung, H., Engelke, K., von Andrian, U.H., Deryugina, E.I., Strongin, A.Y., Bröcker, E.B., and Friedl, P. Compensation mechanism in tumor cell migration: mesenchymal-amoeboid transition after blocking of pericellular proteolysis. J Cell Biol *160*: 267–277, 2003.

25. Pollard, T.D. and Borisy, G.G. Cellular motility driven by assembly and disassembly of actin filaments. Cell *112*: 453–465, 2003.

26. Wang, H.R., Ogunjimi, A.A., Zhang, Y., Ozdamar, B., Bose, R., and Wrana, J.L. Degradation of RhoA by Smurf1 Ubiquitin ligase. Methods Enzymol *406*: 437–447, 2006.

27. Wyckoff, J.B., Pinner, S.E., Gschmeissner, S., Condeelis, J.S., and Sahai, E. ROCK- and myosin-dependent matrix deformation enables protease-independent tumor-cell invasion. In Vivo Curr Biol *16*: 1515–1523, 2006.

28. Sahai, E. and Marshall, C.J. Differing modes of tumour cell invasion have distinct requirements for Rho/ROCK signaling and extracellular proteolysis. Nature Cell Biol *5*: 711–720, 2003.

29. Wyckoff, J.B., Jones, J.G., Condeelis, J.S., and Segall, J.E. A critical step in metastasis: in vivo analysis of intravasation at the primary tumor. Cancer Res *60*: 2504–2511, 2000.

30. Pantel, K., Brakenhoff, R. H., and Brandt, B. Detection, clinical relevance and specific biological properties of disseminating tumour cells. Nat Rev Cancer *8*: 329–340, 2008.

31. Steeg, P.S. Tumor metastasis: mechanistic insights and clinical challenges. Nat Med *12*: 895–904, 2006.

32. Burnet, F.M. The concept of immunological surveillance. Prog Exp Tumor Res *13*: 1–27, 1970.

33. Thomas, L. On immunosurveillance in human cancer. Yale J Biol Med *55*: 329–333, 1982.

34. Bradbury, P.A. and Shepherd, F.A. Immunotherapy for lung cancer. J Thoracic Oncol *3*: S164–S170, 2008.

35. Pardoll, D. Does the immune system see tumors as foreign or self? Annu Rev Immunol *21*: 807–839, 2003.

36. Wood, S.J. Pathogenesis of metastasis formation observed in vivo in the rabbit ear chamber. AMA Arch Pathol *66*: 550–568, 1958.

37. Fidler, I.J. Metastasis: quantitative analysis of distribution and fate of tumor embolila-beled with 125 I-5-iodo-2'-deoxyuridine. J Natl Cancer Inst *45*: 773–782, 1970.

38. Fidler, I.J. and Nicolson, G.L. Fate of recirculating B16 melanoma metastatic variant cells in parabiotic syngeneic recipients. J Natl Cancer Inst *58*: 1867–1872, 1977.

39. Paget, S. The distribution of secondary growths in cancer of the breast. Lancet *1*: 571–573, 1889.

40. Yu, Q., Toole, B.P. and Stamenkovic, I. Induction of apoptosis of metastatic mammary carcinoma cells in vivo by disruption of tumor cell surface CD44 function. J Exp Med *186*: 1985–1996, 1997.

41. Perou, C.M., Sørlie, T., Eisen, M.B., van de Rijn, M., Jeffrey, S.S., Rees, C.A., Pollack, J.R., Ross, D.T., Johnsen, H., Akslen, L.A., Fluge, Ø., Pergamenschikov, A., Williams, C., Zhu, S.X., Lønning, P.E., Børresen-Dale, A.L., Brown, P.O., and Botstein, D. Molecular portraits of human breast tumours. Nature *406*: 747–752, 2000.

42. Ramaswamy, S., Ross, K.N., Lander, E.S., and Golub, T.R. A molecular signature of metastasis in primary solid tumors. Nature Genetics *33*: 49–54, 2002.

43. Welch, D.R., Steeg, P.S., and Rinker-Schaeffer, C.W. Molecular biology of breast metastasis: Genetic regulation of human breast carcinoma metastasis. Breast Cancer Res *2*: 408–416, 2002.

44. Steeg, P.S. Metastasis suppressors alter the signal transduction of cancer cells. Nat Rev Cancer *3*: 55–63, 2003.

45. Ohtaki, T., Shintani, Y., Honda, S., Matsumoto, H., Hori, A., Kanehashi, K., Terao, Y., Kumano, S., Takatsu, Y., Masuda, Y., Ishibashi, Y., Watanabe, T., Asada, M., Yamada, T., Suenaga, M., Kitada, C., Usuki, S., Kurokawa, T., Onda, H., Nishimura, O., Fujino, M. Metastasis suppressor gene KiSS-1 encodes peptide ligand of a G-protein-coupled receptor. Nature *411*: 613–617, 2001.

46. Sahai, E. Illuminating the metastatic process. Nature Rev Cancer *7*: 737–749, 2007.

47. Goodale, D., Phay, C., Postenka, C.O., Keeney, M., and Allan, A.L. Characterization of tumor cell dissemination patterns in preclinical models of cancer metastasis using flow cytometry and laser scanning cytometry. Cytometry Part A 9999: NA, 2008.

48. Sipkins, D.A., Wei, X., Wu, J.W., Runnels, J.M., Côté, D., Means, T.K., Luster, A.D., Scadden, D.T., Lin, C.P. In vivo imaging of specialized bone marrow endothelial micro-domains for tumour engraftment. Nature *435*: 969–973, 2005.

49. Kim, J.W., Wong, C.W., Glodsmith, J.D., Song, C., Fu, W., Allion, M.B., Herlyn, M., Al-Mehdi, A.B., and Muschel, R.J. Rapid apoptosis in the pulmonary vasculature distinguishes non-metastatic from metastatic melanoma cells. Cancer Lett *213*: 203–212, 2004.

50. Jordan, C.T., Guzman, M. L., and Noble, M. Cancer stem cells. New England J Med *355*: 1253–1261, 2006.

51. Pantel, K. and Brakenhoff, R.H. Dissecting the metastatic cascade. Nature Rev Cancer *4*: 448–456, 2004.

52. Goldhirsch, A., Wood, W. C., Gelber, R. D., Coates, A. S., Thuerlimann, B., and Senn, H. J. Meeting highlights: updated international expert consensus on the primary therapy of early breast cancer. J Clin Oncol *21*: 3357–3365, 2003.

53. Raz, D.J., Ray, M.R., Kim, J.Y., He, B., Taron, M., Skrzypski, M., Segal, M., Gandara, D.R., Rosell, R., and Jablons, D.M. A multigene assay is prognostic of survival in patients with early-stage lung adenocarcinoma. Clin Cancer Res. *14*: 5565–5570, 2008.
54. Overall, C.M., and Lopez-Otin, C. Strategies for MMP inhibition in cancer: innovations for the post-trial era. Nat Rev Cancer *2*: 657–672, 2002.
55. Folkman, J. Seminars in medicine of the Beth Israel Hospital, Boston. Clinical applications of research on angiogenesis. N Engl J Med *333*: 1757–1763, 1995.
56. Pander, J., Gelderblom, H., and Guchelaar, H.J. Pharmacogenetics of EGFR and VEGF inhibition. Drug Discovery Today *12*: 1054–1060, 2007.
57. Thatcher, N. First- and second-line treatment of advanced metastatic non-small-cell lung cancer: a global view. BMC Proc. 2: S3, 2008.

Tumor Stem Cells and Metastasis

Jaclyn Y. Hung

Abstract The last decade has seen the emergence of a shift in paradigm in the therapeutic strategies to target cancer. This is based on the existence of a small reservoir of cells within the tumor mass that exhibits the capacity for self-renewal, as well as undergo differentiation to give rise to phenotypically heterogeneous progeny with limited proliferative potential. These stem-like cells likely drive the continued growth of the tumor mass and are capable of disseminating and are subsequently metastasized. Relapse is probably orchestrated by the post-therapy residual drug-resistant "cancer stem cells" that escape treatment. Therefore, the selective targeting of cancer stem cells is supposed to offer radical advances in the treatment and diagnosis of lung cancer. This chapter will discuss the emerging data supporting the validity of this notion and consider the growing evidence that cancer stem cells may contribute to tumor progression, drug resistance, metastasis, and speculates about how taking these cells into consideration may affect the way we treat lung cancer in the future.

Introduction

Despite the advances in diagnosis and the treatment of cancer, lung cancers remain nearly uniformly fatal; 85% of the people who are diagnosed with lung cancer die of the disease within 5 years [1]. This is because at the time of diagnosis, majority of the patients are already beyond cure by surgery or radiotherapy, and a large percentage of those diagnosed with resectable early-stage disease eventually experience recurrence of metastatic disease. While aggressive, treatment-intense protocols do prolong median survival; the overall impact has been mainly on palliation rather than reduction in mortality, with

J.Y. Hung (✉)
Department of Pediatrics, Greehey Children's Cancer Research Institute, University of
Texas Health Science Center, San Antonio, TX, USA
e-mail: hungj@uthscsa.edu

V. Keshamouni et al. (eds.), *Lung Cancer Metastasis*,   47
DOI 10.1007/978-1-4419-0772-1_3, © Springer Science+Business Media, LLC 2009

total cure remaining elusive. Besides, the treatment regimes have a non-specific toxicity profile that exceeds its therapeutic profile.

A key emerging trend in the treatment of patients with cancer is the concept of "Personalized Medicine" consisting of individualized diagnosis and prognosis in combination with targeted therapies – as emphasized by the report from the American Society of Clinical Oncology [2]. The last decade has also seen the emergence of a shift in paradigm in the therapeutic strategies to target cancer. This is based on the existence of "cancer stem cells" (also called cancer-initiating cells) – a conceptual revolution in cancer biology [3–7]. However, the ideas behind the "cancer stem cell hypothesis" are not new and have evolved over the last 150 years. Nonetheless, the recent work of several laboratories prospectively isolating cells with stem cell-like properties has led to these concepts being re-examined more widely. These recent results support the notion that within the tumors, only a small reservoir of cells (termed "cancer stem cells") exhibits the capacity for self-renewal, as well as undergo differentiation to give rise to phenotypically heterogeneous progeny with limited proliferative potential. These cells likely drive the continued growth of the mass and are capable of disseminating and are subsequently metastasized. Relapse is probably orchestrated by the post-therapy residual drug-resistant "cancer stem cells" that escape treatment. It is plausible that existing therapies commonly targeting the bulk mass do not eliminate cancer stem cells. Although a dramatic initial response can often be achieved, if the cancer stem cells are not also effectively eliminated they can eventually regenerate the tumor [8]. Therefore, the selective targeting of "cancer stem cells" is believed to may offer radical advances in the diagnosis and treatment of lung cancer, by attacking the disease at its source.

This chapter will discuss the emerging data supporting the validity of this notion and consider the growing evidence that cancer stem cells may contribute to tumor progression, drug resistance, metastasis and speculates about how taking these cells into consideration may affect the way we treat lung cancer in the future. The amount of data that had been directly derived from studies of lung cancer is as yet quite limited; however, the general paradigms and aspects of cancer stem cells drawn from studies of other cancers provide an adequate review of the role of these cells in lung cancer. Further the implication of this model for drug development and eventually of clinical management of patients will be discussed. The targeted elimination of these cancer stem cells will also be addressed in this chapter. Before proceeding, however, it is important to take into consideration that various aspects of the role of cancer stem cells in solid cancer development and progression are still controversial [9–11].

Cancer Stem Cells

Normal stem cells are defined by their dual capacity to regenerate themselves (self-renewal) and to produce mature cells through differentiation [12]. The "cancer stem cell" hypothesis posits functional heterogeneity within a cancer and the existence of a distinct group of cancer stem cells reminiscent of somatic stem cells. The "cancer stem cell model" proposes that a tumor is similarly sustained by a subpopulation of "cancer stem cells," with a similar ability to perpetuate themselves and the production of progeny for the continued growth of the mass. Three key observations support the existence of a stem-like cell population in a tumor [13]. First, in both hematopoietic malignancies and solid cancers, only a small fraction of tumor mass has the capacity to regenerate a new tumor, operationally demonstrable upon serial transplantation into recipient immunodeficient mice. Second, these cells are characterized by a distinctive profile of surface markers and can be enriched and prospectively isolated through an experimental strategy that sorts the cells based on the expression of surface markers, or lack thereof, or on the efflux of the fluorescent dye Hoechst 33342 (for side population phenotype). Third, secondary or tertiary tumors regenerated by these cells contained mixed populations of tumorigenic and non-tumorigenic cancer cells, thus recapitulating the heterogeneity of the original parent tumor.

The cancer stem cell model is first and best developed in hematopoietic malignancies. A study by Jacob Furth and Morton Kahn in 1937 discovered that a single leukemic cell is able to transfer the systemic disease when transplanted by inoculation into a mouse and thus established the first quantitative assay to determine the frequency of malignant cells within the hematopoietic tumor [14]. Later, in the 1960s, Robert Bruce and Hugo van der Gaag develop a quantitative method to measure the number of murine lymphoma cells capable of proliferating in vivo using a spleen colony-forming assay [15]. They show that only a small subset of primary tissue is able to proliferate in vivo. Another study conducted in 1977 by Anne Hamburger and Sydney Salmon reports that only 1 in 1,000 to 1 in 5,000 cancer cells formed colonies in soft agar assay and establish that not every cancerous cell is capable of tumor initiation [16]. However, the true measures of cancer stem cells are their capacity for self-renewal and exact recapitulation of the original tumor; these studies, rather, measure in vitro proliferation. It is, however, in the initial landmark paper by John Dick and colleagues who provide the first direct evidence for the cancer stem cell model. They described a primitive leukemic cell they termed SCID leukemia-initiating cell that can initiate human acute myeloid leukemia (AML) in a non-obese diabetic (NOD) – severe-combined immunodeficient (SCID) mouse model. These leukemia-initiating cells in AML share a cell-surface ($CD34^+/CD38^-$) phenotype with normal hematopoietic stem cells. They showed that this fraction is highly enriched for leukemia initiation activity in transplanted recipient (0.2–100 stem cells in 10^6 blast cells). By contrast, the $CD34^+/CD38^+$ cells and the majority of the $CD34^-$ cells, which comprised the bulk of the cancers, could not initiate AML. The engrafted AML could be serially purified and transplanted into secondary recipients to generate hierarchical clones of differentiating cells and form AML that is a phenocopy of the original tumor, providing functional evidence for self-renewal [17].

   Using similar approaches (xeno-transplantation followed by serial transplantation) cancer stem cells have subsequently been identified and prospectively isolated from breast and brain cancers, providing the first evidence for cancer stem cells in solid cancers. Clarke and colleagues are the first to provide evidence for the existence of breast cancer stem cells [18]. This work identifies a putative breast cancer stem-like population that is defined by the expression of four cell surface markers (adhesion molecules CD44 and CD24, epithelial-specific antigen, ESA, and a breast/ovarian cancer-specific marker B38.1) and their potential to form tumors after transplantation in the mammary fad-pad of NOD/SCID mice. As few as 200 $CD44^+$ $CD24^{+/-}$ ESA^+ lineage marker (Lin)$^-$ cells are able to generate tumors that are histologically similar to those of the primary breast tumors when injected into NOD/SCID mice models, whereas injection of thousands of cells that have the other phenotype did not form tumors. The tumorigenic subset represented only 2% of the unfractionated bulk breast cancer cells. These tumorigenic cells behave like cancer stem cells in that they can be serially passage from one mouse to another, giving rise to cancer cells with the same phenotype ($CD44^+$ $CD24^{+/-}$ ESA^+ Lin$^-$) and the phenotypically diverse mixed population of non-tumorigenic breast cancer cells. These findings indicate that, like AML, breast cancer cells retain a remnant of stem cells that have the ability of self-renewal to maintain the stem cell pool and can also differentiate into a variety of other cancer cell types [19].
   Similar results for cancers of the central nervous system (CNS) show that a subset of cells expressing the neural stem cell marker CD133 initiates brain cancers [20–22]. Transplantation of these putative neural cancer stem cells into the forebrains of NOD-SCID mice consistently yields tumors and moreover, when injected into mice, only $CD133^+$ cells have the ability to generate heterogeneous tumors phenotypically identical to the tumors from which the stem cells are isolated. Furthermore, these tumors can be serially transplanted. In contrast, cells with the $CD133^-$ phenotype do not form tumors in NOD-SCID. On the basis of this work, cells having the $CD133^+$ phenotype are confirmed as cancer stem cells for CNS tumors [22].

Side Population Phenotype

Subsequently the purification and characterization of cancer stem cells have been reported in many other cancers [23–30]. These cancer-initiating cells have been enriched on the basis of the expression of their unique cell surface markers. However, in human lung cancer, the purification of cancer stem cells has been hampered by the lack of definitive cell surface marker(s). An alternative approach to surface antigens is to use the side population (SP) phenotype [31]. Recent studies have demonstrated that somatic stem cells can be enriched by a "side population" (SP) phenotype [32]. Cells subject to Hoechst 33342 dye staining and fluorescence-activated cell sorting (FACS) analysis can give a profile such that those cells that actively efflux the dye appear as a distinct population of cells on the side of the dual-color emission spectra (blue versus red) FACS profile on a density plot; hence the name "side population" (SP) has been given to these cells. The Hoechst staining profile is a continuum, with no clear-cut separation line between the SP and the non-SP. Therefore, the SP is defined, according to convention, by depletion using Hoechst transporter inhibitors reserpine or verapamil.

This SP phenotype is attributed partly to the activity of various members of the adenosine triphosphate (ATP)-binding cassette (ABC) transporters family such as ABCB1 and ABCG2 that are expressed in normal stem cells [33] and most cancer stem cells. ABCB1 and ABCG2 belong to a family of at least 49 ABC transporters involved in a variety of cellular transport processes. By using the energy of ATP hydrolysis, these transporters actively efflux drugs from cells, thus protecting them from cytotoxic agents. Interestingly, hematopoietic stem cells express high levels of ABCG2, but the gene is turned off in most committed progenitor and mature blood cells.

Goodell et al. first use this method to isolate murine hematopoietic stem cells [34]. In the bone marrow, these SP cells are enriched approximately 1000-fold in hematopoietic stem cell activity in repopulation experiments, which can protect murine recipients from lethal irradiation at low cell doses, thus establishing their functional capacity as hematopoietic stem cells. In addition, SP cells also contribute to both myeloid and lymphoid lineages in the transplant recipients. The SP population is present in bone marrow at a low level (0.02–0.08%) and expresses the murine cell surface markers characteristic (Sca-1$^+$/lin$^{-/low}$) of hematopoietic stem cells. The subsequent isolation of rhesus monkey SP cells demonstrated that a hematopoietic SP is conserved across species. ABCG2 has been identified as a molecular determinant for bone marrow stem cells and proposed as a universal marker for stem cells, although not all reports agree [35, 35a]. In *Abcg2*-knockout mice, the SP is lost, but the mice still have bone marrow stem cells, suggesting that the SP phenotype is a characteristic of the stem cell, but is not crucial for its function. Therefore, the SP phenotype might be a way to identify stem cell populations from various sources independently of cell-type-specific markers, making it an important tool in stem cell characterization and research.

Since its initial application in murine bone marrow hematopoietic stem cells, this Hoechst 33342 dye efflux SP phenotype has been used to sort out presumptive stem cells and progenitors in a diverse range of normal tissues across species including the pancreas [36], prostate [37], lung [38, 39], mammary glands [40, 41], arteries [42], and embryonic stem cells. In many of these studies, it is reported that the SP cells are enriched for stem cell markers and in some studies the SP cells can behave as clonogenic stem cells. These SPs are rare and heterogeneous, varying with tissue type, stage of development, and method of preparation.

Concurrent studies have demonstrated SP cells in human cancer cell lines and primary cancers of different origins, including acute myeloid leukemia [43, 44], neuroblastoma [45], glioma [46], retinoblastoma [47], prostate [48], head and neck [49], liver [50], ovarian [51], thyroid [52], and gastrointestinal [53] cancers. We have recently published that the Hoechst 33342 dye efflux assay can be adapted for the isolation of SP cells from various human lung cancer cell lines and lung tissues from surgical resection [54]. The SP fraction comprise of 0.023–1.08% of cells from human lung cancer tissues and 1.5–6.1% of cells from cell lines and majority of these cells are either in G_0 or in G_1 of the cell cycle. The nature of these SP cells is defined by preferential expression of "stemness" genes *BMI-1* and *NOTCH1* (unpublished data), *hTERT*, and elevated expression of ABC transporters associated with multi-drug resistance. Functional characterization of the SP and non-SP was investigated both in vitro and in vivo. The SP cells are more resistant than non-SP against a number of chemotherapeutic drugs, a number of which, notably cisplatin, gemcitabine, and vinorelbine, are commonly used as first-line therapy for lung cancer. When injected into NOD-SCID mice, SP cells are found to be more tumorigenic than non-SP, thus indicating a significant enrichment of cancer-initiating cells in this small population. Even though the non-SP forms the majority of cells, the tumors initiated from SP cells are larger, very vascular, and required much fewer cells for initiation of the tumor. Hence, the functional importance of the SP is two-fold: they are more significantly enriched in tumorigenicity and are also more resistant to existing chemotherapeutic agents, possibly due to heightened expression of a range of drug resistance transporters. This suggests that the SP will have survival advantage under chemotherapy and can regenerate a tumor leading to refractory/relapsed disease and is likely an important target for more effective therapy.

The propagation of serially passage spheres from primary lung cancer is recently reported [55]. By applying the same conditions that are used for the isolation of human neural stem cells [56], a putative cancer stem-like cell is identified from human lung cancer tissues. These cells express CD133 and have the ability to grow indefinitely as spheres in a serum-free medium containing growth factors, thus having the key characteristics of self-renewal. These lung cancer spheres are also tumorigenic and resistant to chemotherapeutic drugs.

However, both of these studies have limitations. Lung cancer stem cells have not yet been identified directly, although they can be enriched for and propagated in vitro. Nevertheless, for now, the distinct SP phenotype and lung cancer stem cell sphere culture provide an attractive testing model for studying lung cancer-initiating cell biology and a framework for testing potential lung cancer stem cell markers. As well, these models are important tools for developing selective therapies targeting lung cancer stem cells and as predictor of response to treatment.

Origin of Cancer Stem Cells

The existence of cancer stem cells raises an important question regarding the cell of origin for cancer stem cells. However, the origin of cancer stem cell is yet to be resolved [57]. They may originate from the transformation of normal tissue-specific somatic stem cells. The concept that a rare population of tissue stem cells may be the cellular origin of cancer is first proposed by pathologists such as Virchow and Cohnheim about 150 years ago [58, 59]. They observed histological similarities between the embryonic tissue and certain types of cancer such as teratocarcinomas with respect to their enormous capacity for both proliferation and differentiation, albeit aberrant differentiation in the case of tumors. Their observations led to the hypothesis that cancer results from the activation of dormant embryonic tissue remnants – the "embryonal rest hypothesis." Van R. Potter and Barry Pierce revisited these ideas and described cancer as "maturation arrest of tissue-determined stem cells" or "blocked ontogeny" [60]. Somatic stem cells are defined functionally by their dual abilities to self-renew (i.e., divide and produce undifferentiated transit-amplifying daughter cells at an average of $>1/$division) in addition to generating the initial precursors of the specialized end cells characteristics of the tissue, which the stem cell population maintains. Because of its extensive and lifelong turnover, stem cells serve as a tissue reservoir for the slow accumulation of oncogenic mutations and aberrant epigenetic changes that perturb intrinsic mechanisms regulating normal cell proliferation and differentiation leading ultimately to the acquisition of a full-blown malignant phenotype.

Experimental models have identified several types of resident stem cells in the normal lung with proliferative and regenerative potential [61–67]. Although controversial, the stem (or progenitor) cell population of the human lung likely includes the basal cells of the bronchi and bronchioles, Clara cells of the bronchioles, and the type II pneumocytes of the alveoli. The cell types that are exposed to and in which metabolic activation of tobacco-derived carcinogens takes place in the respiratory tract are likely the target cells for DNA damage, tumor initiation, and subsequent development of lung cancer. It is noteworthy that both Clara cells and type II alveolar pneumocytes are the primary sites of xenobiotic metabolism involving the P450 cytochrome enzyme activity in the respiratory epithelium. Implicitly, all known carcinogens in tobacco smoke require metabolic activation for binding to DNA to cause mutations.

Studies suggest that slowly renewing somatic stem cells are located within specific microenvironments (niches) in tissue. The stem cell niche under normal circumstances is a protective environment, but as we age the somatic stem cells of this environment unavoidably suffer cumulative numbers of damaging mutations to their DNA, leading them over the edge to tumorigenesis. Chronic irritation and mucosal injury caused by exposure to cigarette smoke might facilitate trapping of "stem cells" in a state of perpetual activation in an attempt to repair tissue damage, and subsequent genetic changes in the cells or the inability to return to a quiescent period may result in the stem cell progressing to a cancer stem cell [68, 69]. Several stem cell niches that are key in maintaining the epithelial lining of lung tissues have been identified in the proximal and distal airways of mice [70]. Recent studies from a transgenic mouse model that conditionally expresses *K-ras* implicate a population of cells at the region of the bronchiolar-alveolar duct junction that exhibits self-renewal and differentiation, properties characteristics of stem cells as a putative origin of lung adenocarcinomas [71].

Alternatively, cancer stem cells could be the result of transformation events that involve the more mature differentiated cancer cells that acquired stem cell-like functions through a process of de-differentiation [72–75]. Recent findings suggest that cancer stem cells may arise from a rare fusion event [76]. Irrespective of the origin of cancer stem cells, these malignant cells displays stem cell properties, notably the ability to self-renew and to differentiate into a functional hierarchy of tumorigenic and non-tumorigenic cells.

Cancer Stem Cells and Metastasis

Interestingly, the lung cancer SP cells are more invasive than non-SP, suggesting that "stemness" may be related to invasiveness. These stem-like cancer cells are more likely to metastasize, since they are more invasive and angiogenic. The notion of migrating cancer stem cells has many important implications. If cancer stem cells are key players in the metastatic process, then the importance of targeting and neutralizing these cells is even greater. The final stage in malignancy is the metastasis and is the main cause of death for cancer patients. It is known that one of the crucial events to malignancy that occurs before metastasis is the gain of migratory phenotype at the expense of epithelial cell properties. This is referred as the epithelial to mesenchymal transition (see Chapter 4). The EMT is a reprogramming of the epithelial cells that results in the modulation to a mesenchymal pheno- type [77, 78]. It has been speculated that cancer stem cells might undergo EMT and thereby gain migratory and other properties that promote metas- tasis [79]. This concept is proposed as a two-phase process in which "sta- tionary" epithelial cancer stem cells acquire mesenchymal characteristics and become migrating cancer stem cells. The combination of migratory and "stemness" properties integrates both tumor metastasis and initiation con- cepts into one cell and potentially provides an explanation to the tumori- genic progress. Since the putative cancer stem cell is more tumorigenic than other cancer cells, their added increase in mobility enables them to initiate tumors at distant sites from the primary tumor and adds to the importance of developing cancer therapies that target these cells. The EMT is a reversible process; the migratory cancer stem cells with mesenchymal characteristics can revert to an epithelial state at the site of metastasis for the onset of proliferation and secondary tumor formation [80]. Furthermore, invasiveness may also be associated with the interaction between cancer stem cells and their niche [81, 82]. The niche consists of the supporting cells surrounding the cancer stem cells. Notably, studies have shown that EMT and the mesenchymal to epithelial (MET) programs can be triggered through signals from the microenvironment [83].

Kaplan et al. investigated the relationship of niche formation and metastasis [84] and they observed that the initiation of a niche for metastasis was associated with VEGFR1+ hematopoietic progenitor cells derived from bone marrow. Secreted factors from different types of primary tumor cells (melanoma and lung cancer) into conditioned media mobilized these hematopoietic progenitor cells toward future preferred sites of metastasis to form fibronectin-rich cellular clusters. This remodeled the microenvironment of the preferred site into a more favorable, pre-metastatic niche before tumor cells were injected. Blocking the fibronectin-rich clusters by VEGFR1+ antibodies significantly inhibits metastasis. This study suggests that communication between cancer stem cells and target tissue microenvironment at distant sites occurs even before the cancer cells even arrived at its target [79, 85, 86]. The tumor is sustained by the initial pool of cancer stem cells and eventually secrete factors that form the pre-metastatic niche at distinct sites. The metastatic cancer stem cells are directed toward the pre-metastatic niche through chemo-attractants and other homing factors. They then either proliferate into a metastatic lesion or enter a quiescent period until reactivated to promote expansion into a secondary tumor.

Implications for Treatments

While the concept of a "cancer stem cell" is gaining wide acceptance, an alternative stochastic model has been proposed. This model predicts that every cell within the tumor has the intrinsic ability to proliferate extensively, but entry into the cell cycle is a stochastic event with low probability. The model predicts that the tumor is relatively homogeneous, that every cell within the tumor has equal ability to extensively proliferate, metastasize, and regenerate a tumor, and that the stochastic events will cause these cancer-initiating cells to be found in any two sorted cell fractions with equal probability. Existing therapeutic approaches have been based largely on the stochastic model, but the failure of these therapies to cure most solid cancers suggests that the hierarchy or cancer stem cell model may better explain treatment failure. For example, current lung cancer chemotherapy regimens include a platinum compound in combination with taxane analogues, gemcitabine, or vinorelbine. However, most of the patients that respond will relapse, with a median survival of 8–11 months [87]. The current view is that relapse or progression is the result of clonal expansion of drug-resistant malignant stem cells in the original heterogeneous tumor cell population. Whether or not such resistant clones are present de novo or are induced by chemotherapy is not known. However, the Goldie–Coldman hypothesis, proposed more than 20 years ago, suggests that a small percentage of cells in a tumor harbor intrinsic characteristics that make them resistant to treatment [88].

The cancer stem cell hypothesis supports this premise by suggesting that targeting differentiated cells will not achieve long-term remission or cure unless the cancer stem cell phenotype is also targeted. In support of this, it has been reported that human AML CD34$^+$/CD38$^-$ progenitor cells are significantly less sensitive to daunorubicin with respect to decreasing proliferation and the induction of apoptosis when compared with the more committed CD34$^+$/CD38$^+$ cells [89, 89a]. If the drug-resistant clones are indeed orchestrated by the post-therapy residual "cancer stem cells" that escape treatment, then strategies to identify the "drug-resistant clones" may provide the experimental tool to investigate the molecular properties of the clinically relevant malignant cell population. This may in turn result in approaches to devise new molecular targets or combination therapy. By targeting the cancer stem cell, the non-specific therapeutic toxicity seen with conventional chemotherapy and the cancer recurrences, which may arise from drug resistance within the cancer stem cell, may be avoided. Cancer stem cells are more resistant to chemotherapy drugs than the bulk tumor mass due in part to the elevated expression of members of the ABC transporters [90, 91]. Therefore, in non-targeted therapies such as chemotherapy, the co-administration of chemotherapeutics and inhibitors to ABC transporters to sensitize cancer stem cells could be employed as a good defensive measure to multi-drug resistance.

This new model for cancer will also likely impact our understanding of the mechanism of radioresistance [92]. In fact, recent studies have proposed that cancer stem cells can be more resistant to gamma irradiation and also exhibit a difference in apoptotic response. Pharmacological inhibition of c-src tyrosine kinase homologous kinase (CHK), an enzyme involved in the activation of ataxia telangiectasia mutated (ATM) DNA repair pathway, renders the glioblastoma stem cells sensitive to radiation [93].

Cancer stem cells are likely defined by how they act in context [81] and angiogenesis, the formation of new blood vessel is critical in providing the blood supply of the cancer stem cells to support tumor growth [94]. For example, the lung SP cells form larger and more vascular tumors than do non-SP [54]. In glioblastoma, the cancer stem cells produce high levels of VEGF than do other glioma cells [95]. Recent data suggest that glioblastoma and various brain cancers exist and are maintained in aberrant rich vasculature stem cell niches [96]. Therefore, therapies designed to inhibit the formation of blood vessels could prove to be effective [97]. Anti-angiogenic drugs such as

Bevacizumab (Avastin) and Cediranib (AZD2171) are already used in clinical trial for lung cancer [98–101] and glioblastomas [102, 103].

In the era of tailored therapies, the cancer stem cell hypothesis suggests new or altered avenues for drug development. Effective eradication of cancers may require the targeting of cancer stem cells and eliminating the cancer stem cells may be the new measure for all future cancer treatments. Thus, cell signaling pathways required for the maintenance of cancer stem cells are candidate "druggability" targets for successful molecular therapy of cancer. There is evidence that activated Notch, Wnt, Hedgehog, and Bmi-1 may be important players in certain types of lung cancer. Studies have shown that these genes are involved in the regulation of stem cells and may also play a role in cancer stem cells. To suppress or eliminate cancer stem cells, these are potential targets to be explored. These targets may synergize with preclinical agents such as gamma-secretase and cyclopamine to increase efficacy.

Telomerase is upregulated in cancer stem cells [104] and SP of lung cancer [54]. Emerging data suggest that normal stem cells may have longer telomeres compared with cancer stem cell [105]; thus there may be a window of opportunity to potentially target both lung cancer stem cells and more mature cancer cells using telomerase-based therapies, hopefully sparing the normal stem cell [105–107].

Finally, the cancer stem cell model has significant implications for the design of future studies for early detection, risk assessment for metastasis, and improving prognostic information. A recent study showed that a 186 "invasive" gene signature obtained from gene expression profiling of breast cancer stem cells was associated with a poor prognosis and with increased risk of metastasis that has been reported not only in breast cancer but also in several tumor types, including lung cancer [108]. These studies support the view that the identification of cancer stem cell markers may provide valuable predictive and prognostic information and of clinical relevance. The gene signature associated with cancer stem cells could be validated for clinical use, for example, stratifying patients into good and poor prognostics group. Thus, lung cancer patients with poor prognosis could be targeted for more aggressive chemotherapy and novel targeted therapy strategies, while those patients with relatively favorable prognosis are spared from the non-specific therapeutic toxicities.

In conclusion, the ability to isolate enriched cancer stem cell populations is a major step forward, which could open the door to future studies where mechanisms involved in cancer stem cells can be investigated, which hopefully will yield new diagnostic markers and targets, which will ultimately help in the treatment of lung and other cancer. Implementation of the cancer stem cell concept should offer a real possibility of long-term cure rather than current palliative therapy for this challenging disease.

Acknowledgments I would like to recognize support from the Canadian Institute of Health Research, British Columbia Lung Association, and the British Columbia Cancer Agency.

These sources have no role in the preparation of this chapter. I would like to thank Alvin V. Ng and Maria M. Ho for their hard work and contributions. I apologize to colleagues whose work I could not cite due to space limitation.

References

1. Jemal, A., R. Siegel, E. Ward, T. Murray, J. Xu, C. Smigal, and M.J. Thun. 2006. Cancer statistics, 2006. *CA Cancer J Clin* 56(2):106–30.
2. Ozols, R.F., R.S. Herbst, Y.L. Colson, J. Gralow, J. Bonner, W.J. Curran, Jr., B.L. Eisenberg, P.A. Ganz, B.S. Kramer, M.G. Kris, M. Markman, R.J. Mayer, D. Raghavan, G.H. Reaman, R. Sawaya, R.L. Schilsky, L.M. Schuchter, J.W. Sweetenham, L.T. Vahdat, and R.J. Winn. 2007. Clinical cancer advances 2006: major research advances in cancer treatment, prevention, and screening – a report from the American Society of Clinical Oncology. *J Clin Oncol* 25(1):146–62.
3. Clarke, M.F., J.E. Dick, P.B. Dirks, C.J. Eaves, C.H. Jamieson, D.L. Jones, J.Visvader, I.L. Weissman, and G.M. Wahl. 2006. Cancer stem cells – perspectives on current status and future directions: AACR Workshop on cancer stem cells. *Cancer Res* 66(19):9339–44.
4. Marx, J. 2007. Molecular biology. Cancer's perpetual source? *Science* 317(5841):1029–31.
5. Jordan, C.T., M.L. Guzman, and M. Noble. 2006. Cancer stem cells. *N Engl J Med* 355(12):1253–61.
6. Ward, R.J., and P.B. Dirks. 2007. Cancer Stem Cells: At the Headwaters of Tumor Development. *Annu Rev Pathol* 2:175–189.
7. Wicha, M.S., S. Liu, and G. Dontu. 2006. Cancer stem cells: an old idea – a paradigm shift. *Cancer Res* 66(4):1883–90; discussion 1895–6.
8. Michor, F., T.P. Hughes, Y. Iwasa, S. Branford, N.P. Shah, C.L. Sawyers, and M.A. Nowak. 2005. Dynamics of chronic myeloid leukaemia. *Nature* 435(7046):1267–70.
9. Hill, R.P. 2006. Identifying cancer stem cells in solid tumors: case not proven. *Cancer Res* 66(4):1891–5; discussion 1890.
10. Hill, R.P. and R. Perris. 2007. "Destemming" cancer stem cells. *J Natl Cancer Inst* 99(19):1435–40.
11. Kelly, P.N., A. Dakic, J.M. Adams, S.L. Nutt, and A. Strasser. 2007. Tumor growth need not be driven by rare cancer stem cells. *Science* 317(5836):337.
12. Seaberg, R.M. and D. van der Kooy. 2003. Stem and progenitor cells: the premature desertion of rigorous definitions. *Trends Neurosci* 26(3):125–31.
13. Dalerba, P., R.W. Cho, and M.F. Clarke. 2007. Cancer stem cells: models and concepts. *Annu Rev Med* 58:267–84.
14. Furth, J. and J.B. Kahn Jr. 1936. The transmission of leukaemia of mice with a single cell. *Am J cancer* 31:276–82.
15. Bruce, W.R. and H. Van Der Gaag. 1963. A quantitative assay for the number of Murine Lymphoma cells capable of proliferation in vivo. *Nature* 199:79–80.
16. Hamburger, A.W. and S.E. Salmon. 1977. Primary bioassay of human tumor stem cells. *Science* 197(4302):461–3.
17. Bonnet, D. and J.E. Dick. 1997. Human acute myeloid leukemia is organized as a hierarchy that originates from a primitive hematopoietic cell. *Nat Med* 3(7):730–7.
18. Al-Hajj, M., M.S. Wicha, A. Benito-Hernandez, S.J. Morrison, and M.F. Clarke. 2003. Prospective identification of tumorigenic breast cancer cells. *Proc Natl Acad Sci U S A* 100(7):3983–8.
19. Dick, J.E. 2003. Breast cancer stem cells revealed. *Proc Natl Acad Sci U S A* 100(7):3547–9.
20. Hemmati, H.D., I. Nakano, J.A. Lazareff, M. Masterman-Smith, D.H. Geschwind, M. Bronner-Fraser, and H.I. Kornblum. 2003. Cancerous stem cells can arise from pediatric brain tumors. *Proc Natl Acad Sci U S A* 100(25):15178–83.

21. Ignatova, T.N., V.G. Kukekov, E.D. Laywell, O.N. Suslov, F.D. Vrionis, and D.A. Steindler. 2002. Human cortical glial tumors contain neural stem-like cells expressing astroglial and neuronal markers in vitro. *Glia* 39(3):193–206.

22. Singh, S.K., C. Hawkins, I.D. Clarke, J.A. Squire, J. Bayani, T. Hide, R.M. Henkelman, M.D. Cusimano, and P.B. Dirks. 2004. Identification of human brain tumour initiating cells. *Nature* 432(7015):396–401.

23. Collins, A.T., P.A. Berry, C. Hyde, M.J. Stower, and N.J. Maitland. 2005. Prospective identification of tumorigenic prostate cancer stem cells. *Cancer Res* 65(23):10946–51.

24. Dalerba, P., S.J. Dylla, I.K. Park, R. Liu, X. Wang, R.W. Cho, T. Hoey, A. Gurney, E. H. Huang, D.M. Simeone, A.A. Shelton, G. Parmiani, C. Castelli, and M.F. Clarke. 2007. Phenotypic characterization of human colorectal cancer stem cells. *Proc Natl Acad Sci U S A* 104(24):10158–63.

25. Gibbs, C.P., V.G. Kukekov, J.D. Reith, O. Tchigrinova, O.N. Suslov, E.W. Scott, S.C. Ghivizzani, T.N. Ignatova, and D.A. Steindler. 2005. Stem-like cells in bone sarcomas: implications for tumorigenesis. *Neoplasia* 7(11):967–76.

26. Li, C., D.G. Heidt, P. Dalerba, C.F. Burant, L. Zhang, V. Adsay, M. Wicha, M.F. Clarke, and D.M. Simeone. 2007. Identification of pancreatic cancer stem cells. *Cancer Res* 67(3):1030–7.

27. Ma, S., K.W. Chan, L. Hu, T.K. Lee, J.Y. Wo, I.O. Ng, B.J. Zheng, and X.Y. Guan. 2007. Identification and characterization of tumorigenic liver cancer stem/progenitor cells. *Gastroenterology* 132(7):2542–56.

28. Prince, M.E., R. Sivanandan, A. Kaczorowski, G.T. Wolf, M.J. Kaplan, P. Dalerba, I.L. Weissman, M.F. Clarke, and L.E. Ailles. 2007. Identification of a subpopulation of cells with cancer stem cell properties in head and neck squamous cell carcinoma. *Proc Natl Acad Sci U S A* 104(3):973–8.

29. Ricci-Vitiani, L., D.G. Lombardi, E. Pilozzi, M. Biffoni, M. Todaro, C. Peschle, and R. De Maria. 2007. Identification and expansion of human colon-cancer-initiating cells. *Nature* 445(7123):111–5.

30. Fang, D., T.K. Nguyen, K. Leishear, R. Finko, A.N. Kulp, S. Hotz, P.A. Van Belle, X. Xu, D.E. Elder, and M. Herlyn. 2005. A tumorigenic subpopulation with stem cell properties in melanomas. *Cancer Res* 65(20):9328–37.

31. Challen, G.A., and M.H. Little. 2006. A side order of stem cells: the SP phenotype. *Stem Cells* 24(1):3–12.

32. Hadnagy, A., L. Gaboury, R. Beaulieu, and D. Balicki. 2006. SP analysis may be used to identify cancer stem cell populations. *Exp Cell Res* 312(19):3701–10.

33. Bunting, K.D. 2002. ABC transporters as phenotypic markers and functional regulators of stem cells. *Stem Cells* 20(1):11–20.

34. Goodell, M.A., K. Brose, G. Paradis, A.S. Conner, and R.C. Mulligan. 1996. Isolation and functional properties of murine hematopoietic stem cells that are replicating in vivo. *J Exp Med* 183(4):1797–806.

35. Zhou, S., J.D. Schuetz, K.D. Bunting, A.M. Colapietro, J. Sampath, J.J. Morris, I. Lagutina, G.C. Grosveld, M. Osawa, H. Nakauchi, and B.P. Sorrentino. 2001. The ABC transporter Bcrp1/ABCG2 is expressed in a wide variety of stem cells and is a molecular determinant of the side-population phenotype. *Nat Med* 7(9): 1028–34.

35a. Scharenberg, C.W., M.A. Harkey, B. Torok-Storb. 2002. The *ABCG2* transporter is an efficient Hoechst 33342 efflux pump and is preferentially expressed by immature human hematopoietic progenitors. *Blood* 99(2):507–12.

36. Zhang, L., J. Hu, T.P. Hong, Y.N. Liu, Y.H. Wu, and L.S. Li. 2005. Monoclonal side population progenitors isolated from human fetal pancreas. *Biochem Biophys Res Commun* 333(2):603–8.

37. Bhatt, R.I., M.D. Brown, C.A. Hart, P. Gilmore, V.A. Ramani, N.J. George, and N.W. Clarke. 2003. Novel method for the isolation and characterisation of the putative prostatic stem cell. *Cytometry A* 54(2):89–99.

38. Reynolds, S.D., H. Shen, P.R. Reynolds, T. Betsuyaku, J.M. Pilewski, F. Gambelli, M. Di Giuseppe, L.A. Ortiz, and B.R. Stripp. 2007. Molecular and functional properties of lung SP cells. *Am J Physiol Lung Cell Mol Physiol* 292(4):L972–83.

39. Summer, R., D.N. Kotton, X. Sun, B. Ma, K. Fitzsimmons, and A. Fine. 2003. Side population cells and Bcrp1 expression in lung. *Am J Physiol Lung Cell Mol Physiol* 285(1):L97–104.

40. Alvi, A.J., H. Clayton, C. Joshi, T. Enver, A. Ashworth, M.M. Vivanco, T.C. Dale, and M.J. Smalley. 2003. Functional and molecular characterisation of mammary side population cells. *Breast Cancer Res* 5(1):R1–8.

41. Clarke, R.B., K. Spence, E. Anderson, A. Howell, H. Okano, and C.S. Potten. 2005. A putative human breast stem cell population is enriched for steroid receptor-positive cells. *Dev Biol* 277(2):443–56.

42. Sainz, J., A. Al Haj Zen, G. Caligiuri, C. Demerens, D. Urbain, M. Lemitre, and A. Lafont. 2006. Isolation of "side population" progenitor cells from healthy arteries of adult mice. *Arterioscler Thromb Vasc Biol* 26(2):281–6.

43. Feuring-Buske, M., and D.E. Hogge. 2001. Hoechst 33342 efflux identifies a subpopulation of cytogenetically normal CD34(+)CD38(–) progenitor cells from patients with acute myeloid leukemia. *Blood* 97(12):3882–9.

44. Wulf, G.G., R.Y. Wang, I. Kuehnle, D. Weidner, F. Marini, M.K. Brenner, M. Andreeff, and M.A. Goodell. 2001. A leukemic stem cell with intrinsic drug efflux capacity in acute myeloid leukemia. *Blood* 98(4):1166–73.

45. Hirschmann-Jax, C., A.E. Foster, G.G. Wulf, J.G. Nuchtern, T.W. Jax, U. Gobel, M.A. Goodell, and M.K. Brenner. 2004. A distinct "side population" of cells with high drug efflux capacity in human tumor cells. *Proc Natl Acad Sci U S A* 101(39):14228–33.

46. Kondo, T., T. Setoguchi, and T. Taga. 2004. Persistence of a small subpopulation of cancer stem-like cells in the C6 glioma cell line. *Proc Natl Acad Sci U S A* 101(3):781–6.

47. Seigel, G.M., L.M. Campbell, M. Narayan, and F. Gonzalez-Fernandez. 2005. Cancer stem cell characteristics in retinoblastoma. *Mol Vis* 11:729–37.

48. Patrawala, L., T. Calhoun, R. Schneider-Broussard, J. Zhou, K. Claypool, and D.G. Tang. 2005. Side population is enriched in tumorigenic, stem-like cancer cells, whereas ABCG2+ and ABCG2– cancer cells are similarly tumorigenic. *Cancer Res* 65(14):6207–19.

49. Chen, J.S., F.S. Pardo, J. Wang-Rodriguez, T.S. Chu, J.P. Lopez, J. Aguilera, X. Altuna, R.A. Weisman, and W.M. Ongkeko. 2006. EGFR regulates the side population in head and neck squamous cell carcinoma. *Laryngoscope* 116(3):401–6.

50. Chiba, T., K. Kita, Y.W. Zheng, O. Yokosuka, H. Saisho, A. Iwama, H. Nakauchi, and H. Taniguchi. 2006. Side population purified from hepatocellular carcinoma cells harbors cancer stem cell-like properties. *Hepatology* 44(1):240–51.

51. Szotek, P.P., R. Pieretti-Vanmarcke, P.T. Masiakos, D.M. Dinulescu, D. Connolly, R. Foster, D. Dombkowski, F. Preffer, D.T. Maclaughlin, and P.K. Donahoe. 2006. Ovarian cancer side population defines cells with stem cell-like characteristics and Mullerian Inhibiting Substance responsiveness. *Proc Natl Acad Sci U S A* 103(30):11154–9.

52. Mitsutake, N., A. Iwao, K. Nagai, H. Namba, A. Ohtsuru, V. Saenko, and S. Yamashita. 2007. Characterization of side population in thyroid cancer cell lines: cancer stem-like cells are enriched partly but not exclusively. *Endocrinology* 148(4):1797–803.

53. Haraguchi, N., T. Utsunomiya, H. Inoue, F. Tanaka, K. Mimori, G.F. Barnard, and M. Mori. 2006. Characterization of a side population of cancer cells from human gastrointestinal system. *Stem Cells* 24(3):506–513.

54. Ho, M.M., A.V. Ng, S. Lam, and J.Y. Hung. 2007. Side population in human lung cancer cell lines and tumors is enriched with stem-like cancer cells. *Cancer Res* 67(10):4827–33.

55. Eramo, A., F. Lotti, G. Sette, E. Pilozzi, M. Biffoni, A. Di Virgilio, C. Conticello, L. Ruco, C. Peschle, and R. De Maria. 2008. Identification and expansion of the tumorigenic lung cancer stem cell population. *Cell Death Differ* 15(3):504–514.

56. Reynolds, B.A., and S. Weiss. 1992. Generation of neurons and astrocytes from isolated cells of the adult mammalian central nervous system. *Science* 255(5052):1707–10.
57. Bjerkvig, R., B.B. Tysnes, K.S. Aboody, J. Najbauer, and A.J. Terzis. 2005. Opinion: the origin of the cancer stem cell: current controversies and new insights. *Nat Rev Cancer* 5(11):899–904.
58. Cohnheim, J. 1867. Ueber entzundung und eiterung. *Path. Anat. Physiol. Klin. Med.* 40:1–79.
59. Virchow, R. 1855. *Virchows Arch. Pathol. Anat. Physiol. Klin. Med.* 3:23.
60. Sell, S., and G.B. Pierce. 1994. Maturation arrest of stem cell differentiation is a common pathway for the cellular origin of teratocarcinomas and epithelial cancers. *Lab Invest* 70(1):6–22.
61. Emura, M. 2002. Stem cells of the respiratory tract. *Paediatr Respir Rev* 3(1):36–40.
62. Giangreco, A., K.R. Groot, and S.M. Janes. 2007. Lung cancer and lung stem cells: strange bedfellows? *Am J Respir Crit Care Med* 175(6):547–53.
63. Giangreco, A., S.D. Reynolds, and B.R. Stripp. 2002. Terminal bronchioles harbor a unique airway stem cell population that localizes to the bronchoalveolar duct junction. *Am J Pathol* 161(1):173–82.
64. Gomperts, B.N., and R.M. Strieter. 2007. Stem cells and chronic lung disease. *Annu Rev Med* 58:285–98.
65. Griffiths, M.J., D. Bonnet, and S.M. Janes. 2005. Stem cells of the alveolar epithelium. *Lancet* 366(9481):249–60.
66. Kotton, D.N., and A. Fine. 2008. Lung stem cells. *Cell Tissue Res* 331(1):145–56.
67. Lane, S., H.J. Rippon, and A.E. Bishop. 2007. Stem cells in lung repair and regeneration. *Regen Med* 2(4):407–15.
68. Beachy, P.A., S.S. Karhadkar, and D.M. Berman. 2004. Tissue repair and stem cell renewal in carcinogenesis. *Nature* 432(7015):324–31.
69. Beachy, P.A., S.S. Karhadkar, and D.M. Berman. 2004. Mending and malignancy. *Nature* 431(7007):402.
70. Engelhardt, J.F. 2001. Stem cell niches in the mouse airway. *Am J Respir Cell Mol Biol* 24(6):649–52.
71. Kim, C.F., E.L. Jackson, A.E. Woolfenden, S. Lawrence, I. Babar, S. Vogel, D. Crowley, R.T. Bronson, and T. Jacks. 2005. Identification of bronchoalveolar stem cells in normal lung and lung cancer. *Cell* 121(6):823–35.
72. Cozzio, A., E. Passegue, P.M. Ayton, H. Karsunky, M.L. Cleary, and I.L. Weissman. 2003. Similar MLL-associated leukemias arising from self-renewing stem cells and short-lived myeloid progenitors. *Genes Dev* 17(24):3029–35.
73. Jamieson, C.H., L.E. Ailles, S.J. Dylla, M. Muijtjens, C. Jones, J.L. Zehnder, J. Gotlib, K. Li, M.G. Manz, A. Keating, C.L. Sawyers, and I.L. Weissman. 2004. Granulocyte-macrophage progenitors as candidate leukemic stem cells in blast-crisis CML. *N Engl J Med* 351(7):657–67.
74. Krivtsov, A.V., D. Twomey, Z. Feng, M.C. Stubbs, Y. Wang, J. Faber, J.E. Levine, J. Wang, W.C. Hahn, D.G. Gilliland, T.R. Golub, and S.A. Armstrong. 2006. Transformation from committed progenitor to leukaemia stem cell initiated by MLL-AF9. *Nature* 442(7104):818–22.
75. Passegue, E., C.H. Jamieson, L.E. Ailles, and I.L. Weissman. 2003. Normal and leukemic hematopoiesis: are leukemias a stem cell disorder or a reacquisition of stem cell characteristics? *Proc Natl Acad Sci U S A* 100(Suppl 1):11842–9.
76. Duelli, D., and Y. Lazebnik. 2003. Cell fusion: a hidden enemy? *Cancer Cell* 3(5): 445–8.
77. Thiery, J.P. 2002. Epithelial-mesenchymal transitions in tumour progression. *Nat Rev Cancer* 2(6):442–54.
78. Thiery, J.P. 2003. Epithelial-mesenchymal transitions in development and pathologies. *Curr Opin Cell Biol* 15(6):740–6.
79. Brabletz, T., A. Jung, S. Spaderna, F. Hlubek, and T. Kirchner. 2005. Opinion: migrating cancer stem cells – an integrated concept of malignant tumour progression. *Nat Rev Cancer* 5(9):744–9.

80. Chaffer, C.L., J.P. Brennan, J.L. Slavin, T. Blick, E.W. Thompson, and E.D. Williams. 2006. Mesenchymal-to-epithelial transition facilitates bladder cancer metastasis: role of fibroblast growth factor receptor-2. *Cancer Res* 66(23):11271–8.

81. Bissell, M.J. and M.A. Labarge. 2005. Context, tissue plasticity, and cancer: are tumor stem cells also regulated by the microenvironment? *Cancer Cell* 7(1):17–23.

82. Li, L. and W.B. Neaves. 2006. Normal stem cells and cancer stem cells: the niche matters. *Cancer Res* 66(9):4553–7.

83. Tse, J.C. and R. Kalluri. 2007. Mechanisms of metastasis: epithelial-to-mesenchymal transition and contribution of tumor microenvironment. *J Cell Biochem* 101(4):816–29.

84. Kaplan, R.N., R.D. Riba, S. Zacharoulis, A.H. Bramley, L. Vincent, C. Costa, D.D. MacDonald, D.K. Jin, K. Shido, S.A. Kerns, Z. Zhu, D. Hicklin, Y. Wu, J.L. Port, N. Altorki, E.R. Port, D. Ruggero, S.V. Shmelkov, K.K. Jensen, S. Rafii, and D. Lyden. 2005. VEGFR1-positive haematopoietic bone marrow progenitors initiate the pre-metastatic niche. *Nature* 438(7069):820–7.

85. Li, F., B. Tiede, J. Massague, and Y. Kang. 2007. Beyond tumorigenesis: cancer stem cells in metastasis. *Cell Res* 17(1):3–14.

86. Tu, S.M., S.H. Lin, and C.J. Logothetis. 2002. Stem-cell origin of metastasis and heterogeneity in solid tumours. *Lancet Oncol* 3(8):508–13.

87. Schiller, J.H., D. Harrington, C.P. Belani, C. Langer, A. Sandler, J. Krook, J. Zhu, and D.H. Johnson. 2002. Comparison of four chemotherapy regimens for advanced non-small-cell lung cancer. *N Engl J Med* 346(2):92–8.

88. Goldie, J.H. and A.J. Coldman. 1979. A mathematic model for relating the drug sensitivity of tumors to their spontaneous mutation rate. *Cancer Treat Rep* 63(11–12):1727–33.

89. Costello, R.T., F. Mallet, B. Gaugler, D. Sainty, C. Arnoulet, J.A. Gastaut, and D. Olive. 2000. Human acute myeloid leukemia CD34 + /CD38– progenitor cells have decreased sensitivity to chemotherapy and Fas-induced apoptosis, reduced immunogenicity, and impaired dendritic cell transformation capacities. *Cancer Res* 60(16):4403–11.

89a. Guzman, M.L., C.F. Swiderski, D.S. Howard, B.A. Grimes, R.M. Rossi, S.J. Szilvassy, and C.T. Jordan. 2002. Preferential induction of apoptosis for primary human leukemic stem cells. *Proc Natl Acad Sci USA* 99(25):16220–5.

90. Dean, M., T. Fojo, and S. Bates. 2005. Tumour stem cells and drug resistance. *Nat Rev Cancer* 5(4):275–84.

91. Donnenberg, V.S., and A.D. Donnenberg. 2005. Multiple drug resistance in cancer revisited: the cancer stem cell hypothesis. *J Clin Pharmacol* 45(8):872–7.

92. Diehn, M., and M.F. Clarke. 2006. Cancer stem cells and radiotherapy: new insights into tumor radioresistance. *J Natl Cancer Inst* 98(24):1755–7.

93. Bao, S., Q. Wu, R.E. McLendon, Y. Hao, Q. Shi, A.B. Hjelmeland, M.W. Dewhirst, D.D. Bigner, and J.N. Rich. 2006. Glioma stem cells promote radioresistance by preferential activation of the DNA damage response. *Nature* 444(7120):756–60.

94. Gilbertson, R.J., and J.N. Rich. 2007. Making a tumour's bed: glioblastoma stem cells and the vascular niche. *Nat Rev Cancer* 7(10):733–6.

95. Bao, S., Q. Wu, S. Sathornsumetee, Y. Hao, Z. Li, A.B. Hjelmeland, Q. Shi, R.E. McLendon, D.D. Bigner, and J.N. Rich. 2006. Stem cell-like glioma cells promote tumor angiogenesis through vascular endothelial growth factor. *Cancer Res* 66(16):7843–8.

96. Calabrese, C., H. Poppleton, M. Kocak, T.L. Hogg, C. Fuller, B. Hamner, E.Y. Oh, M.W. Gaber, D. Finklestein, M. Allen, A. Frank, I.T. Bayazitov, S.S. Zakharenko, A. Gajjar, A. Davidoff, and R.J. Gilbertson. 2007. A perivascular niche for brain tumor stem cells. *Cancer Cell* 11(1):69–82.

97. Folkman, J. 2002. Role of angiogenesis in tumor growth and metastasis. *Semin Oncol* 29(6 Suppl 16):15–8.

98. Cao, C., J.M. Albert, L. Geng, P.S. Ivy, A. Sandler, D.H. Johnson, and B. Lu. 2006. Vascular endothelial growth factor tyrosine kinase inhibitor AZD2171 and fractionated radiotherapy in mouse models of lung cancer. *Cancer Res* 66(23):11409–15.

99. Herbst, R.S., D.H. Johnson, E. Mininberg, D.P. Carbone, T. Henderson, E.S. Kim, G. Blumenschein, Jr., J.J. Lee, D.D. Liu, M.T. Truong, W.K. Hong, H. Tran, A. Tsao, D. Xie, D.A. Ramies, R. Mass, S. Seshagiri, D.A. Eberhard, S.K. Kelley, and A. Sandler. 2005. Phase I/II trial evaluating the anti-vascular endothelial growth factor monoclonal antibody bevacizumab in combination with the HER-1/epidermal growth factor receptor tyrosine kinase inhibitor erlotinib for patients with recurrent non-small-cell lung cancer. *J Clin Oncol* 23(11):2544–55.

100. Johnson, D.H., L. Fehrenbacher, W.F. Novotny, R.S. Herbst, J.J. Nemunaitis, D.M. Jablons, C.J. Langer, R.F. DeVore, IIIrd, J. Gaudreault, L.A. Damico, E. Holmgren, and F. Kabbinavar. 2004. Randomized phase II trial comparing bevacizumab plus carboplatin and paclitaxel with carboplatin and paclitaxel alone in previously untreated locally advanced or metastatic non-small-cell lung cancer. *J Clin Oncol* 22(11):2184–91.

101. Vokes, E., R. Herbst, and A. Sandler. 2006. Angiogenesis inhibition in the treatment of lung cancer. *Clin Adv Hematol Oncol* 4(11 Suppl 23):1-10; quiz 11-2.

102. Batchelor, T.T., A.G. Sorensen, E. di Tomaso, W.T. Zhang, D.G. Duda, K.S. Cohen, K.R. Kozak, D.P. Cahill, P.J. Chen, M. Zhu, M. Ancukiewicz, M.M. Mrugala, S. Plotkin, J. Drappatz, D.N. Louis, P. Ivy, D.T. Scadden, T. Benner, J.S. Loeffler, P.Y. Wen, and R.K. Jain. 2007. AZD2171, a pan-VEGF receptor tyrosine kinase inhibitor, normalizes tumor vasculature and alleviates edema in glioblastoma patients. *Cancer Cell* 11(1):83–95.

103. Vredenburgh, J.J., A. Desjardins, J.E. Herndon, IInd, J.M. Dowell, D.A. Reardon, J.A. Quinn, J.N. Rich, S. Sathornsumetee, S. Gururangan, M. Wagner, D.D. Bigner, A.H. Friedman, and H.S. Friedman. 2007. Phase II trial of bevacizumab and irinotecan in recurrent malignant glioma. *Clin Cancer Res* 13(4):1253–9.

104. Phatak, P., J.C. Cookson, F. Dai, V. Smith, R.B. Gartenhaus, M.F. Stevens, and A.M. Burger. 2007. Telomere uncapping by the G-quadruplex ligand RHPS4 inhibits clonogenic tumour cell growth in vitro and in vivo consistent with a cancer stem cell targeting mechanism. *Br J Cancer* 96(8):1223–33.

105. Shay, J.W., and W.N. Keith. 2008. Targeting telomerase for cancer therapeutics. *Br J Cancer* 98(4):677–83.

106. Sun, S., J.H. Schiller, M. Spinola, and J.D. Minna. 2007. New molecularly targeted therapies for lung cancer. *J Clin Invest* 117(10):2740–50.

107. Harley, C.B. 2008. Telomerase and cancer therapeutics. *Nat Rev Cancer* 8(3):167–79.

108. Liu, R., X. Wang, G.Y. Chen, P. Dalerba, A. Gurney, T. Hoey, G. Sherlock, J. Lewicki, K. Shedden, and M.F. Clarke. 2007. The prognostic role of a gene signature from tumorigenic breast-cancer cells. *N Engl J Med* 356(3):217–26.

Epithelial–Mesenchymal Transition as a Mechanism of Metastasis

Katia Savary, Stefan Termén, Sylvie Thuault, Venkateshwar Keshamouni, and Aristidis Moustakas

Abstract Mammalian embryonic cells form adhering cell sheets interconnected via various intercellular junctional complexes. Gastrulation and later stages of histo- and organogenesis depend on changes in developmental stage, such as epithelial–mesenchymal transition (EMT), whereby adherent cells disintegrate their intercellular contacts, organize their motility apparatus, and move to new locations in the developing body. EMT generates transitory mesenchymal cells, which can differentiate into myofibroblasts or pericytes (in the case of endothelial–mesenchymal transition (EndMT)), or feed the progenitor pools of cell lineages (e.g., blood, muscle, bone, adipose, and neuronal). EMT is guided by cues from extracellular signaling factors including mitogens, transforming growth factor β, Notch, and Wnt. The signaling molecules can cooperate or act sequentially to initiate transcriptional programs that involve many transcriptional regulators. Changes in gene expression lead to a reprogramming of epithelial protein components and the generation of the mesenchymal progenitor stage. EMT can also contribute to the progression of cancer, when the same growth factor pathways reawaken embryonic transcriptional programs otherwise silenced in adult life. Induction of cancer cell EMT generates rare transitory mesenchymal cells that support tumor growth, remodel the tumor microenvironment, and facilitate tissue invasiveness and metastasis. In that sense, cancer cells undergoing EMT have some of the capacities that one would expect from the so-called "tumor-initiating cells." This makes EMT an attractive problem for medical research with new therapeutic implications.

A. Moustakas (✉)
Ludwig Institute for Cancer Research, Biomedical Center, Uppsala University,
Uppsala, Sweden
e-mail: aris.moustakas@licr.uu.se

V. Keshamouni et al. (eds.), *Lung Cancer Metastasis*,
DOI 10.1007/978-1-4419-0772-1_4, © Springer Science+Business Media, LLC 2009

General and Embryonic Aspects of EMT

Cell polarization in epithelial tissues is responsible for the organization of stable adherens and tight junctions, desmosomes, and gap junctions. Such junctions segregate the apical and basolateral parts of the cell and also define the routes of intercellular communication. This architecture is dynamic. The process of epithelial-to-mesenchymal transition (EMT) disintegrates or reorganizes the adhesion complexes, favoring more labile cell–cell adhesion and communication with the extracellular matrix via focal adhesions [1–3]. The general features of EMT include the downregulation/disorganization of the epithelial proteins in adherens junctions, tight junctions or the cytokeratin filament network, and the upregulation of mesenchymal proteins such as fibronectin, fibroblast-specific protein 1, α-smooth muscle actin, vimentin, and N-cadherin. EMT proceeds by establishing a mesenchymal proteome inside and outside the changing cell, thus aiding its capacity to migrate and penetrate through organized tissues. In addition to embryonic development, EMT plays critical roles during the pathogenesis of disease, such as metastatic cancer and fibrosis of the lung, kidney, and liver [2–5].

EMT is a transitory state of cell differentiation which prepares cells for further developmental remodeling. Accordingly, EMT can be reversed so that mesenchymal progenitor cells differentiate into epithelial cells, especially after migration and homing into new sites within an embryo or an adult organism. Such a process is called mesenchymal–epithelial transition (MET) and occurs during embryogenesis, tumor progression, and healing of fibrotic tissue [3, 4]. Finally, processes functionally similar to EMT take place during vascular remodeling and are called endothelial–mesenchymal transitions (EndMT) [6]. Similar processes also affect the survival and differentiation of embryonic and adult stem cells as we discuss later.

EMT, MET, and EndMT are differentiation programs operating under the control of common and developmentally important signaling pathways [7, 8] (Fig. 1). These include the receptor tyrosine kinase (RTK) pathways initiated by mitogens like hepatocyte growth factor (HGF), fibroblast growth factor (FGF), and vascular endothelial growth factor (VEGF); the receptor serine/threonine kinase (RS/TK) pathways initiated by transforming growth factor β (TGFβ) family members; the Notch receptor; and furthermore the Wnt and Sonic hedgehog (Shh) family pathways. The main role of all such signaling mechanisms is to regulate gene expression and establish a group of transcription factors, which in turn elicit the phenotypic change outlined as EMT. Known transcriptional mediators of EMT include the zinc finger factors Snail1 and Snail2; the ZEB family factors ZEB1 and ZEB2; and the basic helix-loop-helix (bHLH) factors E47, E2-2, and Twist together with the inhibitors of differentiation/DNA binding (Id) [9] (Fig. 1). In this chapter, we summarize the current view on the signaling pathways and the transcription factor programs that regulate EMT. We highlight the role of EMT in tumor progression and metastasis.

Fig. 1 Overview of the major actors involved in the process of EMT. TGFβ, Notch, Wnt, HGF, and FGF signaling pathways induce EMT. Each ligand uses a specific plasma membrane receptor (shown in *ovals*) and intracellular transducer. These signaling pathways regulate a set of transcription factors such as members of the Snail zinc finger family, the ZEB family, the bHLH family members Twist, and E47/E12 (shown in a *rectangle*). These factors then repress expression of epithelial markers such as E-cadherin and induce expression of mesenchymal markers such as vimentin (described in the table; *arrows* indicate how gene expression is regulated), leading to changes in cell morphology and migratory-invasive capacities. The cuboidal, polarized epithelial cells generate via EMT elongated or star-like mesenchymal cells with an increased capacity to invade through the matrix

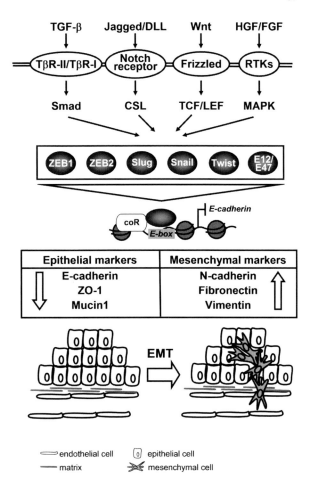

During embryogenesis, EMT enables cells to populate and establish tissues in distant embryonic regions, while during malignant tumor progression EMT empowers cancer cells with metastatic potential. In vivo evidence of EMT has been extensively documented during embryogenesis. Here, we summarize the requirement of EMT at different stages and locations of the developing embryo with the aim to compare these physiological EMT processes to those involved in the pathogenesis of fibrosis or cancer in the adult.

EMT Induces Mesoderm Formation During Gastrulation

Early-stage embryos are composed of two major cell layers, the ectoderm (or epiblast) and the primitive endoderm (or hypoblast). Following gastrulation, a third intermediate cell layer, the mesoderm, is formed. While gastrulation in amphibians and fish involves movements of epithelial cell sheets, in birds and mammals it involves the convergence of epiblast cells at the midline of the embryonic disc and their ingression through the primitive streak to form the underlying mesoderm and the definitive endoderm [10]. This ingression is highly dependent on EMT since it requires that single epiblastic cells delaminate and migrate through the epiblast layer. FGF promotes this EMT process by binding to its tyrosine kinase receptor. Indeed, embryos with mutated FGF8 and its receptor FGFR1 display gastrulation defects in which the mesoderm fails to form or migrate away from the primitive streak [11–13]. Snail1, Snail2, and ZEB2 mediate the effects of FGF on EMT during gastrulation by directly repressing the expression of E-cadherin and inducing N-cadherin [14–17]. This crucial developmental role for Snail family members is also highlighted by the *Snail1* mouse knockout, which is embryonic lethal due to mesodermal defects during gastrulation [18]. Another potent inducer of EMT during gastrulation is Wnt, as targeted null mutation of *Wnt3a* impairs the formation of paraxial mesoderm in the gastrulating mouse embryo [19]. Wnt3a signals via β-catenin and its nuclear partner LEF-1 to maintain the expression of the mesodermal marker brachyury during gastrulation [20].

EMT Induces Formation of Neural Crest Cells

Neural crest cells show multipotency, are capable of some self-renewing decisions, and are often considered as stem cells (21a). They constitute an important transitory tissue, characteristic of vertebrate embryos, and derive from the ectoderm at the end of the neurulation stage [21]. These cells arise from the dorsal region of the neural tube or "neural plate" about the site and period of its closure and delaminate from the neuroepithelium consecutively to an EMT process [22]. During this EMT some of the neuroepithelial cells change shape and properties acquiring a highly motile mesenchymal phenotype crucial for their subsequent series of migrations throughout the embryonic body [23]. They give rise to an amazing array of ectoderm-derived cell types, comprising almost all of the peripheral neurons and glial cells, the melanocytes, vascular smooth muscle and cranial cells, depending on the signals they receive during their migration and their final location in the body. Moreover, the ability of neural crest cells to respond to their microenvironment is easily reactivated in their descendants during post-natal life, leading to the development of highly invasive tumors such as melanomas or gliomas. In this context, understanding the signaling pathways that control early neural crest cell development, especially EMT, may help to understand similar processes involved in tumor metastasis and possibly in cancer stem cell biology.

The EMT signals that control neural crest formation have been studied primarily in avian and *Xenopus* models. Among these signals, bone morphogenetic protein (BMP), Wnt, and FGF signaling pathways play critical roles in inducing neural crest cell specification and delamination from the neural tube [21, 22]. These morphogenetic factors regulate early expression of Snail family transcription factors, cell adhesion molecules, cytoskeletal regulators, and extracellular matrix components implicated in the delamination and early migration events of the neural crest cells [24]. The current model of neural crest formation proposes that a precise gradient of BMP spatially restricted to the border of the neural plate operates together with active Notch signaling. Afterward the anterior neural folds receive FGF, Wnt, and retinoic acid signals, resulting in delamination of neural crest cells.

EMT in Palate Formation

The development of the palate during the 6th–9th week of human gestation starts with the formation of two palatal shelves on the maxillary prominences. The elevated palatal shelves fuse together to form one continuous structure with the medial edge epithelium, which results in the formation of the roof of the mouth or "hard palate." This fusion requires a specialized EMT process which is mainly attributed to the action of TGFβ3, since mice lacking the *Tgfb3* gene exhibit a failure of secondary palate development known as the "cleft palate phenotype." TGFβ3 mediates mouse palatal EMT via the Smad pathway, which leads to upregulation of the transcription factor LEF1, a protein best known for mediating Wnt signaling pathways in different tissue contexts [25]. A recent analysis of the functions of *Snai1* and *Snai2* genes during mouse development showed that approximately 50% of *Snai2*$^{-/-}$ mice present a cleft palate phenotype at birth, and the penetrance of this phenotype increases to 100% when crossed to a *Snai1* heterozygous background [26]. These findings emphasize again the importance of Snail genes during palatal EMT.

EMT in Heart Morphogenesis

In chicken and mouse, the heart valve and septa form after a prominent EMT process in which intracardial cells respond in a sequential manner to Notch signaling. Notch induces TGFβ2 expression, which then further induces Snail1 expression and subsequent repression of E-cadherin (reviewed in [27]). In epithelial cell models in vitro, TGFβ1 induces transcription of Notch family ligands like Jagged1 and Delta-like4, which then activate Notch signaling [28, 29]. The coordinate action of TGFβ and Notch is therefore required for the establishment of EMT and of cell cycle arrest in epithelial cells of the epidermis.

Epithelial and Mesenchymal Reciprocal Interactions in Embryonic Lung Morphogenesis

Reciprocal interactions between epithelial cells (derived from the foregut endoderm) and surrounding mesenchyme (derived from the splanchnic mesoderm) are essential in different aspects of lung development (morphogenesis, vasculogenesis, and maturation) [30]. During lung morphogenesis, these interactions lead to patterning of the respiratory tree through a process of tubular branching similar to the one observed during kidney morphogenesis, which includes epithelial extension, epiboly, sheet closure, and EMT. As suggested initially by grafting experiments [31], and then by gene mutations in the mouse (reviewed in [32]), mesenchymal cells deliver paracrine factors that modify epithelial cell movements, proliferation, and differentiation during lung morphogenesis. Some of these factors are also implicated in the development of pathologies such as lung carcinoma or fibrosis of the adult organ.

These factors include members of the FGF, TGFβ, Shh, epidermal growth factor (EGF), and platelet-derived growth factor (PDGF) families. As a general rule, FGF, EGF, or PDGF signaling through RTK receptors tends to promote proliferation and differentiation, whereas TGFβ or BMP signaling through RS/TK receptors tends to oppose these effects [30]. Glucocorticoids and retinoids, hormones that increase cyclic AMP formation, also play important roles in branching morphogenesis, alveolar development, and cellular differentiation but will not be further discussed here.

Factors Secreted by the Mesenchyme

Among the key mediators of these mesenchymal–epithelial interactions are FGF family members. Particularly, the importance of FGF10 in lung morphogenesis has been revealed by the absence of bronchi and lungs in mouse embryos homozygous for a deletion in the *Fgf10* gene [33, 34]. FGF10 produced by the mesenchyme surrounding the lung buds binds to FGFR2 that is uniformly expressed in the endoderm and increases epithelial cell motility and proliferation, thus promoting lung bud extension (outgrowth of the epithelium) [35]. Another member of the FGF family, FGF7, or keratinocyte growth factor, KGF, is produced by the mesenchyme early in lung development and binds to the same FGFR2 receptor. FGF7 appears to be important in lung development by acting as a proliferation factor for the lung epithelium [36].

Factors Secreted by the Epithelium

Various members of the TGFβ superfamily play different roles during lung morphogenesis. *Tgfb3* knockout mice display abnormal lung development [37], and exposure of lung primordia to exogenous TGFβ1 decreases branching morphogenesis and formation of saccular buds in vitro and in vivo [38, 39]. This inhibitory effect of TGFβ ligands on lung branching morphogenesis is a consequence of activation of the TGFβ receptor TGFβRII and its downstream signaling effectors, Smad2, Smad3, and Smad4, since abrogation of signaling by these proteins results in increased embryonic lung branching morphogenesis in vitro [40, 41].

BMP4, another member of the TGFβ superfamily, is highly expressed in the lung bud epithelium and to a lesser extent in the mesenchyme [42]. BMP4 inhibits epithelial cell proliferation and induces differentiation at the tips of the end buds that facilitates branching [43]. As BMP4 is secreted in response to FGF10, it partially counteracts the effects of FGF10 on epithelial cell motility and proliferation both spatially and temporally.

Sonic hedgehog is secreted by the foregut endoderm and at high levels in the epithelial regions where branching occurs [42, 44]. Shh signals via the patched-smoothened receptor complex located at the mesenchyme [45], where it stimulates mesenchyme proliferation and decreases FGF10 production [46, 47]. An inappropriate expression of Shh in the lung epithelium results in increased epithelial and mesenchymal proliferation and a lack of functional alveoli in transgenic mice [48]. Moreover, $Shh^{-/-}$ mutant mouse embryos lack the dorsoventral separation of the esophagus and trachea and display abnormal lungs due to an absence of branching morphogenesis and reduced mesenchymal proliferation. Downstream of the patched-smoothened receptor complex, Shh effects are mediated by Gli transcription factors. Indeed, all three transcription factors (Gli1, Gli2, and Gli3) are expressed in the lung mesenchyme in different spatiotemporal patterns during lung development and play essential roles in the development of the trachea, esophagus, and lungs [49]. Moreover, the similarities in the tracheal/esophageal phenotypes of the $Gli2^{-/-}$, $Gli2^{-/-}/Gli3^{+/-}$ double-knockout and $Shh^{-/-}$ mouse embryos suggest that transcription factors Gli2 and Gli3 mediate the effects of Shh on the development of these structures [49, 50]. Transgenic mouse studies also suggest that Gli1 may mediate Shh regulation of *patched* expression [50]. Finally, it is also interesting to note that the defects in lung morphogenesis and tracheal/esophageal separation in $Shh^{-/-}$ and in $Gli2^{-/-}/Gli3^{+/-}$ double-knockout embryos are highly similar to those observed in the double-knockout mice for retinoic acid receptors ($Rar\alpha1^{-/-}/Rar\beta2^{-/-}$), suggesting an interrelationship of Shh, Gli, and RA signaling pathways in lung development.

Factors Secreted by the Mesenchyme and the Epithelium

EGF is produced by epithelial and mesenchymal cells in the developing lung. Targeted deletion of the gene encoding the EGF receptor (EGFR) in mice was found to have highly variable effects on lung morphogenesis depending on the genetic background, and the mice died either at an embryonic stage or soon after birth, due to a general growth retardation [51]. However, neonatal $EGFR^{-/-}$ mice often show evidence of lung immaturity which results in visible respiratory distress. The lungs of these mutant mice have impaired branching and deficient alveolization and septation [52].

Similarly, PDGF-A, which is produced by the developing lung epithelium and binds to the PDGFαR in the mesenchyme, plays a critical role in alveologenesis by regulating proliferation and migration of smooth muscle cells surrounding developing alveoli [53]. Indeed, whereas the targeted deletion of the *PDGF-B* gene in mice had no apparent effects on lung development, mice homozygous for targeted deletion of the *PDGF-A* gene have some defects due to abnormal septation [53].

To conclude, it is apparent that major signaling pathways involving several RTKs, Notch, Wnt, and TGFβ family members provide primary input to various embryonic EMT events that are critical during the patterning of many organs and tissues.

EMT in the Context of Cancer Progression

One of the earliest changes in the transformation of epithelial cells toward a carcinoma phenotype is the loss of cell–cell adhesions and cell polarity, which also constitutes the first step in the EMT program (Fig. 2).

Receptor Tyrosine Kinase Signaling in the Establishment of EMT

The oncogenic pathways involving RTK signaling are involved in regulating those cell–cell interactions formed by tight junctions and adherens junctions, which are critical for the stability and function of epithelial sheets [54]. It has been suggested that RTK activation participates in the EMT program by rendering the tight junction leaky and thus allowing access of TGFβ to its receptor, one subunit of which would otherwise remain segregated in the tight junction [55]. This reflects the current idea of an integrated action by various signaling proteins that control the EMT process. In fact, growth factors that activate RTK receptors were the first extracellular molecules that were identified as promoters of EMT through activation of the extracellular-regulated kinase (Erk) members of the MAPK signaling cascade. For instance, HGF that signals via the RTK c-Met initiates a complex signaling cascade that involves the recruitment of several adaptor proteins and the activation of signal transducers including the Erk MAP kinases. HGF signaling results in important modifications of the extracellular matrix (ECM) through induction of several ECM proteins and MMPs, which change cell–ECM and cell–cell interactions through regulation of integrin and cadherin expression and function [56].

EMT in Lung Cancer cells

A549 control   **A549 72 h TGF-β**

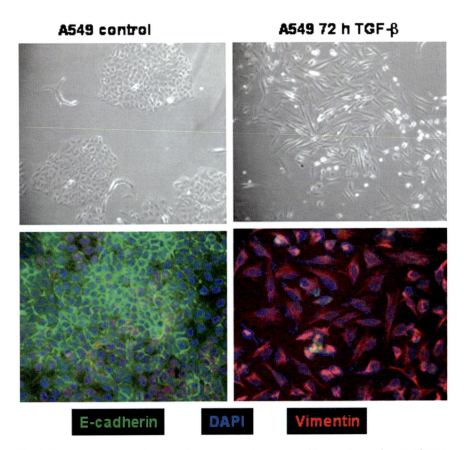

E-cadherin   DAPI   Vimentin

Fig. 2 Phase-contrast and immunofluorescence microscopy of human lung adenocarcinoma A549 cells. Epithelial cell clusters become mesenchymal, elongated, and migratory cells in response to TGFβ1 for 72 h. The adherens junction marker E-cadherin decorates the polarized lung epithelial cells, while the mesenchymal intermediate filament marker vimentin decorates the migratory elongated cells. Nuclei are counterstained using 4′,6′-diamidino-2-phenylindole (DAPI)

Constitutive Erk activation was shown to be essential for complete EMT in both in vitro and in vivo models of epithelial tumor metastasis [57–61]. Recent data suggest that HGF also activates EMT through regulation of the transcription factor Snail1 [62]. Similarly, FGF mediates EMT via activation of its RTK receptor [63] and possibly by enhancing TGFβ signaling. Indeed, recent work in *Xenopus* embryos showed that FGF signaling promotes mesodermal differentiation by enhancing embryonic TGFβ/nodal signaling [64]. In this case, FGF binding to its receptor leads to activation of FGFR/MAPK signaling that induces p53 N-terminal phosphorylation, enabling the interaction of p53 with the TGFβ-activated Smads in the nucleus. Critical gene targets of this regulatory cascade that mediate the EMT response remain to be elucidated.

In addition to Erk MAPKs, phosphatidylinositol-3′-kinase (PI3K) is also a key inducer of EMT downstream of RTK receptors. However, PI3K is activated not only by growth factors but also by integrin receptors and small GTPases of the Rho family that control cytoskeletal organization, and thus it integrates various extracellular signals [65, 66]. Finally, RTKs stimulate the p38 MAPK, whose implication in EMT during embryogenesis was recently highlighted. During gastrulation, FGF/Snail1 and p38/p38-interacting protein (p38IP) pathways act independently but eventually converge to downregulate E-cadherin expression leading to EMT, the former at the mRNA and the latter at the protein level [67]. In this example, both pathways play important roles since disruption of either FGF/Snail1 or p38/p38IP in the mouse results in defective gastrulation.

TGFβ as a Central Regulator of EMT

Whereas the above-mentioned oncogenic pathways involving RTKs play major roles at the early stages of EMT, additional signals were shown to be necessary for the establishment of a full EMT program that results in the mesenchymal and migratory phenotype characteristic of invasive carcinoma cells (Fig. 1). Critical evidence that EMT induced by oncogenic stimuli depends on TGFβ signaling comes from the observation that TGFβ inhibitors are capable of blocking EMT induced by oncogenes like *ras* or *raf* in various models of carcinoma. Interestingly, TGFβ inhibitors also block invasiveness and metastasis [59, 60, 68–70]. TGFβ1 has been described as a potent inducer of EMT in various epithelial cells derived from normal breast, proximal tubules of the kidney, lens, and more recently lung alveoli [71–73]. Moreover, TGFβ establishes a link between the cell cycle and the EMT program, although this link seems to be cell type dependent. In vitro, TGFβ arrests the epithelial cell cycle at the early G1 phase, while inducing EMT [72]. In vivo, carcinomas secrete abnormally high amounts of TGFβ, which acts on the surrounding stromal cells, and thus provokes loss of growth suppressive and pro-apoptotic responses to TGFβ via the action of stromal-derived cytokines, which can also induce EMT [74]. Mechanistically, the ability of TGFβ to induce cytostasis and apoptosis or survival and EMT was shown to depend on the stage of the cell cycle of the responding epithelial cell [75]. In other words, EMT was associated with the G1/S transition whereas apoptosis with the G2/M transition, an interesting scenario worth examining in vivo during cancer progression. Using novel fluorescent probes that mark the cell cycle stage in culture and in live animals, it has once again been confirmed that migratory and invasive cells that undergo EMT are arrested in the G1 phase of the cell cycle and thus it is definitively established that carcinoma cell migration and EMT do not involve concomitant cell proliferation [76].

TGFβ signals through type I and type II RS/TK receptors and via a so-called canonical intracellular pathway that involves the Smad effectors, which regulate transcription of many genes that play critical roles in the control of cell proliferation, apoptosis, differentiation, EMT, and cell migration [77]. The role of Smad proteins during TGFβ-induced EMT has been amply demonstrated. We have shown that EMT could be induced by signaling pathways of the TGFβ/activin branch that activate Smad2/Smad3, whereas pathways of the BMP branch that activate Smad1/Smad5/Smad8 have opposite effects on EMT in normal mammary and lens epithelial cells [72, 78, 79]. In mouse models expressing either mutant Smad proteins that block endogenous Smad signaling, Smad-specific RNA interference (RNAi), tissue-specific Smad knockouts or a mutant TGFβ type I receptor that retains kinase activity but cannot activate Smad2 or Smad3, TGFβ-induced EMT was effectively blocked (reviewed in [80]). For example, Smad4 is indispensable for the transcriptional mechanism that downregulates E-cadherin expression in response to TGFβ [81]. RNAi experiments targeting Smad4 in cultured cell models and tissue-specific knock-out of Smad4 in the mammary gland and the pancreas have all confirmed an important role of Smad4 in the EMT of these epithelial tissue types [82–84]. On the other hand, Smad2 and Smad3 are thought to play different roles depending on the developmental context. For example, mouse liver-specific inactivation of Smad2 and Smad3 confirmed that Smad3 but not Smad2 was required for EMT in hepatocytes [85]. In contrast, Smad2 seemed to counteract the EMT response, preventing hepatocyte de-differentiation. In another model of human kidney tubular epithelial cells, the decrease in E-cadherin was Smad3-dependent, whereas the increase in MMP2 was Smad2-dependent, and the induction of α-smooth muscle actin (α-SMA) was dependent on both Smad2 and Smad3 [86]. In addition, Smad signaling induces ligands of the Notch and Wnt pathways, which are further required for the establishment of EMT [87].

Besides the canonical Smad pathway, TGFβ activates Erk and p38 MAPKs, PI3K, and small GTPases of the Ras and Rho family that contribute to both gene regulation and cytoplasmic signaling involved in cell motility, apoptosis, and EMT [88]. Some selected examples include the serine/threonine protein kinase A (PKA), which is required for TGFβ1-induced apoptosis and EMT together with STAT3 [89]. Furthermore, some of the non-Smad signaling pathways establish cross talks with the canonical Smad pathway. For instance, there is evidence for cross talk between the integrin receptors and the TGFβ for the activation of the p38 MAPK, which in turn contributes to EMT [90, 91]. Integrin-linked kinase (ILK) gene expression can be induced by Smad signaling [92] and ILK contributes to TGFβ-induced EMT [93]. This is also the case for NF-κB activation, which cooperates functionally with Smad signaling during EMT [94]. In conclusion, non-Smad and Smad signals activated by TGFβ participate in the establishment of the EMT program that generates the mesenchymal phenotype characteristic of invasive carcinoma cells.

Downstream of these TGFβ signaling pathways a plethora of genes are involved in EMT as shown in vitro by genome-wide expression analyses and in vivo using models of invasive carcinoma [72, 95–99]. Among these downstream genes, we can distinguish the direct targets of TGFβ, which encode transcription factors that control the EMT differentiation switch, from the genes that define the phenotypic changes associated with EMT.

A Transcriptional Program Governing EMT

In most cell types, it is accepted that TGFβ induces expression of the transcription factors Snail1, Snail2, Twist, and other bHLH proteins, which are potent repressors of all genes that contribute to the epithelial phenotype, and particularly of genes implicated in cell–cell interactions such as *E-cadherin, claudins, connexins, occludin,* and *ZO-family* genes [100]. Moreover, microarray screens have identified regulators of actin dynamics downstream of TGFβ, such as the guanine exchange factor NET1, which leads to sustained activation of Rho GTPases and thus supports actin reorganization, and various tropomyosin genes [101, 102].

Snail1 expression is induced by TGFβ via both Smad3-dependent and Erk MAPK-dependent signaling [103, 104]. Downstream of the TGFβ/Smad signaling pathway, our group identified the high mobility group factor HMGA2 as a new regulator of EMT in mammary epithelial cells [105]. Interestingly, this regulator of mesenchymal differentiation is also highly expressed in a number of tumors. HMGA2 also induces expression of the transcriptional regulators Snail1, Snail2, Twist, and represses expression of Id2. Id proteins bind to bHLH transcription factors and prevent them from binding to DNA. Ids have been shown to inhibit EMT and to be repressed by the TGFβ/Smads pathway [79, 106]. For example, Id2 repression by TGFβ allows the bHLH factors E12/E47 to bind to and repress the *E-cadherin* promoter at its E-box motif [79, 106]. On the other hand, the BMP/Smad pathway strongly induces and stabilizes the Id proteins and consequently preserves epithelial differentiation [79, 107]. In agreement with this molecular model, BMP induces MET in a dominant fashion relative to TGFβ, which mediates EMT [4, 79, 108, 109]. These opposite effects of BMP and TGFβ seem to rely mainly on the levels of Ids in epithelial cells.

In addition to the above-mentioned transcription factors, the two-handed zinc finger/homeodomain proteins ZEB1 and ZEB2 interact with Smads to form repressor complexes on the E-box region of the *E-cadherin* gene but also on other genes [110–112]. Finally, the bHLH proteins E12/E47 and Twist and high-mobility group box-containing proteins (e.g., LEF-1) become involved in the EMT response to TGFβ, which as described above, often involves the intimate cross talk with other pathways such as PDGF and Wnt [9, 25, 99, 113, 114].

As previously mentioned, EMT is a multistep program and the loss of epithelial adhesion molecules does not necessarily lead to a complete EMT. Downregulation of epithelial markers should be accompanied by an upregulation of mesenchymal markers such as α-SMA, fibronectin, vimentin, and MMP. This again involves Smad- and non-Smad pathways of TGFβ activation. Interestingly, some of the transcription factors that are responsible for downregulation of the epithelial markers seem to be required for the induction of the mesenchymal phenotype. For example, Snail1 induces expression of fibronectin or vitronectin [100]. This is, however, not the case for Id2 which represses E-cadherin but fails to induce α-SMA, fibronectin, or MMP2 when overexpressed [115]. Possibly the two most clear demonstrations of transcription factors that mediate the mesenchymal program of differentiation during EMT known so far are the forkhead family protein FoxC2, whose expression can be induced by TGFβ, albeit in an indirect manner that involves long time periods [116], and the fibroblast-specific protein (FSP1) that is transcriptionally induced by other factors such as CArG box-binding factor-A (CBF-A) and KRAB-associated protein 1 (KAP-1) [117]. Further dissection of the mesenchymal differentiation program during EMT is therefore amply warranted.

EMT and Lung Cancer

Lung cancer is the leading cause of cancer death in the United States, with 80% of patients dying of this disease [118]. Sadly, this is virtually unchanged over the past 20 years [119]. Lung cancer is difficult to cure because it has an ability to metastasize early in the lungs and to distant organs, and similarly to most other cancers, the vast majority of lung cancer-related mortality is due to metastatic disease. It follows that there is a great need to understand the process of metastasis in lung cancer in detail.

In order to metastasize, lung cancer cells must change from an epithelial to a mesenchymal phenotype, because mesenchymal cells are empowered with migratory and invasive capacities. The role of EMT during lung cancer progression, unlike many other types of advanced solid tumors, is not yet fully established, despite some prominent emerging cases that we discuss here. Lung tumor cells often secrete TGFβ in an autocrine fashion, which could serve as a driving force toward EMT. The general hypothesis states that lung tumors should gain this ability usually in later stages of cancer development, so there is a chance that lung cancer EMT is discovered in time to effectively treat the patient with EMT inhibitors. But in order to achieve that, we need to understand the process of EMT in lung tumors better. Facts have now started to emerge in the literature.

In A549 lung adenocarcinoma cells that retain characteristics of alveolar type II epithelial cells, TGFβ1 induced EMT by downregulating E-cadherin and upregulating fibronectin, MMP-2, connective tissue growth factor (CTGF) and collagens, decreasing cell-to-cell contact, and causing elongation [120]. Smad2 siRNA knockdown diminished the EMT process as expected. Using the same A549 cell model and a quantitative differential proteomic analysis to compare TGFβ-treated and untreated cells, for the first time it was shown that TGFβ treatment enhanced the migratory and invasive abilities of these cells [121] (Fig. 2). Hallmark EMT markers were up- or downregulated as expected and elongation and cell scattering were observed. Although not identified in the screen itself, p53 is proposed as a node in the network of proteins that orchestrate the EMT response. p53 is known to be involved in TGFβ signaling [122], but its role in EMT has not been investigated.

In a final study of lung A549 adenocarcinomas, among several growth factors investigated, TGFβ1 induced cell elongation the most, while EGF induced the most extensive cell scattering [123], the latter being in agreement with a previous study [124]. In addition and similar to breast and pancreatic cells, plating A549 cells on collagen I induced EMT, which was dependent on Smad signaling. Monitoring TGFβ production revealed that expression of TGFβ1 and TGFβ2 was unchanged, while TGFβ3 was upregulated and secreted by A549 cells in an autocrine fashion. Inhibitor studies identified PI3K and ERK pathways to be activated in the TGFβ3 induction by collagen I, and the same was true for TGFβ3 induction by EGF. The major conclusion from these studies is that interaction of cells with collagen I and with growth factors in the ECM activates both RTK and integrin receptor pathways. These pathways converge on downstream PI3K and ERK signaling pathways to induce autocrine secretion of TGFβ3 which activates the TGFβ receptors to induce EMT via Smads. Similar to adenocarcinoma cells in vitro, immortalized normal epithelial cells (HPL1) isolated from human lung have also been shown to undergo a robust EMT phenotypic response after exposure to various TGFβ and activin isoforms, which occurs concomitantly to the growth arrest response of these cells [72, 125]. However, to this date, no specific signaling pathways or transcriptional regulators have been analyzed in such more normal lung epithelial cell models.

Signs of EMT during lung cancer progression have been described in an in vivo rat model of silica-induced carcinogenesis [126]. In this model, the development of tumors and their protein expression over time could be followed. In the adenocarcinomas and squamous cell carcinomas developed by the host animals, expression of adherens junction components E-cadherin, α-, and β-catenin was significantly reduced compared to the normal and hyperplastic bronchiolar epithelium, but type II pneumocytes, expressed very low levels of these proteins in the normal state. Expression of tight junction protein ZO-1 also went down in this model comparing normal and diseased states of epithelial cells. Mesenchymal markers N-cadherin and the class III intermediate filament vimentin, not normally expressed in lung epithelial cells, were expressed in one third of the tumors studied and were always co-expressed with epithelial markers. Interestingly, these mesenchymal markers were not expressed in preneoplastic lesions, thus appearing at a rather late stage of tumor development.

These reports have begun to address the important issue of EMT in lung cancer and hold some very promising results. However, more studies are needed, especially using animal models of lung cancer that focus either on primary tumor growth or on lung cancer metastasis. Such future studies may allow us to better address the signaling pathways that need to be targeted specifically in the lung in order to prevent this dangerous tumor cell fate.

EMT and Tumor–Stromal Interactions

Since the very early days of cancer research pathologists described a common morphological pattern between the tumor stroma and stromal reactions known to occur during wound healing and inflammatory disorders [127]. It therefore becomes increasingly accepted that a comparison between wound healing, inflammation, and cancer has a direct impact on the understanding of the complex biology of tumor stroma [128]. Fibroblast-like cells enriched in the tumor stroma resemble smooth muscle cells and thus have common phenotypic features, including contractile properties, with the specialized fibroblasts in the granulation tissue generated during the wound healing process. The intermediate phenotype of such cells that is between smooth muscle cells and fibroblasts coined their name "myofibroblasts," whose biology is better understood in the context of inflammatory processes [127]. Such activated myofibroblasts do not only participate in pathological processes, but seem to contribute to the normal physiology of diverse adult tissues. Since not all fibroblast-like cells abundant in the tumor stroma are myofibroblasts, i.e., express α-SMA, a more inclusive term for all fibroblasts within a tumor is cancer-associated fibroblasts (CAFs), irrespective of their origin and phenotype. TGFβ is a key mediator of myofibroblast differentiation in vitro and in vivo and is therefore considered to play a central role in tumor stroma formation [74]. While TGFβ acting in a paracrine manner is best known for its tumor-promoting effects (see above), two recent studies provide evidence for the opposite. Namely, when the TGFβ type II receptor was specifically knocked out from fibroblasts, the otherwise phenotypically inconspicuous mice developed neoplastic lesions in the prostate and the forestomach after a few weeks, suggesting that paracrine TGFβ could indirectly suppress tumorigenesis [129]. Furthermore, in TGFβ receptor-negative fibroblasts from such mice, when co-injected with mammary carcinoma cells into nude mice, the resulting tumors exhibited enhanced growth due to more rapid angiogenesis, increased cell proliferation, and decreased apoptosis [130]. Thus, TGFβ seems to act in a manner that it remodels the tumor environment, possibly based on the central action of CAFs. The cellular mechanism by which CAFs influence tumor progression via the TGFβ pathway remains not yet fully understood.

HGF is known to be secreted from stromal cells of various tumors, while the HGF receptor, c-Met, is expressed by carcinoma cells [131, 132]. HGF and c-Met are well-known markers of advanced cancer that exhibits poor prognosis [133, 134]. TGFβ and PDGF are primary upstream regulators of HGF secretion by tumor mesenchymal cells. A two-way paracrine mechanism between fibroblasts and carcinoma cells seems to link the actions of TGFβ and HGF [135]. In these experiments, TGFβ or conditioned medium from cancer cell lines can induce differentiation of primary fibroblasts to myofibroblasts, leading to enhanced HGF secretion. HGF then acted on the squamous carcinoma cells enhancing their invasiveness. On the other hand, a more established role of TGFβ is to suppress HGF secretion [136]. These examples underline the complexity of paracrine actions taking place within the tumor microenvironment. Despite that, the commonalities between signaling events in the tumor stroma and in tissues suffering from chronic inflammation are remarkable.

Histologically, tissue fibrosis is defined by the overgrowth, hardening, and/or scarring of various tissues and is attributed to excess deposition of extracellular matrix components including collagen, as a result of tissue injury or a variety of stress stimuli including persistent infections, autoimmune reactions, allergic responses, chemical insults, or radiation. Although therapeutic treatments typically target the inflammatory response, the mechanisms driving fibrogenesis are likely to be distinct from those regulating inflammation and some studies have even suggested that ongoing inflammation is needed to reverse established and progressive fibrosis. Numerous molecules have been identified as important regulators of fibrosis and are being investigated as potential targets of antifibrotic drugs, including cytokines, chemokines, angiogenic factors, growth factors, peroxisome proliferator-activated receptors, acute phase proteins, caspases, and components of the renin–angiotensin–aldosterone system [137]. Increasing evidence supports the idea that EMT is also an important process that promotes fibrosis in various adult tissues, including the lungs [138–141]. It is therefore possible that EMT represents one of the common biological mechanisms that link cancer progression to chronic inflammation and fibrosis [5].

The myofibroblast is believed to play a central role during the pathogenesis of lung fibrosis. Once activated, myofibroblasts acquire a spindle or stellate morphology with intracytoplasmic stress fibers, a contractile phenotype, and express mesenchymal markers such as α-SMA and collagen and become major contributors to the secreted extracellular matrix [142]. Myofibroblasts also participate in the structural remodeling and the destruction of alveocapillary units associated with the development of lung fibrosis [143]. Various different mechanisms can activate these myofibroblasts such as paracrine signals derived from lymphocytes and macrophages and pathogen-associated molecular patterns derived from pathogenic organisms that interact with pattern recognition receptors (i.e., Toll-like receptors).

These myofibroblasts can be generated from various cell types. The most obvious source of myofibroblasts is resident lung fibroblasts [144]. These locally produced myofibroblasts were originally believed to be the primary producers of ECM components following injury. Now we know that fibroblasts can originate from multiple tissues besides the lung. They differentiate from circulating bone marrow-derived progenitors, also called "fibrocytes" due to their fibroblast/ myofibroblast-like phenotype (they express CD34, CD45, and type I collagen) [144–148]. They may also derive from alveolar epithelial cells that have undergone EMT [148–150]. Recently it was even demonstrated that endothelial–mesenchymal transition (EndMT) can generate myofibroblasts from endothelial cells in both fibrotic and tumor-associated tissues [6, 150]. In this context, blockade of all sources of myofibroblast production, including EMT, appears crucial for efficient treatment of lung fibrosis. However, this is a difficult task as myofibroblasts are derived from so many different cell types.

In vitro evidence clearly demonstrates that TGFβ easily induces EMT in cultured epithelial cells of kidney, liver, and lung. In addition, TGFβ1 is typically expressed at sites of epithelial degeneration and adjacent fibrogenesis in vivo, and inhibition of TGFβ signaling (e.g., Smad3 knockout) typically preserves tissues and prevents scarring [151]. Therefore, it is logical to think that TGFβ-induced EMT is important during fibrosis, even if this concept needs more experimental support. Finally, the connections between chronic inflammatory conditions and tumor progression may strongly rely on the regulatory processes that control EMT and its reverse phase, MET.

EMT and Cancer Stem Cell Biology

Embryonic stem cells (ESC) are pluripotent cells derived from the inner cell mass/ epiblast of preimplantation embryos [152, 153]. ESCs can differentiate into the three primary germ layers. Similar to what has been described in mouse embryonic stem cells [154], recent data have demonstrated that human embryonic stem cell can also undergo EMT [155]. This EMT is associated with a membranous E- to N-cadherin switch concurrent with an upregulation of the E-cadherin repressor proteins Snail1, Snail2, and ZEB2 and of the matrix metalloproteases MMP-2 and MMP-9. As MMPs regulate cell surface E- cadherin protein levels by proteolytic cleavage [156], MMP upregulation constitutes an alternative, non-transcriptional way to downregulate the adherens junction. Notably, in addition to repressing E-cadherin expression, Snail1 may also play a role in survival of stem cells (reviewed by [100]).

While ESCs are capable of undergoing EMT, recent work raises the exciting possibility that EMT may affect the process of generation of breast cancer stem cells or alternatively their survival [157]. The importance of cancer stem cells in supporting late stages of cancer progression and also providing malignant cell populations that resist to the therapeutic effects of radiation or chemotherapy is becoming increasingly established (see Chapter 3). Despite this, the origin of cancer stem cells remains largely unknown [158]. Breast epithelial cells stably expressing the transcriptional regulators of EMT, Snail1, and Twist provide populations that are enriched in stem cells, and when primed to develop tumors in mice, such EMT-prone cells establish more aggressive tumors with productive metastases [157]. This is consistent with the recent finding that co-cultures of mesenchymal stem cells with tumor cells promote dramatically tumor progression and the process of metastasis [159, 160]. It is therefore possible that the mesenchymal stem cells that empower associated tumor cells with metastatic potential are themselves derived from epithelial precursors via EMT. However, whether such cells represent real stem cells remains unclear. The fact that the breast epithelial cells derived from the stable overexpression of Snail1 and Twist proliferate efficiently and give rise to tumors [157] suggests that EMT might enrich for a transit-amplifying population of progenitor cells rather than generating true stem cells. The ability of mesenchymal cells produced via EMT to fully differentiate to various cell lineages, the hallmark of stem cell biology, remains currently unexplored. In any case, this new exciting link between EMT and tumor stem cell survival provides fresh ideas to the problem of how tumor stroma regulates cancer progression and possibly raises the process of EMT as a central generator of cancer cell types that possess the most dangerous characteristics of malignancy.

How Relevant Is EMT to Cancer Progression and Metastasis?

In recent years it has become increasingly clear that during cancer progression, tumor cells make the choice of reactivating some of their embryonic developmental potential. EMT is a central element of this reawakened developmental program and serves the need of spatial expansion of tumor cells as they over-proliferate and colonize new tissues in the body [1, 7, 161]. The mechanisms of origin of the tumor cells that are capable of undergoing EMT remain largely elusive. However, connections between the so-called cancer stem cells and the EMT phenotype have been made [157, 162, 163]. If this is true, EMT in the tumor context essentially represents mesenchymal differentiation from tumor epithelial stem cells. This idea is compatible with studies of embryonic stem cells that are capable of undergoing EMT in vitro [164]. In fact, a recent report on a mouse model of hepatocellular carcinoma progression and metastasis suggests that sequential signal transduction from TGFβ, which induces PDGF secretion and PDGF receptor activation, cooperates with β-catenin signaling to produce a small population of carcinoma cells that seem to act as cancer stem cells [165].

The hypothesis that EMT during cancer progression may primarily affect the rare cancer stem cells is compatible with the low-frequency observation of transitory mesenchymal cells within or near the mass of a growing tumor that becomes invasive and metastatic. Based on the difficulty to observe such rare cell types using classical histochemical techniques, many oncologists and tumor pathologists have disputed the relevance of EMT in cancer [166]. A more objective view of the role of EMT during advanced tumor progression and metastasis has considered the fact that EMT can be transient and reversible and that it represents only one of the steps required by carcinomas to establish productive expansion via invasiveness and intravasation to the neighboring vasculature [167]. This is also compatible with the ability of epithelial cell sheets to migrate without the need for disseminating single migratory cells [168]. However, mechanisms such as epithelial sheet migration do not exclude the presence or significance of EMT as discussed here. Despite the apparent difficulties in studying tumor-related EMT in human tumor biopsies, recent advances in imaging technology and transgenic mouse models have clearly demonstrated that EMT does occur in vivo during cancer progression [169], and thus it cannot be disregarded by oncologists and tumor pathologists anymore.

Conclusions

Over the past few years, the understanding of the molecular and cellular biology of the EMT process has increased significantly. Extracellular protein factors, signaling pathways, and transcriptional regulators are now appreciated for their contribution to EMT. A future challenge remains in the understanding of complex signaling networks operating during EMT in vivo. Additional important regulators of EMT are also expected to be discovered in the years to come. The possible connection between EMT and the role of cancer stem cells in cancer progression will require long-term investigation. Especially, these processes deserve special attention in the context of lung tumorigenesis and progression, as this important and specific field of cancer research lags behind on the EMT front. Finally, EMT-focused studies also promise the generation of new anti-cancer and anti-fibrosis drugs, a major task of modern cancer research.

Acknowledgments Due to space limitations, only selected literature is cited. Funding of the authors' work is provided by the Ludwig Institute for Cancer Research, the Atlantic Philanthropies/Ludwig Institute for Cancer Research Clinical Discovery Program, the Swedish Cancer Society, the Swedish Research Council and the Marie Curie Research Training Network (RTN) "EpiPlastCarcinoma" under the European Union FP6 program. We thank Carl-Henrik Heldin for his continuous support and all other members of the TGFβ signaling group for their contributions to the scientific work emanating from our laboratory.

References

1. Hay, E.D. The mesenchymal cell, its role in the embryo, and the remarkable signaling mechanisms that create it. Dev. Dyn. 233: 706–720, 2005.
2. Berx, G., E. Raspe, G. Christofori, J.P. Thiery, and J.P. Sleeman. Pre-EMTing metastasis? Recapitulation of morphogenetic processes in cancer. Clin. Exp. Metastasis 24: 587–597, 2007.
3. Hugo, H., M.L. Ackland, T. Blick, M.G. Lawrence, J.A. Clements, E.D. Williams, and E.W. Thompson. Epithelial–mesenchymal and mesenchymal–epithelial transitions in carcinoma progression. J. Cell. Physiol. 213: 374–383, 2007.

4. Zeisberg, M. and R. Kalluri. The role of epithelial-to-mesenchymal transition in renal fibrosis. J. Mol. Med. 82: 175–181, 2004.

5. Radisky, D.C., P.A. Kenny, and M.J. Bissell. Fibrosis and cancer: Do myofibroblasts come also from epithelial cells via EMT? J. Cell. Biochem. 101: 830–839, 2007.

6. Zeisberg, E.M., S. Potenta, L. Xie, M. Zeisberg, and R. Kalluri. Discovery of endothelial to mesenchymal transition as a source for carcinoma-associated fibroblasts. Cancer Res. 67: 10123–10128, 2007.

7. Huber, M.A., N. Kraut, and H. Beug. Molecular requirements for epithelial-mesenchymal transition during tumor progression. Curr. Opin. Cell Biol. 17: 548–558, 2005.

8. Moustakas, A. and C.-H. Heldin. Signaling networks guiding epithelial-mesenchymal transitions during embryogenesis and cancer progression. Cancer Sci. 98: 1512–1520, 2007.

9. Peinado, H., D. Olmeda, and A. Cano. Snail, Zeb and bHLH factors in tumour progression: an alliance against the epithelial phenotype? Nat. Rev. Cancer 7: 415–428, 2007.

10. Keller, R., L. Davidson, A. Edlund, T. Elul, M. Ezin, D. Shook, and P. Skoglund. Mechanisms of convergence and extension by cell intercalation. Philos. Trans. R. Soc. Lond. B. Biol. Sci. 355: 897–922, 2000.

11. Deng, C.-X., A. Wynshaw-Boris, M.M. Shen, C. Daugherty, D.M. Ornitz, and P. Leder. Murine FGFR-1 is required for early postimplantation growth and axial organization. Genes Dev. 8: 3045–3057, 1994.

12. Yamaguchi, T.P., K. Harpal, M. Henkemeyer, and J. Rossant. fgfr-1 is required for embryonic growth and mesodermal patterning during mouse gastrulation. Genes Dev. 8: 3032–3044, 1994.

13. Sun, X., E.N. Meyers, M. Lewandoski, and G.R. Martin. Targeted disruption of Fgf8 causes failure of cell migration in the gastrulating mouse embryo. Genes Dev. 13: 1834–1846, 1999.

14. Batlle, E., E. Sancho, C. Franci, D. Dominguez, M. Monfar, J. Baulida, and A. Garcia De Herreros. The transcription factor snail is a repressor of E-cadherin gene expression in epithelial tumour cells. Nat. Cell Biol. 2: 84–89, 2000.

15. Cano, A., M.A. Perez-Moreno, I. Rodrigo, A. Locascio, M.J. Blanco, M.G. del Barrio, F. Portillo, and M.A. Nieto. The transcription factor snail controls epithelial-mesenchymal transitions by repressing E-cadherin expression. Nat. Cell Biol. 2: 76–83, 2000.

16. Ciruna, B. and J. Rossant. FGF signaling regulates mesoderm cell fate specification and morphogenetic movement at the primitive streak. Dev. Cell 1: 37–49, 2001.

17. Sheng, G., M. dos Reis, and C.D. Stern. Churchill, a zinc finger transcriptional activator, regulates the transition between gastrulation and neurulation. Cell 115: 603–613, 2003.

18. Carver, E.A., R. Jiang, Y. Lan, K.F. Oram, and T. Gridley. The mouse snail gene encodes a key regulator of the epithelial-mesenchymal transition. Mol. Cell. Biol. 21: 8184–8188, 2001.

19. Takada, S., K.L. Stark, M.J. Shea, G. Vassileva, J.A. McMahon, and A.P. McMahon. Wnt-3a regulates somite and tailbud formation in the mouse embryo. Genes Dev. 8: 174–189, 1994.

20. Galceran, J., S.C. Hsu, and R. Grosschedl. Rescue of a Wnt mutation by an activated form of LEF-1: regulation of maintenance but not initiation of Brachyury expression. Proc. Natl. Acad. Sci. USA 98: 8668–8673, 2001.

21. Barrallo-Gimeno, A. and M.A. Nieto. Evolution of the neural crest. Adv. Exp. Med. Biol. 589: 235–244, 2006.

21a. LaBonne, C., and M. Bronner-Fraser. Induction and patterning of the neural crest, a stem cell-like precursor population. J. Neurobiol. 36: 175–189, 1998.

22. Kalcheim, C. Mechanisms of early neural crest development: from cell specification to migration. Int. Rev. Cytol. 200: 143–196, 2000.

23. Halloran, M.C. and J.D. Berndt. Current progress in neural crest cell motility and migration and future prospects for the zebrafish model system. Dev. Dyn. 228: 497–513, 2003.

24. LaBonne, C. and M. Bronner-Fraser. Snail-related transcriptional repressors are required in Xenopus for both the induction of the neural crest and its subsequent migration. Dev. Biol. 221: 195–205, 2000.

25. Nawshad, A., D. LaGamba, and E.D. Hay. Transforming growth factor β (TGFβ) signalling in palatal growth, apoptosis and epithelial mesenchymal transformation (EMT). Arch. Oral Biol. 49: 675–689, 2004.

26. Murray, S.A., K.F. Oram, and T. Gridley. Multiple functions of Snail family genes during palate development in mice. Development 134: 1789–1797, 2007.

27. Person, A.D., S.E. Klewer, and R.B. Runyan. Cell biology of cardiac cushion development. Int. Rev. Cytol. 243: 287–335, 2005.

28. Zavadil, J., L. Cermak, N. Soto-Nieves, and E.P. Böttinger. Integration of TGF-β/Smad and Jagged1/Notch signalling in epithelial-to-mesenchymal transition. EMBO J. 23: 1155–1165, 2004.

29. Niimi, H., K. Pardali, M. Vanlandewijck, C.-H. Heldin, and A. Moustakas. Notch signaling is necessary for epithelial growth arrest by TGF-b. J. Cell Biol. 176: 695–707, 2007.

30. Chuang, P.T. and A.P. McMahon. Branching morphogenesis of the lung: new molecular insights into an old problem. Trends Cell Biol. 13: 86–91, 2003.

31. Shannon, J.M. Induction of alveolar type II cell differentiation in fetal tracheal epithelium by grafted distal lung mesenchyme. Dev. Biol. 166: 600–614, 1994.

32. Cardoso, W.V. and J. Lü. Regulation of early lung morphogenesis: questions, facts and controversies. Development 133: 1611–1624, 2006.

33. Min, H., D.M. Danilenko, S.A. Scully, B. Bolon, B.D. Ring, J.E. Tarpley, M. DeRose, and W.S. Simonet. Fgf-10 is required for both limb and lung development and exhibits striking functional similarity to Drosophila branchless. Genes Dev. 12: 3156–3161, 1998.

34. Sekine, K., H. Ohuchi, M. Fujiwara, M. Yamasaki, T. Yoshizawa, T. Sato, N. Yagishita, D. Matsui, Y. Koga, N. Itoh, and S. Kato. Fgf10 is essential for limb and lung formation. Nat. Genet. 21: 138–141, 1999.

35. Weaver, M., N.R. Dunn, and B.L. Hogan. Bmp4 and Fgf10 play opposing roles during lung bud morphogenesis. Development 127: 2695–2704, 2000.

36. Cardoso, W.V., A. Itoh, H. Nogawa, I. Mason, and J.S. Brody. FGF-1 and FGF-7 induce distinct patterns of growth and differentiation in embryonic lung epithelium. Dev. Dyn. 208: 398–405, 1997.

37. Kaartinen, V., J.W. Voncken, C. Shuler, D. Warburton, D. Bu, N. Heisterkamp, and J. Groffen. Abnormal lung development and cleft palate in mice lacking TGF-β 3 indicates defects of epithelial-mesenchymal interaction. Nat. Genet. 11: 415–421, 1995.

38. Serra, R., R.W. Pelton, and H.L. Moses. TGF β1 inhibits branching morphogenesis and N-myc expression in lung bud organ cultures. Development 120: 2153–2161, 1994.

39. Zhou, L., C.R. Dey, S.E. Wert, and J.A. Whitsett. Arrested lung morphogenesis in transgenic mice bearing an SP-C-TGF-β 1 chimeric gene. Dev. Biol. 175: 227–238, 1996.

40. Zhao, J., D. Bu, M. Lee, H.C. Slavkin, F.L. Hall, and D. Warburton. Abrogation of transforming growth factor-β type II receptor stimulates embryonic mouse lung branching morphogenesis in culture. Dev. Biol. 180: 242–257, 1996.

41. Zhao, J., M. Lee, S. Smith, and D. Warburton. Abrogation of Smad3 and Smad2 or of Smad4 gene expression positively regulates murine embryonic lung branching morphogenesis in culture. Dev. Biol. 194: 182–195., 1998.

42. Bitgood, M.J. and A.P. McMahon. Hedgehog and Bmp genes are coexpressed at many diverse sites of cell-cell interaction in the mouse embryo. Dev. Biol. 172: 126–138, 1995.

43. Bellusci, S., R. Henderson, G. Winnier, T. Oikawa, and B.L. Hogan. Evidence from normal expression and targeted misexpression that bone morphogenetic protein (Bmp-4) plays a role in mouse embryonic lung morphogenesis. Development 122: 1693–1702, 1996.

44. Hogan, B.L. Morphogenesis. Cell 96: 225–233., 1999.

45. Murone, M., A. Rosenthal, and F.J. de Sauvage. Sonic hedgehog signaling by the patched-smoothened receptor complex. Curr. Biol. 9: 76–84, 1999.

46. Litingtung, Y., L. Lei, H. Westphal, and C. Chiang. Sonic hedgehog is essential to foregut development. Nat. Genet. 20: 58–61, 1998.

47. Pepicelli, C.V., P.M. Lewis, and A.P. McMahon. Sonic hedgehog regulates branching morphogenesis in the mammalian lung. Curr. Biol. 8: 1083–1086, 1998.
48. Bellusci, S., Y. Furuta, M.G. Rush, R. Henderson, G. Winnier, and B.L. Hogan. Involvement of Sonic hedgehog (Shh) in mouse embryonic lung growth and morphogenesis. Development 124: 53–63, 1997.
49. Motoyama, J., H. Heng, M.A. Crackower, T. Takabatake, K. Takeshima, L.C. Tsui, and C. Hui. Overlapping and non-overlapping Ptch2 expression with Shh during mouse embryogenesis. Mech. Dev. 78: 81–84, 1998.
50. Grindley, J.C., S. Bellusci, D. Perkins, and B.L. Hogan. Evidence for the involvement of the Gli gene family in embryonic mouse lung development. Dev. Biol. 188: 337–348, 1997.
51. Threadgill, D.W., A.A. Dlugosz, L.A. Hansen, T. Tennenbaum, U. Lichti, D. Yee, C. LaMantia, T. Mourton, K. Herrup, R.C. Harris, et al. Targeted disruption of mouse EGF receptor: effect of genetic background on mutant phenotype. Science 269: 230–234, 1995.
52. Miettinen, P.J., D. Warburton, D. Bu, J.S. Zhao, J.E. Berger, P. Minoo, T. Koivisto, L. Allen, L. Dobbs, Z. Werb, and R. Derynck. Impaired lung branching morphogenesis in the absence of functional EGF receptor. Dev. Biol. 186: 224–236, 1997.
53. Leveen, P., M. Pekny, S. Gebre-Medhin, B. Swolin, E. Larsson, and C. Betsholtz. Mice deficient for PDGF B show renal, cardiovascular, and hematological abnormalities. Genes Dev. 8: 1875–1887, 1994.
54. Aranda, V., T. Haire, M.E. Nolan, J.P. Calarco, A.Z. Rosenberg, J.P. Fawcett, T. Pawson, and S.K. Muthuswamy. Par6-aPKC uncouples ErbB2 induced disruption of polarized epithelial organization from proliferation control. Nat. Cell Biol. 8: 1235–1245, 2006.
55. Carraway, C.A. and K.L. Carraway. Sequestration and segregation of receptor kinases in epithelial cells: implications for ErbB2 oncogenesis. Sci. STKE 2007: re3, 2007.
56. Rosario, M. and W. Birchmeier. How to make tubes: signaling by the Met receptor tyrosine kinase. Trends Cell Biol. 13: 328–335, 2003.
57. Schramek, H., E. Feifel, E. Healy, and V. Pollack. Constitutively active mutant of the mitogen-activated protein kinase kinase MEK1 induces epithelial dedifferentiation and growth inhibition in madin-darby canine kidney-C7 cells. J. Biol. Chem. 272: 11426–11433, 1997.
58. Montesano, R., J.V. Soriano, G. Hosseini, M.S. Pepper, and H. Schramek. Constitutively active mitogen-activated protein kinase kinase MEK1 disrupts morphogenesis and induces an invasive phenotype in Madin-Darby canine kidney epithelial cells. Cell Growth Differ. 10: 317–332, 1999.
59. Lehmann, K., E. Janda, C.E. Pierreux, M. Rytomaa, A. Schulze, M. McMahon, C.S. Hill, H. Beug, and J. Downward. Raf induces TGFβ production while blocking its apoptotic but not invasive responses: a mechanism leading to increased malignancy in epithelial cells. Genes Dev. 14: 2610–2622, 2000.
60. Janda, E., K. Lehmann, I. Killisch, M. Jechlinger, M. Herzig, J. Downward, H. Beug, and S. Grünert. Ras and TGFβ cooperatively regulate epithelial cell plasticity and metastasis: dissection of Ras signaling pathways. J. Cell Biol. 156: 299–313., 2002.
61. Oft, M., R.J. Akhurst, and A. Balmain. Metastasis is driven by sequential elevation of H-ras and Smad2 levels. Nat. Cell Biol. 4: 487–494., 2002.
62. Grotegut, S., D. von Schweinitz, G. Christofori, and F. Lehembre. Hepatocyte growth factor induces cell scattering through MAPK/Egr-1-mediated upregulation of Snail. Embo J 25: 3534–45, 2006.
63. Savagner, P., K.M. Yamada, and J.P. Thiery. The zinc-finger protein slug causes desmosome dissociation, an initial and necessary step for growth factor-induced epithelial-mesenchymal transition. J. Cell Biol. 137: 1403–1419, 1997.
64. Cordenonsi, M., M. Montagner, M. Adorno, L. Zacchigna, G. Martello, A. Mamidi, S. Soligo, S. Dupont, and S. Piccolo. Integration of TGF-β and Ras/MAPK signaling through p53 phosphorylation. Science 315: 840–843, 2007.

65. Irie, H.Y., R.V. Pearline, D. Grueneberg, M. Hsia, P. Ravichandran, N. Kothari, S. Natesan, and J.S. Brugge. Distinct roles of Akt1 and Akt2 in regulating cell migration and epithelial-mesenchymal transition. J. Cell Biol. 171: 1023–1034, 2005.
66. Larue, L. and A. Bellacosa.Epithelial-mesenchymal transition in development and cancer: role of phosphatidylinositol 3' kinase/AKT pathways. Oncogene 24: 7443–7454, 2005.
67. Zohn, I.E., Y. Li, E.Y. Skolnik, K.V. Anderson, J. Han, and L. Niswander. p38 and a p38-interacting protein are critical for downregulation of E-cadherin during mouse gastrulation. Cell 125: 957–69, 2006.
68. Oft, M., K.H. Heider, and H. Beug. TGFβsignaling is necessary for carcinoma cell invasiveness and metastasis. Curr. Biol. 8: 1243–1252., 1998.
69. Portella, G., S.A. Cumming, J. Liddell, W. Cui, H. Ireland, R.J. Akhurst, and A. Balmain. Transforming growth factor β is essential for spindle cell conversion of mouse skin carcinoma in vivo: implications for tumor invasion. Cell Growth Differ. 9: 393–404., 1998.
70. Gotzmann, J., H. Huber, C. Thallinger, M. Wolschek, B. Jansen, R. Schulte-Hermann, H. Beug, and W. Mikulits. Hepatocytes convert to a fibroblastoid phenotype through the cooperation of TGF-β1 and Ha-Ras: steps towards invasiveness. J. Cell Sci. 115: 1189–1202, 2002.
71. Miettinen, P.J., R. Ebner, A.R. Lopez, and R. Derynck. TGF-β induced transdifferentiation of mammary epithelial cells to mesenchymal cells: involvement of type I receptors. J. Cell Biol. 127: 2021–2036., 1994.
72. Valcourt, U., M. Kowanetz, H. Niimi, C.-H. Heldin, and A. Moustakas. TGF-β and the Smad signaling pathway support transcriptomic reprogramming during epithelial-mesenchymal cell transition. Mol. Biol. Cell 16: 1987–2002, 2005.
73. Willis, B.C., J.M. Liebler, K. Luby-Phelps, A.G. Nicholson, E.D. Crandall, R.M. du Bois, and Z. Borok. Induction of epithelial-mesenchymal transition in alveolar epithelial cells by transforming growth factor-β1: potential role in idiopathic pulmonary fibrosis. Am. J. Pathol. 166: 1321–1332, 2005.
74. Bierie, B. and H.L. Moses.: Tumour microenvironment: TGFβ the molecular Jekyll and Hyde of cancer. Nat. Rev. Cancer 6: 506–520, 2006.
75. Yang, Y., X. Pan, W. Lei, J. Wang, and J. Song. Transforming growth factor-β1 induces epithelial-to-mesenchymal transition and apoptosis via a cell cycle-dependent mechanism. Oncogene 25: 7235–7244, 2006.
76. Sakaue-Sawano, A., H. Kurokawa, T. Morimura, A. Hanyu, H. Hama, H. Osawa, S. Kashiwagi, K. Fukami, T. Miyata, H. Miyoshi, T. Imamura, M. Ogawa, H. Masai, and A. Miyawaki. Visualizing spatiotemporal dynamics of multicellular cell-cycle progression. Cell 132: 487–498, 2008.
77. Massagué, J., J. Seoane, and D. Wotton. Smad transcription factors. Genes Dev. 19: 2783–2810, 2005.
78. Piek, E., A. Moustakas, A. Kurisaki, C.-H. Heldin, and P. ten Dijke. TGF-β type I receptor/ALK-5 and Smad proteins mediate epithelial to mesenchymal transdifferentiation in NMuMG breast epithelial cells. J. Cell Sci. 112: 4557–4568, 1999.
79. Kowanetz, M., U. Valcourt, R. Bergström, C.-H. Heldin, and A. Moustakas. Id2 and Id3 define the potency of cell proliferation and differentiation responses to transforming growth factor β and bone morphogenetic protein. Mol. Cell. Biol. 24: 4241–4254, 2004.
80. Pardali, K. and A. Moustakas. Actions of TGF-β as tumor suppressor and pro-metastatic factor in human cancer. Biochim. Biophys. Acta 1775: 21–62, 2007.
81. Takano, S., F. Kanai, A. Jazag, H. Ijichi, J. Yao, H. Ogawa, N. Enomoto, M. Omata, and A. Nakao. Smad4 is Essential for Down-regulation of E-cadherin Induced by TGF-β in Pancreatic Cancer Cell Line PANC-1. J. Biochem. (Tokyo) 141: 345–351, 2007.
82. Li, W., W. Qiao, L. Chen, X. Xu, X. Yang, D. Li, C. Li, S.G. Brodie, M.M. Meguid, L. Hennighausen, and C.-X. Deng. Squamous cell carcinoma and mammary abscess

formation through squamous metaplasia in Smad4/Dpc4 conditional knockout mice. Development 130: 6143–6153, 2003.

83. Bardeesy, N., K.H. Cheng, J.H. Berger, G.C. Chu, J. Pahler, P. Olson, A.F. Hezel, J. Horner, G.Y. Lauwers, D. Hanahan, and R.A. DePinho. Smad4 is dispensable for normal pancreas development yet critical in progression and tumor biology of pancreas cancer. Genes Dev. 20: 3130–3146, 2006.

84. Deckers, M., M. van Dinther, J. Buijs, I. Que, C. Lowik, G. van der Pluijm, and P. ten Dijke. The tumor suppressor Smad4 is required for transforming growth factor β-induced epithelial to mesenchymal transition and bone metastasis of breast cancer cells. Cancer Res. 66: 2202–2209, 2006.

85. Ju, W., A. Ogawa, J. Heyer, D. Nierhof, L. Yu, R. Kucherlapati, D.A. Shafritz, and E.P. Böttinger. Deletion of Smad2 in mouse liver reveals novel functions in hepatocyte growth and differentiation. Mol. Cell. Biol. 26: 654–667, 2006.

86. Phanish, M.K., N.A. Wahab, P. Colville-Nash, B.M. Hendry, and M.E. Dockrell. The differential role of Smad2 and Smad3 in the regulation of pro-fibrotic TGFβ1 responses in human proximal-tubule epithelial cells. Biochem J. 393: 601–607, 2006.

87. Zavadil, J. and E.P. Böttinger. TGF-β and epithelial-to-mesenchymal transitions. Oncogene 24: 5764–5774, 2005.

88. Moustakas, A. and C.-H. Heldin. Non-Smad TGF-β signals. J. Cell Sci. 118: 3573–3584, 2005.

89. Yang, Y., X. Pan, W. Lei, J. Wang, J. Shi, F. Li, and J. Song. Regulation of Transforming Growth Factor-β1-Induced Apoptosis and Epithelial-to-Mesenchymal Transition by Protein Kinase A and Signal Transducers and Activators of Transcription 3. Cancer Res. 66: 8617–8624, 2006.

90. Bhowmick, N.A., R. Zent, M. Ghiassi, M. McDonnell, and H.L. Moses. Integrin β1 signaling is necessary for transforming growth factor-β activation of p38 MAPK and epithelial plasticity. J. Biol. Chem. 276: 46707–713, 2001.

91. Bates, R.C., D.I. Bellovin, C. Brown, E. Maynard, B. Wu, H. Kawakatsu, D. Sheppard, P. Oettgen, and A.M. Mercurio. Transcriptional activation of integrin β6 during the epithelial-mesenchymal transition defines a novel prognostic indicator of aggressive colon carcinoma. J. Clin. Invest. 115: 339–347, 2005.

92. Li, Y., J. Yang, C. Dai, C. Wu, and Y. Liu. Role for integrin-linked kinase in mediating tubular epithelial to mesenchymal transition and renal interstitial fibrogenesis. J. Clin. Invest. 112: 503–516, 2003.

93. Lee, Y.I., Y.J. Kwon, and C.K. Joo. Integrin-linked kinase function is required for transforming growth factor β-mediated epithelial to mesenchymal transition. Biochem. Biophys. Res. Commun. 316: 997–1001, 2004.

94. Shim, J.H., C. Xiao, A.E. Paschal, S.T. Bailey, P. Rao, M.S. Hayden, K.Y. Lee, C. Bussey, M. Steckel, N. Tanaka, G. Yamada, S. Akira, K. Matsumoto, and S. Ghosh. TAK1, but not TAB1 or TAB2, plays an essential role in multiple signaling pathways in vivo. Genes Dev. 19: 2668–2681, 2005.

95. Zavadil, J., M. Bitzer, D. Liang, Y.C. Yang, A. Massimi, S. Kneitz, E. Piek, and E.P. Böttinger. Genetic programs of epithelial cell plasticity directed by transforming growth factor-b. Proc. Natl. Acad. Sci. USA 98: 6686–6691, 2001.

96. Jechlinger, M., S. Grunert, I.H. Tamir, E. Janda, S. Ludemann, T. Waerner, P. Seither, A. Weith, H. Beug, and N. Kraut. Expression profiling of epithelial plasticity in tumor progression. Oncogene 22: 7155–7169, 2003.

97. Kang, Y., P.M. Siegel, W. Shu, M. Drobnjak, S.M. Kakonen, C. Cordon-Cardo, T.A. Guise, and J. Massagué. A multigenic program mediating breast cancer metastasis to bone. Cancer Cell 3: 537–549, 2003.

98. Xie, L., B.K. Law, M.E. Aakre, M. Edgerton, Y. Shyr, N.A. Bhowmick, and H.L. Moses. Transforming growth factor β-regulated gene expression in a mouse mammary gland epithelial cell line. Breast Cancer Res. 5: R187–198, 2003.

99. LaGamba, D., A. Nawshad, and E.D. Hay. Microarray analysis of gene expression during epithelial-mesenchymal transformation. Dev. Dyn. 234: 132–142, 2005.

100. Barrallo-Gimeno, A. and M.A. Nieto. The Snail genes as inducers of cell movement and survival: implications in development and cancer. Development 132: 3151–3161, 2005.

101. Shen, X., J. Li, P.P. Hu, D. Waddell, J. Zhang, and X.-F. Wang. The activity of guanine exchange factor NET1 is essential for transforming growth factor-β-mediated stress fiber formation. J. Biol. Chem. 276: 15362–15368., 2001.

102. Bakin, A.V., A. Safina, C. Rinehart, C. Daroqui, H. Darbary, and D.M. Helfman. A critical role of tropomyosins in TGF-β regulation of the actin cytoskeleton and cell motility in epithelial cells. Mol. Biol. Cell 15: 4682–4694, 2004.

103. Peinado, H., M. Quintanilla, and A. Cano. Transforming growth factor β-1 induces snail transcription factor in epithelial cell lines: mechanisms for epithelial mesenchymal transitions. J. Biol. Chem. 278: 21113–21123, 2003.

104. Sato, M., Y. Muragaki, S. Saika, A.B. Roberts, and A. Ooshima. Targeted disruption of TGF-β1/Smad3 signaling protects against renal tubulointerstitial fibrosis induced by unilateral ureteral obstruction. J. Clin. Invest. 112: 1486–1494, 2003.

105. Thuault, S., U. Valcourt, M. Petersen, G. Manfioletti, C.-H. Heldin, and A. Moustakas. Transforming growth factor-β employs HMGA2 to elicit epithelial-mesenchymal transition. J. Cell Biol. 174: 175–183, 2006.

106. Kondo, M., E. Cubillo, K. Tobiume, T. Shirakihara, N. Fukuda, H. Suzuki, K. Shimizu, K. Takehara, A. Cano, M. Saitoh, and K. Miyazono. A role for Id in the regulation of TGF-β-induced epithelial-mesenchymal transdifferentiation. Cell Death Differ. 11: 1092–1101, 2004.

107. Kang, Y., C.R. Chen, and J. Massagué. A self-enabling TGFβ response coupled to stress signaling. Smad engages stress response factor ATF3 for Id1 repression in epithelial cells. Mol. Cell 11: 915–926, 2003.

108. Zeisberg, M., A.A. Shah, and R. Kalluri. Bone morphogenic protein-7 induces mesenchymal to epithelial transition in adult renal fibroblasts and facilitates regeneration of injured kidney. J. Biol. Chem. 280: 8094–8100, 2005.

109. Saika, S., K. Ikeda, O. Yamanaka, K.C. Flanders, Y. Ohnishi, Y. Nakajima, Y. Muragaki, and A. Ooshima. Adenoviral gene transfer of BMP-7, Id2, or Id3 suppresses injury-induced epithelial-to-mesenchymal transition of lens epithelium in mice. Am. J. Physiol. Cell Physiol. 290: <PAGES>C282–C289</PAGES>, 2006.

110. Comijn, J., G. Berx, P. Vermassen, K. Verschueren, L. van Grunsven, E. Bruyneel, M. Mareel, D. Huylebroeck, and F. van Roy. The two-handed E box binding zinc finger protein SIP1 downregulates E- cadherin and induces invasion. Mol. Cell 7: 1267–1278., 2001.

111. Peinado, H., F. Portillo, and A. Cano. Transcriptional regulation of cadherins during development and carcinogenesis. Int. J. Dev. Biol. 48: 365–375, 2004.

112. Vandewalle, C., J. Comijn, B. De Craene, P. Vermassen, E. Bruyneel, H. Andersen, E. Tulchinsky, F. Van Roy, and G. Berx. SIP1/ZEB2 induces EMT by repressing genes of different epithelial cell-cell junctions. Nucleic Acids Res. 33: 6566–6578, 2005.

113. Eger, A., A. Stockinger, J. Park, E. Langkopf, M. Mikula, J. Gotzmann, W. Mikulits, H. Beug, and R. Foisner. β-Catenin and TGFβ signalling cooperate to maintain a mesenchymal phenotype after FosER-induced epithelial to mesenchymal transition. Oncogene 23: 2672–2680, 2004.

114. Martinez-Alvarez, C., M.J. Blanco, R. Perez, M.A. Rabadan, M. Aparicio, E. Resel, T. Martinez, and M.A. Nieto. Snail family members and cell survival in physiological and pathological cleft palates. Dev. Biol. 265: 207–218, 2004.

115. Li, Y., J. Yang, J.H. Luo, S. Dedhar, and Y. Liu. Tubular epithelial cell dedifferentiation is driven by the helix-loop-helix transcriptional inhibitor Id1. J. Am. Soc. Nephrol. 18: 449–460, 2007.

116. Mani, S.A., J. Yang, M. Brooks, G. Schwaninger, A. Zhou, N. Miura, J.L. Kutok, K. Hartwell, A.L. Richardson, and R.A. Weinberg. Mesenchyme Forkhead 1 (FOXC2) plays a key role in metastasis and is associated with aggressive basal-like breast cancers. Proc. Natl. Acad. Sci. USA 104: 10069–10074, 2007.

117. Venkov, C.D., A.J. Link, J.L. Jennings, D. Plieth, T. Inoue, K. Nagai, C. Xu, Y.N. Dimitrova, F.J. Rauscher, and E.G. Neilson. A proximal activator of transcription in epithelial-mesenchymal transition. J. Clin. Invest. 117: 482–491, 2007.

118. Spira, A. and D.S. Ettinger. Multidisciplinary management of lung cancer. N. Engl. J. Med. 350: 379–392, 2004.

119. Carney, D.N. Lung cancer–time to move on from chemotherapy. N. Engl. J. Med. 346: 126–128, 2002.

120. Kasai, H., J.T. Allen, R.M. Mason, T. Kamimura, and Z. Zhang. TGF-β1 induces human alveolar epithelial to mesenchymal cell transition (EMT). Respir. Res. 6: 56, 2005.

121. Keshamouni, V.G., G. Michailidis, C.S. Grasso, S. Anthwal, J.R. Strahler, A. Walker, D.A. Arenberg, R.C. Reddy, S. Akulapalli, V.J. Thannickal, T.J. Standiford, P.C. Andrews, and G.S. Omenn. Differential protein expression profiling by iTRAQ-2DLC-MS/MS of lung cancer cells undergoing epithelial-mesenchymal transition reveals a migratory/invasive phenotype. J. Proteome Res. 5: 1143–1154, 2006.

122. Cordenonsi, M., S. Dupont, S. Maretto, A. Insinga, C. Imbriano, and S. Piccolo. Links between tumor suppressors: p53 is required for TGF-β gene responses by cooperating with Smads. Cell 113: 301–314, 2003.

123. Shintani, Y., M. Maeda, N. Chaika, K.R. Johnson, and M.J. Wheelock. Collagen I promotes epithelial-to-mesenchymal transition in lung cancer cells via transforming growth factor-β signaling. Am. J. Respir. Cell. Mol. Biol. 38: 95–104, 2008.

124. Lu, Z., S. Ghosh, Z. Wang, and T. Hunter. Downregulation of caveolin-1 function by EGF leads to the loss of E-cadherin, increased transcriptional activity of β-catenin, and enhanced tumor cell invasion. Cancer Cell 4: 499–515, 2003.

125. Masuda, A., M. Kondo, T. Saito, Y. Yatabe, T. Kobayashi, M. Okamoto, M. Suyama, and T. Takahashi. Establishment of human peripheral lung epithelial cell lines (HPL1) retaining differentiated characteristics and responsiveness to epidermal growth factor, hepatocyte growth factor, and transforming growth factor β1. Cancer Res. 57: 4898–4904, 1997.

126. Blanco, D., S. Vicent, E. Elizegi, I. Pino, M.F. Fraga, M. Esteller, U. Saffiotti, F. Lecanda, and L.M. Montuenga. Altered expression of adhesion molecules and epithelial-mesenchymal transition in silica-induced rat lung carcinogenesis. Lab Invest. 84: 999–1012, 2004.

127. Powell, D.W., R.C. Mifflin, J.D. Valentich, S.E. Crowe, J.I. Saada, and A.B. West. Myofibroblasts. I. Paracrine. cells important in health and disease. Am. J. Physiol. 277: <PAGES>C1–9</PAGES>, 1999.

128. Balkwill, F. and A. Mantovani. Inflammation and cancer: back to Virchow? Lancet 357: 539–545, 2001.

129. Bhowmick, N.A., A. Chytil, D. Plieth, A.E. Gorska, N. Dumont, S. Shappell, M.K. Washington, E.G. Neilson, and H.L. Moses. TGF-β signaling in fibroblasts modulates the oncogenic potential of adjacent epithelia. Science 303: 848–851, 2004.

130. Cheng, N., N.A. Bhowmick, A. Chytil, A.E. Gorksa, K.A. Brown, R. Muraoka, C.L. Arteaga, E.G. Neilson, S.W. Hayward, and H.L. Moses. Loss of TGF-β type II receptor in fibroblasts promotes mammary carcinoma growth and invasion through upregulation of TGF-β-, MSP- and HGF-mediated signaling networks. Oncogene 24: 5053–5068, 2005.

131. Nakamura, T., K. Matsumoto, A. Kiritoshi, and Y. Tano. Induction of hepatocyte growth factor in fibroblasts by tumor-derived factors affects invasive growth of tumor cells: in vitro analysis of tumor-stromal interactions. Cancer Res. 57: 3305–3313, 1997.

132. Gmyrek, G.A., M. Walburg, C.P. Webb, H.M. Yu, X. You, E.D. Vaughan, G.F. Vande Woude, and B.S. Knudsen. Normal and malignant prostate epithelial cells differ in their response to hepatocyte growth factor/scatter factor. Am. J. Pathol. 159: 579–590, 2001.

133. Beviglia, L., K. Matsumoto, C.S. Lin, B.L. Ziober, and R.H. Kramer. Expression of the c-Met/HGF receptor in human breast carcinoma: correlation with tumor progression. Int. J. Cancer 74: 301–309, 1997.

134. Masuya, D., C. Huang, D. Liu, T. Nakashima, K. Kameyama, R. Haba, M. Ueno, and H. Yokomise. The tumour-stromal interaction between intratumoral c-Met and stromal hepatocyte growth factor associated with tumour growth and prognosis in non-small-cell lung cancer patients. Br. J. Cancer 90: 1555–1562, 2004.

135. Lewis, M.P., K.A. Lygoe, M.L. Nystrom, W.P. Anderson, P.M. Speight, J.F. Marshall, and G.J. Thomas. Tumour-derived TGF-β1 modulates myofibroblast differentiation and promotes HGF/SF-dependent invasion of squamous carcinoma cells. Br. J. Cancer 90: 822–832, 2004.

136. Joseph, H., A.E. Gorska, P. Sohn, H.L. Moses, and R. Serra. Overexpression of a kinase-deficient transforming growth factor-β type II receptor in mouse mammary stroma results in increased epithelial branching. Mol. Biol. Cell 10: 1221–1234., 1999.

137. Wynn, T.A. Cellular and molecular mechanisms of fibrosis. J. Pathol. 214: 199–210, 2008.

138. Iwano, M., D. Plieth, T.M. Danoff, C. Xue, H. Okada, and E.G. Neilson. Evidence that fibroblasts derive from epithelium during tissue fibrosis. J. Clin. Invest. 110: 341–350, 2002.

139. Yang, J. and Y. Liu. Blockage of tubular epithelial to myofibroblast transition by hepatocyte growth factor prevents renal interstitial fibrosis. J. Am. Soc. Nephrol. 13: 96–107, 2002.

140. Kalluri, R. and E.G. Neilson.Epithelial-mesenchymal transition and its implications for fibrosis. J. Clin. Invest. 112: 1776–1784, 2003.

141. Saika, S., S. Kono-Saika, Y. Ohnishi, M. Sato, Y. Muragaki, A. Ooshima, K.C. Flanders, J. Yoo, M. Anzano, C.Y. Liu, W.W. Kao, and A.B. Roberts. Smad3 signaling is required for epithelial-mesenchymal transition of lens epithelium after injury. Am. J. Pathol. 164: 651–663, 2004.

142. Schurch, W., T.A. Seemayer, and G. Gabbiani.: The myofibroblast a quarter century after its discovery. Am. J. Surg. Pathol. 22: 141–147, 1998.

143. Phan, S.H. The myofibroblast in pulmonary fibrosis. Chest 122: 286S–289S, 2002.

144. Singh, S.R. and I.P. Hall. Airway myofibroblasts and their relationship with airway myocytes and fibroblasts. Proc. Am. Thorac. Soc. 5: 127–132, 2008.

145. Direkze, N.C., K. Hodivala-Dilke, R. Jeffery, T. Hunt, R. Poulsom, D. Oukrif, M.R. Alison, and N.A. Wright. Bone marrow contribution to tumor-associated myofibroblasts and fibroblasts. Cancer Res. 64: 8492–8495, 2004.

146. Forbes, S.J., F.P. Russo, V. Rey, P. Burra, M. Rugge, N.A. Wright, and M.R. Alison. A significant proportion of myofibroblasts are of bone marrow origin in human liver fibrosis. Gastroenterology 126: 955–963, 2004.

147. Ebihara, Y., M. Masuya, A.C. Larue, P.A. Fleming, R.P. Visconti, H. Minamiguchi, C.J. Drake, and M. Ogawa. Hematopoietic origins of fibroblasts: II. In vitro studies of fibroblasts, CFU-F, and fibrocytes. Exp. Hematol. 34: 219–229, 2006.

148. Quan, T.E., S.E. Cowper, and R. Bucala. The role of circulating fibrocytes in fibrosis. Curr. Rheumatol. Rep. 8: 145–150, 2006.

149. Willis, B.C., R.M. duBois, and Z. Borok. Epithelial origin of myofibroblasts during fibrosis in the lung. Proc. Am. Thorac. Soc. 3: 377–382, 2006.

150. Zeisberg, E.M., O. Tarnavski, M. Zeisberg, A.L. Dorfman, J.R. McMullen, E. Gustafsson, A. Chandraker, X. Yuan, W.T. Pu, A.B. Roberts, E.G. Neilson, M.H. Sayegh, S. Izumo, and R. Kalluri. Endothelial-to-mesenchymal transition contributes to cardiac fibrosis. Nat. Med. 13: 952–961, 2007.

151. Hu, B., Z. Wu, and S.H. Phan. Smad3 mediates transforming growth factor-β-induced β-smooth muscle actin expression. Am. J. Respir. Cell Mol. Biol. 29: 397–404, 2003.

152. Reubinoff, B.E., M.F. Pera, C.Y. Fong, A. Trounson, and A. Bongso. Embryonic stem cell lines from human blastocysts: somatic differentiation in vitro. Nat. Biotechnol. 18: 399–404, 2000.

153. Smith, A.G. Embryo-derived stem cells: of mice and men. Annu. Rev. Cell Dev. Biol. 17: 435–462, 2001.

154. Spencer, H.L., A.M. Eastham, C.L. Merry, T.D. Southgate, F. Perez-Campo, F. Soncin, S. Ritson, R. Kemler, P.L. Stern, and C.M. Ward. E-cadherin inhibits cell surface localization of the pro-migratory 5T4 oncofetal antigen in mouse embryonic stem cells. Mol. Biol. Cell 18: 2838–2851, 2007.

155. Eastham, A.M., H. Spencer, F. Soncin, S. Ritson, C.L. Merry, P.L. Stern, and C.M. Ward. Epithelial-mesenchymal transition events during human embryonic stem cell differentiation. Cancer Res. 67: 11254–11262, 2007.

156. Cavallaro, U. and G. Christofori. Cell adhesion and signalling by cadherins and Ig-CAMs in cancer. Nat. Rev. Cancer 4: 118–132, 2004.

157. Mani, S.A., W. Guo, M.J. Liao, E.N. Eaton, A. Ayyanan, A.Y. Zhou, M. Brooks, F. Reinhard, C.C. Zhang, M. Shipitsin, L.L. Campbell, K. Polyak, C. Brisken, J. Yang, and R.A. Weinberg. The epithelial-mesenchymal transition generates cells with properties of stem cells. Cell 133: 704–715, 2008.

158. Lobo, N.A., Y. Shimono, D. Qian, and M.F. Clarke. The biology of cancer stem cells. Annu. Rev. Cell Dev. Biol. 23: 675–699, 2007.

159. Dalerba, P. and M.F. Clarke. Cancer stem cells and tumor metastasis: first steps into uncharted territory. Cell Stem Cell 1: 241–242, 2007.

160. Karnoub, A.E., A.B. Dash, A.P. Vo, A. Sullivan, M.W. Brooks, G.W. Bell, A.L. Richardson, K. Polyak, R. Tubo, and R.A. Weinberg. Mesenchymal stem cells within tumour stroma promote breast cancer metastasis. Nature 449: 557–563, 2007.

161. Thiery, J.-P. and J.P. Sleeman. Complex networks orchestrate epithelial-mesenchymal transitions. Nat. Rev. Mol. Cell. Biol. 7: 131–142, 2006.

162. Prindull, G. Hypothesis: cell plasticity, linking embryonal stem cells to adult stem cell reservoirs and metastatic cancer cells? Exp. Hematol. 33: 738–746, 2005.

163. Ben-Porath, I., M.W. Thomson, V.J. Carey, R. Ge, G.W. Bell, A. Regev, and R.A. Weinberg. An embryonic stem cell-like gene expression signature in poorly differentiated aggressive human tumors. Nat. Genet. 40: 499–507, 2008.

164. Ullmann, U., P. In't Veld, C. Gilles, K. Sermon, M. De Rycke, H. Van de Velde, A. Van Steirteghem, and I. Liebaers. Epithelial-mesenchymal transition process in human embryonic stem cells cultured in feeder-free conditions. Mol. Hum. Reprod. 13: 21–32, 2007.

165. Fischer, A.N., E. Fuchs, M. Mikula, H. Huber, H. Beug, and W. Mikulits. PDGF essentially links TGF-β signaling to nuclear β-catenin accumulation in hepatocellular carcinoma progression. Oncogene In press, 2006.

166. Tarin, D., E.W. Thompson, and D.F. Newgreen. The fallacy of epithelial mesenchymal transition in neoplasia. Cancer Res. 65: 5996–6000; discussion 6000-1, 2005.

167. Christiansen, J.J. and A.K. Rajasekaran. Reassessing epithelial to mesenchymal transition as a prerequisite for carcinoma invasion and metastasis. Cancer Res. 66: 8319–8326, 2006.

168. Wicki, A., F. Lehembre, N. Wick, B. Hantusch, D. Kerjaschki, and G. Christofori. Tumor invasion in the absence of epithelial-mesenchymal transition: podoplanin-mediated remodeling of the actin cytoskeleton. Cancer Cell 9: 261–272, 2006.

169. Trimboli, A.J., K. Fukino, A. de Bruin, G. Wei, L. Shen, S.M. Tanner, N. Creasap, T.J. Rosol, M.L. Robinson, C. Eng, M.C. Ostrowski, and G. Leone. Direct evidence for epithelial-mesenchymal transitions in breast cancer. Cancer Res. 68: 937–945, 2008.

Mechanisms of Tumor Cell Migration and Invasion in Lung Cancer Metastasis

Charles Kumar Thodeti and Kaustabh Ghosh

Abstract Cancer metastasis is a multistep process that involves tumor cell migration and invasion through tumor stroma, intravasation into and extravasation out of the blood vessels, and accumulation at a distant organ site. These events arise from concomitant alterations in the genetic, chemical, and physical state of tumor cells and its microenvironment. This chapter will, however, focus on the molecular determinants of tumor cell migration and invasion, with special emphasis on the cross talk between extracellular matrix, integrin receptors, matrix metalloproteases, and Rho GTPases, all of which undergo dynamic regulation to ultimately modulate cell shape and tension and, thereby, their migratory and invasive behavior. Elucidating these molecular mechanisms will likely identify key players in the metastatic process, which can be exploited to develop novel therapeutic strategies for the treatment for lung cancer.

Introduction

To metastasize, a tumor cell has to degrade the basement membrane (BM), invade the stromal extracellular matrix (ECM) through simultaneous degradation and synthesis of ECM components, intravasate into the neovessels, and finally extravasate from the blood stream at a remote organ site. Acquisition of an invasive phenotype is essential for tumor cells to successfully navigate through the multistep process of metastasis. Invasive phenotype is characterized by both the loss of cell–cell interactions and increased cellular migration. Effective cell migration requires the seamless integration of localized signaling events with global cellular architecture. Cell migration is a complex, cyclical physiochemical process that involves (a) protrusion of leading edge-forming lamellipodium due to the changes in the membrane tension and actin

C.K. Thodeti (✉)
Vascular Biology Program, Children's Hospital/Harvard Medical School,
Boston, MA 02115, USA
e-mail: charles.thodeti@childrens.harvard.edu

V. Keshamouni et al. (eds.), *Lung Cancer Metastasis*,
DOI 10.1007/978-1-4419-0772-1_5, © Springer Science+Business Media, LLC 2009

polymerization; (b) cell attachment to the extracellular matrix and formation of focal adhesions at cell front; (c) detachment of trailing edge by disassembly of focal adhesion; and finally (d) contraction of actin cytoskeleton leading to the forward movement of cell body [1, 2]. Migration requires the concerted effort of a number of molecules such as integrins, ion channels, cell adhesion molecules, soluble cytokines and growth factors, matrix-degrading proteases, and Rho GTPases that converge onto the activation of several cytoskeletal proteins [1–5]. This chapter will cover molecular determinants and mechanisms that coordinately orchestrate a robust actin cytoskeletal reorganization in a way that promotes cancer cell migration and invasion, leading to metastasis.

Basement Membrane

The tumor epithelial cells are separated from the stroma by basement membrane (BM), an amorphous, thick sheet-like structure that binds these tumor cells [6, 7]. BM is mainly composed of type IV collagen, laminin, heparan sulfate proteoglycans, and enactin [8–11], which together form a highly cross-linked network through disulfide and nondisulfide bridges. The BM not only supports adhesion of epithelial cells but also conveys signals to promote their growth, differentiation, and motility. Although the BM appears similar in different tissues, their molecular composition is often tissue specific. In tumors, BM is less cross-linked compared to normal tissue, which makes it more susceptible to proteolysis [12, 13], with the cleaved BM fragments further promoting tumor cell invasion. For example, laminin-5 in the tumor BM, but not in normal quiescent BM, undergoes degradation to expose a cryptic pro-migratory site that stimulates tumor cell migration [14].

Tumor Extracellular Matrix

Extracellular matrix (ECM) is the molecular network outside the cells that supports cell adhesion and function, in addition to providing a structural support to the tissue. The major components of ECM are collagen, fibronectin, laminin, perlecan, decorin, hyaluronan, and syndecan [3]. These ECM molecules have specific recognition sites for cell adhesion receptors (such as integrins), and binding to these receptors promotes cell adhesion, growth, differentiation, and apoptosis. For example, integrins $\alpha5\beta1$ bind specifically to the RGD (Arg-Gly-Asp) sequence in the 10th domain of the FN III repeat [15, 16] and support key cell functions. Notably, the ECM not only supports cell adhesion through the binding of integrin receptors but also transmits external forces into the cells and resists internally generated contractile (tensile) forces. This force balance between cell tension and ECM resistance, which can be altered through changes in ECM stiffness, regulates cell spreading and migration [17–19].

In contrast to normal ECM, tumor ECM is stiffer and consists of a dense cross-linked fibrin matrix, in addition to the regular ECM components such as fibronectin, collagens (predominantly type I), and proteoglycans [20]. The stiffness of tumor ECM increases as a result of continuous remodeling of matrix components by stromal fibroblasts, which alters the type of and increases the cross-linking between different ECM components. Because of its higher stiffness, the tumor ECM can resist the increase in mechanical forces that results from an expanding tumor mass. Extravasation of plasma components from leaky blood vessels and formation of perivascular fibrin gels further raises interstitial pressure, and thus ECM stiffness, which may feed back to enhance integrin-mediated Rho/ROCK (Rho-associated kinase) activities or contractility in tumor cells [21]. In addition to regulating cell spreading and proliferation, ECM rigidity also influences cell migration. In a seminal study, stiffer ECM was shown to reduce migration speed through an increase in cell adhesion strength, while cell migration was significantly increased on compliant ECM [22]. Thus, the physicality of the tumor ECM plays a critical role in regulating cell migration and cancer metastasis.

Matrix Metalloproteinases

Matrix metalloproteinases (MMPs) are a family of 21 multidomain, multifunctional proteins that can cleave ECM components to alter the overall ECM structure and mechanics and promote cell migration [3, 23–25]. In general, MMPs are covalently bound to the plasma membrane, but some can also be secreted into the extracellular space (such as MMP-2, MMP-7, and MMP-9), which then associate with cell surface receptors such as integrins [26] and CD44 [27–29]. MMPs are secreted as inactive zymogens and can be activated by proteinases either inside the cells through a furin-like serine protease or outside the cell by a multimeric protein complex comprised of other MMPs or serine proteases [25]. Some integrins can activate MMPs by recruiting them to the leading edge of an invading cell [26]. MMPs are also known to cleave cell adhesion receptors like E-cadherin and CD44, which allow epithelial–mesenchymal transition and cell migration by breaking the cell–cell or cell–ECM contacts, respectively [30, 31]. However, the MMP activity is held in check by endogenous inhibitors such as tissue inhibitors of metalloproteases (TIMPs) or α2-macroglobulin, which prevent excessive ECM degradation and tissue instability [3, 25, 32–34].

Evidence for the role of MMPs in cancer progression came from both knockout and transgenic mice of MMPs. Compared to wild-type mice, colonization of tumor cells into lung tissue is reduced in MMP-2 or MMP-9 knockout mice, while overexpression of MMP-1, MMP-3, and MMP-9 enhanced cancer susceptibility and progression [31, 35–38]. Expression of a number of MMPs was reported in various human cancers, and levels of MMPs are well correlated with increases in tumor metastasis of tumor [3, 25]. MMP-9 is highly expressed in NSCLC and implicated in tumor angiogenesis and metastasis [39], while MMP-1 expression was shown to be associated with the early onset of lung cancer [40]. Zhu et al. [41] further showed that a single polymorphism in MMP-1 was sufficient to enhance susceptibility to lung cancer [41]. Another interesting study showed that gaseous nitric oxide increased human lung cancer cell migration, invasion, and metastasis through the activation of MMP-2 [42].

More detailed studies have revealed that MMPs in human cancers are secreted by both tumor cells and surrounding stromal cells [3, 25]. Irrespective of their source of origin, MMPs cleave a number of ECM substrates and increase tumor cell invasion. In fact, MMP-dependent proteolysis of ECM presents new substrate for tumor cell adhesion and migration, the first steps in metastasis. For example, MMP-2-dependent cleavage of laminin-5 produces a fragment that increased tumor cell motility through the exposure of a cryptic pro-migratory site [14, 43]. To invade, tumor cells must form invadopodia, and MMP-2 and MMP-9 were shown to be involved in this process through their recruitment to the site of invadopodia formation via binding to $\alpha v \beta 3$ integrin or CD44, respectively [26–29]. MMP-9 was also reported to be localized with CD44 at the rear end of migrating cells, where it presumably helps CD44 detachment that is required for effective cell migration [27].

Cleavage by MMPs changes not only the ECM composition but also its local physical properties. As cells can sense and respond to alterations in its microscale mechanostructural environment by adjusting the level of intracellular tension (contractility) and adhesion strength (to obtain a new force equilibrium), variations in the physicality of tumor ECM can cause tumor cells to modulate the levels of integrin and Rho GTPase activity, the primary mechanosensing elements of a cell [21, 44–46]. However, integrins and Rho are also critically involved in cell migration, thus suggesting that MMP activity can influence tumor cell invasion and metastasis through regulation of cellular mechanotransduction [19, 45].

Integrins

Tumor cells adhere to their surrounding ECM through integrin receptors, the cell surface glycoproteins that exist as heterodimers of noncovalently linked α and β subunits. There are 18 α subunits and 8 β subunits of integrins that together form almost 25 different integrin receptors, each exhibiting distinct ligand specificity. Structurally, each integrin subunit consists of an extracellular domain, a transmembrane domain, and a short cytoplasmic domain. Integrins exist in an inactive closed conformation, and when bound to specific amino acid sequences found within ECM molecules (e.g., RGD) during the initial steps of cell–ECM adhesion, it undergoes conformational changes that permit it to activate intracellular signaling pathways, a process known as "integrin activation" [47, 48]. Integrins do not have intrinsic kinase activity; however, integrin activation via its binding to ECM ligands induces recruitment of cytoskeletal adaptor proteins to the cytoplasmic tail of integrin, which facilitates formation of focal adhesions that, in turn, activate downstream kinases such as FAK, PKC, AKT, and Rho family GTPases [49–51]. Integrins, however, also can be activated by "inside-out signaling" involving activation of cytoplasmic signaling molecules, such as protein kinase C [52, 53], rap-1 [54, 55], and R-Ras [56, 57], which produce activating conformational changes in integrins from inside the cell.

Notably, integrins also act as bidirectional force transducers, i.e., they sense and transduce external ECM-generated mechanical forces into intracellular biochemical signals and simultaneously transmit intracellularly generated tensile (contractile) forces onto the ECM [18, 19, 46, 58, 59]. The balance between the cell-based (internal) and ECM-based (external) mechanical forces regulates cell shape distortion, which can independently dictate whether a cell will undergo growth, differentiation, death, or migration [18, 60, 61]. Integrins transduce these mechanical signals into intracellular biochemistry (in a process called "mechanotransduction") via focal adhesions, macromolecular complexes arising from integrin activation and clustering [18, 19]. These focal adhesions are further strengthened by the intracellular contractile forces generated by the actomyosin machinery (Fig. 1) [62, 63]. Focal adhesions can contain more than 50 cytoskeletal adaptor and signaling proteins, whose dynamics regulates cell adhesion and migration [64, 65]. A recent interesting work shows that the shape and size of focal adhesions can influence directed cell migration by precisely regulating where new cell membrane protrusions would occur [66].

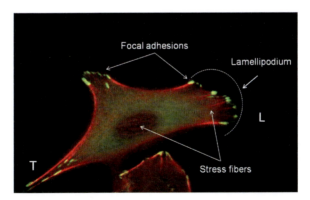

Fig. 1 The structural framework of a motile cancer cell. A549 lung cancer cells were cultured on 2D substrates and stained with phalloidin and a monoclonal antibody against vinculin to visualize actin (*red*) and focal adhesions (*green*), respectively. The image shows a typical motile cell with clearly visible lamellipodium-like structures (*dashed line*) at the leading edge (L), actin-rich stress fibers spanning the length of the cell, and distinct focal adhesions at both leading and trailing (T) edges

Importantly, integrins not only relay mechanical forces across the cell membrane and activate other signaling molecules but also respond to forces by causing rapid activation of additional integrins. For instance, flow-induced shear stress activates αVβ3 integrins in endothelial cells through a signaling complex consisting of vascular endothelial growth factor (VEGF), VE-cadherin, and platelet endothelial cell adhesion molecule (PECAM) [67]. Separately, cyclic strain has been found to activate β1 integrins through a mechanosensitive calcium channel TRPV4 [132]. Although the two mechanisms of integrin activation utilize distinct signaling pathways, they converge at the level of PI3-kinase (phosphoinositide-3 kinase) activation, which is required for both shear stress- and cyclic strain-induced integrin activation. Furthermore, ECM stiffness can also influence integrin expression and activation and thereby cell adhesion and migration [68–70]. In this regard, Paszek et al. [21] demonstrated that matrix rigidity can alone cause hyperactivation and clustering of integrins in mammary epithelial cells, leading to high cellular tension and disruption of normal tissue morphogenesis before progressing to malignancy [21]. Indeed, past reports have shown that integrin expression and activation are altered in various stiff tumors [71]. Specifically, in squamous cell lung carcinoma, α2β1 and α1β1 integrins levels have been shown to be highly elevated, which correlate with an increased tendency to metastasize [72].

The activated integrins can regulate cell migration and invasion through various mechanisms such as regulation of focal adhesions dynamics, activation of intracellular kinases (viz., FAK and PI3 kinases) [65, 71], and recruitment of proteases to the sites of cellular attachment [26]. Indeed, invasive tumors exhibit high levels of FAK activity compared to benign tumors [73, 74]. PI3 kinase activity has also been shown to play a critical role in promoting tumor cell invasiveness through the activation of specific Rho GTPases, viz., Rac and Cdc42 [75]. Furthermore, integrins are known to interact with MMPs within a multimeric complex and localize their proteolytic activity to the leading edge of invasive tumor cells [26, 76]. Thus, integrins can influence tumor cell migration and invasion through their binding to tumor ECM as well as by regulating ECM stiffness through MMP-mediated remodeling. The integrin-dependent regulation of cell behavior is mediated through specific intracellular signaling pathways that ultimately lead to the increase in Rho GTPase activation.

E-Cadherins and Connexins

In addition to binding to ECM via integrins, epithelial cells also associate with one another via adherens junctions (AJ) and tight junctions, which are important for overall stability and polarity of the epithelial layer. E-cadherins are the major components of AJs that stabilize the epithelium through homophilic interactions in the extracellular space and cytoskeletal linkage, which involves actin binding to the β-catenin/α-catenin/p120 catenin complex, via the cytoplasmic tail [77]. Furthermore, maintenance of epithelial integrity by the E-cadherin/ catenin complex has been shown to involve repression of Rho activity via the activation of Rac and Cdc42 [78–80]. Consequently, downregulation or loss of E-cadherin, as demonstrated in a number of epithelial cancers, results in the loss of epithelial stability and polarity, thereby leading to epithelial–mesenchymal transition (EMT) and invasion of cancer cells (see Chapter 4) [77, 81].

Intercellular communications are also mediated by the intercellular channels called gap junctions that directly connect the cytoplasm of adjacent cells. Gap junctions are composed of two connexons, which in turn are made up of proteins called connexins [82]. Incidentally, upregulation of connexins has been shown to be implicated in increased invasion of breast, prostate, and skin cancers [83–86], although the exact correlation between connexin function and expression in metastasis has not been clearly identified. In contrast, downregulation of connexin32 is correlated with lung cancer metastasis [87], further highlighting the vital, albeit complex, role connexins play in cancer cell metastasis.

Rho GTPases

Rho GTPases belong to Ras family of oncogenes and are implicated as pivotal regulators of several signaling networks that are activated by a wide variety of receptors, including integrins. These GTPases affect many aspects of cell behavior, including cell tension and migration [88]. Rho GTPase family mainly includes Cdc42, Rac, and Rho that are widely known to control the formation of filopodia, lamellipodia, and stress fibers (Fig. 1), respectively, which are required for cell migration [89]. Interestingly, Rho GTPases, which lack intrinsic GTPase activity, are activated upon association with guanine nucleotide exchange factors (GEFs) that substitute the bound GDP with GTP, whereas they can be inactivated by GTPase activating proteins (GAPs) that restore the GDP-bound state [88]. Importantly, the activation of Rho family members results in their translocation from the cytosol to the plasma membrane and subsequent interaction with target molecules called effectors. For example, Cdc42 and Rac induce membrane protrusions through the activation of one of their effectors, p21-activated kinase(PAK), that, in turn, activates actin polymerization by modulating LIM kinase/cofilin pathways [88]. Rho, on the other hand, activates ROCK and promotes myosin light-chain phosphorylation, which is required for increased stress fiber formation, cell contractility, and cell migration [89].

Rho GTPases are activated by both soluble factors secreted by tumor stroma as well as by physical forces applied through tumor ECM [88]. For example, lysophosphatidic acid (LPA) mediates signaling to Rho through a seven transmembrane G-protein coupled receptor (GPCR), which activates $G_{\alpha 12/13}$ subunits and recruits RGS domain containing Rho GEFs to activate Rho at the cell membrane. Notably, different factors may activate Rho GTPases through distinct signaling pathways. For instance, growth factors such as EGF and PDGF activate Rho GTPases (Rac) through PI3-kinase-dependent production of phosphatidylinositol-3,4,5-trisphosphate (PIP3), which recruits Rac GEFs to the cell membrane to promote membrane protrusions necessary for cell migration [89]. Integrin binding to the ECM, on the other hand, results in the activation of a number of kinases and adaptor proteins at focal adhesions, such as FAK, Src, and p130 CAS, which further activate GEFs associated with Rac, Rho, and Cdc42, leading to activation of Rho GTPases [89, 90]. Importantly, matrix stiffness can also promote integrin activation and concomitant FA assembly that, in turn, enhances Rho activity [21]. In addition to matrix stiffness, application of exogenous force (such as flow-induced shear stress and cyclic stress) can also activate Rho through the activation and clustering of integrins [21, 91] (Thodeti, unpublished results). Upon activation, Rho causes an increase in cell contractility and tension [44], which further clusters integrins [62], thus creating a self-sustaining mechanical feedback loop of Rho activation and cell tension that ultimately regulates cells shape and migration [19, 21, 44].

Although mutations in Rho GTPases have not been reported in tumors (except for RhoH), they play a crucial role in tumorigenesis likely through alterations in its activity and/or expression [5]. Reports suggest the elevation of Rho activity and expression in lung, breast, colon, pancreas tumors as well as head and neck squamous cell carcinoma [92–94]. Furthermore, elevated levels of ROCK activity, a downstream effector of Rho, have been correlated with high incidence of metastasis and poor prognosis of patients with inflammatory breast cancer [95]. In another study, detailed genomic analysis has revealed an essential role for RhoC in tumor invasion and metastasis [96]. Furthermore, Rho/ROCK-dependent MLCK (myosin light-chain kinase) activity has been shown to be critical for E1AF/PEA3 (an ETS family transcription factor frequently overexpressed in NSCLCs)-induced increase in lung tumor cell invasion [97]. The influence of Rho GTPases in tumor cell invasion was further highlighted from studies where lung carcinoma cells expressing a tumor suppressor gene, the fragile histidine triad (FHIT), exhibited a dramatic inhibition in cell migration and invasion via the downregulation of RhoC expression [98]. Furthermore, expression of dominant negative mutants of Rho and Rac inhibited migration and invasion of both human and mouse lung tumor cells [99].

Mechanistically, Rho GTPases promote tumor cell metastasis by (a) disrupting cell–cell contacts and polarity of epithelial cells, (b) enhancing matrix degradation and remodeling, and (c) increasing cell motility [5]. For example, Rac1 controls cell polarity through its association with par6 (polarity protein6) and inhibition of Rac1 activity leads to loss of polarity [88]. The CdC42-PAK pathway is also implicated in the regulation of lung tumor cell polarity through the action of tumor suppressor LKB1, which is mutated in almost 30% of NSCLCs [100]. Furthermore, Rho and ROCK also promote TGF-β-induced loss of adherence junctions that is required for the invasive behavior, while Rac is shown to be required for Ras-induced loss of cell–cell contacts [101]. ROCK is also known to induce redistribution of proteins such as ezrin (a cytoskeleton linker protein) as well as adherens junction and ECM-binding proteins, thus enabling cell invasion [102]. Rho, on the other hand, stimulates human osteocarcinoma cell invasion through activation of MMP-2, which degrades the ECM [103]. Importantly, siRNA knockdown of RhoC or a ROCK inhibitor (Y-27632) reduces MMP-9 expression and tumor cell invasion and metastasis [104]. In a separate study, knockdown of Rac1 expression, together with downregulation of Par6alpha and PKC (protein kinase C) iota, inhibited MMP-10 expression and invasion of NSCLC cells [105].

Rho GTPases can also promote tumor cell migration by mediating cytoskeletal linkage with cell surface ECM receptors. For example, RhoA can facilitate increased association of adaptor protein ezrin with CD44 receptors through ROCK-mediated phosphorylation [106]. Rac1, on the other hand, increases the association of ezrin and CD44 by inhibiting the antagonist of ezrin, NF2 (neurofibromin 2) [107]. Interestingly, the expression of both ezrin and CD44 was shown to be increased in metastatic tumor cells [108, 109]. Thus, Rho GTPases regulate tumor cell migration and invasion not only via MMP-mediated ECM degradation but also by facilitating physical changes between and within tumor cells, as manifested by the breakdown of cell–cell contacts and association of cytoskeletal proteins with cell surface receptors. Through such mechanism, Rho GTPases successfully integrate physical cues from tumor ECM (stiffness and exogenous forces) and transduce them into intracellular biochemical signaling via the integrin-containing focal adhesion complexes, thus leading to increased cell contractility and migration.

Actin-Binding Proteins

Cell motility is dependent on the polymerization of actin cytoskeleton and actomyosin contraction that are mediated by a number of actin-binding molecules including cofilin and filamin, and kinases and phosphatases that regulate myosin phosphorylation [110]. Of these molecules, cofilin has recently assumed greater significance with regard to its role in cancer cell motility and invasion [111]. Cofilin is an actin-severing protein whose expression is typically associated with highly invasive and migratory phenotype seen in a number of cancers [111]. For example, cofilin1 expression was shown to be upregulated in TGF-β-induced epithelial–mesenchymal transition (EMT) of lung cancer A549 cells, thus implicating a role of cofilin1 in invasive phenotype of cancer cells [112, 113]. Further analyses revealed an increase in cofilin mRNA stability in response to TGF-β, which was shown to contribute toward the observed increase in mRNA and protein expression. Importantly, cofilin must be expressed at an optimal level to promote cell motility; too high or too low levels can, in fact, inhibit the migratory phenotype [111]. In addition to its overall expression levels, the spatiotemporal regulation of cofilin activity also influences directed cancer cell migration in response to growth factors such as EGF [114, 115].

Filamin is another actin-binding protein whose expression appears to be altered in cancers and correlated with invasiveness. For example, downregulation of filamin A has been shown to increase prostate cancer cell motility [116]. In contrast, filamin A expression was shown to be increased during TGF-β-induced EMT of A549 lung cancer cells, although the functional role of filamin A in EMT is yet to be ascertained [113]. Notably, the calpain-mediated cleavage of filamin A plays a key role in the migratory phenotype, as evidenced by more recent studies where nuclear translocation of a 90 kDa filamin A fragment was shown to be inversely correlated with prostate cancer metastasis [117, 118].

Methods to Study Cancer Cell Invasion and Metastasis

Given the critical role of tumor cell invasion and metastasis in cancer development and progression, it becomes imperative that we devise appropriate methods to delineate the processes underlying these key cellular phenotypes. To address this, several approaches have been adopted, including the two-dimensional (2D) Boyden Chamber/Transwell assay [119, 120]. Despite being the most widely used in vitro technique [42, 86, 99, 121–123], this assay is limited by its inability to truly mimic the more complex 3D tissue microenvironment that cancer cells in vivo must interact with en route to blood vessel intravasation. To overcome this problem, 3D collagen gel assays have been developed wherein cells are embedded in collagen gels and their invasion observed through acquisition of multiplanar time lapse confocal images [124, 125]. Furthermore, to mimic the in vivo extravasation of metastatic tumor cells at a remote organ site, the 3D collagen gel assay has been subsequently modified through addition of an endothelial cell layer [126]. Importantly, greater advancements in optical imaging techniques, such as the establishment of "intravital imaging," have led to direct observations of cancer cell metastasis in vivo. These imaging techniques include noninvasive tissue-/whole body-level measurements using fluorescence reflectance imaging, bioluminescence, and Raman spectroscopy or invasive techniques that employ confocal or epifluorescence imaging [127].

Conclusions and Clinical Perspective

There is increasing evidence now suggesting that in addition to the genetic and chemical composition of the tumor cells and the stroma, the physical environment of tumor ECM also has a significant effect on tumor metastasis. This arises from force-induced regulation of integrins and Rho and their cross talk with matrix-degrading MMPs that, together, influence cell migration and invasion. Importantly, such mechanical signaling can also cross talk with the canonical biochemical signaling pathways, resulting in the creation of a self-sustaining feedback mechanism that continuously alters ECM mechanostructural properties in favor of cell invasion. Thus, development of pharmacological inhibitors that specifically target the mechanical signaling via integrins, MMPs, and Rho could potentially inhibit lung cancer metastasis by normalizing the abnormal mechanotransduction induced by tumor ECM. Preclinical evaluation and development of antagonists of several such inhibitory molecules are currently undergoing, and a few of them have even entered into clinical trials. For example, preliminary results from phase III trials of MMP inhibitors such as BAY 12-9566 and prinomastat did not show beneficial effects against lung cancer [3]. This can be explained, at least in part, by the fact that MMP activity is required for the generation of endogenous anti-angiogenic substrates such as endostatin and tumstatin which inhibit tumor progression [128, 129], and therefore blocking MMP activity could inhibit the production of these molecules allowing tumor growth. However, integrin antagonists volociximab and cilengitide showed encouraging safety profiles in phase I trials and are now under evaluation in phase II trials for lung cancer [130, 131]. It will be interesting to see which one of these molecules is effective in keeping tumor metastasis in check. The efficacy of these anticancer molecules may be further enhanced using nanotechnological methods that promote targeted delivery of these selected molecules specifically to the tumor site. More recently, a novel biomaterial-based approach for cancer therapy has been suggested that proposes to employ injectable biomimetic materials that can target metastatic tumor site, self-assemble into scaffolds, and provide an optimal mechanostructural environment that can normalize tumor cell mechanosensing and, thus, prevent metastasis [45].

References

1. Friedl, P. and K. Wolf, *Tumour-cell invasion and migration: diversity and escape mechanisms*. Nat Rev Cancer, 2003, **3**(5): 362–74.
2. Hood, J.D. and D.A. Cheresh, *Role of integrins in cell invasion and migration*. Nat Rev Cancer, 2002, **2**(2): 91–100.
3. Egeblad, M. and Z. Werb, *New functions for the matrix metalloproteinases in cancer progression*. Nat Rev Cancer, 2002, **2**(3): 161–74.
4. Monteith, G.R. et al., *Calcium and cancer: targeting Ca2+ transport*. Nat Rev Cancer, 2007, **7**(7): 519–30.
5. Sahai, E. and C.J. Marshall, *RHO-GTPases and cancer*. Nat Rev Cancer, 2002, **2**(2): 133–42.
6. Kalluri, R., *Basement membranes: structure, assembly and role in tumour angiogenesis*. Nat Rev Cancer, 2003, **3**(6): 422–33.
7. Vracko, R., *Basal lamina scaffold-anatomy and significance for maintenance of orderly tissue structure*. Am J Pathol, 1974, **77**(2): 314–46.
8. Paulsson, M., *Basement membrane proteins: structure, assembly, and cellular interactions*. Crit Rev Biochem Mol Biol, 1992, **27**(1–2): 93–127.

9. Schittny, J.C. and P.D. Yurchenco, *Basement membranes: molecular organization and function in development and disease.* Curr Opin Cell Biol, 1989, **1**(5): 983–8.
10. Yurchenco, P.D., S. Smirnov, and T. Mathus, *Analysis of basement membrane self-assembly and cellular interactions with native and recombinant glycoproteins.* Methods Cell Biol, 2002, **69**: 111–44.
11. Yurchenco, P.D. et al., *Models for the self-assembly of basement membrane.* J Histochem Cytochem, 1986, **34**(1): 93–102.
12. Kalluri, R. et al., *Isoform switching of type IV collagen is developmentally arrested in X-linked Alport syndrome leading to increased susceptibility of renal basement membranes to endoproteolysis.* J Clin Invest, 1997, **99**(10): 2470–8.
13. Wisdom, B.J. Jr. et al., *Type IV collagen of Engelbreth–Holm–Swarm tumor matrix: identification of constituent chains.* Connect Tissue Res, 1992, **27**(4): 225–34.
14. Giannelli, G. et al., *Induction of cell migration by matrix metalloprotease-2 cleavage of laminin-5.* Science, 1997, **277**(5323): 225–8.
15. Ruoslahti, E. and M.D. Pierschbacher, *New perspectives in cell adhesion: RGD and integrins.* Science, 1987, **238**(4826): 491–7.
16. Takagi, J., *Structural basis for ligand recognition by RGD (Arg-Gly-Asp)-dependent integrins.* Biochem Soc Trans, 2004, **32**(Pt3): 403–6.
17. Ingber, D., *Extracellular matrix and cell shape: potential control points for inhibition of angiogenesis.* J Cell Biochem, 1991, **47**(3): 236–41.
18. Ingber, D.E., *Integrins, tensegrity, and mechanotransduction.* Gravit Space Biol Bull, 1997, **10**(2): 49–55.
19. Ingber, D.E., *Cellular mechanotransduction: putting all the pieces together again.* FASEB J, 2006, **20**(7): 811–27.
20. Dvorak, H.F., *Tumors: wounds that do not heal. Similarities between tumor stroma generation and wound healing.* N Engl J Med, 1986, **315**(26): 1650–9.
21. Paszek, M.J. et al., *Tensional homeostasis and the malignant phenotype.* Cancer Cell, 2005, **8**(3): 241–54.
22. Lauffenburger, D.A. and A.F. Horwitz, *Cell migration: a physically integrated molecular process.* Cell, 1996, **84**(3): 359–69.
23. Noel, A., M. Jost, and E. Maquoi, *Matrix metalloproteinases at cancer tumor–host interface.* Semin Cell Dev Biol, 2008, **19**(1): 52–60.
24. Rydlova, M. et al., *Biological activity and clinical implications of the matrix metalloproteinases.* Anticancer Res, 2008, **28**(2B): 1389–97.
25. Sternlicht, M.D. and Z. Werb, *How matrix metalloproteinases regulate cell behavior.* Annu Rev Cell Dev Biol, 2001, **17**: 463–516.
26. Brooks, P.C. et al., *Localization of matrix metalloproteinase MMP-2 to the surface of invasive cells by interaction with integrin alpha v beta 3.* Cell, 1996, **85**(5): 683–93.
27. Yu, Q. and I. Stamenkovic, *Localization of matrix metalloproteinase 9 to the cell surface provides a mechanism for CD44-mediated tumor invasion.* Genes Dev, 1999, **13**(1): 35–48.
28. Yu, Q. and I. Stamenkovic, *Cell surface-localized matrix metalloproteinase-9 proteolytically activates TGF-beta and promotes tumor invasion and angiogenesis.* Genes Dev, 2000, **14**(2): 163–76.
29. Yu, W.H. et al., *CD44 anchors the assembly of matrilysin/MMP-7 with heparin-binding epidermal growth factor precursor and ErbB4 and regulates female reproductive organ remodeling.* Genes Dev, 2002, **16**(3): 307–23.
30. Kajita, M. et al., *Membrane-type 1 matrix metalloproteinase cleaves CD44 and promotes cell migration.* J Cell Biol, 2001, **153**(5): 893–904.
31. Sternlicht, M.D. et al., *The stromal proteinase MMP3/stromelysin-1 promotes mammary carcinogenesis.* Cell, 1999, **98**(2): 137–46.
32. Sottrup-Jensen, L., *Alpha-macroglobulins: structure, shape, and mechanism of proteinase complex formation.* J Biol Chem, 1989, **264**(20): 11539–42.

33. Sottrup-Jensen, L. and H. Birkedal-Hansen, *Human fibroblast collagenase–alpha-macro-globulin interactions. Localization of cleavage sites in the bait regions of five mammalian alpha-macroglobulins.* J Biol Chem, 1989, **264**(1): 393–401.
34. Sottrup-Jensen, L. et al., *The alpha-macroglobulin bait region. Sequence diversity and localization of cleavage sites for proteinases in five mammalian alpha-macroglobulins.* J Biol Chem, 1989, **264**(27): 15781–9.
35. Coussens, L.M. et al., *MMP-9 supplied by bone marrow-derived cells contributes to skin carcinogenesis.* Cell, 2000, **103**(3): 481–90.
36. Ha, H.Y. et al., *Overexpression of membrane-type matrix metalloproteinase-1 gene induces mammary gland abnormalities and adenocarcinoma in transgenic mice.* Cancer Res, 2001, **61**(3): 984–90.
37. Itoh, T. et al., *Experimental metastasis is suppressed in MMP-9-deficient mice.* Clin Exp Metastasis, 1999, **17**(2): 177–81.
38. Itoh, T. et al., *Reduced angiogenesis and tumor progression in gelatinase A-deficient mice.* Cancer Res, 1998, **58**(5): 1048–51.
39. Martins, S.J. et al., *Prognostic relevance of TTF-1 and MMP-9 expression in advanced lung adenocarcinoma.* Lung Cancer, 2008.
40. Sauter, W. et al., *Matrix metalloproteinase 1 (MMP1) is associated with early-onset lung cancer.* Cancer Epidemiol Biomarkers Prev, 2008, **17**(5): 1127–35.
41. Zhu, Y. et al., *A single nucleotide polymorphism in the matrix metalloproteinase-1 promoter enhances lung cancer susceptibility.* Cancer Res, 2001, **61**(21): 7825–9.
42. Chen, J.H. et al., *Gaseous nitrogen oxide promotes human lung cancer cell line A549 migration, invasion, and metastasis via iNOS-mediated MMP-2 production.* Toxicol Sci, 2008, **106**(2): 364–75.
43. Xu, J. et al., *Proteolytic exposure of a cryptic site within collagen type IV is required for angiogenesis and tumor growth in vivo.* J Cell Biol, 2001, **154**(5): 1069–79.
44. Huang, S. and D.E. Ingber, *Cell tension, matrix mechanics, and cancer development.* Cancer Cell, 2005, **8**(3): 175–6.
45. Ingber, D.E., *Can cancer be reversed by engineering the tumor microenvironment?* Semin Cancer Biol, 2008, **18**(5): 356–64.
46. Alenghat, F.J. and D.E. Ingber, *Mechanotransduction: all signals point to cytoskeleton, matrix, and integrins.* Sci STKE, 2002, 2002(119): PE6.
47. Woodside, D.G., S. Liu, and M.H. Ginsberg, *Integrin activation.* Thromb Haemost, 2001, **86**(1): 316–23.
48. Shimaoka, M., J. Takagi, and T.A. Springer, *Conformational regulation of integrin structure and function.* Annu Rev Biophys Biomol Struct, 2002, **31**: 485–516.
49. Hynes, R.O., *Integrins: a family of cell surface receptors.* Cell, 1987, **48**(4): 549–54.
50. Hynes, R.O., *Integrins: bidirectional, allosteric signaling machines.* Cell, 2002, **110**(6): 673–87.
51. Schwartz, M.A., *Integrin signaling revisited.* Trends Cell Biol, 2001, **11**(12): 466–70.
52. Ng, T. et al., *PKCalpha regulates beta1 integrin-dependent cell motility through association and control of integrin traffic.* EMBO J, 1999, **18**(14): 3909–23.
53. Thodeti, C.K. et al., *ADAM12/syndecan-4 signaling promotes beta 1 integrin-dependent cell spreading through protein kinase Calpha and RhoA.* J Biol Chem, 2003, **278**(11): 9576–84.
54. Bos, J.L., *Linking Rap to cell adhesion.* Curr Opin Cell Biol, 2005, **17**(2): 123–8.
55. Bos, J.L. et al., *The role of Rap1 in integrin-mediated cell adhesion.* Biochem Soc Trans, 2003, **31**(Pt 1): 83–6.
56. Berrier, A.L. et al., *Activated R-ras, Rac1, PI 3-kinase and PKCepsilon can each restore cell spreading inhibited by isolated integrin beta1 cytoplasmic domains.* J Cell Biol, 2000, **151**(7): 1549–60.
57. Zhang, Z. et al., *Integrin activation by R-ras.* Cell, 1996, **85**(1): 61–9.
58. Lele, T.P., C.K. Thodeti, and D.E. Ingber, *Force meets chemistry: analysis of mechanochemical conversion in focal adhesions using fluorescence recovery after photobleaching.* J Cell Biochem, 2006, **97**(6): 1175–83.

59. Parker, K.K. and D.E. Ingber, *Extracellular matrix, mechanotransduction and structural hierarchies in heart tissue engineering*. Philos Trans R Soc Lond B Biol Sci, 2007, **362**(1484): 1267–79.
60. Chen, C.S. et al., *Geometric control of cell life and death*. Science, 1997, **276**(5317): 1425–8.
61. Ingber, D.E. et al., *Cell shape, cytoskeletal mechanics, and cell cycle control in angiogenesis*. J Biomech, 1995, **28**(12): 1471–84.
62. Chrzanowska-Wodnicka, M. and K. Burridge, *Rho-stimulated contractility drives the formation of stress fibers and focal adhesions*. J Cell Biol, 1996, **133**(6): 1403–15.
63. Riveline, D. et al., *Focal contacts as mechanosensors: externally applied local mechanical force induces growth of focal contacts by an mDia1-dependent and ROCK-independent mechanism*. J Cell Biol, 2001, **153**(6): 1175–86.
64. Bershadsky, A., M. Kozlov, and B. Geiger, *Adhesion-mediated mechanosensitivity: a time to experiment, and a time to theorize*. Curr Opin Cell Biol, 2006, **18**(5): 472–81.
65. Zamir, E. and B. Geiger, *Molecular complexity and dynamics of cell–matrix adhesions*. J Cell Sci, 2001, **114**(Pt 20): 3583–90.
66. Xia, N. et al., *Directional control of cell motility through focal adhesion positioning and spatial control of Rac activation*. FASEB J, 2008, **22**(6): 1649–59.
67. Tzima, E. et al., *A mechanosensory complex that mediates the endothelial cell response to fluid shear stress*. Nature, 2005, **437**(7057): 426–31.
68. Delcommenne, M. and C.H. Streuli, *Control of integrin expression by extracellular matrix*. J Biol Chem, 1995, **270**(45): 26794–801.
69. Lo, C.M. et al., *Cell movement is guided by the rigidity of the substrate*. Biophys J, 2000, **79**(1): 144–52.
70. Yeung, T. et al., *Effects of substrate stiffness on cell morphology, cytoskeletal structure, and adhesion*. Cell Motil Cytoskeleton, 2005, **60**(1): 24–34.
71. Guo, W. and F.G. Giancotti, *Integrin signalling during tumour progression*. Nat Rev Mol Cell Biol, 2004, **5**(10): 816–26.
72. Chen, F.A. et al., *Clones of tumor cells derived from a single primary human lung tumor reveal different patterns of beta 1 integrin expression*. Cell Adhes Commun, 1994, **2**(4): 345–57.
73. Owens, L.V. et al., *Overexpression of the focal adhesion kinase (p125FAK) in invasive human tumors*. Cancer Res, 1995, **55**(13): 2752–5.
74. Weiner, T.M. et al., *Expression of focal adhesion kinase gene and invasive cancer*. Lancet, 1993, **342**(8878): 1024–5.
75. Keely, P.J. et al., *Cdc42 and Rac1 induce integrin-mediated cell motility and invasiveness through PI(3)K*. Nature, 1997, **390**(6660): 632–6.
76. Deryugina, E.I. et al., *Functional activation of integrin alpha V beta 3 in tumor cells expressing membrane-type 1 matrix metalloproteinase*. Int J Cancer, 2000, **86**(1): 15–23.
77. Yilmaz, M. and G. Christofori, *EMT, the cytoskeleton, and cancer cell invasion*. Cancer Metastasis Rev, 2009, **28**(1–2): 15–33.
78. Noren, N.K. et al., *p120 catenin regulates the actin cytoskeleton via Rho family GTPases*. J Cell Biol, 2000, **150**(3): 567–80.
79. Noren, N.K. et al., *Cadherin engagement regulates Rho family GTPases*. J Biol Chem, 2001, **276**(36): 33305–8.
80. Wildenberg, G.A. et al., *p120-catenin and p190RhoGAP regulate cell–cell adhesion by coordinating antagonism between Rac and Rho*. Cell, 2006, **127**(5): 1027–39.
81. Cavallaro, U. and G. Christofori, *Cell adhesion and signalling by cadherins and Ig-CAMs in cancer*. Nat Rev Cancer, 2004, **4**(2): 118–32.
82. Czyz, J., *The stage-specific function of gap junctions during tumourigenesis*. Cell Mol Biol Lett, 2008, **13**(1): 92–102.
83. Kamibayashi, Y. et al., *Aberrant expression of gap junction proteins (connexins) is associated with tumor progression during multistage mouse skin carcinogenesis in vivo*. Carcinogenesis, 1995, **16**(6): 1287–97.

84. Kanczuga-Koda, L. et al., *Increased expression of connexins 26 and 43 in lymph node metastases of breast cancer*. J Clin Pathol, 2006, **59**(4): 429–33.
85. Miekus, K. et al., *Contact stimulation of prostate cancer cell migration: the role of gap junctional coupling and migration stimulated by heterotypic cell-to-cell contacts in determination of the metastatic phenotype of Dunning rat prostate cancer cells*. Biol Cell, 2005, **97**(12): 893–903.
86. Zhang, W. et al., *Increased invasive capacity of connexin43-overexpressing malignant glioma cells*. J Neurosurg, 2003, **99**(6): 1039–46.
87. Shimizu, K. et al., *Reduced expression of the Connexin26 gene and its aberrant DNA methylation in rat lung adenocarcinomas induced by N-nitrosobis(2-hydroxypropyl)a-mine*. Mol Carcinog, 2006, **45**(9): 710–4.
88. Hall, A. and C.D. Nobes, *Rho GTPases: molecular switches that control the organization and dynamics of the actin cytoskeleton*. Philos Trans R Soc Lond B Biol Sci, 2000, **355**(1399): 965–70.
89. Burridge, K. and K. Wennerberg, *Rho and Rac take center stage*. Cell, 2004, **116**(2): 167–79.
90. DeMali, K.A., K. Wennerberg, and K. Burridge, *Integrin signaling to the actin cytoskeleton*. Curr Opin Cell Biol, 2003, **15**(5): 572–82.
91. Tzima, E. et al., *Activation of integrins in endothelial cells by fluid shear stress mediates Rho-dependent cytoskeletal alignment*. EMBO J, 2001, **20**(17): 4639–47.
92. Fritz, G., I. Just, and B. Kaina, *Rho GTPases are over-expressed in human tumors*. Int J Cancer, 1999, **81**(5): 682–7.
93. Schnelzer, A. et al., *Rac1 in human breast cancer: overexpression, mutation analysis, and characterization of a new isoform, Rac1b*. Oncogene, 2000, **19**(26): 3013–20.
94. van Golen, K.L. et al., *RhoC GTPase, a novel transforming oncogene for human mammary epithelial cells that partially recapitulates the inflammatory breast cancer phenotype*. Cancer Res, 2000, **60**(20): 5832–8.
95. Paszek, M.J. and V.M. Weaver, *The tension mounts: mechanics meets morphogenesis and malignancy*. J Mammary Gland Biol Neoplasia, 2004, **9**(4): 325–42.
96. Clark, E.A. et al., *Genomic analysis of metastasis reveals an essential role for RhoC*. Nature, 2000, **406**(6795): 532–5.
97. Hakuma, N. et al., *E1AF/PEA3 activates the Rho/Rho-associated kinase pathway to increase the malignancy potential of non-small-cell lung cancer cells*. Cancer Res, 2005, **65**(23): 10776–82.
98. Jayachandran, G. et al., *Fragile histidine triad-mediated tumor suppression of lung cancer by targeting multiple components of the Ras/Rho GTPase molecular switch*. Cancer Res, 2007, **67**(21): 10379–88.
99. Shimada, T. et al., *Adenoviral transfer of rho family proteins to lung cancer cells ameliorates cell proliferation and motility and increases apoptotic change*. Kobe J Med Sci, 2007, **53**(3): 125–34.
100. Zhang, S. et al., *The tumor suppressor LKB1 regulates lung cancer cell polarity by mediating cdc42 recruitment and activity*. Cancer Res, 2008, **68**(3): 740–8.
101. Bhowmick, N.A. et al., *Transforming growth factor-beta1 mediates epithelial to mesenchymal transdifferentiation through a RhoA-dependent mechanism*. Mol Biol Cell, 2001, **12**(1): 27–36.
102. Croft, D.R. et al., *Conditional ROCK activation in vivo induces tumor cell dissemination and angiogenesis*. Cancer Res, 2004, **64**(24): 8994–9001.
103. Matsumoto, Y. et al., *Small GTP-binding protein, Rho, both increased and decreased cellular motility, activation of matrix metalloproteinase 2 and invasion of human osteosarcoma cells*. Jpn J Cancer Res, 2001, **92**(4): 429–38.
104. Xue, F. et al., *Blockade of Rho/Rho-associated coiled coil-forming kinase signaling can prevent progression of hepatocellular carcinoma in matrix metalloproteinase-dependent manner*. Hepatol Res, 2008, **38**(8): 810–817.

105. Frederick, L.A. et al., *Matrix metalloproteinase-10 is a critical effector of protein kinase Ciota-Par6alpha-mediated lung cancer.* Oncogene, 2008, **27**(35): 4841–53.
106. Matsui, T. et al., *Rho-kinase phosphorylates COOH-terminal threonines of ezrin/radixin/moesin (ERM) proteins and regulates their head-to-tail association.* J Cell Biol, 1998, **140**(3): 647–57.
107. Shaw, R.J. et al., *The Nf2 tumor suppressor, merlin, functions in Rac-dependent signaling.* Dev Cell, 2001, **1**(1): 63–72.
108. Akisawa, N. et al., *High levels of ezrin expressed by human pancreatic adenocarcinoma cell lines with high metastatic potential.* Biochem Biophys Res Commun, 1999, **258**(2): 395–400.
109. Khanna, C. et al., *Metastasis-associated differences in gene expression in a murine model of osteosarcoma.* Cancer Res, 2001, **61**(9): 3750–9.
110. Olson, M.F. and E. Sahai, *The actin cytoskeleton in cancer cell motility.* Clin Exp Metastasis, 2009, **26**(4): 273–87.
111. Wang, W., R. Eddy, and J. Condeelis, *The cofilin pathway in breast cancer invasion and metastasis.* Nat Rev Cancer, 2007, **7**(6): 429–40.
112. Keshamouni, V.G. et al., *Temporal quantitative proteomics by iTRAQ 2D-LC-MS/MS and corresponding mRNA expression analysis identify post-transcriptional modulation of actin-cytoskeleton regulators during TGF-beta-Induced epithelial–mesenchymal transition.* J Proteome Res, 2009, **8**(1): 35–47.
113. Keshamouni, V.G. et al., *Differential protein expression profiling by iTRAQ-2DLC-MS/MS of lung cancer cells undergoing epithelial–mesenchymal transition reveals a migratory/invasive phenotype.* J Proteome Res, 2006, **5**(5): 1143–54.
114. Mouneimne, G. et al., *Spatial and temporal control of cofilin activity is required for directional sensing during chemotaxis.* Curr Biol, 2006, **16**(22): 2193–205.
115. van Rheenen, J. et al., *EGF-induced PIP2 hydrolysis releases and activates cofilin locally in carcinoma cells.* J Cell Biol, 2007, **179**(6): 1247–59.
116. Varambally, S. et al., *Integrative genomic and proteomic analysis of prostate cancer reveals signatures of metastatic progression.* Cancer Cell, 2005, **8**(5): 393–406.
117. Feng, Y. and C.A. Walsh, *The many faces of filamin: a versatile molecular scaffold for cell motility and signalling.* Nat Cell Biol, 2004, **6**(11): 1034–8.
118. Bedolla, R.G. et al., *Nuclear versus cytoplasmic localization of filamin A in prostate cancer: immunohistochemical correlation with metastases.* Clin Cancer Res, 2009, **15**(3): 788–96.
119. Boyden, S., *The chemotactic effect of mixtures of antibody and antigen on polymorphonuclear leucocytes.* J Exp Med, 1962, **115**: 453–66.
120. Zigmond, S.H., *Ability of polymorphonuclear leukocytes to orient in gradients of chemotactic factors.* J Cell Biol, 1977, **75**(2 Pt 1): 606–16.
121. Goncharova, E.A., D.A. Goncharov, and V.P. Krymskaya, *Assays for in vitro monitoring of human airway smooth muscle (ASM) and human pulmonary arterial vascular smooth muscle (VSM) cell migration.* Nat Protoc, 2006, **1**(6): 2933–9.
122. Von Offenberg Sweeney, N. et al., *Cyclic strain-mediated regulation of vascular endothelial cell migration and tube formation.* Biochem Biophys Res Commun, 2005, **329**(2): 573–82.
123. Thodeti CK, F.C., Nielsen CK, Holck P, Sundberg C, Kveiborg M, Mahalingam Y, Albrechtsen R, Couchman JR, Wewer UM., *Hierarchy of ADAM12 binding to integrins in tumor cells.* Exp Cell Res, 2005, **309**: 438–50.
124. Dittmar, T. et al., *Induction of cancer cell migration by epidermal growth factor is initiated by specific phosphorylation of tyrosine 1248 of c-erbB-2 receptor via EGFR.* FASEB J, 2002, **16**(13): 1823–5.
125. Niggemann, B. et al., *Tumor cell locomotion: differential dynamics of spontaneous and induced migration in a 3D collagen matrix.* Exp Cell Res, 2004, **298**(1): 178–87.
126. Brandt, B. et al., *3D-extravasation model – selection of highly motile and metastatic cancer cells.* Semin Cancer Biol, 2005, **15**(5): 387–95.

127. Sahai, E., *Illuminating the metastatic process.* Nat Rev Cancer, 2007, **7**(10): 737–49.
128. Folkman, J., *Antiangiogenesis in cancer therapy–endostatin and its mechanisms of action.* Exp Cell Res, 2006, **312**(5): 594–607.
129. Maeshima, Y. et al., *Identification of the anti-angiogenic site within vascular basement membrane-derived tumstatin.* J Biol Chem, 2001, **276**(18): 15240–8.
130. Albert, J.M. et al., *Integrin alpha v beta 3 antagonist Cilengitide enhances efficacy of radiotherapy in endothelial cell and non-small-cell lung cancer models.* Int J Radiat Oncol Biol Phys, 2006, **65**(5): 1536–43.
131. Kuwada, S.K., *Drug evaluation: Volociximab, an angiogenesis-inhibiting chimeric monoclonal antibody.* Curr Opin Mol Ther, 2007, **9**(1): 92–8.
132. Thodeti, C.K., et al., *TRPV4 channels mediate cyclic strain-induced endothelial cell reorientation through integrin-to-integrin signaling.* Circ Res. 2009, **104**(9): 1123–30.

Immunologic Mechanisms in Lung Carcinogenesis and Metastasis

Jay M. Lee, Jane Yanagawa, Saswati Hazra, Sherven Sharma, Tonya Walser, Edward Garon, and Steven M. Dubinett

Abstract Progression and metastasis of cancer proceeds in the context of a host response that includes interactions with immune cells that can both attenuate and paradoxically promote the process of metastasis. Growing evidence demonstrating the role of the inflammatory response in carcinogenesis is shedding light on a functional relationship between the host immune system and the malignant neoplasm. The interaction between neoplasm and the immune system can be described with the concepts of (1) cancer immunosurveillance, (2) cancer immunoediting, (3) complicity of the host cellular networks in lung tumorigenesis, and (4) tumor-mediated immunosuppression. Understanding the molecular mechanisms involved in inflammation and lung carcinogenesis provides insight for new drug development that target reversible, non-mutational events in the chemoprevention and treatment of lung cancer.

Introduction

The acquisition of genetic mutations facilitates cancer development and the malignant phenotype and is critically linked to acquiring cellular properties associated with the malignant phenotype and metastatic spread. While genetic changes are important in cellular transformation into neoplastic cells, the inflammatory response in the tumor microenvironment is a significant contributor to tumor progression. This complex interaction between the neoplastic epithelial cells and the stromal inflammatory response is essential in malignant progression to metastasis. The functional relationship between inflammation, host immune system, and cancer is a more widely accepted concept due to the growing evidence that demonstrates the role of inflammatory response of immune cells in carcinogenesis [1–3]. The interaction between neoplasm and

J.M. Lee (✉)
Division of Cardiothoracic Surgery, Department of Surgery, UCLA Lung Cancer Research Program, Jonsson Comprehensive Cancer Center, David Geffen School of Medicine at UCLA, Los Angeles, CA 90095, USA
e-mail: jaymoonlee@mednet.ucla.edu

V. Keshamouni et al. (eds.), *Lung Cancer Metastasis*,
DOI 10.1007/978-1-4419-0772-1_6, © Springer Science+Business Media, LLC 2009

inflammation/immune system can be described with the concepts of (1) cancer immunosurveillance, (2) cancer immunoediting, (3) complicity of the host cellular networks in lung tumorigenesis, and (4) tumor-mediated immunosuppression. The understanding of molecular mechanisms involved in inflammation and lung carcinogenesis provides insight for new drug development that target reversible, non-mutational events in the chemoprevention and treatment of lung cancer.

Cancer Immunosurveillance

Paul Ehrlich first proposed the concept of the immune system-mediated suppression of tumor growth of cancer cells nearly 100 years ago [4], and Frank Macfarlane Burnet is credited with formulating the idea of cancer immunosurveillance with the introduction of the "clonal selection theory" in 1957 [5–7]. This concept suggested that the immune system recognized and destroyed clones of transformed cells before growth into clinically evident tumors [8]. A critical cornerstone of the cancer immunosurveillance hypothesis was subsequently demonstrated when mice were immunized against syngeneic tumor transplants that had been induced by chemical carcinogens or viruses [9]. Subsequent introduction of live tumor cells into the immunized mouse resulted in rejection of the tumor transplant. These studies were the initial findings that implied the existence of tumor-specific antigens. This hypothesis was eventually validated in a variety of more modern murine models in which immune deficiencies were noted to be associated with an increase in spontaneous as well as induced neoplasms [10]. The evidence that cancer immunosurveillance may be operative in humans is exemplified in studies that document an increase in cancer incidence among immunosuppressed organ transplant recipients [9, 11, 12]. In a study of heart transplant recipients, Pham and colleagues reported a prevalence of lung cancer that was 25-fold higher than the general population [11]. Dickson et al. reported a 6.9% incidence of de novo primary lung cancer in the native lung in single-lung transplant recipients, which was characterized by an aggressive and frequently fatal course, and the history of tobacco-related lung disease significantly increased the risk of developing bronchogenic cancer after transplantation [12]. These results demonstrated that single lung transplant patients had a significantly greater risk for developing lung cancer than the general non-transplanted population and double-lung transplant recipients [12]. In addition, histopathologic evidence demonstrating the presence of inflammatory infiltrates in areas surrounding tumors and the finding of lymphocytic proliferation in tumor draining lymph nodes further support the existence of cancer immunosurveillance.

More recently, Dieu-Nosjean et al. reported the existence of tumor-induced bronchus-associated lymphoid tissue within NSCLC tumors [13]. These tertiary lymphoid structures are composed of mature dendritic cell (DC) clusters adjacent to B-cell follicles and exhibit features of an ongoing immune response. The authors found that increased density of these intratumoral mature DCs correlated with better outcome. In murine tumor models, DCs transduced to secrete CCL21, a protein involved in leukocyte chemotaxis and activation, have been shown to result in the generation of tumor-specific T cells and tumor regression [14]. These studies suggest that manipulation of such natural immunologic mechanisms of tumor rejection have great potential for therapy. A phase I trial to assess the intratumoral administration of CCL21-secreting human DCs to treat advanced lung cancer is already underway at UCLA [15].

Cancer Immunoediting

Although the hypothesis of cancer immunosurveillance is supported by a wealth of compelling evidence from murine and human studies [6, 8–12], the process of cancer immunosurveillance has evolved into a more current concept termed "immunoediting" by Schreiber and colleagues [6, 8–10]. Given that immunocompetent individuals still develop malignancies despite the presence of an intact immune system and certain cancers are capable of escaping immune recognition and destruction, a complex interaction between the cancer cells and the host immune system may result in changing tumor immunogenicity. This is the fundamental basis of cancer immunoediting [6].

Prior to the detection of a clinically apparent lung cancer, there is an extensive interaction between the transformed cells and the host immune and inflammatory responses that may select for cancerous cells with the ability to survive in a competent immune environment. The ability of cancer cells to evade immune recognition may occur with acquisition of genetic mutations that facilitate the development of the malignant phenotype and subsequent tumor formation. These mutations may be critically linked to acquiring cellular properties associated with carcinogenesis, such as apoptosis resistance, unregulated proliferation, invasion, metastasis, and angiogenesis. Although both humoral (antibody) and cell-mediated immune (T lymphocyte) responses to the tumor have been demonstrated, the anti-tumor immune response has traditionally been understood as a cell-mediated process involving the presentation of tumor-associated antigens by antigen presenting cells (APC) to the T lymphocytes, resulting in the generation of immune effector cells with the ability to destroy cancerous cells [16]. Although anti-tumor humoral responses have been shown to exist in tumor-bearing hosts, protection of the host from tumor progression has not been convincing [16]. As APC take up tumor antigens, the adaptive immune system may be alerted as the tumor antigen is presented to T cells. Investigators have detected tumor-specific humoral and cellular responses in patients with lung cancer indicating that the host immune system has recognized the tumor [17, 18]. This immune recognition process through both humoral and cell-mediated mechanisms may result in the destruction of immunogenic tumor cells expressing a specific tumor antigen and result in the selection of immune-resistant and less immunogenic cancer cells. These remaining cells may possess properties to evade the immune system that include (1) failure to express major histocompatibility complex (MHC) which is required for immune effector cells to recognize processed tumor antigens and mediate cancer cell killing, (2) expression of poorly immunogenic antigen epitopes, or (3) production of immunosuppressive cytokines that suppress the anti-tumor immune responses. Thus, cancer immunoediting involves immuno-surveillance via a immune-mediated tumor cell selection process that leads to alterations in the immunogenicity of the cancer, and this incomplete tumor destruction results in a population of cancer cells with the ability to evade immune recognition and eradication [10]. Ultimately, these selected tumor cells resist immune and inflammatory responses, demonstrate the ability for progressive tumor growth, and result in a clinically detectable lung cancer.

Complicity of Host Cellular Networks in Lung Tumorigenesis

Although the ability of tumor cells to escape the immune effector contributes to cancer development, the pulmonary environment presents a unique milieu in which lung carcinogenesis proceeds in complicity with the host cellular network. Because inflammation appears to play an important role in the pathogenesis of lung cancer, a thorough understanding of lung cancer pathogenesis requires consideration of the tumor microenvironment (TME) and the inflammatory pathways operative in carcinogenesis [19].

The tobacco-induced pulmonary cellular network presents a unique environment in which carcinogenesis proceeds in complicity with surrounding lung inflammatory, structural, and stromal cells. The commonalities in smoking, COPD, and lung cancer begin with the profound alterations induced by cigarette smoke, which contains known carcinogens as well as high levels of reactive oxygen species (ROS). The ready induction of ROS following tobacco smoke exposure leads to impairment of epithelial and endothelial cell function as well as inflammation. The ongoing inflammatory processes in COPD may be persistent even following smoking cessation and have been quantified and related to disease progression [20]. As COPD progresses, the percentage of the airways that contain macrophages, neutrophils, T cells, B cells, and lymphoid aggregates containing follicles increases [20].

The pulmonary diseases that are associated with the greatest risk for lung cancer are characterized by abundant and deregulated inflammation [21–23]. Among the cytokines, growth factors, and mediators released in these lung diseases and the developing TME, IL-1β, PGE2, and TGF-β have been found to have deleterious properties that simultaneously pave the way for both destruction of specific host cell-mediated immune responses against tumor antigens and epithelial mesenchymal transition (EMT) [24–28].

EMT is the developmental shift from a polarized, epithelial phenotype to a highly motile mesenchymal phenotype (see Chapter 4) [29]. While this process is essential in embryogenesis and organ development, EMT is also critically involved in much adult pathology, including cancer, chronic inflammation, and fibrosis [29, 30]. Although EMT is a tightly regulated phenomenon during embryonic development [31], in cancer progression this process is unregulated with selective elements of the process amplified and other aspects circumvented [32].

The connection between inflammation and EMT progression in lung cancer development and resistance to therapy has recently been emphasized [24, 33]. For example, IL-1β and PGE2 have the capacity to decrease E-cadherin expression and promote EMT. These inflammatory mediators have the capacity to upregulate the zinc-finger E-box-binding transcriptional repressors of E-cadherin including Zeb1, Snail, and Slug, thus leading to EMT progression [24, 34]. Recent work from Robert Weinberg's laboratory suggests a direct link between EMT and gain of epithelial stem cell properties [35]. Thus, inflammation may impact stem cell properties via EMT-dependent events in the pathogenesis of lung cancer. While EMT-induced alterations have been widely implicated in the epithelial malignancy metastatic process, the work of Mani et al. [35] suggests that the EMT genetic program may also regulate early events in carcinogenesis, therefore implicating the inflammatory pulmonary environment in both lung cancer initiation and progression. The fact that tobacco and tobacco-specific carcinogens may be involved by directly or indirectly promoting EMT adds additional importance to these relationships. For example, Yoshino et al. [36] found that benzo[a]pyrene induced EMT-related genes in lung cancer cells; while fibronectin and Twist were induced, E-cadherin expression was decreased. In support of these findings, and in the context of another tobacco-induced malignancy, Fondrevelle et al. [37] found that the expression of Twist was influenced by smoking status in bladder cancer patients. Tobacco-specific carcinogen 4-(n-methyl-n-nitrosamino)-1-(3-pyridyl)-1-butanone (NNK) has also been found to promote EMT via induction of E-cadherin transcriptional repressors in human bronchial epithelial cells [38].

Thus lung cancer develops in a host environment in which the deregulated inflammatory response promotes tumor progression.

Tumor-Mediated Immunosuppression

It was originally hypothesized more than 30 years ago that specialized T cell subpopulations existed to suppress immune responses [39]. North and others pursued this avenue of investigation within the context of tumor immunity [40–43]. However, these early studies in the field of suppressor T cells were stymied by an inability to characterize the cellular and molecular mechanisms responsible for the observed suppressive phenomena. There has been a renewed interest in the study of T-cell-mediated suppression of immunity that has been accompanied by the identification of regulatory T cells. Although a variety of T regulatory cells have been described [44], much attention has focused on the specific activities of those that have been referred to as "naturally occurring" CD4 + CD25^{high} T regulatory cells [45, 46] and hereafter will be referred to as CD4 + CD25 + T reg cells. Although investigators had pursued this topic for many years, the groundbreaking studies of Sakaguchi et al. [47] have been viewed as initiating a renaissance in T reg cell research; these, as well as more recent results, have led to the characterization of the CD4 + CD25 + T cell population as "professional suppressor cells" [45]. These studies revealed that transfer of CD25-depleted CD4 cells to nude mice recipients resulted in the spontaneous development of autoimmune disease [47]. Reconstitution of CD4 + CD25 + cells within a limited period after transfer of CD4 + CD25– cells prevented the autoimmune disease in a dose-dependent fashion. These initial studies indicated that CD4 + CD25 + cells contribute to the maintenance of self-tolerance by downregulating immune response to self and non-self-antigens; elimination or reduction of CD4 + CD25 + cells ablated this general suppression, and thereby not only enhanced immune responses to non-self-antigens but also elicited autoimmune responses to certain self-antigens [47]. Subsequent studies have revealed that these cells are both hyporesponsive and suppressive and can act through an APC-independent pathway [47–50]. The CD4 + CD25 + cells were found to require TCR-dependent activation for induction of suppressor activity [50]. The thymic origin of CD4 + CD25 + T reg cells has been documented [51, 52]. As originally hypothesized by Shevach [53] and subsequently demonstrated by Jordan et al. [54], the derivation of T reg cells in the thymus appears to occur through a process referred to as "altered negative selection." More recently it has been appreciated that T reg cells can differentiate from activated human PBL CD4 + CD25– cells in the periphery [55, 56]. Although many aspects of this peripheral T reg cell differentiation pathway have not yet been defined, it may be pivotal in limiting immune responses to human cancer.

The active immune suppression induced by the tumor has been well docu-mented in lung cancer and other malignancies [57]. Tumor-reactive T cells have been shown to accumulate in lung cancer tissues but fail to respond [58, 59]. In fact, a high proportion of NSCLC tumor-infiltrating lymphocytes (TIL) are CD4 + CD25^{high} T regulatory (T reg) cells [60]. Tumor cells may contribute to promoting immune suppression by directing surrounding inflammatory cells to release suppressive cytokines in the tumor milieu, augmenting the trafficking of suppressor cells to the tumor site, and/or promoting differentiation of effector lymphocytes to a T reg cell phenotype [61, 62]. Liu et al. recently demonstrated that tumor cells could directly convert CD4 + CD25– T cells to T reg cells through the production of high levels of TGF-β, suggesting a possible mechan-ism through which tumor cells evade the immune system [63]. One major impediment to effective therapy is our inadequate understanding of how lung cancer cells escape immune surveillance and inhibit anti-tumor immunity [64]. In previous studies an immune suppressive network in NSCLC that is due to overexpression of tumor cyclooxygenase 2 (COX-2) has been defined. COX-2 isoenzyme activity is significantly increased in cancerous tissues compared to their normal counterparts in several malignancies and studies document this overexpression in human lung cancer [65]. In murine lung cancer models specific genetic or pharmacological inhibition of COX-2 in vivo led to significant tumor regression [66]. Although COX-2 metabolites have been identified as mediators of immunosuppression, the specific molecular and cellular pathways in the COX-2-dependent immune suppressive network are now being defined. Particular attention has recently focused on defining the pathways whereby COX-2 and its metabolite prostaglandin E2 (PGE2) inhibit immune responses in lung cancer by promoting T regulatory cell activity. PGE2 promotes the CD4 + CD25 + T regulatory phenotype and increases the expression of the forkhead transcription factor FOXP3 that is known to program the development and function of T reg cells. This pivotal relationship is currently under investigation in the laboratory utilizing human cells in vitro as well as in patients with lung cancer. Based on the results of pre-clinical murine models [67] and human cells in vitro [26], clinical studies are now evaluating the optimal biological dose of a COX-2 inhibitor, celecoxib, to decrease FOXP3 and T regulatory function in patients with lung cancer.

COX-2

Cyclooxygenase (also referred to as prostaglandin endoperoxidase or prostaglandin G hydroperoxide synthase) is the rate-limiting enzyme for the production of eicosanoids, prostaglandins (PGs) and thromboxanes (TX), from free arachidonic acid, which is released from the membrane phospholipids by phospholipase A2 [68]. Cyclooxygenase is bound to the cytosolic side of the endoplasmic reticulum and cell membrane [69]. It is a bifunctional enzyme, with fatty acid cyclooxygenase (COX) activity producing PGG2 from arachidonic acid and two O_2 molecules and PG hydroperoxidase (HOX) activity in which PGG2 undergoes a two-electron reduction to PGH2 [70, 71]. PGH2 is converted to final products by isomerases and individual prostaglandin (PG) synthases that are often expressed in a cell type-dependent manner. Three forms of COX have now been described [72–74]. COX-1 is constitutively expressed in most cells and tissues; its activity appears to depend entirely on substrate availability. Alternatively, an inducible isoenzyme, COX-2, acts as an immediate early gene expressed in response to cytokines, growth factors, and other stimuli. All COX isoforms share the same structural features including a hydrophobic channel that allows the arachidonic acid bearing a constrained hairpin configuration to access the COX catalytic site [70, 71].

Thromboxanes and prostacyclins are short-lived molecules with half-lives on the order of seconds, whereas prostaglandins (PGs) have half-lives within the range of tens of minutes to hours [75, 76]. Interacting with their cell surface

G-protein (heterotrimeric GTP-binding protein)-coupled receptors (GPCR), PGs serve as autocrine and paracrine mediators of "housekeeping" functions, including the regulation of renal water and sodium metabolism, stomach acid secretion, parturition, and homeostasis. It has been shown that in certain experimental settings some PGs, especially PGJ2, are able to bind nuclear receptors such as PPAR-gamma [77]. At least nine PG receptors have been identified to date, four of which bind PGE2 and two bind PGD2. There are individual receptors for PGF2-alpha, PGI2, and TxA2 [69]. Among other PGs, PGE2 is a major COX-2 metabolite abundantly present in the cancer micro-environment, and it is an important mediator of immune regulation [78], epithelial cell growth and invasion [79], as well as epithelial survival [80].

COX-2 and Lung Cancer

Several studies have demonstrated high-level constitutive COX-2 expression in human NSCLC [65, 81–89]. In the initial report describing COX-2 in human lung cancer, Huang et al. assessed COX-2 expression in NSCLC and normal adjacent lung tissue of resected specimens by immunohistochemistry [65]. All of the 15 tumor specimens (8 adenocarcinomas and 7 squamous cell carcinomas) showed cytoplasmic staining for COX-2 in tumor cells. In contrast, adjacent normal lung showed no COX-2 staining in the alveolar lining epithelium, but demonstrated positive cytoplasmic staining often in alveolar macrophages and occasionally in bronchiolar epithelium. Wolff et al. showed with immunohistochemistry that COX-2 was expressed in 19 of 21 adenocarcinomas and in all 11 squamous cell carcinomas studied [82]. Hida et al. reported that COX-2 overexpression was seen in approximately 70% of lung adenocarcinomas [87]. The level of staining appeared to be less in squamous cell carcinomas than in the adenocarcinomas. Hida et al. reported that COX-2 expression was documented in one-third of atypical adenomatous hyperplasias and carcinomas in situ which support the role of COX-2 throughout the progression from pre-malignant lesion to the metastatic phenotype [87]. In addition, the same study demonstrated a greater proportion of lung cancer cells staining positively in lymph node metastases compared to the corresponding primary tumor [87]. In the report from Tsubochi and colleagues, there was a significant association between COX-2 expression and lymph node metastasis in patients with adenocarcinomas, but evaluation of squamous cell carcinomas did not demonstrate this relationship [86].

Other studies have corroborated and expanded on these initial findings further documenting the importance of COX-2 in lung cancer [83–85, 88, 89]. Khuri et al. evaluated COX-2 expression in specimens from 160 stage I NSCLC patients by in situ hybridization and reported that COX-2 overexpression appears to portend a shorter survival among patients with early-stage NSCLC [83]. The strength of COX-2 expression was associated with both a decreased overall survival rate (p = 0.001) and a diminished disease-free survival rate (p = 0.022) [83]. Tsubochi et al. showed the relationship between COX-2 expression and poor prognosis in stage I adenocarcinomas [86]. Other reports have associated tumor COX-2 overexpression with poor prognosis as well independent of TNM stage in surgically resected NSCLC [83]. These reports, together with other studies documenting an increase in COX-2 expression in precursor lesions [81, 82], a common polymorphism in the COX-2 gene associated with increased risk of lung cancer [90], and epidemiological studies that indicate a decreased incidence of lung cancer in patients who regularly take aspirin [91], all support the involvement of COX-2 in the pathogenesis of lung cancer.

Mounting evidence indicates that tumor COX-2 activity has a multi-faceted role in conferring the malignant and metastatic phenotype of lung cancer. Although multiple genetic alterations are necessary for lung cancer invasion and metastasis, COX-2 may be a central element in orchestrating this process [62, 86, 87, 89] and has been implicated in apoptosis resistance [80, 92], angiogenesis [93, 94], decreased host immunity [26, 66], and enhanced invasion and metastasis [95, 96]. These newly discovered molecular mechanisms in the pathogenesis of lung cancer provide novel opportunities for targeted therapies in NSCLC carcinogenesis [97, 98]. COX-2 is one of the targets under investigation for lung cancer therapy and chemoprevention [99, 100].

COX-2 Downstream Signaling: Prostanoid Receptors

The prostanoid receptors are in the superfamily of G-protein-coupled receptors (GPCR). PGE2 exerts its multiple effects through four GPCR designated as EP1, EP2, EP3, and EP4 [74]. Studies of the receptor subtypes have shown that the EP1 receptor acts via G_q protein and upon activation increases cellular Ca^{2+} levels. Studies indicate EP1 receptors can be localized not only on the cell membrane but also on the nuclear membrane [101]. The EP2 and EP4 receptor signaling is mediated by G_s G-proteins and leads to activation of adenylate cyclase and elevated cAMP synthesis. In contrast, EP3 signaling through G_i inhibits adenylate cyclase and cAMP synthesis [102].

The EP_4 receptor is critically involved in inducing the expression of COX-2 and PGE_2 synthase [103]. We have previously demonstrated the importance of PGE2 and its signaling through the EP4 receptor in mediating NSCLC invasiveness and shown that genetic inhibition of tumor COX-2 led to diminished matrix metalloproteinase (MMP)-2, CD44, and EP4 receptor expression and invasion [96]. These findings indicate that PGE2 regulates COX-2-dependent, CD44- and MMP-2-mediated invasion in NSCLC via EP receptor signaling [96]. Yang and colleagues revealed in a murine model that tumor metastasis to the lung was significantly reduced when treated with a specific EP4 antagonist or when EP4 receptor expression was knocked down in the tumor cells using

RNA interference technology [104]. In addition, the host EP4 receptors contribute to tumor metastasis and tumor growth with decreased metastasis and tumor growth in EP4 receptor knockout animals [104]. Further evidence supporting the role of prostanoid receptors in lung carcinogenesis was shown by the fibronectin-mediated stimulation of human lung carcinoma cell proliferation through the PGE_2 receptor subtype EP4 [105]. Thus, blocking the COX-2-dependent PGE2 production or activity by targeting the downstream signaling pathway of COX-2, such as EP4 receptor, may produce more profound anticancer effects than COX-2 inhibition alone. This could be the basis for new approaches in chemoprevention or treatment of NSCLC.

Reversal of Epithelial–Mesenchymal Transition

EMT requires alterations in cell morphology, adhesion, and migration [30]. These cellular changes result in variable expression of proteins which serve as EMT markers. Decreased E-cadherin level is a hallmark feature of EMT, which allows reduction in cell-to-cell adhesion and enhances migratory capacity [30]. We have previously shown a COX-2-dependent transcriptional regulation of E-cadherin expression and cellular aggregation in NSCLC, and a reciprocal relationship between COX-2 and E-cadherin, as well as ZEB1 and E-cadherin [24]. COX-2 and PGE2 expression resulted in significant reduction in E-cadherin via a ZEB1 and Snail transcriptional factor-mediated mechanism and inhibition of COX-2 resulted in rescue of E-cadherin expression [24]. Thus, therapies targeting the COX pathway may diminish the propensity for tumor metastasis in NSCLC by blocking the PGE_2-mediated induction of E-cadherin transcriptional repressors. This newly defined pathway for transcriptional regulation of E-cadherin in NSCLC has important implications for chemoprevention and treatment of NSCLC using COX-2 inhibitors in combination with other agents. For example, E-cadherin expression in NSCLC has recently been implicated as a marker of sensitivity to epidermal growth factor receptor (EGFR) tyrosine kinase inhibitors (TKI) [106]. Concordantly, low-serum E-cadherin levels have also been found to correlate with response to combination therapy with erlotinib and celecoxib in patients with NSCLC [107]. By enhancing E-cadherin expression, COX-2 inhibitors may therefore augment sensitivity to EGFR TKI therapy [108].

Histone deacetylase (HDAC) inhibitors may be another strategy to increase E-cadherin and overcome EGFR inhibitor resistance in patients with lung cancer. Transcriptional repressor, ZEB1, inhibits E-cadherin expression by recruiting HDAC. Witta et al. have shown that E-cadherin transfection into a gefitinib-resistant line increased its sensitivity to gefitinib, and pretreating resistant cell lines with an HDAC inhibitor induced E-cadherin and EGFR [109]. This resulted in enhanced growth inhibition and apoptosis effect of gefitinib similar to that in gefitinib-sensitive NSCLC cell lines [109]. Thus, combined HDAC inhibitor and gefitinib treatment may represent a potential strategy to overcome resistance to EGFR TKI.

Bone morphogenetic protein-7 (BMP-7), also known as osteogenic protein-1, is a member of the transforming growth factor-β (TGF-β) superfamily [110–112]. It is expressed during embryonic development and plays an important role in organogenesis [111, 112]. BMP-7 production is highest in the kidney, and its genetic deletion in murine studies revealed severe impairment in eye, skeletal, and kidney development [110]. In the embryonic lung, BMP-5 and BMP-7 expression has been detected in the mesenchyme and endoderm, respectively, and BMP-4 expression has been restricted to the distal epithelial cells and the adjacent mesenchyme [113]. TGF-β is a major regulator and inducer of EMT [30]. Zeisberg et al. have reported that BMP-7 reverses the TGF-β1-induced EMT by re-induction of E-cadherin through a Smad-dependent mechanism in renal tubular epithelial cells and mammary ductal epithelial cells [114]. In addition, administration of BMP-7 led to repair of severely damaged renal tubular epithelial cells and reversal of chronic renal injury [114]. These results provide evidence of the complex interaction between BMP-7 and TGF-β1 in the regulation of EMT and imply a potential role of BMP-7 as a therapeutic target in reversing EMT in carcinogenesis.

Interaction Between COX-2 and EGFR Signaling

Inflammation and receptor tyrosine kinase signaling pathways form complex networks with multiple overlapping modules that have proven to contribute to malignant phenotypes [33]. COX-2/PGE2 and EGFR cross-signaling has been one of the most extensively studied relationships between these pathways. Studies demonstrating that EGFR and COX-2 can interact to regulate cellular proliferation, migration, and invasion [79, 115–118] have triggered interest in evaluating the combination of COX-2 and EGFR inhibition in NSCLC. Coffey et al. [117] demonstrated that the activation of EGFR by transforming growth factor alpha stimulates COX-2 production resulting in increased release of PGE2 and increased mitogenesis. They also showed that COX-2 inhibition in a human colon cancer cell line led to attenuation of TGF-α activity. Another study [118] evaluated the effects of PGE2 on EGFR activation in a colon cancer cell line. PGE2 induced increased phosphorylation of EGFR and Erk 1/2, leading to cell proliferation. Inactivation of EGFR TK with selective inhibitors resulted in decreased PGE2-related Erk activation, decreased c-fos mRNA production, and decreased cell proliferation. In addition, EGFR inhibitors have been associated with a decrease in the production of angiogenic factors such as IL-8 and VEGF [119, 120]. This has also been found to be a mechanism of angiogenesis inhibition by COX-2 inhibitors [121, 122]. When studied in combination in a familial adenomatous polyposis (FAP) mouse model, treatment with EKB-785 (an EGFR TKI) and sulindac (a COX inhibitor) resulted in a 95–97% reduction in the incidence of colonic polyps [123]. Consistent with these findings, the co-expression of EGFR and COX-2 in human cervical cancer specimens portends a poor prognosis with increased recurrences [124]. Recently, Chen et al. [125] reported that the combination of an EGFR TKI with celecoxib either additively or synergistically inhibited growth of squamous cell carcinoma of the head and neck (SCCHN), significantly induced G1 arrest and apoptosis, and suppressed capillary formation of endothelium. Furthermore, the combination showed strong reduction of EGFR, Erk1/2, and Akt phosphorylation in SCCHN cells as compared with the single agents [125]. Importantly, we have recently found a novel mechanism of PGE2-induced EGFR TKI resistance in NSCLC mediated through an EGFR-independent activation of the MAPK/Erk signaling pathway [79]. In these investigations, we demonstrate that PGE2 is able to completely overcome the growth inhibitory activity of EGFR TKIs in approximately 40% of NSCLC cell lines.

COX-2 Clinical Trials

Based on these findings, recent studies have been conducted evaluating combined inhibition of the EGFR and COX-2 pathways in patients with NSCLC. Gadgeel et al. [126] reported a phase II study of gefitinib and celecoxib in patients with platinum refractory NSCLC. Patients received gefitinib 250 mg daily and celecoxib 400 mg twice daily. The response rate to the combination of celecoxib and gefitinib was similar to that observed with gefitinib alone. O'Byrne [127] recently reported a phase I/II trial of combination therapy with gefitinib (250 mg/day) and rofecoxib (50 mg/day) in patients with platinum-pretreated relapsed NSCLC. Gefitinib combined with rofecoxib was found to provide disease control rates equivalent to that expected with single-agent gefitinib. The lack of beneficial effect of combined EGFR TKI and COX-2 inhibitor therapy from these studies raises the question of whether higher dosage may have a critical effect on efficacy.

Reckamp et al. conducted a phase I trial evaluating escalating doses of celecoxib (200–800 mg twice daily) in combination with a fixed dose of erlotinib (150 mg/day) in late-stage NSCLC patients and established an optimal biological dose (OBD) of 600 mg twice daily, as defined by the maximal decrease in urinary prostaglandin E-M (PGE-M) [108]. This study revealed an acceptable toxicity profile with combination therapy and demonstrated a disease control rate above that expected for erlotinib alone. Based on these results, a phase II trial is planned to assess combination therapy with celecoxib at 600 mg twice daily and erlotinib versus single-agent erlotinib. The use of COX-2 inhibitors at the optimal biological dose may improve efficacy of combination therapy and may explain the lack of benefit in some trials in which a lower dose of COX-2 inhibitors was used. Although the use of COX-2 inhibitors at the optimal biological dose may promote responses to combination therapy, there may be associated toxicities with the use of COX-2 inhibitors. Gridelli et al. [128] evaluated the addition of rofecoxib (50 mg/day) to cisplatin and gemcitabine in stage IV or IIIB NSCLC subjects. The groups receiving rofecoxib were closed early due to safety issues surrounding the higher frequency of cardiac ischemia in subjects that received rofecoxib at 50 mg/day [128]. In a cumulative meta-analysis of 18 randomized controlled trials and 11 observational studies, Juni et al. reported on the increased risk of myocardial infarction in subjects who received rofecoxib [129]. Other reports have shown that rofecoxib exhibits a greater risk of cardiovascular toxicity as compared to celecoxib and may be dose dependent [130]. Solomon et al. found that rofecoxib was associated with a greater incidence of cardiovascular toxicity compared to celecoxib and NSAIDS and that patients taking rofecoxib at >25 mg doses were associated with higher risk than lower doses [130]. These studies suggest that COX-2 inhibitors may have differing cardiovascular risk and dose may also determine safety profile. It is unclear if cardiac ischemia will occur at a higher risk with short-term usage of COX-2 inhibitors alone or in combination with targeted therapies or conventional chemotherapy.

Several ongoing clinical trials are evaluating COX-2 inhibitors as adjuvants to chemotherapy in patients with advanced NSCLC. Lilenbaum and colleagues reported a phase II trial of irinotecan/docetaxel or irinotecan/gemcitabine with or without celecoxib to determine if COX-2 inhibition may enhance the efficacy of these chemotherapeutic agents [131]. Patients were randomly assigned to receive irinotecan 60 mg/m^2 and docetaxel 35 mg/m^2, or irinotecan 100 mg/m^2 and gemcitabine 1,000 mg/m^2, with or without celecoxib 400 mg twice daily, for four cycles [131]. The median survival was 6.31 months for patients treated with celecoxib and 8.99 months for those treated with chemotherapy alone, and the 1-year survival rates were 24 and 36%, respectively [131]. COX-2 inhibition did not appear to enhance efficacy of this chemotherapeutic regimen.

However, critical to the interpretation of these studies and to the design of future studies is the consideration of patient selection. Chan A et al. [132] compared the use of aspirin on the relative risk of colorectal cancer in relation to the expression of COX-2 in the tumor. The authors found that the regular use of aspirin only reduces the risk of colorectal cancers that overexpress COX-2 but not in those with either weak or absent expression of COX-2. Similarly, a randomized phase II trial [133] to assess whether there was benefit with dual eicosanoid inhibition or with either agent (celecoxib or zileuton) alone in addition to chemotherapy found an advantage only for celecoxib and chemotherapy in patients with moderate to high tumor expression of COX-2. These studies illustrate the importance of a more individualized approach to therapy that ideally minimizes the risk–benefit ratio and improves efficacy in future clinical trials.

Targeted Prevention

Crucial to the development of preventive strategies are the elucidation of the molecular mechanisms leading to the transformation of normal tissues to cancer and ways to stratify patients' risk.

Inflammatory pathways are believed to play an important role in lung cancer initiation [134]. CXCR2 and its ligands, which are associated with inflammatory and proangiogenic functions, is one such pathway implicated in the development of lung cancer. In a murine model where mice develop lung adenocarcinoma due to somatic activation of the KRAS oncogene, vascular endothelial cells and neutrophils with high expression of CXCR2 and CXCR2 ligands were found in pre-malignant alveolar lesions. Importantly, CXCR2 inhibition blocked the expansion of early alveolar neoplastic lesions [135].

Several reports have also documented high constitutive expression of COX-2 in precursor lesions in addition to established lung cancers, leading to studies that have focused on the potential role of COX-2 inhibitors in chemoprevention. Mao et al. reported on the feasibility of celecoxib as a chemopreventive agent for lung cancer by administering heavy current smokers with a 6-month course of oral celecoxib and performing serial bronchoscopies with bronchoalveolar lavage and biopsy [136]. Treatment with celecoxib significantly reduced the Ki-67 labeling index in smokers by 35% (p = 0.016) and increased the expression of nuclear survivin by 23% (p = 0.036) without significantly changing that of cytoplasmic survivin [136]. These findings support the hypothesis that oral administration of celecoxib is capable of modulating Ki-67 labeling index in the bronchial tissue of active smokers at high risk for developing lung cancers [136]. Larger randomized, placebo-controlled clinical trials are underway to determine efficacy of COX-2 inhibitors in preventing the development of bronchogenic carcinoma [100, 137].

Another potential pathway linking inflammation and lung cancer progression is the expression of the transcription factor Snail. Best known as an inducer of EMT, inflammatory mediators (including TGF-β, IL-1β, and PGE2) have been shown to upregulate Snail [24, 34, 138]. Elevated levels of Snail exist in both human lung cancers and pre-malignant lesions, and Snail overexpression enhances diverse malignant phenotypes in NSCLC cell lines as well as in immortalized human bronchial epithelial cell lines [139, 140].

Factors such as these that play a pathologic role across the spectrum of carcinogenesis – from premalignancy to advanced disease – hold unique potential as targets for therapy. For example, 30% of lung cancer patients after resection of early disease develop recurrence. In this population, targeting these factors could potentially treat patients for any remnant of the cancer they already have while simultaneously preventing the cancer they are at risk of developing.

Advances in risk assessment play a crucial role in the development of preventive measures. For example, COPD has long been well established to be associated with lung cancer risk [141], and recent studies emphasize the integral role of inflammation as a potential central shared pathway in the pathogenesis of COPD and lung cancer [134]. This opens an intriguing field of investigation to assess the capacity of agents that limit inflammation in patients with COPD to serve as lung cancer chemoprevention. For example, a cohort study has already suggested that inhaled corticosteroids may have a role in lung cancer prevention in patients who have COPD [142]. By studying another high-risk group for lung cancer – current and ex-smokers – radiographic assessments of emphysema and spirometric evaluation of airflow obstruction have been correlated to lung cancer risk in this population, providing potential clinical and imaging parameters for lung cancer risk assessment [143]. Such assessments direct the appropriate attention and potential chemopreventive measures to the people who need it most.

Conclusion

Lung carcinogenesis is a complex process involving the acquisition of genetic mutations that lead to cancer development and the malignant phenotype. These mutations are critically linked to interrelated steps in tumorigenesis including apoptosis resistance, unregulated proliferation, invasion, angiogenesis, and metastasis. While genetic changes are essential in cellular transformation into neoplastic cells, the stromal inflammatory response in the tumor microenvironment has equally a significant role in cancer progression and metastasis. This complex interaction between the neoplasm and the host immune system can be described by the concepts of (1) cancer immunosurveillance, (2) cancer immunoediting, (3) complicity of the host cellular networks in lung tumorigenesis, and (4) tumor-mediated immunosuppression.

Elucidation of the molecular mechanisms involved in these cellular changes provides opportunities to develop innovative therapies. COX-2 has been implicated in apoptosis resistance, angiogenesis, decreased host immunity, and enhanced invasion and metastasis and thus has a pivotal role in carcinogenesis. COX-2 is one of the targets under investigation for lung cancer therapy and chemoprevention. Furthermore, targeting the downstream signaling pathways of COX-2 may produce more profound effects than COX-2 inhibition alone, and thus strategies to antagonize the prostanoid receptors, such as EP4, are potential candidate targets in cancer prevention and therapy.

EMT in cancer is an unregulated process in a host environment with deregulated inflammatory response that degrades CMI and permits lung cancer progression. Understanding transcriptional regulation of key features in EMT, such as the downregulation of E-cadherin, has important implications for chemoprevention and treatment of NSCLC using COX-2 inhibitors in combination with other agents. COX-2 inhibition enhances tumor E-cadherin expression and may therefore augment sensitivity to other anti-tumor agents, such as EGFR TKI therapy. Based on these observations, several ongoing clinical trials are currently evaluating COX-2 inhibitors as adjuvants to chemotherapy in patients with advanced NSCLC and to determine efficacy of COX-2 inhibitors in prevention of bronchogenic carcinoma. In addition, the reversal of EMT has been a focus of intense investigation. As further understanding of the complex interaction between BMP-7 and TGF-β in the regulation of EMT is required, strategies to enhance BMP-7 expression are potential therapeutic targets to reverse EMT in lung carcinogenesis. Strategies to inhibit transcriptional repressors such as Snail may also prove to be an effective method to combat EMT-related malignant phenotypes.

Given the immunosuppressive environment in the tumor, investigators are attempting to reverse these events by stimulating host immune responses against tumor antigens in lung cancer. Both TGF-β and PGE2 are among the mediators that promote the CD4 + CD25 + T regulatory phenotype and increase the expression of the forkhead transcription factor FOXP3 that is known to program the development and function of T reg cells. These pivotal relationships are currently under investigation in the laboratory, and clinical studies are underway currently to evaluate the optimal biological dose of a COX-2 inhibitor, celecoxib, to decrease FOXP3 and T regulatory function in patients with lung cancer.

In summary, the elucidation of molecular mechanisms involved in inflammation and lung carcinogenesis, in combination with the appropriate attention to patient selection and risk assessment, will provide insight for new drug developments that target the reversible, non-mutational events that contribute to tumor progression in lung cancer.

References

1. DeNardo, D.G., M. Johansson, and L.M. Coussens. Immune cells as mediators of solid tumor metastasis. Cancer Metastasis Rev 27: 11–8, 2008.
2. de Visser, K.E., A. Eichten, and L.M. Coussens. Paradoxical roles of the immune system during cancer development. Nat Rev Cancer 6: 24–37, 2006.
3. Balkwill, F., K.A. Charles, and A. Mantovani. Smoldering and polarized inflammation in the initiation and promotion of malignant disease. Cancer Cell 7: 211–7, 2005.
4. Schwartz, R.S. Paul Ehrlich's magic bullets. N Engl J Med 350: 1079–80, 2004.
5. Fenner, F. and G. Ada Frank. MacFarlane Burnet: two personal views. Nat Immunol 8: 111–3, 2007.
6. Dunn, G.P., L.J. Old, and R.D. Schreiber. The immunobiology of cancer immunosurveillance and immunoediting. Immunity 21: 137–48, 2004.
7. Burnet, F.M. The Clonal Selection Theory of Acquired Immunity. London: Cambridge University Press, 1959.
8. O'Mahony, D. and S. Kummar, and M.E. Gutierrez. Non-small-cell lung cancer vaccine therapy: a concise review. J Clin Oncol 23: 9022–8, 2005.
9. Dunn, G.P., L.J. Old, and R.D. Schreiber. The three Es of cancer immunoediting. Annu Rev Immunol 22: 329–60, 2004.
10. Dunn, G.P., A.T. Bruce, H. Ikeda, L.J. Old, and R.D. Schreiber. Cancer immunoediting: from immunosurveillance to tumor escape. Nat Immunol 3: 991–8, 2002.
11. Pham, S.M., R.L. Kormos, R.J. Landreneau, A. Kawai, I. Gonzalez-Cancel, R.L. Hardesty, B.G. Hattler, and B.P. Griffith. Solid tumors after heart transplantation: lethality of lung cancer. Ann Thorac Surg 60: 1623–6, 1995.
12. Dickson, R.P., R.D. Davis, J.B. Rea, and S.M. Palmer. High frequency of bronchogenic carcinoma after single-lung transplantation. J Heart Lung Transplant 25: 1297–301, 2006.

13. Dieu-Nosjean, M.C., M. Antoine, C. Danel, D. Heudes, M. Wislez, V. Poulot, N. Rabbe, L. Laurans, E. Tartour, L. de Chaisemartin, S. Lebecque, W.H. Fridman, and J. Cadranel. Long-term survival for patients with non-small-cell lung cancer with intratumoral lymphoid structures. J Clin Oncol 26: 4410–7, 2008.
14. Kirk, C.J., D. Hartigan-O'Connor, and J.J. Mule. The dynamics of the T-cell antitumor response: chemokine-secreting dendritic cells can prime tumor-reactive T cells extranodally. Cancer Res 61: 8794–802, 2001.
15. Baratelli, F., H. Takedatsu, S. Hazra, K. Peebles, J. Luo, P.S. Kurimoto, G. Zeng, R.K. Batra, S. Sharma, S.M. Dubinett, and J.M. Lee. Pre-clinical characterization of GMP grade CCL21-gene modified dendritic cells for application in a phase I trial in non-small cell lung cancer. J Transl Med 6: 38, 2008.
16. Korst, R.J. and R.G. Crystal. Active, specific immunotherapy for lung cancer: hurdles and strategies using genetic modification. Ann Thorac Surg 76: 1319–26, 2003.
17. Ichiki, Y., M. Takenoyama, M. Mizukami, T. So, M. Sugaya, M. Yasuda, T. Hanagiri, K. Sugio, and K. Yasumoto. Simultaneous cellular and humoral immune response against mutated p53 in a patient with lung cancer. J Immunol 172: 4844–50, 2004.
18. Glassy, M.C., J. Yasutomi, and K. Koda. Lessons learned about the therapeutic potential of the natural human immune response to lung cancer. Expert Opin Investig Drugs 8: 995–1006, 1999.
19. Walser, T.C., X. Cui, J. Yanagawa, J.M. Lee, E. Heinrich, G. Lee, S. Sharma, and S.M. Dubinett. Smoking and lung cancer: The role of inflammation. Proceedings of the American Thoracic Society, 2008.
20. Hogg, J.C., F. Chu, S. Utokaparch, R. Woods, W.M. Elliott, L. Buzatu, R.M. Cherniack, R.M. Rogers, F.C. Sciurba, H.O. Coxson, and P.D. Pare. The nature of small-airway obstruction in chronic obstructive pulmonary disease. N Engl J Med 350: 2645–53, 2004.
21. Taraseviciene-Stewart, L. and N.F. Voelkel. Molecular pathogenesis of emphysema. J Clin Invest 118: 394–402, 2008.
22. O'Donnell, R., D. Breen, S. Wilson, and R. Djukanovic. Inflammatory cells in the airways in COPD. Thorax 61: 448–54, 2006.
23. Sevenoaks, M.J. and R.A. Stockley. Chronic Obstructive Pulmonary Disease, inflammation and co-morbidity–a common inflammatory phenotype? Respir Res 7: 70, 2006.
24. Dohadwala, M., S.C. Yang, J. Luo, S. Sharma, R.K. Batra, M. Huang, Y. Lin, L. Goodglick, K. Krysan, M.C. Fishbein, L. Hong, C. Lai, R.B. Cameron, R.M. Gemmill, H.A. Drabkin, and S.M. Dubinett. Cyclooxygenase-2-dependent regulation of E-cadherin: prostaglandin E(2) induces transcriptional repressors ZEB1 and snail in non-small cell lung cancer. Cancer Res 66: 5338–45, 2006.
25. Charuworn, B. Inflammation-mediated promotion of EMT in NSCLC: IL-1beta mediates a MEK/Erk- and JNK/SAPK-dependent down-regulation of E-cadherin. (American Thoracic Society 2006).
26. Baratelli, F., Y. Lin, L. Zhu, S.C. Yang, N. Heuze-Vourc'h, G. Zeng, K. Reckamp, M. Dohadwala, S. Sharma, and S.M. Dubinett. Prostaglandin E2 induces FOXP3 gene expression and T regulatory cell function in human CD4+ T cells. J Immunol 175: 1483–90, 2005.
27. Keshamouni, V.G., G. Michailidis, C.S. Grasso, S. Anthwal, J.R. Strahler, A. Walker, D. A. Arenberg, R.C. Reddy, S. Akulapalli, V.J. Thannickal, T.J. Standiford, P.C. Andrews, and G.S. Omenn. Differential protein expression profiling by iTRAQ-2DLC-MS/MS of lung cancer cells undergoing epithelial-mesenchymal transition reveals a migratory/invasive phenotype. J Proteome Res 5: 1143–54, 2006.
28. Leng, Q., Z. Bentwich, and G. Borkow. Increased TGF-beta, Cbl-b and CTLA-4 levels and immunosuppression in association with chronic immune activation. Int Immunol 18: 637–44, 2006.
29. Huber, M.A., N. Kraut, and H. Beug. Molecular requirements for epithelial-mesenchymal transition during tumor progression. Curr Opin Cell Biol 17: 548–58, 2005.

30. Lee, J.M., S. Dedhar, R. Kalluri, and E.W. Thompson. The epithelial-mesenchymal transition: new insights in signaling, development, and disease. J Cell Biol *172*: 973–81, 2006.

31. Thiery, J.P. Epithelial-mesenchymal transitions in development and pathologies. Curr Opin Cell Biol *15*: 740–6, 2003.

32. Dasari, V., M. Gallup, H. Lemjabbar, I. Maltseva, and N. McNamara. Epithelial-mesenchymal transition in lung cancer: is tobacco the "smoking gun"? Am J Respir Cell Mol Biol *35*: 3–9, 2006.

33. Krysan, K., J.M. Lee, M. Dohadwala, B.K. Gardner, K.L. Reckamp, E. Garon, M. St John, S. Sharma, and S.M. Dubinett. Inflammation, epithelial to mesenchymal transition, and epidermal growth factor receptor tyrosine kinase inhibitor resistance. J Thorac Oncol *3*: 107–10, 2008.

34. Heinrich, E., M. Dohadwala, B. Charuworn, and S. Dubinett. Inflammation-dependent regulation of epithelial-mesenchymal transition in non-small cell lung cancer: the role of interleukin-1b. (Proceedings of the American Association for Cancer Research: 2008).

35. Mani, S.A., W. Guo, M.J. Liao, E.N. Eaton, A. Ayyanan, A.Y. Zhou, M. Brooks, F. Reinhard, C.C. Zhang, M. Shipitsin, L.L. Campbell, K. Polyak, C. Brisken, J. Yang, and R.A. Weinberg. The epithelial-mesenchymal transition generates cells with properties of stem cells. Cell *133*: 704–15, 2008.

36. Yoshino, I., T. Kometani, F. Shoji, A. Osoegawa, T. Ohba, H. Kouso, T. Takenaka, T. Yohena, and Y. Maehara. Induction of epithelial-mesenchymal transition-related genes by benzo[a]pyrene in lung cancer cells. Cancer *110*: 369–74, 2007.

37. Fondrevelle, M.E., B. Kantelip, R.E. Reiter, D.K. Chopin, J.P. Thiery, F. Monnien, H. Bittard, and H. Wallerand. The expression of Twist has an impact on survival in human bladder cancer and is influenced by the smoking status. Urologic Oncology, 2008.

38. Lee, G., M. Dohadwala, and S. Dubinett. Chronic exposure to Tobacco-Specific 4-(N-methyl-N-nitrosamino)-1-(3-pyridyl)-1-butanone (NNK) Induces Epithelial-to-Mesenchymal Transition in Non-small Cell Lung Cancer (Proceedings of the American Thoracic Society, 2008).

39. Gershon, R.K. and K. Kondo. Cell interactions in the induction of tolerance: the role of thymic lymphocytes. Immunology *18*: 723–37, 1970.

40. Dye, E.S. and R.J. North. T cell-mediated immunosuppression as an obstacle to adoptive immunotherapy of the P815 mastocytoma and its metastases. J Exp Med *154*: 1033–42, 1981.

41. Berendt, M.J. and R.J. North. T-cell-mediated suppression of anti-tumor immunity. An explanation for progressive growth of an immunogenic tumor. J Exp Med *151*: 69–80, 1980.

42. DiGiacomo, A. and R.J. North. T cell suppressors of antitumor immunity. The production of Ly-1-,2+ suppressors of delayed sensitivity precedes the production of suppressors of protective immunity. J Exp Med *164*: 1179–92, 1986.

43. Rakhmilevich, A.L. and R.J. North. Elimination of CD4+ T cells in mice bearing an advanced sarcoma augments the antitumor action of interleukin-2. Cancer Immunol Immunother *38*: 107–12, 1994.

44. Antony, P.A. and N.P. Restifo. Do CD4+ CD25+ immunoregulatory T cells hinder tumor immunotherapy? J Immunother *25*: 202–6, 2002.

45. Shevach, E.M. Certified professionals: CD4(+)CD25(+) suppressor T cells. J Exp Med *193*: F41–6, 2001.

46. Maloy, K.J. and F. Powrie. Regulatory T cells in the control of immune pathology. Nat Immunol *2*: 816–22, 2001.

47. Sakaguchi, S., N. Sakaguchi, M. Asano, M. Itoh, and M. Toda. Immunologic self-tolerance maintained by activated T cells expressing IL-2 receptor alpha-chains (CD25). Breakdown of a single mechanism of self-tolerance causes various autoimmune diseases. J Immunol *155*: 1151–64, 1995.

48. Thornton, A.M. and E.M. Shevach. Suppressor effector function of CD4+CD25+ immunoregulatory T cells is antigen nonspecific. J Immunol *164*: 183–90, 2000.
49. Takahashi, T., Y. Kuniyasu, M. Toda, N. Sakaguchi, M. Itoh, M. Iwata, J. Shimizu, and S. Sakaguchi. Immunologic self-tolerance maintained by CD25+CD4+ naturally anergic and suppressive T cells: induction of autoimmune disease by breaking their anergic/suppressive state. Int Immunol *10*: 1969–80, 1998.
50. Thornton, A.M. and E.M. Shevach. CD4+CD25+ immunoregulatory T cells suppress polyclonal T cell activation in vitro by inhibiting interleukin 2 production. J Exp Med *188*: 287–96, 1998.
51. Itoh, M., T. Takahashi, N. Sakaguchi, Y. Kuniyasu, J. Shimizu, F. Otsuka, and S. Sakaguchi. Thymus and autoimmunity: production of CD25+CD4+ naturally anergic and suppressive T cells as a key function of the thymus in maintaining immunologic self-tolerance. J Immunol *162*: 5317–26, 1999.
52. Papiernik, M., M.L. de Moraes, C. Pontoux, F. Vasseur, and C. Penit. Regulatory CD4 T cells: expression of IL-2R alpha chain, resistance to clonal deletion and IL-2 dependency. Int Immunol *10*: 371–8, 1998.
53. Shevach, E.M. Regulatory T cells in autoimmmunity*. Annu Rev Immunol *18*: 423–49, 2000.
54. Jordan, M.S., A. Boesteanu, A.J. Reed, A.L. Petrone, A.E. Holenbeck, M.A. Lerman, A. Naji, and A.J. Caton. Thymic selection of CD4+CD25+ regulatory T cells induced by an agonist self-peptide. Nat Immunol *2*: 301–6, 2001.
55. Sakaguchi, S. The origin of FOXP3-expressing CD4+ regulatory T cells: thymus or periphery. J Clin Invest *112*: 1310–2, 2003.
56. Walker, M.R., D.J. Kasprowicz, V.H. Gersuk, A. Benard, M. Van Landeghen, J.H. Buckner, and S.F. Ziegler. Induction of FoxP3 and acquisition of T regulatory activity by stimulated human CD4+CD25- T cells. J Clin Invest *112*: 1437–43, 2003.
57. Sogn, J.A. Tumor immunology: the glass is half full. Immunity *9*: 757–63, 1998.
58. Yoshino, I., T. Yano, M. Murata, T. Ishida, K. Sugimachi, G. Kimura, and K. Nomoto. Tumor-reactive T-cells accumulate in lung cancer tissues but fail to respond due to tumor cell-derived factor. Cancer Res *52*: 775–81, 1992.
59. Batra, R.K., Y. Lin, S. Sharma, M. Dohadwala, J. Luo, M. Pold, and S.M. Dubinett. Non-small cell lung cancer-derived soluble mediators enhance apoptosis in activated T lymphocytes through an I kappa B kinase-dependent mechanism. Cancer Res *63*: 642–6, 2003.
60. Woo, E.Y., H. Yeh, C.S. Chu, K. Schlienger, R.G. Carroll, J.L. Riley, L.R. Kaiser, and C.H. June. Cutting edge: Regulatory T cells from lung cancer patients directly inhibit autologous T cell proliferation. J Immunol *168*: 4272–6, 2002.
61. Alleva, D.G., C.J. Burger, and K.D. Elgert. Tumor-induced regulation of suppressor macrophage nitric oxide and TNF-alpha production. Role of tumor-derived IL-10, TGF-beta, and prostaglandin E2. J Immunol *153*: 1674–86, 1994.
62. Huang, M., S. Sharma, J.T. Mao, and S.M. Dubinett. Non-small cell lung cancer-derived soluble mediators and prostaglandin E2 enhance peripheral blood lymphocyte IL-10 transcription and protein production. J Immunol *157*: 5512–20, 1996.
63. Liu, V.C., L.Y. Wong, T. Jang, A.H. Shah, I. Park, X. Yang, Q. Zhang, S. Lonning, B.A. Teicher, and C. Lee. Tumor evasion of the immune system by converting CD4+CD25- T cells into CD4+CD25+ T regulatory cells: role of tumor-derived TGF-beta. J Immunol *178*: 2883–92, 2007.
64. Finke, J. and R. Bukowski, eds., Lung Cancer and Immune Dysfunction (Humana Press, 2004): 335–348.
65. Huang, M., M. Stolina, S. Sharma, J. Mao, L. Zhu, P. Miller, J. Wollman, H. Herschman, and S. Dubinett. Non-small cell lung cancer cyclooxygenase-2-dependent regulation of cytokine balance in lymphocytes and macrophages: up-regulation of interleukin 10 and down-regulation of interleukin 12 production. Cancer Res *58*: 1208–1216, 1998.

66. Stolina, M., S. Sharma, Y. Lin, M. Dohadwala, B. Gardner, J. Luo, L. Zhu, M. Kronenberg, P.W. Miller, J. Portanova, J.C. Lee, and S.M. Dubinett. Specific inhibition of cyclooxygenase 2 restores antitumor reactivity by altering the balance of IL-10 and IL-12 synthesis. J Immunol *164*: 361–70, 2000.

67. Sharma, S., S.C. Yang, L. Zhu, K. Reckamp, B. Gardner, F. Baratelli, M. Huang, R.K. Batra, and S.M. Dubinett. Tumor cyclooxygenase-2/prostaglandin E2-dependent promotion of FOXP3 expression and CD4+ CD25+ T regulatory cell activities in lung cancer. Cancer Res *65*: 5211–20, 2005.

68. Katori, M. and M. Majima. Cyclooxygenase-2: its rich diversity of roles and possible application of its selective inhibitors. Inflamm Res *49*: 367–92, 2000.

69. Funk, C.D. Prostaglandins and leukotrienes: advances in eicosanoid biology. Science *294*: 1871–5, 2001.

70. FitzGerald, G.A. COX-2 and beyond: Approaches to prostaglandin inhibition in human disease. Nat Rev Drug Discov *2*: 879–90, 2003.

71. Malkowski, M.G., S.L. Ginell, W.L. Smith, and R.M. Garavito. The productive conformation of arachidonic acid bound to prostaglandin synthase. Science *289*: 1933–7, 2000.

72. Chandrasekharan, N.V., H. Dai, K.L. Roos, N.K. Evanson, J. Tomsik, T.S. Elton, and D.L. Simmons. COX-3, a cyclooxygenase-1 variant inhibited by acetaminophen and other analgesic/antipyretic drugs: cloning, structure, and expression. Proc Natl Acad Sci USA *99*: 13926–31, 2002.

73. Smith, W.L., D.L. DeWitt, and R.M. Garavito. Cyclooxygenases: structural, cellular, and molecular biology. Annu Rev Biochem *69*: 145–82, 2000.

74. Dubois, R.N., S.B. Abramson, L. Crofford, R.A. Gupta, L.S. Simon, L.B. Van De Putte, and P.E. Lipsky. Cyclooxygenase in biology and disease. FASEB J *12*: 1063–73, 1998.

75. Aoyama, T., Y. Yui, H. Morishita, and C. Kawai. Prostaglandin I2 half-life regulated by high density lipoprotein is decreased in acute myocardial infarction and unstable angina pectoris. Circulation *81*: 1784–91, 1990.

76. Ishihara, O., M.H. Sullivan, and M.G. Elder. Differences of metabolism of prostaglandin E2 and F2 alpha by decidual stromal cells and macrophages in culture. Eicosanoids *4*: 203–7, 1991.

77. Kliewer, S.A., J.M. Lenhard, T.M. Willson, I. Patel, D.C. Morris, and J.M. Lehmann. A prostaglandin J2 metabolite binds peroxisome proliferator-activated receptor gamma and promotes adipocyte differentiation. Cell *83*: 813–9, 1995.

78. Riedl, K., K. Krysan, M. Pold, H. Dalwadi, N. Heuze-Vourc'h, M. Dohadwala, M. Liu, X. Cui, R. Figlin, J.T. Mao, R. Strieter, S. Sharma, and S.M. Dubinett. Multifaceted roles of cyclooxygenase-2 in lung cancer. Drug Resist Updat *7*: 169–84, 2004.

79. Krysan, K., K. Reckamp, S. Sharma, M. Dohadwala, and S. Dubinett. PGE2 activates MAPK/Erk pathway in non-small cell lung cancer cells in an EGF receptor-independent manner. Cancer Res *65*: 6275–81, 2005.

80. Tsujii, M. and R. Dubois. Alterations in cellular adhesion and apoptosis in epithelial cells overexpressing prostaglandin endoperoxide synthase-2. Cell *83*: 493–501, 1995.

81. Hosomi, Y., T. Yokose, Y. Hirose, R. Nakajima, K. Nagai, Y. Nishiwaki, and A. Ochiai. Increased cyclooxygenase 2 (COX-2) expression occurs frequently in precursor lesions of human adenocarcinoma of the lung. Lung Cancer *30*: 73–81, 2000.

82. Wolff, H., K. Saukkonen, S. Anttila, A. Karjalainen, H. Vainio, and A. Ristimaki. Expression of cyclooxygenase-2 in human lung carcinoma. Cancer Res *58*: 4997–5001, 1998.

83. Khuri, F.R., H. Wu, J.J. Lee, B.L. Kemp, R. Lotan, S.M. Lippman, L. Feng, W.K. Hong, and X.-C. Xu. Cyclooxygenase-2 overexpression is a marker of poor prognosis in stage I non-small cell lung cancer. Clin Cancer Res *7*: 861–7, 2001.

84. Soslow, R.A., A.J. Dannenberg, D. Rush, B.M. Woerner, K.N. Khan, J. Masferrer, and A.T. Koki. COX-2 is expressed in human pulmonary, colonic, and mammary tumors. Cancer *89*: 2637–45, 2000.

85. Hasturk, S., B. Kemp, S.K. Kalapurakal, J.M. Kurie, W.K. Hong, and J.S. Lee. Expression of cyclooxygenase-1 and cyclooxygenase-2 in bronchial epithelium and nonsmall cell lung carcinoma. Cancer 94: 1023–31, 2002.

86. Tsubochi, H., N. Sato, M. Hiyama, M. Kaimori, S. Endo, Y. Sohara, and T. Imai. Combined analysis of cyclooxygenase-2 expression with p53 and Ki-67 in nonsmall cell lung cancer. Ann Thorac Surg 82: 1198–204, 2006.

87. Hida, T., Y. Yatabe, H. Achiwa, H. Muramatsu, K. Kozaki, S. Nakamura, M. Ogawa, T. Mitsudomi, T. Sugiura, and T. Takahashi. Increased expression of cyclooxygenase 2 occurs frequently in human lung cancers, specifically in adenocarcinomas. Cancer Res 58: 3761–4, 1998.

88. Brabender, J., J. Park, R. Metzger, P.M. Schneider, R.V. Lord, A.H. Holscher, K.D. Danenberg, and P.V. Danenberg. Prognostic significance of cyclooxygenase 2 mRNA expression in non-small cell lung cancer. Ann Surg 235: 440–3, 2002.

89. Achiwa, H., Y. Yatabe, T. Hida, T. Kuroishi, K. Kozaki, S. Nakamura, M. Ogawa, T. Sugiura, T. Mitsudomi, and T. Takahashi. Prognostic significance of elevated cyclooxygenase 2 expression in primary, resected lung adenocarcinomas. Clin Cancer Res 5: 1001–5, 1999.

90. Campa, D., S. Zienolddiny, V. Maggini, V. Skaug, A. Haugen, and F. Canzian. Association of a common polymorphism in the cyclooxygenase 2 gene with risk of non-small cell lung cancer. Carcinogenesis 25: 229–35, 2004.

91. Schreinemachers, D.M. and R.B. Everson. Aspirin use and lung, colon, and breast cancer incidence in a prospective study. Epidemiology 5: 138–46, 1994.

92. Krysan, K., H. Dalwadi, S. Sharma, M. Pold, and S. Dubinett. Cyclooxygenase 2-dependent expression of survivin is critical for apoptosis resistance in non-small cell lung cancer. Cancer Res 64: 6359–62, 2004.

93. Leahy, K.M., A.T. Koki, and J.L. Masferrer. Role of cyclooxygenases in angiogenesis. Curr Med Chem 7: 1163–70, 2000.

94. Gately, S. The contributions of cyclooxygenase-2 to tumor angiogenesis. Cancer Metastasis Rev 19: 19–27, 2000.

95. Dohadwala, M., R.K. Batra, J. Luo, Y. Lin, K. Krysan, M. Pold, S. Sharma, and S.M. Dubinett. Autocrine/paracrine prostaglandin E2 production by non-small cell lung cancer cells regulates matrix metalloproteinase-2 and CD44 in cyclooxygenase-2-dependent invasion. J Biol Chem 277: 50828–33, 2002.

96. Dohadwala, M., J. Luo, L. Zhu, Y. Lin, G.J. Dougherty, S. Sharma, M. Huang, M. Pold, R.K. Batra, and S.M. Dubinett. Non-small cell lung cancer cyclooxygenase-2-dependent invasion is mediated by CD44. J Biol Chem 276: 20809–12, 2001.

97. Dy, G.K. and A.A. Adjei. Novel targets for lung cancer therapy: part II. J Clin Oncol 20: 3016–28, 2002.

98. Dy, G.K. and A.A. Adjei. Novel targets for lung cancer therapy: part I. J Clin Oncol 20: 2881–94, 2002.

99. Dubinett, S., S. Sharma, M. Huang, M. Dohadwala, M. Pold, and J. Mao., Cyclooxygenase-2 in lung cancer, in Progressive Experimental Tumor Research, ed. Bertino, J.R. (Basel: Basel Karger, 2003).

100. Lee, J.M., J.T. Mao, K. Krysan, and S.M. Dubinett. Significance of cyclooxygenase-2 in prognosis, targeted therapy and chemoprevention of NSCLC. Future Oncol 3: 149–53, 2007.

101. Bhattacharya, M., K.G. Peri, G. Almazan, A. Ribeiro-da-Silva, H. Shichi, Y. Durocher, M. Abramovitz, X. Hou, D.R. Varma, and S. Chemtob. Nuclear localization of prostaglandin E2 receptors. Proc Natl Acad Sci USA 95: 15792–7, 1998.

102. Breyer, R.M., C.R. Kennedy, Y. Zhang, and M.D. Breyer. Structure-function analyses of eicosanoid receptors. Physiologic and therapeutic implications. Ann N Y Acad Sci 905: 221–31, 2000.

103. Fujino, H. and J.W. Regan. Prostanoid receptors and phosphatidylinositol 3-kinase: a pathway to cancer? Trends Pharmacol Sci 24: 335–40, 2003.

104. Yang, L., Y. Huang, R. Porta, K. Yanagisawa, A. Gonzalez, E. Segi, D.H. Johnson, S. Narumiya, and D.P. Carbone. Host and direct antitumor effects and profound reduction in tumor metastasis with selective EP4 receptor antagonism. Cancer Res 66: 9665–72, 2006.

105. Han, S., J.D. Ritzenthaler, B. Wingerd, H.N. Rivera, and J. Roman. Extracellular matrix fibronectin increases prostaglandin E2 receptor subtype EP4 in lung carcinoma cells through multiple signaling pathways: the role of AP-2. J Biol Chem 282: 7961–72, 2007.

106. Lippman, S.M., N. Gibson, K. Subbaramaiah, and A.J. Dannenberg. Combined targeting of the epidermal growth factor receptor and cyclooxygenase-2 pathways. Clin Cancer Res 11: 6097–9, 2005.

107. Reckamp, K.L., B.K. Gardner, R.A. Figlin, D. Elashoff, K. Krysan, M. Dohadwala, J. Mao, S. Sharma, L. Inge, A. Rajasekaran, and S.M. Dubinett. Tumor response to combination celecoxib and erlotinib therapy in non-small cell lung cancer is associated with a low baseline matrix metalloproteinase-9 and a decline in serum-soluble E-cadherin. J Thorac Oncol 3: 117–24, 2008.

108. Reckamp, K.L., K. Krysan, J.D. Morrow, G.L. Milne, R.A. Newman, C. Tucker, R.M. Elashoff, S.M. Dubinett, and R.A. Figlin. A phase I trial to determine the optimal biological dose of celecoxib when combined with erlotinib in advanced non-small cell lung cancer. Clin Cancer Res 12: 3381–8, 2006.

109. Witta, S.E., R.M. Gemmill, F.R. Hirsch, C.D. Coldren, K. Hedman, L. Ravdel, B. Helfrich, R. Dziadziuszko, D.C. Chan, M. Sugita, Z. Chan, A. Baron, W. Franklin, H. A. Drabkin, L. Girard, A.F. Gazdar, J.D. Minna, and P.A. Bunn., Jr. Restoring E-cadherin expression increases sensitivity to epidermal growth factor receptor inhibitors in lung cancer cell lines. Cancer Res 66: 944–50, 2006.

110. Hogan, B.L. Bone morphogenetic proteins in development. Curr Opin Genet Dev 6: 432–8, 1996.

111. Okada, H. and R. Kalluri. Recapitulation of kidney development paradigms by BMP-7 reverses chronic renal injury. Clin Exp Nephrol 9: 100–1, 2005.

112. Kopp, J.B. BMP-7 and the proximal tubule. Kidney Int 61: 351–2, 2002.

113. Bellusci, S., R. Henderson, G. Winnier, T. Oikawa, and B.L. Hogan. Evidence from normal expression and targeted misexpression that bone morphogenetic protein (Bmp-4) plays a role in mouse embryonic lung morphogenesis. Development 122: 1693–702, 1996.

114. Zeisberg, M., J. Hanai, H. Sugimoto, T. Mammoto, D. Charytan, F. Strutz, and R. Kalluri. BMP-7 counteracts TGF-beta1-induced epithelial-to-mesenchymal transition and reverses chronic renal injury. Nat Med 9: 964–8, 2003.

115. Shao, J., B.M. Evers, and H. Sheng. Prostaglandin E2 synergistically enhances receptor tyrosine kinase-dependent signaling system in colon cancer cells. J Biol Chem 279: 14287–93, 2004.

116. Buchanan, F.G., D. Wang, F. Bargiacchi, and R.N. DuBois. Prostaglandin E2 regulates cell migration via the intracellular activation of the epidermal growth factor receptor. J Biol Chem 278: 35451–7, 2003.

117. Coffey, R.J., C.J. Hawkey, L. Damstrup, R. Graves-Deal, V.C. Daniel, P.J. Dempsey, R. Chinery, S.C. Kirkland, R.N. DuBois, T.L. Jetton, and J.D. Morrow. Epidermal growth factor receptor activation induces nuclear targeting of cyclooxygenase-2, basolateral release of prostaglandins, and mitogenesis in polarizing colon cancer cells. Proc Natl Acad Sci USA 94: 657–62, 1997.

118. Pai, R., B. Soreghan, I.L. Szabo, M. Pavelka, D. Baatar, and A.S. Tarnawski. Prostaglandin E2 transactivates EGF receptor: a novel mechanism for promoting colon cancer growth and gastrointestinal hypertrophy. Nat Med 8: 289–93, 2002.

119. Yang, X.D., X.C. Jia, J.R. Corvalan, P. Wang, and C.G. Davis. Development of ABX-EGF, a fully human anti-EGF receptor monoclonal antibody, for cancer therapy. Crit Rev Oncol Hematol 38: 17–23, 2001.

120. Hirata, A., S. Ogawa, T. Kometani, T. Kuwano, S. Naito, M. Kuwano, and M. Ono. ZD1839 (Iressa) induces antiangiogenic effects through inhibition of epidermal growth factor receptor tyrosine kinase. Cancer Res 62: 2554–60, 2002.

121. Pold, M., L.X. Zhu, S. Sharma, M.D. Burdick, Y. Lin, P.P. Lee, A. Pold, J. Luo, K. Krysan, M. Dohadwala, J.T. Mao, R.K. Batra, R.M. Strieter, and S.M. Dubinett. Cyclooxygenase-2-dependent expression of angiogenic CXC chemokines ENA-78/CXC Ligand (CXCL) 5 and interleukin-8/CXCL8 in human non-small cell lung cancer. Cancer Res 64: 1853–60, 2004.

122. Williams, C.S., M. Tsujii, J. Reese, S.K. Dey, and R.N. DuBois. Host cyclooxygenase-2 modulates carcinoma growth. J Clin Invest 105: 1589–94, 2000.

123. Torrance, C.J., P.E. Jackson, E. Montgomery, K.W. Kinzler, B. Vogelstein, A. Wissner, M. Nunes, P. Frost, and C.M. Discafani. Combinatorial chemoprevention of intestinal neoplasia. Nat Med 6: 1024–8, 2000.

124. Kim, G.E., Y.B. Kim, N.H. Cho, H.C. Chung, H.R. Pyo, J.D. Lee, T.K. Park, W.S. Koom, M. Chun, and C.O. Suh. Synchronous coexpression of epidermal growth factor receptor and cyclooxygenase-2 in carcinomas of the uterine cervix: a potential predictor of poor survival. Clin Cancer Res 10: 1366–74, 2004.

125. Chen, Z., X. Zhang, M. Li, Z. Wang, H.S. Wieand, J.R. Grandis, and D.M. Shin. Simultaneously targeting epidermal growth factor receptor tyrosine kinase and cyclooxygenase-2, an efficient approach to inhibition of squamous cell carcinoma of the head and neck. Clin Cancer Res 10: 5930–9, 2004.

126. Gadgeel, S.M., J.C. Ruckdeschel, E.I. Heath, L.K. Heilbrun, R. Venkatramana-moorthy, and A. Wozniak. Phase II study of gefitinib, an epidermal growth factor receptor tyrosine kinase inhibitor (EGFR-TKI), and celecoxib, a cyclooxygenase-2 (COX-2) inhibitor, in patients with platinum refractory non-small cell lung cancer (NSCLC). J Thorac Oncol 2: 299–305, 2007.

127. O'Byrne, K.J., S. Danson, D. Dunlop, N. Botwood, F. Taguchi, D. Carbone, and M. Ranson. Combination therapy with gefitinib and rofecoxib in patients with platinum-pretreated relapsed non small-cell lung cancer. J Clin Oncol 25: 3266–73, 2007.

128. Gridelli, C., C. Gallo, A. Ceribelli, V. Gebbia, T. Gamucci, F. Ciardiello, F. Carozza, A. Favaretto, B. Daniele, D. Galetta, S. Barbera, F. Rosetti, A. Rossi, P. Maione, F. Cognetti, A. Testa, M. Di Maio, A. Morabito, and F. Perrone. Factorial phase III randomised trial of rofecoxib and prolonged constant infusion of gemcitabine in advanced non-small-cell lung cancer: the GEmcitabine-COxib in NSCLC (GECO) study. Lancet Oncol 8: 500–12, 2007.

129. Juni, P., L. Nartey, S. Reichenbach, R. Sterchi, P.A. Dieppe, and M. Egger. Risk of cardiovascular events and rofecoxib: cumulative meta-analysis. Lancet 364: 2021–9, 2004.

130. Solomon, D.H., S. Schneeweiss, R.J. Glynn, Y. Kiyota, R. Levin, H. Mogun, and J. Avorn. Relationship between selective cyclooxygenase-2 inhibitors and acute myocardial infarction in older adults. Circulation 109: 2068–73, 2004.

131. Lilenbaum, R., M.A. Socinski, N.K. Altorki, L.L. Hart, R.S. Keresztes, S. Hariharan, M.E. Morrison, R. Fayyad, and P. Bonomi. Randomized phase II trial of docetaxel/irinotecan and gemcitabine/irinotecan with or without celecoxib in the second-line treatment of non-small-cell lung cancer. J Clin Oncol 24: 4825–32, 2006.

132. Chan, A.T., S. Ogino, and C.S. Fuchs. Aspirin and the risk of colorectal cancer in relation to the expression of COX-2. N Engl J Med 356: 2131–42, 2007.

133. Edelman, M.J., D. Watson, X. Wang, C. Morrison, R.A. Kratzke, S. Jewell, L. Hodgson, A.M. Mauer, A. Gajra, G.A. Masters, M. Bedor, E.E. Vokes, and M.J. Green. Eicosanoid modulation in advanced lung cancer: cyclooxygenase-2 expression is a positive predictive factor for celecoxib + chemotherapy – Cancer and Leukemia Group B Trial 30203. J Clin Oncol 26: 848–55, 2008.

134. Lee, J.M., J. Yanagawa, K.A. Peebles, S. Sharma, J.T. Mao, and S.M. Dubinett. Inflammation in lung carcinogenesis: new targets for lung cancer chemoprevention and treatment. Crit Rev Oncol Hematol 66: 208–17, 2008.

135. Wislez, M., N. Fujimoto, J.G. Izzo, A.E. Hanna, D.D. Cody, R.R. Langley, H. Tang, M.D. Burdick, M. Sato, J.D. Minna, L. Mao, I. Wistuba, R.M. Strieter, and J.M. Kurie. High expression of ligands for chemokine receptor CXCR2 in alveolar epithelial neoplasia induced by oncogenic kras. Cancer Res 66: 4198–207, 2006.

136. Mao, J.T., M.C. Fishbein, B. Adams, M.D. Roth, L. Goodglick, L. Hong, M. Burdick, E.R. Strieter, C. Holmes, D.P. Tashkin, and S.M. Dubinett. Celecoxib decreases Ki-67 proliferative index in active smokers. Clin Cancer Res 12: 314–20, 2006.

137. Mao, J.T., X. Cui, K. Reckamp, M. Liu, K. Krysan, H. Dalwadi, S. Sharma, S. Hazra, R. Strieter, B. Gardner, and S.M. Dubinett. Chemoprevention strategies with cyclooxygenase-2 inhibitors for lung cancer. Clin Lung Cancer 7: 30–9, 2005.

138. Peebles, K.A., J.M. Lee, J.T. Mao, S. Hazra, K.L. Reckamp, K. Krysan, M. Dohadwala, E.L. Heinrich, T.C. Walser, X. Cui, F.E. Baratelli, E. Garon, S. Sharma, and S.M. Dubinett. Inflammation and lung carcinogenesis: applying findings in prevention and treatment. Expert Rev Anticancer Ther 7: 1405–21, 2007.

139. Walser, T.C., J. Yanagawa, J. Luo, M. Liu, L. Goodglick, L. Hong, M.C. Fishbein, J.D. Minna, J.W. Shay, R.M. Strieter, and S. Dubinett. Snail-induced and EMT-mediated early lung cancer development: Promotion of invasion and expansion of stem cell populations (Seventh Annual AACR International Conference, Frontiers in Cancer Prevention Research: 2008).

140. Yanagawa, J., T.C. Walser, L. Zhu, J. Luo, L. Hong, M.C. Fishbein, L. Goodglick, R. M. Strieter, S. Sharma, and S. Dubinett. The zinc-finger E-box-binding transcriptional repressor Snail promotes tumor progression and angiogenesis in non-small cell lung cancer (Seventh Annual AACR International Conference, Frontiers in Cancer Prevention Research: 2008).

141. Skillrud, D.M., K.P. Offord, and R.D. Miller. Higher risk of lung cancer in chronic obstructive pulmonary disease. A prospective, matched, controlled study. Ann Intern Med 105: 503–7, 1986.

142. Parimon, T., J.W. Chien, C.L. Bryson, M.B. McDonell, E.M. Udris, and D.H. Au. Inhaled corticosteroids and risk of lung cancer among patients with chronic obstructive pulmonary disease. Am J Respir Crit Care Med 175: 712–9, 2007.

143. Wilson, D.O., J.L. Weissfeld, A. Balkan, J.G. Schragin, C.R. Fuhrman, S.N. Fisher, J. Wilson, J.K. Leader, J.M. Siegfried, S.D. Shapiro, and F.C. Sciurba. Association of radiographic emphysema and airflow obstruction with lung cancer. Am J Respir Crit Care Med 178: 738–44, 2008.

Angiogenesis and Angiogenic Diversity in Lung Cancer Metastasis

Douglas A. Arenberg

Abstract Angiogenesis is a pervasive biological phenomenon that is at the core of many physiologic and pathologic processes. To be sustained, the increase in metabolic activity brought on with tissue proliferation *must* be accompanied by a proportional increase in blood supply. When pre-existing vasculature is insufficient to meet the demands of the proliferating cell population, signals for angiogenesis are generated by resident and infiltrating cells. Angiogenesis is a vital part of tumor biology and occurs in response to a wide range of molecular signals within the tumor microenvironment, and these signals need not arise directly from the tumor cell. This has given rise to the notion of diversity of the angiogenic mechanisms or a unique angiogenic signature of each tumor's microenvironment [7, 8]. This chapter will focus on the basic cellular mechanisms of angiogenesis, followed by a discussion of various factors that are involved in lung cancer angiogenesis, and the clinical implications of the diversity of angiogenic pathways in cancer.

Introduction

Of all the malignant cells in a primary tumor, a small fraction is able to metastasize to a distant organ. In this respect, the process of metastasis can be thought of as a natural subcloning experiment, which selects for those cells within the tumor capable of performing all the tasks of the metastatic process. Fidler summarized the sequential but overlapping steps of the metastatic cascade in the Clowes Memorial Award Lecture in 1990 [1]. While significant knowledge has been added to the field in the nearly two decades since then, much of what he said then still applies today. In particular he noted that the ability to promote angiogenesis is one of several critical tasks of the metastatic cell.

D.A. Arenberg (✉)
Division of Pulmonary and Critical Care, Department of Medicine, University
of Michigan, Ann Arbor, MI 48109-5642, USA
e-mail: darenber@umich.edu

V. Keshamouni et al. (eds.), *Lung Cancer Metastasis*,
DOI 10.1007/978-1-4419-0772-1_7, © Springer Science+Business Media, LLC 2009

Angiogenesis is a vital part of tumor biology, and while it appears to be essential for metastasis to occur, direct evidence in support of this is difficult to find. In part this is because most assays for metastasis rely on the development of large visible tumors, and these require angiogenesis to develop even after the tumor cell has metastasized. Some evidence suggests that angiogenesis is not, in fact, required for individual cells to metastasize [2, 3]. On the other hand, there is good experimental evidence that the onset of angiogenesis in the tumor microenvironment precedes the invasion of malignant cells into the stroma [4]. There is strong evidence implying that lymphangiogenesis is required for the process of lymphatic metastasis [5, 6]. Regardless of the mixed evidence in this respect, animal studies clearly show that *inhibition* of angiogenesis can maintain metastatic tumor deposits in a dormant state [2, 3]. Since metastatic disease is the primary cause of death in most cases of lung cancer, the discussion of angiogenesis, its mechanisms, and potential targets is essential in any consideration of lung cancer metastasis.

Angiogenesis is a pervasive biological phenomenon that is at the core of many physiologic and pathologic processes. To be sustained, the increase in metabolic activity brought on with tissue proliferation *must* be accompanied by a proportional increase in blood supply. When pre-existing vasculature is insufficient to meet the demands of the proliferating cell population, signals for angiogenesis are generated by resident and infiltrating cells. Angiogenesis occurs in response to a wide range of molecular signals within the tumor microenvironment, and these signals need not arise directly from the tumor cell. This has given rise to the notion of diversity of the angiogenic mechanisms or a unique angiogenic signature of each tumor's microenvironment [7, 8]. This chapter will focus on the basic cellular mechanisms of angiogenesis, followed by a discussion of various factors that are involved in lung cancer angiogenesis, and the clinical implications of the diversity of angiogenic pathways in cancer.

The Sequence of Events in Physiologic Angiogenesis

The absolute dependence of tissue on adequate blood supply suggests several characteristics of angiogenesis. First, the vascular system must be able to rapidly respond to increased tissue needs with increased microvasculature. Second, because of the high metabolic cost of angiogenesis, under basal conditions, the process must be tightly controlled, occurring only when necessary. Indeed, endothelial cells are normally quiescent, but during the angiogenic response, they become activated. The rate of normal capillary endothelial cell turnover is typically measured in months or years [7, 8]. However, when microvasculature endothelial cells are stimulated in vivo, they degrade their basement membrane, migrate directionally, divide, organize into functioning capillaries, and deposit new basal lamina all within a matter of days. These steps are not sequential. Rather, they represent an orchestration of overlapping events necessary to return injured tissue to homeostasis.

The angiogenic signal. The signal(s) which initiate angiogenesis vary with the condition which requires angiogenesis and may be organ specific [9]. During the wound response, angiogenic factors may be released through platelet degranulation [10] or proteolytic digestion of extracellular matrix [11]. The importance of these mechanisms may lie in the fact that they do not require new protein synthesis and may occur rapidly in response to tissue injury [12]. In pathologic angiogenesis, many different cells may be the source of angiogenic signals, including tumor cells [13], fibroblasts [14], endothelial cells [15, 16], epithelial cells [17], or activated macrophages [18–20]. Embryonic angiogenesis is activated by genes which are transcribed in response to hypoxia and hypoglycemia [21]. Importantly, the signal for angiogenesis may also be initiated by loss of inhibitory signals, rather than simply requiring a positive stimulus [22].

Endothelial detachment. For endothelium to invade into the surrounding matrix, cells must detach from their tight association with neighboring endothelial cells. These cell–cell appositions, called adherens junctions, are composed of cadherin family proteins. Vascular–endothelial cadherin (VE-cadherin, or cadherin 5) is highly specific for endothelial cells [23] and associates with the cytoskeleton through β-catenin, and plakoglobin [24, 25]. One of the earliest events in the angiogenic response is alteration of the adherens junction complexes, leading to increased pericellular permeability, and detachment of the endothelial cell from its neighboring cells [26].

Proteolysis and cell migration. The loss of tight cell–cell adhesion results in leakage of plasma and deposition of a primordial matrix rich in fibrinogen and fibrin. In order to form new vessels, the existing basement membrane and surrounding fibrin matrix must be degraded. Hiraoka et al. used a mouse aortic ring explants to study the role of proteolytic pathways in vessel invasion into three-dimensional fibrin gels. This model is characterized by both vessel-tube formation and perivascular mesenchymal cell invasion. They demonstrated that matrix metalloprotease (MMP) inhibitors blocked endothelial cell tube formation without inhibiting invasion of perivascular mesenchymal cells. The plasminogen activation system was not necessary for endothelial tubes to invade the fibrin matrix [27]. Expression of membrane-type 1 MMP (MT1-MMP) was sufficient to confer fibrin-invasive capacity to "invasion-null" cells, and its expression had to be confined to the cell surface (as opposed to a soluble form) [27]. These observations were derived from well-defined systems of pure or nearly pure fibrin gels. Invasion into perivascular matrix in vivo may be more complex, requiring other proteolytic enzymes or pathways as well. Proteolytic activity may also release angiogenic growth factors which are sequestered in the basement membrane [11, 15].

After proteolysis, angiogenic endothelial cells must migrate through an extracellular matrix consisting of a variety of components, including fibrin, fibronectin, vitronectin, and hyaluronan as well as other glycosaminoglycans [28]. Locomotion through this environment requires cell–matrix adhesion which occurs through cell surface-associated integrins. Reversible integrin-mediated binding to matrix components allows migration along a chemotactic gradient through the extracellular matrix scaffold. Since endothelial cells must respond to injury in all organs and tissues of the body, they must be capable of adherence to a variety of matrix components. The $a_v\beta_3$ and $a_v\beta_5$ integrins are important endothelial cell adhesion molecules which display appropriately promiscuous binding profiles and are both involved in angiogenesis [29, 30]. The importance of this cell–matrix interaction in angiogenesis is demonstrated by work showing that specific inhibition of integrin binding in angiogenic endothelium leads to apoptosis of the endothelial cell [29, 30].

Cell proliferation. While DNA synthesis occurs early in the angiogenic response, vascular sprouting can occur in the absence of endothelial cell proliferation [31]. However, when proliferation is inhibited, the angiogenic response does not progress beyond this earliest stage of neovascularization [31]. Maintenance of the angiogenic response requires an increase in the number of endothelial cells to provide adequate capillary perfusion. While some angiogenic factors are only chemotactic for endothelial cells [32], most are endothelial cell mitogens also [32, 33]. The signaling pathways which control cell proliferation are separable from those which lead to other aspects of the angiogenic response and may be dependent on the degree of cell–matrix adhesion [34]. In vitro studies demonstrate that endothelial cell proliferation occurs in conditions of increased cell–matrix adhesiveness, whereas cells plated on poorly adhesive substrates undergo growth arrest and lose viability. In contrast, intermediate levels of adhesiveness promoted differentiation into tube-like structures [34]. One might visualize that these in vitro findings have a correlate with wound repair in vivo. The primordial matrix of an early wound is rich in plasma proteins which provide an abundant source of extracellular matrix to which endothelial cells may adhere, thus promoting cell migration and proliferation. However, as a wound matures, the primordial matrix is altered, and the composition of matrix proteins evolves. Fibroblasts deposit type III collagen, and phagocytic cells remove debris, perhaps leading to reduced adhesiveness of the matrix and promoting capillary tube formation [12, 35–38].

Tube formation. The integrity of the circulatory system must be maintained once capillary endothelial cells invade neoplastic tissue. This requires the formation of functioning capillaries with tight cell–cell adhesion. In addition to the importance of cadherin 5 and the adherens junction, tube formation requires the function of CD31 (platelet endothelial cell adhesion molecule; PECAM-1) [39]. CD31 is a membrane glycoprotein and a member of the immunoglobulin supergene family that can mediate both heterotypic and homotypic adhesion [40]. Inhibition of in vitro and in vivo angiogenesis by neutralizing antibodies to CD31 shows the importance of this interaction [41].

Vessel maturation. After the formation of a continuous capillary tube, the final step in forming a new blood vessel is the deposition of a basement membrane. Inhibition of collagen biosynthesis prevents in vitro formation of capillary-like tubes and inhibits an in vivo model of angiogenesis [42]. Once a vessel is formed, it is stabilized by the presence of pericytes which reduce vascular permeability and protect vessels from apoptotic signals [43]. Pericytes migrate to, and stabilize blood vessels through a mechanism that involves the angiopoietin-1/Tie-2 ligand receptor interactions as well as the cytokine platelet-derived growth factor (PDGF-BB) [44]. In many tumors, vessels lack pericyte coverage [45]. This may reflect the fact that mature, pericyte-coated vessels are less susceptible to angiogenic signals. However, given that pericytes are critical in stabilizing blood vessels and that pericyte-coated vessels are resistant to apoptotic signals, the role of pericytes in tumor angiogenesis is likely a "two-edged sword" [46–48]. Further research into the role of pericytes in tumor angiogenesis should clarify their contribution.

A more novel concept recently introduced in the field of tumor angiogenesis is the discovery of circulating bone marrow-derived endothelial cell precursors (ECP). These circulating cells are recruited to tumors by a mechanism that requires both VEGFR1 and VEGFR2 tyrosine kinase receptors [49]. Investigators have related the number of ECPs to the stage and activity of cancer in a clinical setting [50]. Additionally, an intriguing antiangiogenic strategy directed at eliminating circulating EPCs involves the use of cytotoxic agents in a continuous low dose (lower than would be effective against malignant cells) [51]. The basis for this approach is the knowledge that traditional cytotoxic chemotherapy is effective against angiogenic endothelial cells. The use of intermittent dosing made necessary by dose-limiting toxicities of these drugs results in endothelial recovery during which time any antiangiogenic effect of cytotoxic therapy is presumably lost. A low-dose continuous strategy, referred to as metronomic chemotherapy, has been proven effective as an antiangiogenic strategy in animal models [52]. However, a small but important study of solid tumors from patients who had previously received bone marrow transplants before developing cancer allowed the investigators to determine the source of endothelial cells in the tumor. This approach demonstrated that only a small proportion (<5%) of endothelial cells in solid tumors were marrow (donor) derived [53], suggesting that these cells may not be as critical to human tumor angiogenesis and antiangiogenic "metronomic chemotherapy" may not have the same impact on human cancer as is seen in animal models. Studies of this approach in humans are currently ongoing.

Factors Which Regulate Angiogenesis

The net angiogenic activity in any given tissue reflects the balance of pro- and antiangiogenic influences within the tissue. There is a plethora of proteins and other molecular products that can contribute to this balance either directly or indirectly (Table 1). These include the cytokines, acidic and basic fibroblast growth factor (aFGF, and bFGF), vascular endothelial cell growth factor (VEGF), members of the family of chemotactic cytokines known as CXC

Table 1 A listing of angiogenic (left column) and angiostatic (right column) mediators

Promote angiogenesis	Inhibit angiogenesis
12(*R*)-Hydroxyeicosatrienoic acid (12-HETE)	Angiopoietin-2
Acidic fibroblast growth factors (aFGF)	Angiostatic steroids
Adenosine	Angiostatin
	ELR⁻ CXC chemokines
	CXCL4
Angiogenin	CXCL9
	CXCL10
	CXCL11
Angiopoietin	Endostatin
Angiotensin II	Endothelial–monocyte-activating peptide II (EMAP-II)
Angiotropin	
Basic fibroblast growth factors (bFGF)	Eosinophil major basic protein
Ceruloplasmin	High-molecular-weight hyaluronan
Copper	Interferon α, β, and γ
ELR⁺ CXC chemokines	
CXCL1	
CXCL2	Interleukin-1 (IL-1)
CXCL5	
CXCL8	
Epidermal growth factor (EGF)	Interleukin-4 (IL-4)
Fibrin peptide fragments	Interleukin-12 (IL-12)
	Metalloproteinase and thrombospondin
Fibroblast growth factors	domain-homologues (METH)-1 and -2
Heparin	Nitric oxide
Hepatocyte growth factor (HGF)	
	Placental RNase inhibitor
Hyaluronan fragments	Prostaglandin synthase inhibitor
Interleukin-2 (IL-2)	Protamine
Migration inhibitory factor (MIF)	Retinoids
Nicotinamide	Somatostatin
Platelet-activating factor	Thrombospondin-1
Polyamines	Tissue inhibitors of metalloproteases (TIMPs)
Prostaglandin E_1, E_2	Vasostatin
Soluble E-selectin	Vitamin A
Transforming growth factor (TGF-α and -β)	Vitreous fluids
Tumor necrosis factor-α (TNF-α)	
Vascular endothelial growth factor (VEGF)	

chemokines, and the angiopoietin/TIE ligand–receptor system. Also important are internal peptide fragments of larger peptides identified as potent angiogenesis inhibitors, such as angiostatin and endostatin. Only a fraction of these will be discussed in detail.

Fibroblast growth factors. The fibroblast growth factor (FGF) gene family consists of nine members, the prototypes of which are acidic FGF (aFGF) and basic FGF (bFGF). These two members of the FGF family are distinct in that they lack a classic signal peptide to direct their processing in the Golgi apparatus and eventual secretion [54]. Consequently, little is known of how FGF becomes secreted into the extracellular space. Members of the FGF family which do possess the signal peptide sequence were initially discovered as oncogenic growth factors [55]. Transfection of cells with aFGF mutants containing a signal peptide leads to cell transformation [56, 57]. Thus, the lack of signal sequence in aFGF and bFGF may reflect the evolution of a tighter degree of control over their secretion [56, 57]. FGFs induce endothelial cell migration, proliferation, and tube formation in vitro [58, 59]. The involvement of FGFs in pathologic angiogenesis is inferred by studies of tumor-associated angiogenesis. Basic FGF may influence angiogenesis associated with Kaposi's sarcoma [60], breast cancer [61], and lung cancer [62, 63].

FGF receptors. Specific high-affinity FGF receptors have been cloned and exist in three different isoforms (FGFR-1, -2, and -3) that result from alternative splicing of the FGFR gene transcripts. FGFs also bind to glycosaminoglycans [64], and this low-affinity binding is necessary for FGFs to bind to their high-affinity cell surface receptors [65]. Each receptor has three immunoglobulin (Ig)-like extracellular domains (except for FGFR-2 which has only two Ig domains), a transmembrane domain, and an intracellular tyrosine kinase domain [66]. The alternative extracellular domains confer differing ligand-binding specificity for members of the FGF family [66], and these splice variants are distributed in a tissue-specific manner [67].

Vascular endothelial cell growth factor. Also identified as vascular permeability factor (VPF), VEGF is the initial member of a family of proteins with mitogenic and angiogenic activity [68]. VEGF exists in multiple isoforms (VEGF-189, -165, and -121) distinguished by the amino acid length of the primary structure [69] and resulting from alternative splicing of a single gene product [69]. Additionally, the VEGF family consists of two other closely related members, VEGF B [70] and C [71], which map to different chromosomes [72]. VEGF B and C likely play a critical role in the development of the lymphatic system [73, 74]. VEGF is biologically active as a dimer [75] and requires downstream activity of nitric-oxide synthase and guanylate cyclase to induce angiogenesis via its receptors [76]. While VEGF was initially thought to be an endothelial cell-specific agonist, specific VEGF receptors are also present on monocytes, and VEGF induces migration of these cells [77].

The strongest data demonstrating a role for VEGF in angiogenesis are derived from mice with targeted deletion of either the *VEGF* gene or its receptors. Heterozygous mice with a single null allele for the *VEGF* gene develop abnormal vessels and die at embryonic days 11–12 [78, 79]. Similarly, targeted inactivation of either of the two known receptors for VEGF results in embryonic lethality at days 8–9 [80, 81]. VEGF is also expressed in multiple experimental and "naturally occurring" human tumors including lung cancer

[62, 82]. In preclinical models, neutralizing antibodies to VEGF are effective in inhibiting tumor growth in tumor cell lines expressing VEGF [83–85]. This observation led to the clinical development of a humanized monoclonal antibody against VEGF, bevacizumab. A phase III trial of bevacizumab in combination with standard chemotherapy showed that inhibition of VEGF results in modest improvements in survival and time to progression [86]. As a result this antibody is now approved in the United States for use in advanced non-small cell (nonsquamous) lung cancer.

Among the factors known to regulate expression of VEGF, as well as its receptors, is hypoxia [87], which induces VEGF from a number of cell types [87–89]. A major factor responsible for transcriptional activation of VEGF is the transcription factor HIF-1, which is composed of heterodimers of two subunits, HIF-1α, and the aryl hydrocarbon-receptor nuclear translocator (*arnt*, also known as HIF-1β). Interestingly, embryos from HIF-1α-deficient cells actually express higher levels of VEGF mRNA than do wild-type embryos, and it appears that hypoglycemia induces the expression of VEGF via a non-HIF-1α-dependent mechanism [90]. Murine embryonic stem cells genetically engineered to lack the *arnt/HIF-1β* gene fail to augment VEGF expression in response to hypoxia. Embryos derived from these cells display a developmental phenotype similar to VEGF "knockout" mice [21]. Arnt/HIF-1β is a required factor for the hypoxic induction of VEGF gene transcription. Other studies suggest that hypoxic induction of VEGF expression requires both HIF-1α and arnt/HIF-1β [91].

VEGF receptors. The two known receptors for VEGF, flk-1/KDR and flt-1, are tyrosine kinase transmembrane proteins. The receptors probably mediate different actions of VEGF. For example, studies employing VEGF mutants which retain binding to only one of the two receptors reveal that flk-1/KDR mediates VEGF-induced endothelial cell proliferation [92]. In contrast, migration of monocytes in response to VEGF occurs via the flt-1 VEGF receptor [77]. There are currently several pharmacologic small-molecule inhibitors targeted to these receptors [93, 94]. The structure of these receptors is sufficiently similar to other tyrosine kinase family receptors that many of the pharmacologic inhibitors of these receptors under development end up being classified as "multi-targeted inhibitors," which is almost certainly more by accident than by predesign. Nevertheless, the ability of some small molecular inhibitors to target multiple growth factor receptor tyrosine kinases may prove to be of benefit in the clinical setting [93–95].

Angiostatin and endostatin. These two molecules are potent inhibitors of angiogenesis [3, 96] discovered while studying an interesting phenomenon: the inhibition of metastatic tumor growth by primary tumors [3]. Angiostatin was isolated from the urine of tumor-bearing mice [3]. Mice bearing experimental Lewis lung carcinoma tumors typically developed extensive metastases only after removal of the primary tumor. However, in mice which received injections of purified angiostatin, growth of metastases was inhibited, even after removal of the primary tumor [3]. Using a similar experimental strategy, the same group of investigators also isolated endostatin, a molecule with similar activity in animal models [96].

While neither angiostatin nor endostatin has shown to be effective in human disease, they shared an interesting property in that both are internal fragments of larger peptides with neither angiogenic nor angiostatic properties [3, 96]. Angiostatin is a 38-kDa internal fragment derived from plasminogen, and endostatin is a 20-kDa internal fragment of collagen XVIII [3, 96]. Subsequent studies revealed that macrophage metalloelastase is responsible for the proteolytic cleavage of plasminogen to yield angiostatin [97, 98]. Another endogenous inhibitor of angiogenesis that fits this pattern is PEX, a fragment of matrix metalloprotease-2 (MMP-2) comprising the C-terminal hemopexin-like domain [99]. Among the more exciting findings associated with angiostatin and endostatin is their ability to induce and sustain dormancy of micrometastases via suppression of angiogenesis in animal models of cancer [100].

The angiopoietin/TIE receptor–ligand system. This receptor–ligand system is important in the development of the vascular system and is strongly implicated in pathologic angiogenesis as well. The Tie receptors (Tie-1 and Tie-2) are protein-tyrosine kinases that are expressed in the embryonic yolk sac and in areas of vascular development. Tie-1-deficient animals develop to birth but die perinatally due to a defect in vascular integrity, with resulting hemorrhage and generalized edema [101]. In contrast, embryos deficient in Tie-2 (also known as tek) die at embryonic days 10–11, with the most prominent abnormalities being failure of development of the endothelial lining of the heart and failure of the early vascular system to progress beyond its earliest stages of vessel formation [101].

A search for ligands for this receptor system led to the cloning of angiopoietin-1, which is a specific activating ligand for Tie-2 [102]. Expression of angiopoietin-1 in developing embryos is localized predominantly to the myocardial tissue surrounding the endocardium and later in mesenchymal tissue surrounding the developing vasculature [102]. Angiopoietin-1 is not an endothelial cell mitogen, nor does it induce tube formation in vitro, but it plays a vital role in the remodeling of the vascular system during development [102, 103], perhaps by facilitating communication between endothelium and the surrounding mesenchymal cells. A naturally occurring antagonist for the Tie-2 receptor exists, termed angiopoietin-2, and is expressed in areas of vascular remodeling in embryonic and adult tissues [104]. It appears that the ratio of angiopoietin-1 to angiopoietin-2 is critical for determining the maturity of vessels, with angiopoietin-1 serving as a stabilizing signal and attracting vascular pericytes to developing blood vessels and angiopoietin-2 destabilizing the vessels and facilitating the angiogenic response [105].

In general, cancers are characterized by a higher ratio of angiopoietin-2 to angiopoietin-1 [105] than is corresponding normal tissue. Expression of angiopoietin-2 mRNA is associated with greater vessel density *only* in tumors where VEGF mRNA is coexpressed, and coexpression of both factors is associated with poor survival [106]. Higher serum levels of angiopoietin-2 protein detected in lung cancer patients were associated with advancing stage of disease and worse prognosis as well [107]. Interestingly, angiopoietin-2 expression seems to be enhanced by the tumor-associated cytokine IL-10 [108], which is known to be elevated in lung cancer [109–112]. The interactions between angiopoietin-2, angiopoietin-1, and their receptors pose an interesting potential target for tumor angiogenesis.

CXC chemokines. CXC chemokines are a unique family of cytokines named for their leukocyte chemotactic activity (chemotactic cytokines). With respect to angiogenesis, an important aspect of the CXC chemokine family is that it is composed of many members that display either angiogenic or angiostatic activity (see Table 1) [113–117]. The role of the chemokines in lung cancer, and in angiogenesis in particular, is covered in greater detail in Chapter 8.

Many studies have confirmed the central role of angiogenic CXC chemokines in promoting angiogenesis in lung cancer [113, 118–123]. In human lung cancer tumors, the level of angiogenic CXC chemokine expression in tumor homogenates correlates strongly with the vessel density of the corresponding tissue section [124]. This correlation was much stronger than that for either vascular endothelial cell growth factor (VEGF) or basic fibroblast growth factor (bFGF) [124]. Notably, higher levels of CXC chemokine expression in resected tumors are associated with poorer prognosis after surgical resection [124]. Therefore, it is important to identify mechanisms which increase expression of angiogenic CXC chemokines in tumors. Unfortunately, despite many studies implicating the angiogenic CXC chemokines in solid tumor angiogenesis [121, 123, 125–135], efforts at developing antiangiogenic cancer therapy have so far ignored the role of CXC chemokines.

Clinical Implications of Angiogenic Diversity and Angiogenesis Inhibition in Lung Cancer Metastasis

Antiangiogenic therapy for malignancies is a long sought-after goal of the medical–scientific community. An effective systemic inhibitor of tumor-derived angiogenic activity could theoretically prevent further growth of a primary tumor and halt the development of metastases. A guiding principle in this approach is that tumor endothelium is not genetically abnormal like the malignant cell and therefore not subject to a high rate of mutation; it is unlikely to develop "drug resistance" to angiostatic therapy. This assumption has led some investigators to propose a two-compartment approach to tumor therapy, one targeted at the malignant cells and the other at the endothelial cells [136]. However, the promise of antiangiogenic therapies suggested by animal models has borne little fruit in the clinical context. Perhaps one reason is the diversity of angiogenic mechanisms and the adaptability of the tumor to changes in the angiogenic microenvironment. Cancer is a disease characterized by clinical, histologic, and molecular heterogeneity. Therefore, it is not surprising to find that the molecular profiles of lung cancer angiogenic factors (or the "angiogenic signature") of lung cancer display a similar degree of variability from tumor to tumor [137]. The evidence for this comes from both in vitro and in vivo studies of lung cancer, as well as in observations of the variable response to single-target antiangiogenic agents in clinical use.

Many factors contribute to tumor-associated angiogenic activity in lung cancer including VEGF, bFGF, and the CXC chemokines. There is diversity not only in the molecular factors which promote angiogenesis (or the "angiogenic signature") of a tumor [137–141] but also in the mechanisms by which tumors can induce the production of angiogenic factors. This diversity poses a potential problem for therapeutic targeting of angiogenesis.

If tumors retain the ability to switch their angiogenic phenotype when one pathway is blocked by a "targeted agent," this approach is unlikely to result in sustained inhibition of tumor growth. There is experimental proof that this is indeed the case. Mizukami et al. demonstrated that colon cancer cells induce angiogenic responses through multiple independent pathways [135]. They employed a colon cancer cell line in which hypoxia-inducible factor (HIF-1) was stably knocked down (DLD-1^{HIF-kd}). DLD-1^{HIF-kd} cells had predictably decreased levels of VEGF but increased levels of the angiogenic CXC chemokine CXCL8. In tumor xenografts of DLD-1^{HIF-kd} cells, angiogenesis proceeded by production of CXCL8 as a compensatory pathway. They further demonstrated that the mechanism of compensation involved hypoxia-induced production of hydrogen peroxide (H_2O_2), which subsequently activated NF-κB to induce CXCL8 expression [135]. This H_2O_2-mediated activation of NF-κB was enhanced by the presence of mutant K-ras. Mizukami et al. concluded that K-ras mutations favored the expression of the angiogenic factor CXCL8, particularly in the setting of hypoxia [135].

This is consistent with observations we have made in lung cancer, where K-ras mutant tumors had lower levels of VEGF and higher levels of angiogenic CXC chemokines [137]. Work in our lab has suggested that lung cancer tumors also display angiogenic plasticity [137]. We showed that lung cancer tumors implanted into mice deficient for CXCR2, the receptor for angiogenic CXC chemokines, express higher levels of VEGF [137]. On the other hand, tumors developing in a transgenic mouse with lung-specific overexpression of MIF showed the expected increase in tumor size, number, and levels of tumor-associated CXC chemokines but markedly reduced levels of VEGF (unpublished observations). Angiogenic diversity and plasticity is therefore a critical feature of lung cancer tumors and must be accounted for in devising therapeutic strategies aimed at inhibiting angiogenesis. Indeed, a single agent targeted against VEGF (bevacizumab) has shown measurable but relatively modest survival benefit in patients with lung cancer [86], falling disappointingly short of the promise offered by preclinical observations. The data from studies employing so-called multitargeted agents should provide some additional insights into this problem in a clinical setting [93–95], as one would expect an agent targeting multiple angiogenic mediators to prove more effective than a single target inhibitor. Drug development efforts recognizing the extensive array of factors that promote tumor angiogenesis and aimed at broadening the targets of tumor angiogenesis should also prove to be beneficial.

Summary

Angiogenesis is a complex process that involves the activation of normally quiescent endothelium. Multiple overlapping cellular functions require coordinated orchestration for angiogenesis to proceed normally, making this an area ripe for intervention. The complex control of angiogenesis is illustrated by the ever increasing number of molecules which can affect the response. While research has primarily focused on the discovery of individual angiogenic factors, recent studies have highlighted the importance of endogenous angiostatic factors and on the diversity of angiogenic pathways available to malignant tumors. Since angiogenesis is intricately associated with metastatic tumor growth, additional effective antiangiogenic strategies should be developed and tested for their ability to reduce lung cancer metastasis. There has been remarkable progress in the knowledge of angiogenesis in the last three decades. A nuanced understanding of tumor angiogenic diversity and adaptability will improve our ability to exploit the angiogenic dependence of tumor growth.

References

1. Fidler, I.J. Critical factors in the biology of human cancer metastasis: Twenty-Eighth G.H.A. Clowes Memorial Award Lecture. Cancer Res 50: 6130–38, 1990.
2. Holmgren, L., M.S. O'Reilly, and J. Folkman. Dormancy of micrometastases: balanced proliferation and apoptosis in the presence of angiogenesis suppression [see comments]. Nat Med 1: 149–53, 1995.
3. O'Reilly, M.S., L. Holmgren, Y. Shing, C. Chen, R.A. Rosenthal, M. Moses, W.S. Lane, Y. Cao, E.H. Sage, and J. Folkman. Angiostatin: A novel angiogenesis inhibitor that mediates suppression of metastases by a Lewis lung carcinoma. Cell 79: 315–28, 1994.
4. Brown, J., L. Guidi, A. Schnitt, L.V.D. Water, M. Iruela-Arispe, T. Yeo, K. Tognazzi, and H. Dvorak. Vascular stroma formation in carcinoma in situ, invasive carcinoma, and metastatic carcinoma of the breast. Clin Cancer Res 5: 1041–56, 1999.
5. He, Y., T. Karpanen, and K. Alitalo. Role of lymphangiogenic factors in tumor metastasis. Biochim Biophys Acta 1654: 3–12, 2004.
6. He, Y., K. Kozaki, T. Karpanen, K. Koshikawa, S. Yla-Herttuala, T. Takahashi and K. Alitalo. Suppression of Tumor Lymphangiogenesis and Lymph Node Metastasis by Blocking Vascular Endothelial Growth Factor Receptor 3 Signaling. J Natl Cancer Inst 94: 819–25, 2002.
7. Engerman, R.L., D. Pfaffenenbach, and M.D. Davis. Cell turnover of capillaries. Lab Invest 17: 738–43, 1967.
8. Tannock, I.F. and H.S. Hayashi. The proliferation of capillary and endothelial cells. Cancer Res 32: 77–82, 1972.
9. Auerbach, R. Angiogenesis-inducing factors: a review. Vol. 69, Lymphokines: Academic Press, NY, 1981.

10. Sato, N., J.G. Beitz, J. Kato, M. Yamamoto, J.W. Clark, P. Calabresi, A. Raymond and A.R. Frackelton, Jr. Platelet-derived growth factor indirectly stimulates angiogenesis in vitro. Am J Pathol *142*: 1119–30, 1993.

11. Vlodavsky, I., G. Korner, R. Ishai-Michaeli, P. Bashkin, R. Bar-Shavit and Z. Fuks. Extracellular matrix-resident growth factors and enzymes: possible involvement in tumor metastases and angiogenesis. Canc Metastasis Rev *9*: 203–26, 1990.

12. Clark, R.A. Basics of cutaneous wound repair. J Dermatol Surg Oncol *19*: 693–706, 1993.

13. Gimbrone, M.A., S.B. Leapman, R.S. Cotran and J. Folkman. Tumor dormancy in vivo by prevention of neovascularization. J Exp Med *136*: 261–76, 1972.

14. Anderson, I.C., S.E. Mari, R.J. Broderick, B.P. Mari and M.A. Shipp. The angiogenic factor interleukin 8 is induced in non-small cell lung cancer/pulmonary fibroblast cocultures. Cancer Res *60*: 269–72, 2000.

15. Vlodavski, I., J. Folkman, R. Sullivan, R. Fridman, R. Ishai-Michaeli, J. Sasse and M. Klagsbrun. Endothelial cell-derived basic fibroblast growth factor: synthesis and deposition into subendothelial extracellular matrix. Proc Natl Acad Sci USA *84*: 2292–6, 1987.

16. Strieter, R.M., S.L. Kunkel, H.J. Showell, and R.M. Marks. Monokine-induced gene expression of human endothelial cell-derived neutrophil chemotactic factor. Biochem Biophys Res Commun *156*: 1340–5, 1988.

17. Nickoloff, B.J., R.S. Mitra, J. Varani, V.M. Dixit and P.J. Polverini. Aberrant production of interleukin-8 and thrombospondin-1 by psoriatic keratinocytes mediates angiogenesis. Am J Pathol *144*: 820–8, 1994.

18. Polverini, P.J. and S.J. Leibovich. Induction of neovascularization in vivo and endothelial cell proliferation in vitro by tumor-associated macrophages. Lab. Invest. *51*: 635–42, 1984.

19. White, E.S., D.L. Livant, S. Markwart and D.A. Arenberg. Monocyte–fibronectin interactions, via alpha(5)beta(1) integrin, induce expression of CXC chemokine-dependent angiogenic activity. J Immunol *167*: 5362–6, 2001.

20. White, E.S., S.R.B. Strom, N.L. Wys, and D.A. Arenberg. Non-Small Cell Lung Cancer Cells Induce Monocytes to Increase Expression of Angiogenic Activity. J Immunol *166*: 7549–55, 2001.

21. Maltepe, E., J.V. Schmidt, D. Baunoch, C.A. Bradfield and M.C. Simon. Abnormal angiogenesis and responses to glucose and oxygen deprivation in mice lacking the protein ARNT. Nature *386*: 403–07, 1997.

22. Rastinejad, F., P.J. Polverini, and N.P. Bouck. Regulation of the activity of a new inhibitor of angiogenesis by a cancer suppressor gene. Cell *56*: 345–55, 1989.

23. Lampugnani, M.G., M. Resnati, M. Raiteri, R. Pigott, A. Pisacane, G. Houen, L.P. Ruco and E. Dejana. A novel endothelial-specific membrane protein is a marker of cell–cell contacts. J Cell Biol *118*: 1511–22, 1992.

24. Lampugnani, M.G., M. Corada, L. Caveda, F. Breviario, O. Ayalon, B. Geiger and E. Dejana. The molecular organization of endothelial cell to cell junctions: differential association of plakoglobin, beta-catenin, and alpha-catenin with vascular endothelial cadherin (VE-cadherin). J Cell Biol *129*: 203–17, 1995.

25. Tanihara, H., M. Kido, S. Obata, R.L. Heimark, M. Davidson, T. St John and S. Suzuki. Characterization of cadherin-4 and cadherin-5 reveals new aspects of cadherins. J Cell Sci *107*: 1697–704, 1994.

26. Dejana, E. Endothelial adherens junctions: implications in the control of vascular permeability and angiogenesis. J Clin Invest *98*: 1949–53, 1996.

27. Hiraoka, N., E. Allen, I.J. Apel, M.R. Gyetko and S.J. Weiss. Matrix metalloproteinases regulate neovascularization by acting as pericellular fibrinolysins. Cell *95*: 365–77, 1998.

28. Arnold, F. and D.C. West. Angiogenesis in wound healing. Pharmacol Ther *52*: 407–22, 1991.

29. Brooks, P.C., R.A. Clark, and D.A. Cheresh. Requirement of vascular integrin alpha v beta 3 for angiogenesis. Science *264*: 569–71, 1994.

30. Brooks, P.C., A.M. Montgomery, M. Rosenfeld, R.A. Reisfeld, T. Hu, G. Klier and D.A. Cheresh. Integrin alpha v beta 3 antagonists promote tumor regression by inducing apoptosis of angiogenic blood vessels. Cell *79*: 1157–64, 1994.
31. Sholly, M.M., G.P. Fergusen, H.R. Seibel, J.L. Montour and J.D. Wilson. Mechanisms of neovascularization: vascular sprouting can occur without proliferation of endothelial cells. Lab Invest *51*: 624–34, 1984.
32. Sunderkotter, C., M. Goebeler, K. Schulze-Osthoff, R. Bhardwaj, and C. Sorg. Macrophage-derived angiogenesis factors. Pharmacol Ther *51*: 195–216, 1991.
33. Koolwijk, P., M.G. van Erck, W.J. de Vree, M.A. Vermeer, H.A. Weich, R. Hanemaaijer and V.W. van Hinsbergh. Cooperative effect of TNFalpha, bFGF, and VEGF on the formation of tubular structures of human microvascular endothelial cells in a fibrin matrix. Role of urokinase activity. J Cell Biol *132*: 1177–88, 1996.
34. Ingber, D.E. and J. Folkman. Mechanochemical switching between growth and differentiation during fibroblast growth factor-stimulated angiogenesis in vitro: role of extracellular matrix. J Cell Biol *109*: 317–30, 1989.
35. Davidson, J.M. Wound repair, in *Inflammation: Basic Principles and Clinical Correlates*, ed. Gallin, J.I., I.M. Goldstein and R. Snyderman (New York: Raven Press, Ltd, 1992).
36. French-Constant, C., D.W.L. Van, H.F. Dvorak and R.O. Hynes. Reappearance of an embryonic pattern of fibronectin splicing during wound healing in the adult rat. J Cell Biol *109*: 903–14, 1989.
37. Kurkinen, M., A. Vaheri, P.J. Roberts and S. Stenan. Sequential appearance of fibronectin and collagen in experimental granulation tissue. Lab Invest *43*: 47–51, 1980.
38. Leibovich, S.J. and D.M. Weisman. Macrophages, wound repair and angiogenesis. Prog Clin Biol Res *266*: 131–45, 1988.
39. Matsumura, T., K. Wolff, and P. Petzelbauer. Endothelial cell tube formation depends on cadherin 5 and CD31 interactions with filamentous actin. J Immunol *158*: 3408–16, 1997.
40. DeLisser, H., J. Chilkotowsky, H. Yan, M. Daise, C. Buck, and S. Albelda. Deletions in the cytoplasmic domain of platelet–endothelial cell adhesion molecule-1 (PECAM-1, CD31) result in changes in ligand binding properties. J Cell Biol 124: 195–203, 1994.
41. Delisser, H.M., M. Christofidou-Solomidou, R.M. Strieter, M.D. Burdick, C.S. Robinson, R.S. Wexler, J.S. Kerr, C. Garlanda, J.R. Merwin and S.M. Albelda. Involvement of endothelial PECAM-1/CD31 in angiogenesis. Am J Pathol *151*: 671–7, 1997.
42. Haralabopoulos, G.C., D.S. Grant, H.K. Kleinman, P.I. Lelkes, S.P. Papaioannou and M.E. Maragoudakis. Inhibitors of basement membrane collagen synthesis prevent endothelial cell alignment in matrigel in vitro and angiogenesis in vivo. Lab Invest *71*: 575–82, 1994.
43. Erber, R., A. Thurnher, A.D. Katsen, G. Groth, H. Kerger, H.P. Hammes, M.D. Menger, A. Ullrich and P. Vajkoczy. Combined inhibition of VEGF-and PDGF-signaling enforces tumor vessel regression by interfering with pericyte-mediated endothelial cell survival mechanisms. FASEB J *18*: 338–40, 2004.
44. Benjamin, L.E., I. Hemo, and E. Keshet. A plasticity window for blood vessel remodelling is defined by pericyte coverage of the preformed endothelial network and is regulated by PDGF-B and VEGF. Development *125*: 1591–8, 1998.
45. Abramsson, A., O. Berlin, H. Papayan, D. Paulin, M. Shani and C. Betsholtz. Analysis of mural cell recruitment to tumor vessels. Circulation *105*: 112–7, 2002.
46. Guo, P., B. Hu, W. Gu, L. Xu, D. Wang, H.J. Huang, W.K. Cavenee, and S.Y. Cheng. Platelet-derived growth factor-B enhances glioma angiogenesis by stimulating vascular endothelial growth factor expression in tumor endothelia and by promoting pericyte recruitment. Am J Pathol *162*: 1083–93, 2003.
47. Furuhashi, M., T. Sjoblom, A. Abramsson, J. Ellingsen, P. Micke, H. Li, E. Bergsten-Folestad, U. Eriksson, R. Heuchel, C. Betsholtz, C.H. Heldin, and A. Ostman. Platelet-derived growth factor production by B16 melanoma cells leads to increased pericyte abundance in tumors and an associated increase in tumor growth rate. Cancer Res *64*: 2725–33, 2004.

48. Lehti, K., E. Allen, H. Birkedal-Hansen, K. Holmbeck, Y. Miyake, T.H. Chun and S.J. Weiss. An MT1-MMP-PDGF receptor-beta axis regulates mural cell investment of the microvasculature. Genes Dev 19: 979–91, 2005.
49. Lyden, D., K. Hattori, S. Dias, C. Costa, P. Blaikie, L. Butros, A. Chadburn, B. Heissig, W. Marks and L. Witte. Impaired recruitment of bone-marrow-derived endothelial and hematopoietic precursor cells blocks tumor angiogenesis and growth. Nat Med 7: 1194–201, 2001.
50. Beerepoot, L.V., N. Mehra, J.S.P. Vermaat, B.A. Zonnenberg, M.F.G.B. Gebbink and E.E. Voest. Increased levels of viable circulating endothelial cells are an indicator of progressive disease in cancer patients. Ann Oncol 15: 139–45, 2004.
51. Browder, T., C.E. Butterfield, B.M. Kraling, B. Shi, B. Marshall, M.S. O'Reilly and J. Folkman. Antiangiogenic scheduling of chemotherapy improves efficacy against experimental drug-resistant cancer. Cancer Res 60: 1878–86, 2000.
52. Kerbel, R.S. and B.A. Kamen. The anti-angiogenic basis of metronomic chemotherapy. Nat Rev Cancer 4: 423–36, 2004.
53. Peters, B.A., L.A. Diaz, K. Polyak, L. Meszler, K. Romans, E.C. Guinan, J.H. Antin, D. Myerson, S.R. Hamilton, B. Vogelstein, K.W. Kinzler and C. Lengauer. Contribution of bone marrow-derived endothelial cells to human tumor vasculature. Nat Med 11: 261–62, 2005.
54. Burgess, W.H. and T. Maciag. The heparin-binding (fibroblast) growth factor family of proteins. Annu Rev Biochem 58: 575–606, 1989.
55. Talarico, D. and C. Basilico. The K-fgf/hst oncogene induces transformation through an autocrine mechanism that requires extracellular stimulation of the mitogenic pathway. Mol Cell Biol 11: 1138–45, 1991.
56. Forough, R., Z. Xi, M. MacPhee, S. Friedman, K.A. Engleka, T. Sayers, R.H. Wiltrout and T. Maciag. Differential transforming abilities of non-secreted and secreted forms of human fibroblast growth factor-1. J Biol Chem 268: 2960–8, 1993.
57. Rogelj, S., R.A. Weinberg, P. Fanning and M. Klagsbrun. Basic fibroblast growth factor fused to a signal peptide transforms cells. Nature 331: 173–5, 1988.
58. Connolly, D.T., B.L. Stoddard, N.K. Harakas and J. Feder. Human fibroblast-derived growth factor is a mitogen and chemoattractant for endothelial cells. Biochem Biophys Res Commun 144: 705–12, 1987.
59. Montesano, R., J.D. Vassalli, A. Baird, R. Guillemin and L. Orci. Basic fibroblast growth factor induces angiogenesis in vitro. Proc Natl Acad Sci USA 83: 7297–301, 1986.
60. Ensoli, B., P. Markham, V. Kao, G. Barillari, V. Fiorelli, R. Gendelman, M. Raffeld, G. Zon and R.C. Gallo. Block of AIDS-Kaposi's sarcoma (KS) cell growth, angiogenesis, and lesion formation in nude mice by antisense oligonucleotide targeting basic fibroblast growth factor. A novel strategy for the therapy of KS. J Clin Invest 94: 1736–46, 1994.
61. Lewis, C.E., R. Leek, A. Harris and J.O. McGee. Cytokine regulation of angiogenesis in breast cancer: the role of tumor-associated macrophages. J Leukoc Biol 57: 747–51, 1995.
62. Brattstrom, D., M. Bergqvist, A. Larsson, J. Holmertz, P. Hesselius, L. Rosenberg, O. Brodin and G. Wagenius. Basic fibroblast growth factor and vascular endothelial growth factor in sera from non-small cell lung cancer patients. Anticancer Res 18: 1123–7, 1998.
63. Iwasaki, A., M. Kuwahara, Y. Yoshinaga and T. Shirakusa. Basic fibroblast growth factor (bFGF) and vascular endothelial growth factor (VEGF) levels, as prognostic indicators in NSCLC. Eur J Cardiothorac Surg 25: 443–8, 2004.
64. Friesel, R.E. and T. Maciag. Molecular mechanisms of angiogenesis: fibroblast growth factor signal transduction. Faseb J 9: 919–25, 1995.
65. Yayon, A., M. Klagsbrun, J.D. Esko, P. Leder and D.M. Ornitz. Cell surface, heparin-like molecules are required for binding of basic fibroblast growth factor to its high affinity receptor. Cell 64: 841–8, 1991.
66. Johnson, D.E. and L.T. Williams. Structural and Functional Diversity in the FGF receptor multigene family. Adv Cancer Res 60: 1–40, 1993.

67. Orr-Urtreger, A., M.T. Bedford, T. Burakova, E. Arman, Y. Zimmer, A. Yayon, D. Givol and P. Lonai. Developmental localization of the splicing alternatives of fibroblast growth factor receptor 2 (FGFR2). Dev Biol *158*: 475–86, 1993.
68. Tischer, E., D. Gospodarowicz, R. Mitchell, M. Silva, J. Schilling, K. Lau, T. Crisp, J.C. Fiddes and J.A. Abraham. Vascular endothelial growth factor: a new member of the platelet-derived growth factor gene family. Biochem Biophys Res Commun *165*: 1198–206, 1989.
69. Tischer, E., R. Mitchell, T. Hartman, M. Silva, D. Gospodarowicz, J.C. Fiddes and J.A. Abraham. The human gene for vascular endothelial growth factor. Multiple protein forms are encoded through alternative exon splicing. J Biol Chem *266*: 11947–54, 1991.
70. Olofsson, B., K. Pajusola, A. Kaipainen, G. von Euler, V. Joukov, O. Saksela, A. Orpana, R.F. Pettersson, K. Alitalo and U. Eriksson. Vascular endothelial growth factor B, a novel growth factor for endothelial cells. Proc Natl Acad Sci USA *93*: 2576–81, 1996.
71. Joukov, V., K. Pajusola, A. Kaipainen, D. Chilov, I. Lahtinen, E. Kukk, O. Saksela, N. Kalkkinen and K. Alitalo. A novel vascular endothelial growth factor, VEGF-C, is a ligand for the Flt4 (VEGFR-3) and KDR (VEGFR-2) receptor tyrosine kinases [published erratum appears in EMBO J 1996 Apr 1;15(7):1751]. Embo J *15*: 290–98, 1996.
72. Wei, M.H., N.C. Popescu, M.I. Lerman, M.J. Merrill and D.B. Zimonjic. Localization of the human vascular endothelial growth factor gene, VEGF, at chromosome 6p12. Hum Genet *97*: 794–7, 1996.
73. Jeltsch, M., A. Kaipainen, V. Joukov, X. Meng, M. Lakso, H. Rauvala, M. Swartz, D. Fukumura, R.K. Jain and K. Alitalo. Hyperplasia of lymphatic vessels in VEGF-C transgenic mice. Science *276*: 1423–5, 1997.
74. Kukk, E., A. Lymboussaki, S. Taira, A. Kaipainen, M. Jeltsch, V. Joukov, and K. Alitalo. VEGF-C receptor binding and pattern of expression with VEGFR-3 suggests a role in lymphatic vascular development. Development *122*: 3829–37, 1996.
75. Claffey, K.P., D.R. Senger, and B.M. Spiegelman. Structural requirements for dimerization, glycosylation, secretion, and biological function of VPF/VEGF. Biochim Biophys Acta *1246*: 1–9, 1995.
76. Ziche, M., L. Morbidelli, R. Choudhuri, H.-T. Zhang, S. Donnini and H.J. Granger. Nitric Oxide synthase lies downstream from vascular endothelial growth factor-induced, but not basic fibroblast growth factor-induced angiogenesis. J Clin Invest *99*: 2626–34, 1997.
77. Barleon, B., S. Sozzani, D. Zhou, H.A. Weich, A. Mantovani and D. Marme. Migration of human monocytes in response to vascular endothelial growth factor (VEGF) is mediated via the VEGF receptor flt-1. Blood *87*: 3336–43, 1996.
78. Carmeliet, P., V. Ferreira, G. Breier, S. Pollefeyt, L. Kieckens, M. Gertsenstein, M. Fahrig, A. Vandenhoeck, K. Harpal, C. Eberhardt, C. Declercq, J. Pawling, L. Moons, D. Collen, W. Risau and A. Nagy. Abnormal blood vessel development and lethality in embryos lacking a single VEGF allele. Nature *380*: 435–9, 1996.
79. Ferrara, N., K. Carver-Moore, H. Chen, M. Dowd, L. Lu, K.S. O'Shea, L. Powell-Braxton, K.J. Hillan and M.W. Moore. Heterozygous embryonic lethality induced by targeted inactivation of the VEGF gene. Nature *380*: 439–42, 1996.
80. Fong, G.H., J. Rossant, M. Gertsenstein and M.L. Breitman. Role of the Flt-1 receptor tyrosine kinase in regulating the assembly of vascular endothelium. Nature *376*: 66–70, 1995.
81. Shalaby, F., J. Rossant, T.P. Yamaguchi, M. Gertsenstein, X.F. Wu, M.L. Breitman and A.C. Schuh. Failure of blood-island formation and vasculogenesis in Flk-1- deficient mice. Nature *376*: 62–6, 1995.
82. Ohta, Y., Y. Endo, M. Tanaka, J. Shimizu, M. Oda, Y. Hayashi, Y. Watanabe and T. Sasaki. Significance of vascular endothelial growth factor messenger RNA expression in primary lung cancer. Clin Cancer Res *2*: 1411–6, 1996.

83. Borgstrom, P., K.J. Hillan, P. Sriramarao and N. Ferrara. Complete inhibition of angiogenesis and growth of microtumors by anti-vascular endothelial growth factor neutralizing antibody: novel concepts of angiostatic therapy from intravital videomicroscopy. Cancer Res 56: 4032–9, 1996.

84. Claffey, K.P., L.F. Brown, L.F. del Aguila, K. Tognazzi, K.T. Yeo, E.J. Manseau and H.F. Dvorak. Expression of vascular permeability factor/vascular endothelial growth factor by melanoma cells increases tumor growth, angiogenesis, and experimental metastasis. Cancer Res 56: 172–81, 1996.

85. Kim, J.K., B. Li, J. Winer, M. Armanini, N. Gillett, H.S. Phillips and N. Ferrara. Inhibition of vascular endothelial growth factor-induced angiogenesis suppresses tumor growth in vivo. Nature 362: 841–44, 1993.

86. Sandler, A.B., R. Gray, J. Brahmer, A. Dowlati, J.H. Schiller, M.C. Perry and D.H. Johnson. Randomized phase II/III trial of paclitaxel (P) plus carboplatin (C) with or without bevacizumab (NSC# 704865) in patients with advanced non-squamous non-small cell lung cancer (NSCLC): An Eastern Cooperative Oncology Group (ECOG) Trial-E4599. J Clin Oncol 23: 4–4, 2005.

87. Detmar, M., L.F. Brown, B. Berse, R.W. Jackman, B.M. Elicker, H.F. Dvorak and K.P. Claffey. Hypoxia regulates the expression of vascular permeability factor/vascular endothelial growth factor (VPF/VEGF) and its receptors in human skin. J Invest Dermatol 108: 263–8, 1997.

88. Freeman, M.R., F.X. Schneck, M.L. Gagnon, C. Corless, S. Soker, K. Niknejad, G.E. Peoples and M. Klagsbrun. Peripheral blood T lymphocytes and lymphocytes infiltrating human cancers express vascular endothelial growth factor: a potential role for T cells in angiogenesis. Cancer Res 55: 4140–5, 1995.

89. Brogi, E., T. Wu, A. Namiki and J.M. Isner. Indirect angiogenic cytokines upregulate VEGF and bFGF gene expression in vascular smooth muscle cells, whereas hypoxia upregulates VEGF expression only. Circulation 90: 649–52, 1994.

90. Kotch, L.E., N.V. Iyer, E. Laughner and G.L. Semenza. Defective Vascularization of HIF-1 alpha-Null Embryos Is Not Associated with VEGF Deficiency but with Mesenchymal Cell Death. Dev Biol 209: 254–67, 1999.

91. Forsythe, J.A., B.H. Jiang, N.V. Iyer, F. Agani, S.W. Leung, R.D. Koos and G.L. Semenza. Activation of vascular endothelial growth factor gene transcription by hypoxia-inducible factor 1. Mol Cell Biol 16: 4604–13, 1996.

92. Keyt, B.A., H.V. Nguyen, L.T. Berleau, C.M. Duarte, J. Park, H. Chen and N. Ferrara. Identification of vascular endothelial growth factor determinants for binding KDR and FLT-1 receptors. Generation of receptor-selective VEGF variants by site-directed mutagenesis. J Biol Chem 271: 5638–46, 1996.

93. Giaccone, G. The potential of antiangiogenic therapy in non-small cell lung cancer. Clin Cancer Res 13: 1961–70, 2007.

94. Blumenschein, G. and J.V. Heymach. Angiogenesis inhibitors for lung cancer: clinical developments and future directions. J Thorac Oncol 1: 744–48, 2006.

95. Ardizzoni, A. and M. Tiseo. Combination of target agents: challenges and opportunities. Pisa symposium. J Thorac Oncol 2: S4–S6, 2007.

96. O'Reilly, M.S. T. Boehm, Y. Shing, N. Fukai, G. Vasios, W.S. Lane, E. Flynn, J.R. Birkhead, B.R. Olsen and J. Folkman. Endostatin: an endogenous inhibitor of angiogenesis and tumor growth. Cell 88: 277–85, 1997.

97. Dong, Z., R. Kumar, X. Yang, and I.J. Fidler. Macrophage-derived metalloelastase is responsible for the generation of angiostatin in Lewis lung carcinoma. Cell 88: 801–10, 1997.

98. Dong, Z., J. Yoneda, R. Kumar, and I.J. Fidler. Angiostatin-mediated suppression of cancer metastases by primary neoplasms engineered to produce Granulocyte/Macrophage colony-stimulating factor [In Process Citation]. J Exp Med 188: 755–63, 1998.

99. Brooks, P.C., S. Silletti, T.L. von Schalscha, M. Friedlander and D.A. Cheresh. Disruption of angiogenesis by PEX, a noncatalytic metalloproteinase fragment with integrin binding activity. Cell 92: 391–400, 1998.

100. O'Reilly, M.S. L. Holmgren, C. Chen and J. Folkman. Angiostatin induces and sustains dormancy of human primary tumors in mice. Nat Med 2: 689–92, 1996.

101. Sato, T.N., Y. Tozawa, U. Deutsch, K. Wolburg-Buchholz, Y. Fujiwara, M. Gendron-Maguire, T. Gridley, H. Wolburg, W. Risau and Y. Qin. Distinct roles of the receptor tyrosine kinases Tie-1 and Tie-2 in blood vessel formation. Nature 376: 70–4, 1995.

102. Davis, S., T.H. Aldrich, P.F. Jones, A. Acheson, D.L. Compton, V. Jain, T.E. Ryan, J. Bruno, C. Radziejewski, P.C. Maisonpierre and G.D. Yancopoulos. Isolation of angiopoietin-1, a ligand for the TIE2 receptor, by secretion-trap expression cloning [see comments]. Cell 87: 1161–9, 1996.

103. Suri, C., P.F. Jones, S. Patan, S. Bartunkova, P.C. Maisonpierre, S. Davis, T.N. Sato and G.D. Yancopoulos. Requisite role of angiopoietin-1, a ligand for the TIE2 receptor, during embryonic angiogenesis [see comments]. Cell 87: 1171–80, 1996.

104. Maisonpierre, P.C., C. Suri, P.F. Jones, S. Bartunkova, S.J. Wiegand, C. Radziejewski, D. Compton, J. McClain, T.H. Aldrich, N. Papadopoulos, T.J. Daly, S. Davis, T.N. Sato, and G.D. Yancopoulos. Angiopoietin-2, a natural antagonist for Tie2 that disrupts in vivo angiogenesis [see comments]. Science 277: 55–60, 1997.

105. Tait, C.R. and P.F. Jones. Angiopoietins in tumours: the angiogenic switch. J Pathol 204: 1–10, 2004.

106. Tanaka, F., S. Ishikawa, K. Yanagihara, R. Miyahara, Y. Kawano, M. Li, Y. Otake and H. Wada. Expression of angiopoietins and its clinical significance in non-small cell lung cancer. Cancer Res 62: 7124–9, 2002.

107. Park, J.H., K.J. Park, Y.S. Kim, S.S. Sheen, K.S. Lee, H.N. Lee, Y.J. Oh and S.C. Hwang. Serum angiopoietin-2 as a clinical marker for lung cancer. Chest 132: 200–6, 2007.

108. Hatanaka, H., Y. Abe, M. Naruke, M. Tokunaga, Y. Oshika, T. Kawakami, H. Osada, J. Nagata, J. Kamochi, T. Tsuchida, H. Kijima, H. Yamazaki, H. Inoue, Y. Ueyama and M. Nakamura. Significant correlation between interleukin 10 expression and vascularization through angiopoietin/TIE2 networks in non-small cell lung cancer. Clin Cancer Res 7: 1287–92, 2001.

109. Smith, D.R., S.L. Kunkel, M.D. Burdick, C.M. Wilke, M.B. Orringer, R.I. Whyte and R.M. Strieter. Production of Interleukin-10 by human bronchogenic carcinoma. Am. J. Pathol. 145: 18–25, 1994.

110. Huang, M., J. Wang, P. Lee, S. Sharma, J.T. Mao, H. Meissner, K. Uyemura, R. Modlin, J. Wollman and S.M. Dubinett. Human non-small cell lung cancer cells express a type 2 cytokine pattern. Cancer Res 55: 3847–53, 1995.

111. Huang, M., S. Sharma, J.T. Mao, and S.M. Dubinett. Non-small cell lung cancer-derived soluble mediators and prostaglandin E2 enhance peripheral blood lymphocyte IL-10 transcription and protein production. J Immunol 157: 5512–20, 1996.

112. Huang, M., M. Stolina, S. Sharma, J.T. Mao, L. Zhu, P.W. Miller, J. Wollman, H. Herschman, and S.M. Dubinett. Non-small cell lung cancer cyclooxygenase-2-dependent regulation of cytokine balance in lymphocytes and macrophages: up-regulation of interleukin 10 and down-regulation of interleukin 12 production. Cancer Res 58: 1208–16, 1998.

113. Arenberg, D.A., M.P. Keane, B. DiGiovine, S.L. Kunkel, S.B. Morris, Y.Y. Xue, M.D. Burdick, M.C. Glass, M.D. Iannettoni, and R.M. Strieter. Epithelial–neutrophil activating peptide (ENA-78) is an important angiogenic factor in non-small cell lung cancer. J Clin Invest 102: 465–72, 1998.

114. Smith, D.R., P.J. Polverini, S.L. Kunkel, M.B. Orringer, R.I. Whyte, M.D. Burdick, C.A. Wilke and R.M. Strieter. Inhibition of interleukin 8 attenuates angiogenesis in bronchogenic carcinoma. J Exp Med 179: 1409–15, 1994.

115. Strieter, R.M., S.L. Kunkel, D.A. Arenberg, M.D. Burdick and P.J. Polverini. Interferon gamma-inducible protein 10 (IP-10), a member of the C-X-C chemokine family, is an inhibitor of angiogenesis. Biochem Biophys Res Commun 210: 51–7, 1995.

116. Strieter, R.M., P.J. Polverini, D.A. Arenberg and S.L. Kunkel. The role of CXC chemokines as regulators of angiogenesis. Shock 4: 155–60, 1995.

117. Strieter, R.M., P.J. Polverini, S.L. Kunkel, D.A. Arenberg, M.D. Burdick, J. Kasper, J. Dzuiba, J. Van Damme, A. Walz, D. Marriott, S. Chan, S. Roczniak and A. Shanafelt. The functional role of the ELR motif in CXC chemokine-mediated angiogenesis. J Biol Chem 270: 27348–57, 1995.

118. Arenberg, D.A., S.L. Kunkel, P.J. Polverini, S.B. Morris, M.D. Burdick, M. Glass, D.T. Taub, M.D. Iannetoni, R.I. Whyte, and R.M. Strieter. Interferon-γ-inducible protein 10 (IP-10) is an angiostatic factor that inhibits human non-small cell lung cancer (NSCLC) tumorigenesis and spontaneous metastases. J Exp Med 184: 981–92, 1996.

119. Arenberg, D.A., P.J. Polverini, S.L. Kunkel, A. Shanafelt, J. Hesselgesser, R. Horuk and R.M. Strieter. The role of CXC chemokines in the regulation of angiogenesis in non-small cell lung cancer. J Leukoc Biol 62: 554–62, 1997.

120. Arenberg, D.A., S.L. Kunkel, P.J. Polverini, M. Glass, M.D. Burdick and R.M. Strieter. Inhibition of interleukin-8 reduces tumorigenesis of human non-small cell lung cancer in SCID mice. J Clin Invest 97: 2792–802, 1996.

121. Yuan, A., P.C. Yang, C.J. Yu, W.J. Chen, F.Y. Lin, S.H. Kuo, and K.T. Luh. Interleukin-8 messenger ribonucleic acid expression correlates with tumor progression, tumor angiogenesis, patient survival, and timing of relapse in non-small-cell lung cancer. Am J Respir Crit Care Med 162: 1957–63, 2000.

122. Yuan, A., C.J. Yu, K.T. Luh, S.H. Kuo, Y.C. Lee and P.C. Yang. Aberrant p53 expression correlates with expression of vascular endothelial growth factor mRNA and interleukin-8 mRNA and neoangiogenesis in non-small-cell lung cancer. J Clin Oncol 20: 900–10, 2002.

123. Yatsunami, J., N. Tsuruta, K. Ogata, K. Wakamatsu, K. Takayama, M. Kawasaki, Y. Nakanishi, N. Hara, and S. Hayashi. Interleukin-8 participates in angiogenesis in non-small cell, but not small cell carcinoma of the lung. Cancer Lett 120: 101–8, 1997.

124. White, E.S., K.R. Flaherty, S. Carskadon, A. Brant, M.D. Iannettoni, J. Yee, M.B. Orringer and D.A. Arenberg. Macrophage migration inhibitory factor and CXC chemokine expression in non-small cell lung cancer: role in angiogenesis and prognosis. Clin Cancer Res 9: 853–60, 2003.

125. Chopra, V., T.V. Dinh, and E.V. Hannigan. Serum levels of interleukins, growth factors and angiogenin in patients with endometrial cancer. J Cancer Res Clin Oncol 123: 167–72, 1997.

126. Chopra, V., T.V. Dinh, and E.V. Hannigan. Circulating serum levels of cytokines and angiogenic factors in patients with cervical cancer. Cancer Invest 16: 152–9, 1998.

127. Ferrer, F.A., L.J. Miller, R.I. Andrawis, S.H. Kurtzman, P.C. Albertsen, V.P. Laudone and D.L. Kreutzer. Angiogenesis and prostate cancer: in vivo and in vitro expression of angiogenesis factors by prostate cancer cells. Urology 51: 161–7, 1998.

128. Fujimoto, J., H. Sakaguchi, I. Aoki and T. Tamaya. Clinical implications of expression of interleukin 8 related to angiogenesis in uterine cervical cancers. Cancer Res 60: 2632–5, 2000.

129. Kitadai, Y., Y. Takahashi, K. Haruma, K. Naka, K. Sumii, H. Yokozaki, W. Yasui, N. Mukaida, Y. Ohmoto, G. Kajiyama, I.J. Fidler and E. Tahara. Transfection of interleukin-8 increases angiogenesis and tumorigenesis of human gastric carcinoma cells in nude mice. Br J Cancer 81: 647–53, 1999.

130. Miller, L.J., S.H. Kurtzman, Y. Wang, K.H. Anderson, R.R. Lindquist and D.L. Kreutzer. Expression of interleukin-8 receptors on tumor cells and vascular endothelial cells in human breast cancer tissue. Anticancer Res 18: 77–81, 1998.

131. Shi, Q., J.L. Abbruzzese, S. Huang, I.J. Fidler, Q. Xiong and K. Xie. Constitutive and inducible interleukin 8 expression by hypoxia and acidosis renders human pancreatic cancer cells more tumorigenic and metastatic. Clin Cancer Res 5: 3711–21, 1999.

132. Xu, L., K. Xie, N. Mukaida, K. Matsushima, and I.J. Fidler. Hypoxia-induced elevation in interleukin-8 expression by human ovarian carcinoma cells. Cancer Res 59: 5822–9, 1999.

133. Yoneda, J., H. Kuniyasu, M.A. Crispens, J.E. Price, C.D. Bucana and I.J. Fidler. Expression of angiogenesis-related genes and progression of human ovarian carcinomas in nude mice. J Natl Cancer Inst 90: 447–54, 1998.

134. Wolf, J.S., Z. Chen, G. Dong, J.B. Sunwoo, C.C. Bancroft, D.E. Capo, N.T. Yeh, N. Mukaida and C. Van Waes. IL (interleukin)-1alpha promotes nuclear factor-kappaB and AP-1-induced IL-8 expression, cell survival, and proliferation in head and neck squamous cell carcinomas. Clin Cancer Res 7: 1812–20, 2001.

135. Mizukami, Y., W.S. Jo, E.M. Duerr, M. Gala, J. Li, X. Zhang, M.A. Zimmer, O. Iliopoulos, L.R. Zukerberg, Y. Kohgo, M.P. Lynch, B.R. Rueda and D.C. Chung. Induction of interleukin-8 preserves the angiogenic response in HIF-1alpha-deficient colon cancer cells. Nat Med 11: 992–7, 2005.

136. Folkman, J. Clinical applications of research on angiogenesis. N Eng J Med 333: 1757–63, 1995.

137. McClelland, M.R., S.L. Carskadon, L. Zhao, E.S. White, D.G. Beer, M.B. Orringer, A. Pickens, A.C. Chang and D.A. Arenberg. Diversity of the angiogenic phenotype in non-small cell lung cancer. Am J Respir Cell Mol Biol 36: 343–50, 2007.

138. Kerbel, R.S., J. Yu, J. Tran, S. Man, A. Viloria-Petit, G. Klement, B.L. Coomber and J. Rak. Possible Mechanisms of Acquired Resistance to Anti-angiogenic Drugs: Implications for the Use of Combination Therapy Approaches. Cancer Metastasis Rev 20: 79–86, 2001.

139. Quesada, A.R., M.A. Medina, and E. Alba. Playing only one instrument may be not enough: Limitations and future of the antiangiogenic treatment of cancer. Bioessays 29: 1159–68, 2007.

140. Jung, Y.D., S.A. Ahmad, Y. Akagi, Y. Takahashi, W. Liu, N. Reinmuth, R.M. Shaheen, F. Fan and L.M. Ellis. Role of the tumor microenvironment in mediating response to anti-angiogenic therapy. Cancer Metastasis Rev 19: 147–57, 2000.

141. Taylor, A.P., L. Osorio, R. Craig, J.A. Raleigh, Z. Ying, D.M. Goldenberg, and R.D. Blumenthal. Tumor-specific regulation of angiogenic growth factors and their receptors during recovery from cytotoxic therapy (2002).

Chemokines in Lung Cancer Metastasis

Borna Mehrad, Ellen C. Keeley, and Robert M. Strieter

Abstract Chemokines were first described for their ability to recruit inflammatory leukocytes, but their biological role has now been recognized in many other biological processes, including control of cancer angiogenesis and mediating homing of metastatic cells. In this chapter, we review the role of chemokines in angiogenesis and angiostasis and metastasis in the context of lung cancer.

Introduction

Chemokine ligands are a superfamily of structurally homologous cytokine molecules that share four conserved cysteine residues at their amino terminus. Chemokines are subdivided into CC, CXC, C, and CX_3C families based on the sequence position of amino acids in relation to the first two cysteine residues. The CXC family, defined by separation of the first two cysteine residues by a non-conserved amino acid, is further divided on the basis of presence or absence of a glutamic acid–leucine–arginine (Glu–Leu–Arg or ELR) sequence immediately adjacent to the CXC motif [1–3]. Chemokines were originally described for their chemotactic properties for leukocytes; they have subsequently been recognized as mediators in diverse biological processes relating to cancer development, including angiogenesis and homing of cancer cells to sites of metastasis.

Angiogenic Chemokines: The CXCR2 Ligands

In the complex microenvironment of a tumor, formation of new blood vessels is determined by the complex interplay between angiogenic and angiostatic mediators. Unique among mediators of angiogenesis, CXC chemokine family members that contain the ELR motif are potent promoters of angiogenesis,

R.M. Strieter (✉)
Division of Pulmonary and Critical Care Medicine, Department of Medicine,
University of Virginia, Charlottesville, VA 22908, USA
e-mail: strieter@virginia.edu

V. Keshamouni et al. (eds.), *Lung Cancer Metastasis*,
DOI 10.1007/978-1-4419-0772-1_8, © Springer Science+Business Media, LLC 2009

155

whereas a subset of the ELR-negative CXC chemokine ligands display angiostatic properties [3]. The angiogenic ELR-containing chemokine ligands include
CXCL1, CXCL2, CXCL3, CXCL5, CXCL6, CXCL7, and CXCL8 (Table 1)
and signal their angiogenic effects via the receptor CXCR2 (CD182) [3, 4].

Table 1 Human chemokine family members involved in regulation of angiogenesis

Systematic name	Old nomenclature	Receptor
Angiogenic		
CXCL1	Gro-α	CXCR2
CXCL2	Gro-β	CXCR2
CXCL3	Gro-γ	CXCR2
CXCL5	ENA-78	CXCR2
CXCL6	GCP-2	CXCR2
CXCL7	NAP-2	CXCR2
CXCL8	IL-8	CXCR2
CCL2	MCP-1	CCR2
CCL11	Eotaxin-1	CCR3
CCL16	LEC	CCR1
Angiostatic		
CXCL4	PF-4	CXCR3B*
CXCL4L1	PF-4 variant	CXCR3B*
CXCL9	Mig	CXCR3B
CXCL10	IP-10	CXCR3B
CXCL11	I-TAC	CXCR3B
CXCL14	BRAK	?
CCL21	6Ckine	CXCR3**
Metastases		
CXCL12	SDF-1	CXCR4, ?CXCP7

* additional receptors may be involved; ? undefined receptor; ** applies only
to the mouse ligand.

The angiogenic ELR+ CXC chemokines directly mediate survival, proliferation, and chemotaxis of endothelial cells via autocrine, paracrine, and hor-
monal mechanisms. There is also increasing awareness of cross-talk between
angiogenic mediators of different classes that act in concert to generate the net
angiogenic microenvironment of the tumor. For example, activated neutrophils
release both vascular endothelial cell growth factor (VEGF) and CXCL8 [5].
VEGF-mediated activation of endothelial cells leads to both upregulation of
the anti-apoptotic molecule Bcl-2 and expression of CXCL8 by endothelial
cells. Endothelial cell-derived CXCL8, in turn, is necessary to maintain the
angiogenic phenotype of endothelial cells [6]. Other pathways that promote
CXC chemokine-mediated angiogenesis include the expression of angiogenic
CXC chemokines via NF-kB activation in malignant cells and consequent
enhanced tumor-associated angiogenesis [7–10].

In humans, all ELR+ CXC chemokines can bind and signal via CXCR2, and CXCL6 and CXCL8 additionally bind and signal via another receptor, CXCR1 [11]. While CXCR1 and CXCR2 are both expressed by human endothelial cells [11–13], CXCR2 is the primary functional chemokine receptor in endothelial cell chemotaxis [11, 12]. For example, CXCL8 mediates phosphorylation of extracellular signal-regulated protein kinase (ERK)-1 and ERK-2, rapid stress fiber assembly, chemotaxis, enhanced proliferation and tube formation in endothelial cells, effects that are blocked by immunoneutralization of CXCR2 or by inhibition of ERK-1 and ERK-2 [4]. These in vitro and in vivo studies establish CXCR2 as the critical receptor for ELR+ CXC chemokine-mediated angiogenesis.

The binding of ELR+ CXC chemokine ligands to CXCR2 and the internalization of the ligand–receptor complex is an essential step in initiation of chemotaxis and is also a major mechanism of clearance of ligands [14]. Interestingly, the fate of the CXCR2 receptor is also dependent on the local concentration of ligands: in the setting of low concentrations of ligand, internalized CXCR2 is sequentially targeted to clathrin-coated pits, early endosomes, sorting endosomes, recycling endosomes, and finally to the cell surface [14]. Conversely, prolonged or high concentrations of ELR+ CXC chemokines result in targeting of internalized CXCR2 to late endosome and subsequently to the lysosome for degradation [14].

Several lines of evidence support the role of CXCR2 and its ligands in angiogenesis in the context of non-small cell lung carcinoma (NSCLC). In clinical samples, tumor levels of ELR+ CXC chemokines in patients with non-small cell lung cancer correlated with patient mortality [15, 16]. In studies of CXCR2 in a mouse model of syngeneic lung cancer, tumor cells implanted into CXCR2-deficient mice demonstrated reduced growth, increased tumor-associated necrosis, inhibited tumor-associated angiogenesis and metastatic potential, as compared to the same tumors implanted into wild-type animals [17]. Activating K-ras mutations are common in lung cancer and a recently published transgenic mouse model with a conditional mutant mouse for K-ras demonstrated markedly elevated levels of the CXCR2 ligands CXCL1, CXCL2, and CXCL5 bronchoalveolar lavage fluid [18]. In a related model of spontaneously developing lung adenocarcinoma in mice with somatic activation of the oncogene K-ras, tumors were found to produce high levels of ELR+ CXC chemokines, and neutralization of CXCR2 attenuated the development of pre-malignant lesions and caused apoptosis of endothelial cells, leading to reduced tumor-associated angiogenesis within the lesions [19].

CXCL8 is markedly elevated and contributes to the overall angiogenic activity of non-small cell lung cancer, and NSCLC cell lines that constitutively express CXCL8 displayed greater tumorigenicity that correlated directly with angiogenesis in mouse models [20, 21]. Using an in vivo model system of transplanting human NSCLC in SCID mice, tumor-derived CXCL8 was shown to correlate directly with tumorigenesis [22]. Depletion of CXCL8 in the chimeric mice resulted in reduced tumor growth and metastases associated with reduced tumor angiogenesis [22]. CXCL5, another ELR+ CXC chemokine that mediated angiogenesis via CXCR2, is also expressed in resected NSCLC specimens in levels that exceed CXCL8 [23]. CXCL5 does not affect tumor cell proliferation in vitro, but its neutralization in chimeric mouse models of NSCLC results in reduced tumor growth and metastases, reduced tumor angiogenesis, and increased tumor cell apoptosis [23]. Interestingly, the production of both CXCL5 and CXCL8 by NSCLC cell lines appears to be dependent on tumor expression of COX-2: tumor overexpression of COX-2 results in increased tumor expression of CXCL5 and CXCL8, and specific COX-2 inhibition decreased the production of both chemokines and nuclear translocation of NF-kB [24]. Consistent with this, when COX-2 overexpressing NSCLC tumors were implanted in SCID mice, enhanced tumor growth was inhibited by neutralization of CXCL5 and CXCL8, but not VEGF [24].

Angiostatic Chemokines: CXCR2-Independent Effects

The Duffy antigens are co-dominant alleles expressed on erythrocytes that are recognized clinically as blood group antigens and as receptors for one of the malaria parasites, *Plasmodium vivax* [25]. The Duffy antigens are also promiscuous but are non-signaling chemokine receptors that act as the only decoy receptors for CXC chemokines [26]. In this context, Duffy antigen receptor of chemokines (DARC) binds the angiogenic ELR+ CXC chemokine ligands CXCL1, CXCL5, and CXCL8 [23, 27, 28]. The relevance of DARC in NSCLC was addressed by overexpressing this protein in A549 human lung adenocarcinoma cell line [29]. The transfected cells expressed DARC on their surface and produced similar amounts of mRNA for angiogenic ELR+ CXC chemokines as control cancer cells. When implanted into SCID animals, the resulting tumors displayed reduced cellularity, reduced vascularity, and reduced metastatic potential and paradoxically increased size in vivo [29]. These data suggest that overexpression of DARC in non-small cell tumor cell lines resulted in tumor binding of ELR+ CXC chemokine ligands, thus rendering them unavailable to recruit and stimulate endothelial cells and reduce tumor-associated angiogenesis.

Most of the literature on chemokine regulation of angiogenesis has centered on the role of the CXC family. Several members of the CC chemokine family, including CCL2, CCL11, and CCL16, have also been implicated in angiogenesis. CCL11, a CC chemokine ligand that signals via CCR3, has been shown to mediate chemotaxis of human endothelial cells and blood vessel formation in chick chorioallantoic membrane and Matrigel plugs in vivo and independent of its eosinophil recruiting effects [30]. Similarly, CCL16 has been shown to mediate endothelial chemotaxis in vitro and to promote vessel formation in chick chorioallantoic membrane [31]. In addition, CCL16 induced the production of other angiogenic molecules, including VEGF, CXCL8, and CCL2 from endothelial cells, and the effect on endothelial cells were inhibited by antagonism of CCR1 but not blocking CCR8 or CCR2 [31]. To our knowledge, the role of CCL16 in tumor angiogenesis had not been investigated directly, but the high expression of this chemokine in the liver may be relevant to hepatic metastases.

The most studied CC chemokine ligand implicated in angiogenesis is CCL2: endothelial cells express the CCL2 receptor, CCR2, and demonstrate chemotaxis and tube formation in response to CCL2 in vitro [32, 33]. In vivo, CCL2-mediated angiogenesis has been demonstrated in several systems, including corneal implantation, chick chorioallantoic membrane, Matrigel plug, and sponge implantation models [34–36] and appears to be independent of its induction of leukocyte recruitment [35]. The chemotaxis of endothelial cells by CCL2 is dependent on CCL2-induced overexpression of membrane type 1 metalloproteinase on endothelial cell surfaces [32] and is mediated via the ERK cascade and the transcription factor Ets-1 [37]. The relevance of CCL2-mediated angiogenesis has also been examined in the context of the Lewis lung carcinoma model of non-small cell bronchogenic carcinoma [38]. Implantation of Lewis lung carcinoma cells transduced with IL-1β into syngeneic wild-type recipients resulted in greater infiltration of COX-2-expressing macrophages, greater tumor growth, and tumor-related angiogenesis as compared to cancer cells transduced with a control vector. This effect was abrogated when the cancer cells were implanted into CCL2−/− recipients or when COX-2 was inhibited pharmacologically. Interestingly, the angiogenic effect was also dependent on local expression of VEGF and ELR+ CXC chemokines and was partially inhibited with blockade of CXCR2 [38]. In this model system, the authors concluded that the contribution of CCL2 was to recruit COX-2-expressing macrophages that, in turn, induced angiogenesis via VEGF and ELR+ CXC chemokines [38].

Angiostatic Chemokines: The CXCR3 Ligands

The angiostatic CXC chemokines are all ELR-negative ligands and include CXCL4, CXCL4L1, CXCL9, CXCL10, CXCL11, and CXCL14 [1–3, 39–45] (Table 1). A subset of these angiostatic chemokines, CXCL9-11, are strongly induced by both type I and type II interferons (IFN-α/β and IFN-γ, respectively) and signal via the main angiostatic chemokine receptor, CXCR3, also designated CD183. Human CXCR3 exists in at least three variants, designated CXCR3A, CXCR3B, and CXCR3alt, and generated by alternative splicing of mRNA of a single gene. CXCR3A is the main variant of CXCR3 that mediates influx of leukocytes, including Th1 effector T cells, activated B cells, and NK cells, and its expression is strongly induced by IL-2 [1, 46–51]. Conversely, CXCR3B is the main angiostatic splice variant of CXCR3 and is expressed on endothelial cells [13, 52, 53]. The angiostatic signaling cascade of CXCR3B was recently identified as being dependent on p38 MAP kinase pathway [54].

The final splice variant, CXCR3alt, was most recently described as the result of post-transcriptional exon skipping and has an enhanced response to CXCL11 as compared CXCL9 or CXCL10 [55]. The role of CXCR3alt in angiogenesis and its relationship to CXCR3A and CXCR3B has not been established and awaits further study.

In addition to binding the CXCR3 variants, the ligand CXCL10 also binds extracellular glycosaminoglycans. The interaction between CXCL10 (and also CXCL4) with cell surface heparan sulfate was originally reported to be the primary mechanism by which they inhibit endothelial cell proliferation [56], raising the question of whether the angiostatic properties of CXCL10 are mediated via this mechanism. This issue was addressed when CXCL10 variants with mutated binding sites for CXCR3 or glycosaminoglycans were transfected into a human melanoma cell line [57]. Implantation of the vector-transfected cells into nude mice showed that tumor lines expressing wild-type CXCL10 and CXCL10 mutants with partial or complete loss of glycosaminoglycans binding showed remarkable reduction in tumor growth compared to control vector-transfected tumor cells, whereas tranfectants expressing mutants with loss of CXCR3 binding did not inhibit tumor growth [57]. This work provides strong evidence that tumor growth and tumor-associated angiostasis are specifically dependent on interaction of CXCR3 chemokine ligands with CXCR3, but not glycosaminoglycans.

A number of studies have examined the role of CXCR3 ligands in inhibition of tumor-associated angiogenesis. In a SCID mouse model, CXCL10 production from implanted adenocarcinoma and squamous cell NSCLC cell lines was inversely correlated with tumor growth and was most marked in squamous cell tumors [58]. The appearance of spontaneous lung metastases in SCID mice bearing adenocarcinoma tumors occurred after CXCL10 levels from either the primary tumor or the plasma had reached a nadir [58]. In subsequent experiments, depletion of CXCL10 in squamous cell tumors resulted in an increase in their size [58]. In contrast, reconstitution of intra-tumor CXCL10 in adenocarcinoma tumors reduced both their size and their metastatic potential; this was unrelated to infiltrating neutrophils or mononuclear cells (i.e., macrophages or NK cells) and directly attributable to a reduction in tumor-associated angiogenesis [58]. These findings correlated with data obtained from human tissue samples: In resected tumors from patients with non-small cell bronchogenic carcinoma, CXCL10 levels were higher in the squamous cell carcinoma specimens as compared to adjacent lung tissue or adenocarcinoma samples [58]. The ex vivo tumor angiostatic activity of squamous cell carcinoma samples was attributable to tumor CXCL10 levels, since neutralization of CXCL10 resulted in increased tumor-associated angiogenic activity. In contrast to CXCL10, CXCL9 levels in human specimens of non-small cell carcinoma were not significantly different from that found in normal lung tissue [59]. However, overexpression of CXCL9 resulted in the inhibition of NSCLC tumor growth and metastasis via a decrease in tumor-associated angiogenesis [59]. These findings support the importance of the interferon-inducible ELR-negative CXC chemokines in inhibiting non-small cell carcinoma growth by attenuation of tumor-derived angiogenesis.

CXCL4 (previously designated platelet factor-4) was the first described angiostatic chemokine [60]. CXCL4 inhibits endothelial cell migration, proliferation, and in vivo angiogenesis in response to basic fibroblast growth factor (bFGF) or VEGF [60, 61]. FITC-labeled CXCL4 injected systemically selectively binds to the endothelium only in areas of active angiogenesis [62, 63]. Like CXCL10, CXCL4 signals via CXCR3B and also binds cell surface glycosaminoglycans [64]. The angiostatic activity of CXCL4 is not abrogated in heparan sulfate-deficient cells, and CXCL4 mutants or peptides lacking heparin affinity are capable of inhibiting angiogenesis [64–66], indicating that interaction with cell surface glycosaminoglycans is not essential for these effects. CXCL4 nevertheless also can produce angiostatic properties independent of CXCR3, as discussed later in this chapter. CXCL4 also exists as a non-allelic variant, designated CXCL4L1 or PF-4var, that was recently isolated from activated human platelets [41]. CXCL4L1 differs from CXCL4 in only three amino acids but exhibits a numbers of important differences: CXCL4 is stored in secretory granules and is released in response to protein kinase-C activation, whereas CXCL4L1 is not stored [67]. CXCL4L1 is a more potent angiostatic molecule than CXCL4 in response to angiogenic stimuli, as well as in animal models of melanoma and non-small cell carcinoma in immunocompromised and immunocompetent animals [41, 68, 69].

CXCL14 (previous designation BRAK) is also an ELR-negative angiostatic CXC chemokine ligand [40]. CXCL14 inhibits endothelial cell chemotaxis and in vivo angiogenesis in response to CXCL8, bFGF, and VEGF [40]. Consistent with this biology, CXCL14 is downregulated in many cancers [70–72]. CXCL14 was found to be relatively overexpressed in and around localized prostate cancers as compared to normal or hypertrophic prostate tissue, and transgenic expression of CXCL14 in a prostate cancer line and implantation into immunodeficient mice resulted in impaired cancer growth related to impaired angiogenesis [73], suggesting that, at least in the setting of prostate cancer, CXCL14 might act as an endogenous tumor suppressor via its angiostatic properties.

Finally, murine CCL21, while a CC and not a CXC chemokine ligand, binds and signals via mouse CXCR3. Administration of exogenous mouse CCL21 to SCID mice implanted with A549 lung carcinoma cells resulted in reduced tumor growth and metastases and tumor vascularity [74]. Importantly, mouse CCL21 expression did not influence the proliferation of A549 cells nor affect leukocyte influx into the tumor, and human CCL21 (which does not bind human or murine CXCR3) did not affect tumorigenicity, providing further proof of concept of the role of CXCR3 as mediating an anti-angiogenic phenotype.

CXCR3-Mediated "Immunoangiostasis": Combined Tumor-Mediated and Anti-tumor Th1 Immunity

The literature suggests that CXCR3 ligands mediate two independent anti-tumor effects: The first of these is tumor-specific angiostasis, as described above. The second is recruitment of Th1 polarized leukocytes in the context of anti-tumor cell-mediated immunity. Importantly, the recruitment of these effector leukocytes to the tumor and consequent release of interferons in the tumor microenvironment induces a positive feedback loop engendering further local expression of CXCL9-11, thereby recruiting CXCR3-expressing cells that act as a further source of IFN-γ that, in turn, induce further production of CXCL9-10-11 [1, 46–49, 75]. We have dubbed this combined effect of escalating Th1 immunity and inhibition of angiogenesis "immunoangiostasis" [76, 77].

This paradigm was tested in the context of a mouse model of renal cell carcinoma [76]. The effectiveness of systemic IL-2 therapy in this system was found to be dependent on CXCR3 and resulted in upregulation of CXCR3 on peripheral blood mononuclear cells but, interestingly, downregulation of CXCR3 ligands in the tumor [76]. The anti-tumor effects of systemic IL-2 were enhanced when it was combined with overexpression of the CXCR3 ligand, CXCL9, within the tumor [76]. Consistent with the immunoangiostasis hypothesis, the mechanism for inhibition of tumor growth related to local tumor-associated angiostasis as well as enhanced immunity toward tumor antigens [76]. These findings are similar to the previously reported study of IL-12-mediated regression of renal cell carcinoma in a murine model, where the anti-tumor effect of IL-12 was lost when CXCR3 ligands were depleted [78].

Immunoangiostasis appears to be relevant to non-small cell carcinoma [79, 80]. In models of syngeneic implantation of alveolar cell carcinoma and Lewis lung carcinoma, intra-tumor injection of a recombinant CC chemokine, CCL21, abrogated tumor growth in immunocompetent but not CD4 knockout, CD8 knockout, or SCID recipients, indicating that T-cell-mediated immunity was required for the anti-tumor effect [80]. This effect was associated with intra-tumor expression of IFNγ and CXCL9-10 [80]. Importantly, immunoneutralization of CXCL9, CXCL10, or IFNγ resulted in reduction of all three cytokines, reduced number of intra-tumor CXCR3-expressing T cells, and reduced anti-tumor effects [79].

Angiostatic Chemokines: CXCR3-Independent Effects

As noted above, the ability of CXCL4 to bind to extracellular molecules mediates several of its biological functions. The inhibitory effect of CXCL4 on angiogenesis is, in part, mediated by complex formation with bFGF, VEGF$_{165}$, and CXCL8 [65, 81, 82], as well as by binding the receptors for bFGF and VEGF$_{165}$ [65, 83–85]. In the case of bFGF, heterodimerization with CXCL4 prevents homodimerization of bFGF that is necessary for receptor binding [65, 85]. CXCL4 impairs $VEGF_{165}$ binding to its receptors on endothelial cells by a similar mechanism [84]. In contrast to its interaction with the heparin-binding angiogenic mediators (including bFGF, $VEGF_{165}$, and CXCL8), CXCL4 does not bind non-heparin-binding angiogenic peptides, as exemplified by $VEGF_{121}$ or its receptor [84, 86, 87].

CXCL12 (previously designated stromal cell-derived factor-1) is an ELR-negative CXC chemokine ligand that signals via CXCR4 (also designated CD184). The CXCL12–CXCR4 ligand–receptor pair is important to homing of many progenitor cells and in cancer metastases [88, 89] and has also implicated by some groups as promoting tumor angiogenesis [90–93]. CXCL12 may be involved in upregulating levels of VEGF and bFGF and subcutaneous injection of CXCL12 into mice induces formation of local small blood vessels [92, 93]. However, it has yet to be demonstrated in an in vivo tumor model system that endogenous CXCL12 binding to CXCR4 mediates a significant portion of primary tumor angiogenesis and angiogenesis-dependent tumor growth. The argument in favor of angiogenesis is weakened by the observation that, although many tumor cells express CXCR4, CXCL12 is essentially absent from the tumor environment in breast, non-small cell lung, and renal cell carcinomas [88, 94, 95] and that, in the context of breast and non-small cell carcinoma, CXCL12 or CXCR4 neutralization does not affect tumor size or angiogenesis [88, 94].

Chemokine-Mediated Metastasis

The CXCL12–CXCR4 biological axis is an evolutionarily ancient mechanism for homeostatic homing of progenitor cells [96–99]. The role of this biological axis in mediating metastasis was first demonstrated in breast carcinoma: CXCR4 was found to be highly expressed by the tumor cells at the level of mRNA and as a functional membrane protein and mediated the chemotaxis to CXCL12 in vitro [94]. Moreover, neutralization of CXCR4 in vivo inhibited lung metastases when human breast cancer lines were implanted into SCID mice [94]. CXCR4 has since been noted to be important to tumor cell survival, tumor cell proliferation, and metastasis of cancer cells, including human pancreatic and prostate tumor cell lines, colorectal cancer, and osteosarcoma [100–103].

Both primary human NSCLC cells and cancer cell lines A549 and Calu-6 express CXCR4, but not its ligand CXCL12 [88]. In addition, CXCL12 mediated chemotaxis, calcium mobilization, and activation of mitogen-activated protein kinase p42/44 of A549 cells [88]. As compared to the primary tumor or blood, CXCL12 was found to have higher expression in the following organs: lungs, liver, adrenal glands, and bone marrow, organs that are clinically recognized as sites of metastases [88]. Whereas 65% of tumor cells in the primary tumor site expressed CXCR4, tumor cells at metastasis sites were 99% CXCR4 expressing, suggesting that CXCR4-expressing cells were enriched in the process of metastasis. Finally, immunoneutralization of CXCL12 in a heterotropic SCID model resulted in substantially attenuated metastases to the adrenal glands, liver, lung, and bone marrow but did not result in measurable change in tumor-associated angiogenesis or in vivo growth of primary tumors [88].

Given the importance of CXCR4 in mediating metastases, the mechanism of regulation of CXCR4 in cancer cells is of great interest. Hypoxia-induced expression of the transcription factor hypoxia-inducible factor-1α (HIF-1α) has been found to be critical for expression of CXCR4 [104, 105]. Moreover, in normoxic conditions, the tumor suppressor von Hippel–Lindau (VHL) targets HIF-1α for degradation resulting in attenuated expression of CXCR4 [104, 105]. In contrast, under normoxic conditions, TKR-activated PI3 kinase/AKT/mTor and ERK1/2/MAP kinase pathways can augment the expression of HIF-1α [106–108]. In this context, the combination of hypoxia and EGFR activation markedly upregulates the expression of CXCR4 on non-small cell lung cancer cells via the PI3-K/PTEN/AKT/mTOR pathway activation of HIF-1α [109]. This link between hypoxia-induced HIF-1α and CXCR4 expression provides a novel mechanism to reduce metastases in a variety of cancers.

CXCR7 is a newly described CXC chemokine receptor that binds CXCL11 and CXCL12 [110, 111]. CXCR7 is expressed by several tumor lines, including murine breast and lung carcinoma cell lines and a human breast cancer line, activated endothelial cells, and tumor vasculature [111, 112]. CXCR7 expression was also noted in human prostate cancer samples and corresponded with tumor aggressiveness [113]. In vitro, overexpression of CXCR7 in prostate cancer cell lines resulted in increased basal proliferation and proliferation in response to CXCL12, reduced apoptosis rate, increased adherence to endothelial cell layers, and increased ability to invade matrigel, whereas reduced expression of CXCR7 by siRNA had the opposite effect [113]. CXCR7 appears to mediate tumor growth in several in vivo models: Blockade of CXCR7 with a small molecule inhibitor resulted in reduced tumor growth in several cancer models, including A549 human lung carcinoma xenograft in immunocompromised mice and syngeneic mouse Lewis lung carcinoma models [111], and its overexpression in a human breast cancer line resulted in formation of larger tumors in SCID mice, whereas RNAi knockdown of CXCR7 in murine breast cancer and Lewis lung carcinoma lines resulted in reduced tumor growth in syngeneic models [112]. Interestingly, CXCR7 overexpression also resulted in a number of downstream effects, including CXCL8 and VEGF expression by the tumor cells in vitro and production of larger and more vascular tumors when implanted into SCID mice [113]. Interestingly, recent data suggest an antagonistic relationship between the effects of expression of CXCR4 and CXCR7 [114]. In the context of cancer, overexpressing CXCR4 by transfection in a prostate cancer cell line resulted in reduced expression of CXCR7; similarly, reducing the expression of CXCR4 by siRNA caused enhanced expression of

CXCR7 [113]. In the converse, however, increased or attenuated expression of CXCR7 did not influence CXCR4 expression [113]. In summary, CXCR7 may well play an important role in mediating tumorigenesis in human cancers, but its precise contribution remains to be defined.

Conclusion

The biologic role of chemokines was originally thought to be restricted to recruitment of subpopulations of leukocytes in the context of inflammation, but in the context of cancer, these cytokines display pleiotropic effects including regulation of neovascularization and controlling metastases. These findings support the notion that inhibition of angiogenic or augmentation of angiostatic chemokines or targeting mechanisms of metastases can be studied as novel therapeutic targets in bronchogenic carcinoma.

Acknowledgments This work was supported by NIH grant HL73848 and an American Lung Association Career Investigator Award (Mehrad) and CA87879 and HL66027 (Strieter).

References

1. Luster, A.D. Chemokines–chemotactic cytokines that mediate inflammation. N Engl J Med *338*: 436–45, 1998.
2. Belperio, J.A., M.P. Keane, D.A. Arenberg, C.L. Addison, J.E. Ehlert, M.D. Burdick, and R.M. Strieter. CXC chemokines in angiogenesis. J Leukoc Biol *68*: 1–8, 2000.
3. Strieter, R.M., P.J. Polverini, S.L. Kunkel, D.A. Arenberg, M.D. Burdick, J. Kasper, J. Dzuiba, J.V. Damme, A. Walz, D. Marriott, S.Y. Chan, S. Roczniak, and A.B. Shanafelt. The functional role of the 'ELR' motif in CXC chemokine-mediated angiogenesis. J Biol Chem *270*: 27348–57, 1995.
4. Heidemann, J., H. Ogawa, M.B. Dwinell, P. Rafiee, C. Maaser, H.R. Gockel, M.F. Otterson, D.M. Ota, N. Lugering, W. Domschke, and D.G. Binion. Angiogenic effects of interleukin 8 (CXCL8) in human intestinal microvascular endothelial cells are mediated by CXCR2. J Biol Chem *278*: 8508–15, 2003.
5. Schruefer, R., N. Lutze, J. Schymeinsky, and B. Walzog. Human neutrophils promote angiogenesis by a paracrine feedforward mechanism involving endothelial interleukin-8. Am J Physiol Heart Circ Physiol *288*: H1186–92, 2005.
6. Nor, J.E., J. Christensen, J. Liu, M. Peters, D.J. Mooney, R.M. Strieter, and P.J. Polverini. Up-Regulation of Bcl-2 in microvascular endothelial cells enhances intratumoral angiogenesis and accelerates tumor growth. Cancer Res *61*: 2183–8, 2001.
7. Dong, G., Z. Chen, Z.Y. Li, N.T. Yeh, C.C. Bancroft, and C. Van Waes. Hepatocyte growth factor/scatter factor-induced activation of MEK and PI3K signal pathways contributes to expression of proangiogenic cytokines interleukin-8 and vascular endothelial growth factor in head and neck squamous cell carcinoma. Cancer Res *61*: 5911–8, 2001.
8. Hirata, A., S. Ogawa, T. Kometani, T. Kuwano, S. Naito, M. Kuwano, and M. Ono. ZD1839 (Iressa) induces antiangiogenic effects through inhibition of epidermal growth factor receptor tyrosine kinase. Cancer Res *62*: 2554–60, 2002.

9. Levine, L., J.A. Lucci, 3rd, B. Pazdrak, J.Z. Cheng, Y.S. Guo, C.M. Townsend, Jr., andM.R. Hellmich. Bombesin stimulates nuclear factor kappa B activation and expression of proangiogenic factors in prostate cancer cells. Cancer Res *63*: 3495–502, 2003.

10. Richmond, A. Nf-kappa B, chemokine gene transcription and tumour growth. Nat Rev Immunol *2*: 664–74, 2002.

11. Addison, C.L., T.O. Daniel, M.D. Burdick, H. Liu, J.E. Ehlert, Y.Y. Xue, L. Buechi, A. Walz, A. Richmond, and R.M. Strieter. The CXC chemokine receptor 2, CXCR2, is the putative receptor for ELR(+) CXC chemokine-induced angiogenic activity. J Immunol *165*: 5269–77, 2000.

12. Murdoch, C., P.N. Monk, and A. Finn. Cxc chemokine receptor expression on human endothelial cells. Cytokine *11*: 704–712, 1999.

13. Salcedo, R., J.H. Resau, D. Halverson, E.A. Hudson, M. Dambach, D. Powell, K. Wasserman, and J.J. Oppenheim. Differential expression and responsiveness of chemokine receptors (CXCR1-3) by human microvascular endothelial cells and umbilical vein endothelial cells. Faseb J *14*: 2055–64, 2000.

14. Richmond, A., G.H. Fan, P. Dhawan, and J. Yang. How do chemokine/chemokine receptor activations affect tumorigenesis? Novartis Found Symp 256: 74–89; discussion 89–91, 106–11, 266–9, 2004.

15. White, E.S., K.R. Flaherty, S. Carskadon, A. Brant, M.D. Iannettoni, J. Yee, M.B. Orringer, and D.A. Arenberg. Macrophage migration inhibitory factor and CXC chemokine expression in non-small cell lung cancer: role in angiogenesis and prognosis. Clin Cancer Res *9*: 853–60, 2003.

16. Chen, J.J., P.L. Yao, A. Yuan, T.M. Hong, C.T. Shun, M.L. Kuo, Y.C. Lee, and P.C. Yang. Up-regulation of tumor interleukin-8 expression by infiltrating macrophages: its correlation with tumor angiogenesis and patient survival in non-small cell lung cancer. Clin Cancer Res *9*: 729–37, 2003.

17. Keane, M.P., J.A. Belperio, Y.Y. Xue, M.D. Burdick, and R.M. Strieter. Depletion of CXCR2 inhibits tumor growth and angiogenesis in a murine model of lung cancer. J Immunol *172*: 2853–60, 2004.

18. Ji, H., A.M. Houghton, T.J. Mariani, S. Perera, C.B. Kim, R. Padera, G. Tonon, K. McNamara, L.A. Marconcini, A. Hezel, N. El-Bardeesy, R.T. Bronson, D. Sugarbaker, R.S. Maser, S.D. Shapiro, and K.K. Wong. K-ras activation generates an inflammatory response in lung tumors. Oncogene *25*: 2105–12, 2006.

19. Wislez, M., N. Fujimoto, J.G. Izzo, A.E. Hanna, D.D. Cody, R.R. Langley, H. Tang, M.D. Burdick, M. Sato, J.D. Minna, L. Mao, I. Wistuba, R.M. Strieter, and J.M. Kurie. High expression of ligands for chemokine receptor CXCR2 in alveolar epithelial neoplasia induced by oncogenic kras. Cancer Res *66*: 4198–207, 2006.

20. Yatsunami, J., N. Tsuruta, K. Ogata, K. Wakamatsu, K. Takayama, M. Kawasaki, Y. Nakanishi, N. Hara, and S. Hayashi. Interleukin-8 participates in angiogenesis in non-small cell, but not small cell carcinoma of the lung. Cancer Lett *120*: 101–8, 1997.

21. Smith, D.R., P.J. Polverini, S.L. Kunkel, M.B. Orringer, R.I. Whyte, M.D. Burdick, C.A. Wilke, and R.M. Strieter. IL-8 mediated angiogenesis in human bronchogenic carcinoma. J. Exp. Med. *179*: 1409–1415, 1994.

22. Arenberg, D.A., S.L. Kunkel, M.D. Burdick, P.J. Polverini, and R.M. Strieter. Treatment with anti-IL-8 inhibits non-small cell lung cancer tumor growth (Meeting abstract). J Investig Med *43*: 479A 1995.

23. Arenberg, D.A., M.P. Keane, B. DiGiovine, S.L. Kunkel, S.B. Morris, Y.Y. Xue, M.D. Burdick, M.C. Glass, M.D. Iannettoni, and R.M. Strieter. Epithelial-neutrophil activating peptide (ENA-78) is an important angiogenic factor in non-small cell lung cancer. J Clin Invest *102*: 465–72, 1998.

24. Pold, M., L.X. Zhu, S. Sharma, M.D. Burdick, Y. Lin, P.P. Lee, A. Pold, J. Luo, K. Krysan, M. Dohadwala, J.T. Mao, R.K. Batra, R.M. Strieter, and S.M. Dubinett. Cyclooxygenase-2-dependent expression of angiogenic CXC chemokines ENA-78/CXC

ligand (CXCL) 5 and interleukin-8/CXCL8 in human non-small cell lung cancer. Cancer Res *64*: 1853–60, 2004.

25. Hadley, T.J. and S.C. Peiper. From malaria to chemokine receptor: the emerging physiologic role of the Duffy blood group antigen. Blood *89*: 3077–91, 1997.

26. Locati, M., Y.M. Torre, E. Galliera, R. Bonecchi, H. Bodduluri, G. Vago, A. Vecchi, and A. Mantovani. Silent chemoattractant receptors: D6 as a decoy and scavenger receptor for inflammatory CC chemokines. Cytokine Growth Factor Rev *16*: 679–86, 2005.

27. Arenberg, D.A., S.L. Kunkel, P.J. Polverini, M. Glass, M.D. Burdick, and R.M. Strieter. Inhibition of interleukin-8 reduces tumorigenesis of human non-small cell lung cancer in SCID mice. J Clin Invest *97*: 2792–802, 1996.

28. Moore, B.B., D.A. Arenberg, K. Stoy, T. Morgan, C.L. Addison, S.B. Morris, M. Glass, C. Wilke, Y.Y. Xue, S. Sitterding, S.L. Kunkel, M.D. Burdick, and R.M. Strieter. Distinct CXC chemokines mediate tumorigenicity of prostate cancer cells. Am J Pathol *154*: 1503–12, 1999.

29. Addison, C.L., J.A. Belperio, M.D. Burdick, and R.M. Strieter. Overexpression of the duffy antigen receptor for chemokines (DARC) by NSCLC tumor cells results in increased tumor necrosis. BMC Cancer *4*: 28, 2004.

30. Salcedo, R., H.A. Young, M.L. Ponce, J.M. Ward, H.K. Kleinman, W.J. Murphy, and J.J. Oppenheim. Eotaxin (CCL11) induces in vivo angiogenic responses by human CCR3+ endothelial cells. J Immunol *166*: 7571–8, 2001.

31. Strasly, M., G. Doronzo, P. Capello, D. Valdembri, M. Arese, S. Mitola, P. Moore, G. Alessandri, M. Giovarelli, and F. Bussolino. CCL16 activates an angiogenic program in vascular endothelial cells. Blood *103*: 40–9, 2004.

32. Galvez, B.G., L. Genis, S. Matias-Roman, S.A. Oblander, K. Tryggvason, S.S. Apte, and A.G. Arroyo. Membrane type 1-matrix metalloproteinase is regulated by chemokines monocyte-chemoattractant protein-1/ccl2 and interleukin-8/CXCL8 in endothelial cells during angiogenesis. J Biol Chem *280*: 1292–8, 2005.

33. Weber, K.S., P.J. Nelson, H.J. Grone, and C. Weber. Expression of CCR2 by endothelial cells: implications for MCP-1 mediated wound injury repair and In vivo inflammatory activation of endothelium. Arterioscler Thromb Vasc Biol *19*: 2085–93, 1999.

34. Goede, V., L. Brogelli, M. Ziche, and H.G. Augustin. Induction of inflammatory angiogenesis by monocyte chemoattractant protein-1. Int J Cancer *82*: 765–70, 1999.

35. Salcedo, R., M.L. Ponce, H.A. Young, K. Wasserman, J.M. Ward, H.K. Kleinman, J.J. Oppenheim, and W.J. Murphy. Human endothelial cells express CCR2 and respond to MCP-1: direct role of MCP-1 in angiogenesis and tumor progression. Blood *96*: 34–40, 2000.

36. Barcelos, L.S., A. Talvani, A.S. Teixeira, G.D. Cassali, S.P. Andrade, and M.M. Teixeira. Production and in vivo effects of chemokines CXCL1-3/KC and CCL2/JE in a model of inflammatory angiogenesis in mice. Inflamm Res *53*: 576–84, 2004.

37. Stamatovic, S.M., R.F. Keep, M. Mostarica-Stojkovic, and A.V. Andjelkovic. CCL2 regulates angiogenesis via activation of Ets-1 transcription factor. J Immunol *177*: 2651–61, 2006.

38. Nakao, S., T. Kuwano, C. Tsutsumi-Miyahara, S. Ueda, Y.N. Kimura, S. Hamano, K.H. Sonoda, Y. Saijo, T. Nukiwa, R.M. Strieter, T. Ishibashi, M. Kuwano, and M. Ono. Infiltration of COX-2-expressing macrophages is a prerequisite for IL-1 beta-induced neovascularization and tumor growth. J Clin Invest *115*: 2979–91, 2005.

39. Strieter, R.M., J.A. Belperio, D.A. Arenberg, M.I. Smith, M.D. Burdick, and M.P. Keane. CXC chemokine in angiogenesis. In Universes in delicate balance: Chemokines and the nervous system, eds. Ransohoff, R.M., K. Suzuki, A.E.I. Proudfoot and W. F. Hickey. Amsterdam, The Netherlands: Elsevier Science B.V., 129–48, 2002.

40. Shellenberger, T.D., M. Wang, M. Gujrati, A. Jayakumar, R.M. Strieter, C. Ioannides, C.L. Efferson, A.K. El-Naggar, G.L. Clayman, and M.J. Frederick. BRAK/CXCL14 is a potent inhibitor of angiogenesis and is a chemotactic factor for immature dendritic cells. Cancer Res. *64*: 8262–8270, 2004.

41. Struyf, S., M.D. Burdick, P. Proost, J. Van Damme, and R.M. Strieter. Platelets release CXCL4L1, a nonallelic variant of the chemokine platelet factor-4/CXCL4 and potent inhibitor of angiogenesis. Circ Res 95: 855–7, 2004.

42. Rollins, B.J. Chemokines. Blood 90: 909–28, 1997.

43. Balkwill, F. The molecular and cellular biology of the chemokines. J Viral Hepat 5: 1–14, 1998.

44. Strieter, R.M., J.A. Belperio, R.J. Phillips, and M.P. Keane. Chemokines: angiogenesis and metastases in lung cancer. Novartis Found Symp 256: 173–84; discussion 184–8, 259–69, 2004.

45. Strieter, R.M., J.A. Belperio, R.J. Phillips, and M.P. Keane. CXC chemokines in angiogenesis of cancer. Semin Cancer Biol 14: 195–200, 2004.

46. Moser, B. and P. Loetscher. Lymphocyte traffic control by chemokines. Nat Immunol 2: 123–8, 2001.

47. Loetscher, M., B. Gerber, P. Loetscher, S.A. Jones, L. Piali, I. Clark-Lewis, M. Baggiolini, and B. Moser. Chemokine receptor specific for IP10 and mig: structure, function, and expression in activated T-lymphocytes. J Exp Med 184: 963–9, 1996.

48. Rabin, R.L., M.K. Park, F. Liao, R. Swofford, D. Stephany, and J.M. Farber. Chemokine receptor responses on T cells are achieved through regulation of both receptor expression and signaling. J Immunol 162: 3840–50, 1999.

49. Qin, S., J.B. Rottman, P. Myers, N. Kassam, M. Weinblatt, M. Loetscher, A.E. Koch, B. Moser, and C.R. Mackay. The chemokine receptors CXCR3 and CCR5 mark subsets of T cells associated with certain inflammatory reactions. J Clin Invest 101: 746–54, 1998.

50. Loetscher, M., P. Loetscher, N. Brass, E. Meese, and B. Moser. Lymphocyte-specific chemokine receptor CXCR3: regulation, chemokine binding and gene localization. Eur J Immunol 28: 3696–705, 1998.

51. Beider, K., A. Nagler, O. Wald, S. Franitza, M. Dagan-Berger, H. Wald, H. Giladi, S. Brocke, J. Hanna, O. Mandelboim, M. Darash-Yahana, E. Galun, and A. Peled. Involvement of CXCR4 and IL-2 in the homing and retention of human NK and NK T cells to the bone marrow and spleen of NOD/SCID mice. Blood 102: 1951–8, 2003.

52. Romagnani, P., F. Annunziato, L. Lasagni, E. Lazzeri, C. Beltrame, M. Francalanci, M. Uguccioni, G. Galli, L. Cosmi, L. Maurenzig, M. Baggiolini, E. Maggi, S. Romagnani, and M. Serio. Cell cycle-dependent expression of CXC chemokine receptor 3 by endothelial cells mediates angiostatic activity. J Clin Invest 107: 53–63., 2001.

53. Lasagni, L., M. Francalanci, F. Annunziato, E. Lazzeri, S. Giannini, L. Cosmi, C. Sagrinati, B. Mazzinghi, C. Orlando, E. Maggi, F. Marra, S. Romagnani, M. Serio, and P. Romagnani. An alternatively spliced variant of CXCR3 mediates the inhibition of endothelial cell growth induced by IP-10, Mig, and I-TAC, and acts as functional receptor for platelet factor 4. J Exp Med 197: 1537–49, 2003.

54. Petrai, I., K. Rombouts, L. Lasagni, F. Annunziato, L. Cosmi, R.G. Romanelli, C. Sagrinati, B. Mazzinghi, M. Pinzani, S. Romagnani, P. Romagnani, and F. Marra. Activation of p38(MAPK) mediates the angiostatic effect of the chemokine receptor CXCR3-B. Int J Biochem Cell Biol 40: 1764–74, 2008.

55. Ehlert, J.E., C.A. Addison, M.D. Burdick, S.L. Kunkel, and R.M. Strieter. Identification and Partial Characterization of a Variant of Human CXCR3 Generated by Posttranscriptional Exon Skipping. J Immunol 173: 6234–40, 2004.

56. Luster, A.D., S.M. Greenberg, and P. Leder. The IP-10 chemokine binds to a specific cell surface heparan sulfate site shared with platelet factor 4 and inhibits endothelial cell proliferation. J Exp Med 182: 219–31, 1995.

57. Yang, J. and A. Richmond. The angiostatic activity of interferon-inducible protein-10/CXCL10 in human melanoma depends on binding to CXCR3 but not to glycosaminoglycan. Mol Ther 9: 846–55, 2004.

58. Arenberg, D.A., S.L. Kunkel, P.J. Polverini, S.B. Morris, M.D. Burdick, M.C. Glass, D.T. Taub, M.D. Iannettoni, R.I. Whyte, and R.M. Strieter. Interferon-gamma-inducible

protein 10 (IP-10) is an angiostatic factor that inhibits human non-small cell lung cancer (NSCLC) tumorigenesis and spontaneous metastases. J Exp Med *184*: 981–92, 1996.

59. Addison, C.L., D.A. Arenberg, S.B. Morris, Y.Y. Xue, M.D. Burdick, M.S. Mulligan, M.D. Iannettoni, and R.M. Strieter. The CXC chemokine, monokine induced by interferon-gamma, inhibits non-small cell lung carcinoma tumor growth and metastasis. Hum Gene Ther *11*: 247–61, 2000.

60. Maione, T.E., G.S. Gray, J. Petro, A.J. Hunt, A.L. Donner, S.I. Bauer, H.F. Carson, and R.J. Sharpe. Inhibition of angiogenesis by recombinant human platelet factor-4 and related peptides. Science *247*: 77–9, 1990.

61. Gupta, S.K. and J.P. Singh. Inhibition of endothelial cell proliferation by platelet factor-4 involves a unique action on S phase progression. J Cell Biol *127*: 1121–7, 1994.

62. Hansell, P., T.E. Maione, and P. Borgstrom. Selective binding of platelet factor 4 to regions of active angiogenesis in vivo. Am J Physiol *269*: H829–36, 1995.

63. Borgstrom, P., R. Discipio, and T.E. Maione. Recombinant platelet factor 4, an angiogenic marker for human breast carcinoma. Anticancer Res *18*: 4035–41, 1998.

64. Bikfalvi, A. Platelet factor 4: an inhibitor of angiogenesis. Semin Thromb Hemost *30*: 379–85, 2004.

65. Perollet, C., Z.C. Han, C. Savona, J.P. Caen, and A. Bikfalvi. Platelet factor 4 modulates fibroblast growth factor 2 (FGF-2) activity and inhibits FGF-2 dimerization. Blood *91*: 3289–99, 1998.

66. Bikfalvi, A. and G. Gimenez-Gallego. The control of angiogenesis and tumor invasion by platelet factor-4 and platelet factor-4-derived molecules. Semin Thromb Hemost *30*: 137–44, 2004.

67. Lasagni, L., R. Grepin, B. Mazzinghi, E. Lazzeri, C. Meini, C. Sagrinati, F. Liotta, F. Frosali, E. Ronconi, N. Alain-Courtois, L. Ballerini, G.S. Netti, E. Maggi, F. Annunziato, M. Serio, S. Romagnani, A. Bikfalvi, and P. Romagnani. PF-4/CXCL4 and CXCL4L1 exhibit distinct subcellular localization and a differentially regulated mechanism of secretion. Blood *109*: 4127–34, 2007.

68. Vandercappellen, J., S. Noppen, H. Verbeke, W. Put, R. Conings, M. Gouwy, E. Schutyser, P. Proost, R. Sciot, K. Geboes, G. Opdenakker, J. Van Damme, and S. Struyf. Stimulation of angiostatic platelet factor-4 variant (CXCL4L1/PF-4var) versus inhibition of angiogenic granulocyte chemotactic protein-2 (CXCL6/GCP-2) in normal and tumoral mesenchymal cells. J Leukoc Biol *82*: 1519–30, 2007.

69. Struyf, S., M.D. Burdick, E. Peeters, K. Van den Broeck, C. Dillen, P. Proost, J. Van Damme, and R.M. Strieter. Platelet factor-4 variant chemokine CXCL4L1 inhibits melanoma and lung carcinoma growth and metastasis by preventing angiogenesis. Cancer Res *67*: 5940–8, 2007.

70. Frederick, M.J., Y. Henderson, X. Xu, M.T. Deavers, A.A. Sahin, H. Wu, D.E. Lewis, A.K. El-Naggar, and G.L. Clayman. In vivo expression of the novel CXC chemokine BRAK in normal and cancerous human tissue. Am J Pathol *156*: 1937–50, 2000.

71. Hromas, R., H.E. Broxmeyer, C. Kim, H. Nakshatri, K. Christopherson, 2nd, M. Azam and Y.H. Hou. Cloning of BRAK, a novel divergent CXC chemokine preferentially expressed in normal versus malignant cells. Biochem Biophys Res Commun *255*: 703–6, 1999.

72. Sleeman, M.A., J.K. Fraser, J.G. Murison, S.L. Kelly, R.L. Prestidge, D.J. Palmer, J.D. Watson, and K.D. Kumble. B cell- and monocyte-activating chemokine (BMAC), a novel non-ELR alpha-chemokine. Int Immunol *12*: 677–89, 2000.

73. Schwarze, S.R., J. Luo, W.B. Isaacs, and D.F. Jarrard. Modulation of CXCL14 (BRAK) expression in prostate cancer. Prostate *13*: 13, 2005.

74. Arenberg, D.A., A. Zlotnick, S.R. Strom, M.D. Burdick, and R.M. Strieter. The murine CC chemokine, 6C-kine, inhibits tumor growth and angiogenesis in a human lung cancer SCID mouse model. Cancer Immunol Immunother *49*: 587–92, 2001.

75. Hancock, W.W., B. Lu, W. Gao, V. Csizmadia, K. Faia, J.A. King, S.T. Smiley, M. Ling, N.P. Gerard, and C. Gerard. Requirement of the chemokine receptor CXCR3 for acute allograft rejection. J Exp Med *192*: 1515–20, 2000.
76. Pan, J., M.D. Burdick, J.A. Belperio, Y.Y. Xue, C. Gerard, S. Sharma, S.M. Dubinett, and R.M. Strieter. CXCR3/CXCR3 ligand biological axis impairs RENCA tumor growth by a mechanism of immunoangiostasis. J Immunol *176*: 1456–64, 2006.
77. Strieter, R.M., J.A. Belperio, M.D. Burdick, S. Sharma, S.M. Dubinett and M.P. Keane. CXC chemokines: angiogenesis, immunoangiostasis, and metastases in lung cancer. Ann N Y Acad Sci *1028*: 351–60, 2004.
78. Tannenbaum, C.S., R. Tubbs, D. Armstrong, J.H. Finke, R.M. Bukowski, and T.A. Hamilton. The CXC chemokines IP-10 and Mig are necessary for IL-12-mediated regression of the mouse RENCA tumor. J Immunol *161*: 927–32, 1998.
79. Sharma, S., S.C. Yang, S. Hillinger, L.X. Zhu, M. Huang, R.K. Batra, J.F. Lin, M.D. Burdick, R.M. Strieter, and S.M. Dubinett. SLC/CCL21-mediated anti-tumor responses require IFNgamma, MIG/CXCL9 and IP-10/CXCL10. Mol Cancer *2*: 22, 2003.
80. Sharma, S., M. Stolina, J. Luo, R.M. Strieter, M. Burdick, L.X. Zhu, R.K. Batra, and S. M. Dubinett. Secondary lymphoid tissue chemokine mediates T cell-dependent antitumor responses in vivo. J Immunol *164*: 4558–63, 2000.
81. Dudek, A.Z., I. Nesmelova, K. Mayo, C.M. Verfaillie, S. Pitchford, and A. Slungaard. Platelet factor 4 promotes adhesion of hematopoietic progenitor cells and binds IL-8: novel mechanisms for modulation of hematopoiesis. Blood *101*: 4687–94, 2003.
82. Sulpice, E., M. Bryckaert, J. Lacour, J.O. Contreres, and G. Tobelem. Platelet factor 4 inhibits FGF2-induced endothelial cell proliferation via the extracellular signal-regulated kinase pathway but not by the phosphatidylinositol 3-kinase pathway. Blood *100*: 3087–94, 2002.
83. Sato, Y., M. Abe, and R. Takaki. Platelet factor 4 blocks the binding of basic fibroblast growth factor to the receptor and inhibits the spontaneous migration of vascular endothelial cells. Biochem Biophys Res Commun *172*: 595–600, 1990.
84. Gengrinovitch, S., S.M. Greenberg, T. Cohen, H. Gitay-Goren, P. Rockwell, T.E. Maione, B.Z. Levi, and G. Neufeld. Platelet factor-4 inhibits the mitogenic activity of VEGF121 and VEGF165 using several concurrent mechanisms. J Biol Chem *270*: 15059–65, 1995.
85. Jouan, V., X. Canron, M. Alemany, J.P. Caen, G. Quentin, J. Plouet, and A. Bikfalvi. Inhibition of in vitro angiogenesis by platelet factor-4-derived peptides and mechanism of action. Blood *94*: 984–93, 1999.
86. Houck, K.A., D.W. Leung, A.M. Rowland, J. Winer, and N. Ferrara. Dual regulation of vascular endothelial growth factor bioavailability by genetic and proteolytic mechanisms. J Biol Chem *267*: 26031–7, 1992.
87. Houck, K.A., N. Ferrara, J. Winer, G. Cachianes, B. Li, and D.W. Leung. The vascular endothelial growth factor family: identification of a fourth molecular species and characterization of alternative splicing of RNA. Mol Endocrinol *5*: 1806–14, 1991.
88. Phillips, R.J., M.D. Burdick, M. Lutz, J.A. Belperio, M.P. Keane, and R.M. Strieter. The stromal derived factor-1/CXCL12-CXC chemokine receptor 4 biological axis in non-small cell lung cancer metastases. Am J Respir Crit Care Med *167*: 1676–86, 2003.
89. Mehrad, B., M.P. Keane, B.N. Gomperts, and R.M. Strieter. Circulating progenitor cells in chronic lung disease. Expert Review of Respiratory Medicine *1*: 157–165, 2007.
90. Bachelder, R.E., M.A. Wendt, and A.M. Mercurio. Vascular endothelial growth factor promotes breast carcinoma invasion in an autocrine manner by regulating the chemokine receptor CXCR4. Cancer Res *62*: 7203–6, 2002.
91. Salcedo, R. and J.J. Oppenheim. Role of Chemokines in Angiogenesis: CXCL12/SDF-1 and CXCR4 Interaction, a Key Regulator of Endothelial Cell Responses. Microcirculation *10*: 359–70, 2003.

92. Kijowski, J., M. Baj-Krzyworzeka, M. Majka, R. Reca, L.A. Marquez, M. Christofidou-Solomidou, A. Janowska-Wieczorek, and M.Z. Ratajczak. The SDF-1-CXCR4 axis stimulates VEGF secretion and activates integrins but does not affect proliferation and survival in lymphohematopoietic cells. Stem Cells *19*: 453–66, 2001.

93. Salcedo, R., K. Wasserman, H.A. Young, M.C. Grimm, O.M. Howard, M.R. Anver, H.K. Kleinman, W.J. Murphy, and J.J. Oppenheim. Vascular endothelial growth factor and basic fibroblast growth factor induce expression of CXCR4 on human endothelial cells: In vivo neovascularization induced by stromal-derived factor-1alpha. Am J Pathol *154*: 1125–35, 1999.

94. Muller, A., B. Homey, H. Soto, N. Ge, D. Catron, M.E. Buchanan, T. McClanahan, E. Murphy, W. Yuan, S.N. Wagner, J.L. Barrera, A. Mohar, E. Verastegui, and A. Zlotnik. Involvement of chemokine receptors in breast cancer metastasis. Nature *410*: 50–6, 2001.

95. Schrader, A.J., O. Lechner, M. Templin, K.E. Dittmar, S. Machtens, M. Mengel, M. Probst-Kepper, A. Franzke, T. Wollensak, P. Gatzlaff, J. Atzpodien, J. Buer, and J. Lauber. CXCR4/CXCL12 expression and signalling in kidney cancer. Br J Cancer *86*: 1250–6, 2002.

96. Boldajipour, B., H. Mahabaleshwar, E. Kardash, M. Reichman-Fried, H. Blaser, S. Minina, D. Wilson, Q. Xu, and E. Raz. Control of chemokine-guided cell migration by ligand sequestration. Cell *132*: 463–73, 2008.

97. Doitsidou, M., M. Reichman-Fried, J. Stebler, M. Koprunner, J. Dorries, D. Meyer, C.V. Esguerra, T. Leung, and E. Raz. Guidance of primordial germ cell migration by the chemokine SDF-1. Cell *111*: 647–59, 2002.

98. Knaut, H., C. Werz, R. Geisler, and C. Nusslein-Volhard. A zebrafish homologue of the chemokine receptor Cxcr4 is a germ-cell guidance receptor. Nature *421*: 279–82, 2003.

99. Zou, Y.R., A.H. Kottmann, M. Kuroda, I. Taniuchi, and D.R. Littman. Function of the chemokine receptor CXCR4 in haematopoiesis and in cerebellar development. Nature *393*: 595–9, 1998.

100. Marchesi, F., P. Monti, B.E. Leone, A. Zerbi, A. Vecchi, L. Piemonti, A. Mantovani and P. Allavena. Increased survival, proliferation, and migration in metastatic human pancreatic tumor cells expressing functional CXCR4. Cancer Res *64*: 8420–7, 2004.

101. Arya, M., H.R. Patel, C. McGurk, R. Tatoud, H. Klocker, J. Masters, and M. Williamson. The importance of the CXCL12-CXCR4 chemokine ligand-receptor interaction in prostate cancer metastasis. J Exp Ther Oncol *4*: 291–303, 2004.

102. Kim, J., H. Takeuchi, S.T. Lam, R.R. Turner, H.J. Wang, C. Kuo, L. Foshag, A.J. Bilchik, and D.S. Hoon. Chemokine receptor CXCR4 expression in colorectal cancer patients increases the risk for recurrence and for poor survival. J Clin Oncol *23*: 2744–53, 2005.

103. Perissinotto, E., G. Cavalloni, F. Leone, V. Fonsato, S. Mitola, G. Grignani, N. Surrenti, D. Sangiolo, F. Bussolino, W. Piacibello, and M. Aglietta. Involvement of chemokine receptor 4/stromal cell-derived factor 1 system during osteosarcoma tumor progression. Clin Cancer Res *11*: 490–7, 2005.

104. Schioppa, T., B. Uranchimeg, A. Saccani, S.K. Biswas, A. Doni, A. Rapisarda, S. Bernasconi, S. Saccani, M. Nebuloni, L. Vago, A. Mantovani, G. Melillo, and A. Sica. Regulation of the chemokine receptor CXCR4 by hypoxia. J Exp Med *198*: 1391–402, 2003.

105. Staller, P., J. Sulitkova, J. Lisztwan, H. Moch, E.J. Oakeley, and W. Krek. Chemokine receptor CXCR4 downregulated by von Hippel-Lindau tumour suppressor pVHL. Nature *425*: 307–11, 2003.

106. Semenza, G.L. Targeting HIF-1 for cancer therapy. Nat Rev Cancer *3*: 721–32, 2003.

107. Semenza, G. Signal transduction to hypoxia-inducible factor 1. Biochem Pharmacol *64*: 993–8, 2002.

108. Zhong, H., K. Chiles, D. Feldser, E. Laughner, C. Hanrahan, M.M. Georgescu, J.W. Simons, and G.L. Semenza. Modulation of hypoxia-inducible factor 1alpha

expression by the epidermal growth factor/phosphatidylinositol 3-kinase/PTEN/AKT/
FRAP pathway in human prostate cancer cells: implications for tumor angiogenesis and
therapeutics. Cancer Res *60*: 1541–5, 2000.

109. Phillips, R.J., J. Mestas, M. Gharaee-Kermani, M.D. Burdick, A. Sica, J.A. Belperio,
M.P. Keane, and R.M. Strieter. Epidermal growth factor and hypoxia-induced expression of CXC chemokine receptor 4 on non-small cell lung cancer cells is regulated by the
phosphatidylinositol 3-kinase/PTEN/AKT/mammalian target of rapamycin signaling
pathway and activation of hypoxia inducible factor-1alpha. J Biol Chem *280*: 22473–81,
2005.

110. Balabanian, K., B. Lagane, S. Infantino, K.Y. Chow, J. Harriague, B. Moepps,
F. Arenzana-Seisdedos, M. Thelen, and F. Bachelerie. The chemokine SDF-1/
CXCL12 binds to and signals through the orphan receptor RDC1 in T lymphocytes.
J Biol Chem *280*: 35760–6, 2005.

111. Burns, J.M., B.C. Summers, Y. Wang, A. Melikian, R. Berahovich, Z. Miao, M.E.
Penfold, M.J. Sunshine, D.R. Littman, C.J. Kuo, K. Wei, B.E. McMaster, K. Wright,
M.C. Howard, and T.J. Schall. A novel chemokine receptor for SDF-1 and I-TAC
involved in cell survival, cell adhesion, and tumor development. J Exp Med *203*:
2201–13, 2006.

112. Miao, Z., K.E. Luker, B.C. Summers, R. Berahovich, M.S. Bhojani, A. Rehemtulla,
C.G. Kleer, J.J. Essner, A. Nasevicius, G.D. Luker, M.C. Howard, and T.J. Schall.
CXCR7 (RDC1) promotes breast and lung tumor growth in vivo and is expressed on
tumor-associated vasculature. Proc Natl Acad Sci USA *104*: 15735–40, 2007.

113. Wang, J., Y. Shiozawa, Y. Wang, Y. Jung, K.J. Pienta, R. Mehra, R. Loberg, and
R.S. Taichman. The Role of CXCR7/RDC1 as a Chemokine Receptor for CXCL12/
SDF-1 in Prostate Cancer. J Biol Chem *283*: 4283–94, 2008.

114. Dambly-Chaudiere, C., N. Cubedo, and A. Ghysen. Control of cell migration in the
development of the posterior lateral line: antagonistic interactions between the chemokine receptors CXCR4 and CXCR7/RDC1. BMC Dev Biol *7*: 23, 2007.

Molecular Control of Lymphatic Metastasis in Lung Cancer

Mark M. Fuster and Judith A. Varner

Abstract Lymph node metastasis in lung cancer is a strong independent predictor of poor prognosis, and designation of the tumor "nodal" status is a challenging and central component of the lung carcinoma TNM staging system. In recent years, genetic studies in mouse models as well as pathologic human lung cancer studies have revealed a variety of molecules that may critically regulate thoracic lymph node metastasis. These include important lymphatic endothelial growth factors such as VEGF-C and VEGF-D as well as the pro-angiogenic factors VEGF-A and FGF-2 (often overexpressed by lung carcinoma cells) that stimulate the growth of lymphatic conduit in both the primary tumor and the downstream lymph nodes. This process of pathologic lymphangiogenesis correlates with lymph node metastasis and poor prognosis in lung cancer. Certain families of chemokines also appear to be critical for driving the process of tumor–lymphatic invasion, where the cognate chemokine receptors (e.g., CXCR4 or CCR7) are often overexpressed by carcinoma cells. In addition to lymphatic growth factors and chemokine effectors, a variety of molecules may facilitate interactions of lymphatic endothelial cells with growth factors, chemokines and their receptors, as well as the extracellular matrix. These include proteoglycans and integrins, and their roles in coordinating tumor-lymphatic interactions in the lung carcinoma microenvironment may be critical for lymph node metastasis.

Introduction

The lymphatic system is a low-pressure vascular network of thin-walled blind-ended sacs, lymphatic capillaries, and collecting vessels coupled with a family of secondary immune organs that include lymph nodes, the spleen, and several organ-associated lymphoid patches. The lymphoid organ component of this

M.M. Fuster (✉)
Department of Medicine, Division of Pulmonary and Critical Care, University of California, San Diego; VA San Diego Healthcare System, San Diego, CA, USA
e-mail: mfuster@ucsd.edu

V. Keshamouni et al. (eds.), *Lung Cancer Metastasis*,
DOI 10.1007/978-1-4419-0772-1_9, © Springer Science+Business Media, LLC 2009

173

system, which is critical for immune surveillance and acquired immune responses in local tissues, is positioned in line with the vascular component. In the interstitium surrounding blood capillaries, lymphatic microvasculature serves a critical role in fluid and protein homeostasis by returning plasma ultrafiltrate back to the systemic venous circulation via larger smooth muscle-lined collecting lymphatic vessels.

While playing a central role in normal circulatory physiology, lymphatic vasculature also contributes to highly dynamic processes during certain pathologic states [1]. Lymphatic endothelial cells lining this vasculature play central roles in these processes, some of which include sprouting of new lymphatic vessels from preexisting vessels (lymphangiogenesis), lymphatic intra- and extravasation of immune cells or tumor cells during inflammation or cancer, and lymphatic endothelial hyper- or hypoplasia associated with lymphedema states (see excellent reviews in [2–4]). In lung cancer, two of these pathophysiologic events (tumor lymphangiogenesis and invasion of tumor lymphatic vasculature) contribute to lymphatic tumor progression, with profound effects on lymph node metastasis and prognosis. These processes are governed by a variety of key molecular regulators and biophysical forces that will be discussed herein. In addition, we include the consideration of molecular families that may broadly and simultaneously modulate the actions of multiple major lymphatic endothelial effectors. While the focus of this chapter is on the biology of lymphatic endothelium during the pathogenesis of nodal metastasis in lung cancer, the discussion will highlight the importance of understanding the molecular effectors of this process as a prerequisite for future development of targeted anti-metastasis therapy.

Tumor Lymphangiogenesis in Lung Cancer

Carcinomas utilize the lymphatic circulation as a major portal for metastasis. As part of normal circulatory physiology and homeostasis, the lymphatic system serves to return interstitial fluid along with a variety of low-molecular weight solutes to the blood circulation while playing an essential role in immune defense [1]. In carcinoma, however, lymphatic vasculature associated with the tumor microenvironment provides a conduit for tumor cells to disseminate directly to lymph nodes, a process that strongly correlates with mortality among solid tumors. It is well established, for example, that the (N)odal status in the "TNM" staging classification for lung cancer, a leading cause of cancer death, refers to the extent to which tumor has disseminated to lymph nodes (LN) and constitutes a major determinant of prognosis [5, 6]. Nodal metastasis is a major form of metastatic tumor progression for both non-small cell lung carcinoma (NSCLC) and small cell lung carcinoma (SCLC). Indeed, the overall 5-year survival of surgically treated NSCLC patients drops from 60–80% for clinical-stage I patients to under 50% for clinical-stage II patients, with the only difference between stages being clinical N0 (no LN involvement) versus N1 (peribronchial/hilar LN involvement) disease [6, 7]. Moreover, the TNM system is used for defining treatment and prognosis among most solid tumors, wherein the clinical (or more accurate pathologic-) N-status of the patient often has major impact on the course of management (e.g., use of surgical resection versus the sole use or additional use of combination chemotherapy/radiation treatment). Herein, we review and illustrate the evidence for a variety of biological determinants of nodal metastasis in cancer, with a special focus on lung cancer when/where data are available. We aim to highlight both well-established mechanisms and novel pathways that might represent future targets for novel anti-metastasis therapy.

For many solid tumors, sprouting of lymphatic vessels in the tumor environment, a process known as tumor lymphangiogenesis, increases lymphatic conduit that promotes the ultimate transit of tumor cells to regional nodes and the systemic circulation [8–10]. The process most likely results from sprouting of lymphatic capillaries from preexisting lymphatic vessels in the tumor microenvironment, particularly at the periphery of the primary tumor [11]. Following tumor–lymphatic invasion, this conduit may transmit a "tidal" flow of tumor cells down a pressure gradient directed away from the tumor [9]. Tumor dissemination may be further facilitated by a variety of tumor–lymphatic molecular adhesion interactions [8, 12]. Ultimately, investment of tumors with lymphatic vasculature strongly potentiates lymph node metastasis [13–16], and several effectors of tumor lymphangiogenesis have recently been identified. These include the vascular endothelial growth factors VEGF-C and VEGF-D that interact with the lymphatic endothelial receptor VEGFR-3, a vascular growth receptor that is strongly expressed on lymphatic endothelia [17, 18]. These factors may also interact with VEGFR-2 in addition to VEGFR-2/3 heterodimers and the neuropilin (Nrp2) semaphorin receptor expressed on lymphatic capillaries [19–21], with the relative degrees of affinity for the various receptors dependent on the degree of proteolytic processing [22]. The importance of these effectors has recently been demonstrated in a variety of animal models of cancer, wherein overexpression of VEGF-C or VEGF-D by tumor cells was sufficient to strongly induce lymphangiogenesis and promote lymph node metastasis. Among these are several mouse models for pathologic lymphangiogenesis, with many providing genetic evidence for these important interactions [23–26]. In addition to tumor cells as a source for such pro-lymphangiogenic factors, tumor-infiltrating macrophages derived from circulating bone marrow precursors may also promote both tumor angiogenesis and lymphangiogenesis through the secretion of VEGF-A, VEGF-C, basic fibroblast growth factor (FGF-2), tumor necrosis factor (TNF)-alpha, and other pro-angiogenic as well as pro-lymphangiogenic substances [27, 28].

It is only in recent years that analysis of the lymphatic network within tumors as well as the relationships between carcinoma cells, lymphatic endothelium, and other stromal components in clinical tumor and lymph node specimens has been possible. Identification of molecular markers specific for lymphatic endothelial cells, many of which are now commercially available, has allowed for the application of such analysis to models of lymphatic tumor progression in gene-targeted mice as well as applications to clinical specimens in order to link patterns of lymphatic vessel behavior with tumor production of specific growth factors as well as outcome data. Some of these markers include the transcription factor Prox-1 (expressed early during the process of lymphatic endothelial differentiation), LYVE-1 (the CD44 homolog lymphatic vessel hyaluronan receptor-1), and VEGFR-3 (major receptor for VEGF-C and VEGF-D) [18, 29, 30]. The application of these markers to clinical oncology specimens from a wide number of tumors has revealed a relatively constant pattern that links peri- and sometimes intra-tumoral lymphatic vessel proliferation with lymph node metastasis, and a variety of examples are emerging from the clinical lung cancer literature, as will be reviewed. Beyond this, with such tools in hand, the functional relationships between lymphatic endothelial effectors and lymphatic vasculature in vivo are now being realized in gene-targeted experimental systems.

In clinical oncology, several studies have shown that tumor-cell expression of major pro-lymphangiogenic growth factors such as VEGF-C and VEGF-D correlates with lymph node metastasis and poor prognosis in carcinomas of the lung, breast, colon, prostate, stomach, and head/neck, among others (reviewed in [31]). Specifically in the setting of lung cancer, several studies have demonstrated significant correlations between tumor expression of these growth factors and stimulation of lymphatic metastasis as well as poor prognosis, with direct growth stimulation of tumor lymphatic vasculature as the most probable mechanism [32–38]. The latter would provide a high level of conduit for initiating lymphatic tumor spread at the primary tumor site, and it appears to be consistent with other studies that correlate elevated cognate receptor (i.e., VEGFR-3) expression in NSCLC lymphatic vasculature, lymph node metastasis, and/or poor survival [33, 39, 40]. However, this may not be the only tumor progression mechanism promoted by these growth factors. It also appears that tumor autocrine/paracrine VEGF-C/VEGFR-3 loops may stimulate growth signaling among tumor cells in addition to cross talk between tumor cells and the local lymphatic microvasculature [41, 42]. In addition to this, the major *angiogenic* tumor growth factor, VEGF-A, may also play critical roles in *lymph* angiogenesis through interaction with VEGF receptors on tumor lymphatic endothelial cells [8, 43, 44]. Thus, tumor expression of VEGF-A in lung cancer, which independently correlates with poor outcome [37, 45, 46], may exert its negative prognostic effects through both the inhibition of blood-angiogenesis and effects on *lymphatic* vascular remodeling and proliferation. The latter may even include VEGF-A-dependent lymph node lymphangiogenesis in the downstream/sentinel lymph node *before* tumor metastasizes to the node [47]. At the current time, despite strong evidence for prognostic association, the body of correlative clinical data still makes it difficult to determine the relative degree(s) to which these various VEGF-dependent pro-lymphangiogenic pathways contribute to lymphatic vessel remodeling and lymph node metastasis in lung cancer. This poses challenges upon how such growth factors might be integrated as biomarkers into routine (including array-driven) clinical pathways for lung cancer treatment and prognosis. In some NSCLCs, for example, complex tumor-cell VEGF-C/VEGFR-3 (and VEGFR-2) autocrine/paracrine loops may contribute to lymphangiogenesis, wherein the ratio of VEGF-C to VEGFR-3 expression may be more predictive of lymph node metastasis than the absolute level of tumor VEGF-C mRNA expression [41]. Nevertheless, the weight of clinical evidence points to a strong positive link between degree of lymphatic vessel proliferation in the primary lung cancer, lymph node metastasis, and poor clinical outcome [9, 13, 14, 37].

What molecular mechanisms might stimulate the lymphatic endothelial signaling pathways that mediate lymphangiogenesis in lung cancer? Major stimulation of lymphatic endothelial proliferation during tumor lymphangiogenesis occurs through the activation of homodimeric receptor tyrosine kinases VEGFR-2, VEGFR-3, and even VEGFR-2/3 heterodimers on lymphatic endothelial cells that line lymphatic vasculature predominantly at the periphery of many solid tumors (reviewed in [22]). This activation occurs primarily following receptor binding and stimulation by the soluble effectors VEGF-C and VEGF-D. These major lymphatic endothelial growth factors contain receptor-binding VEGF-homology domains and amino- as well as carboxy-terminal propeptides that are proteolytically cleaved, with differential affinities toward the major lymphatic endothelial receptors VEGFR-3 and VEGFR-2, depending on the degree of cleavage [19, 48]. The major form of receptor activation occurs through VEGFR-3. Activation of the receptor tyrosine kinase leads to major ERK-dependent endothelial proliferation, AKT-dependent endothelial survival, and stimulation of endothelial cell migration [22]. With the release of these factors in the parenchyma of lung carcinomas, major stimulation of lymphangiogenesis and lymph node metastasis may take place.

In addition to growth factor-dependent pathways that stimulate VEGF receptors, a variety of other molecular mechanisms have now been shown to contribute to tumor (as well as developmental) lymphangiogenesis, and a number of these may function either alone or synergistically with VEGF-dependent signaling to stimulate lymphatic metastasis in lung cancer (Table 1). For example, tumor expression of FGF-2 in lung carcinoma correlates with poor prognosis [45, 49], and it has recently been shown that FGF-2 stimulates both blood-angiogenesis and lymphangiogenesis [50–52]. It is also possible that other growth factors that have been established as pro-lymphangiogenic effectors, such as platelet-derived growth factor (PDGF), hepatocyte growth factor (HFG), or members of the insulin-like growth factor (IGF) family [4, 53, 54], might play important roles in stimulating lymphatic vessel sprouting in lung carcinomas. The degree to which other effector molecules involved in the maturation of nascent lymphatic vessels (i.e., the integrin $\alpha9\beta1$, the forkhead transcription factor FOXC2, or the angiopoietin Ang2) [55] contribute to patterning of lymphangiogenic vasculature in lung cancer is unknown.

Table 1 Major molecular effectors of tumor lymphangiogenesis in lung cancer

Molecular effector	Effect on lymphatic vasculature	Possible role(s) in lymphangiogenesis and nodal metastasis in NSCLC	References relevant to lymphangiogenesis in lung cancer
VEGF-C	Major soluble effector of tumor and developmental lymphangiogenesis	– Stimulus released by tumor cells with direct/paracrine stimulation of lymphatic endothelial proliferation (dominant mechanism) – Autocrine tumor-cell stimulation (indirect)	[32, 33, 35, 37, 42]
VEGF-D	Major soluble effector of tumor and developmental lymphangiogenesis	Stimulus released by tumor cells with direct/paracrine stimulation of lymphatic endothelial proliferation	[36, 38]
VEGFR-3 (Flt-4)	Major receptor tyrosine kinase for VEGF-C, VEGF-D on lymphatic vessels	– Receptor stimulation on lymphatic vessels: Initiates major lymphatic endothelial growth signaling and differentiation pathways – Expression on tumor cells mediates autocrine tumor stimulation	[22, 32, 33, 39, 40, 42]
VEGF-A	Soluble effector of both angiogenesis and lymphangiogenesis	– Paracrine lymphatic vessel growth stimulus released by tumor cells – Major effector of blood angiogenesis (possible contribution to hematogenous lymph node metastasis) – Effector of lymph node lymphangiogenesis downstream from primary tumor	[34, 37, 45]
VEGFR-2 (Flk-1; KDR)	– Receptor tyrosine kinase for VEGF-A on lymphatic (and blood) vessels – Receptor tyrosine kinase for appropriately processed VEGF-C and VEGF-D on lymphatic vessels	– Receptor stimulation on lymphatic (and blood) vasculature: Initiates major endothelial growth signaling and differentiation pathways – Expression on tumor cells mediates autocrine tumor stimulation – May heterodimerize with VEGFR-3, with signaling possible by VEGF-A, VEGF-C, VEGF-D	[22, 36, 56, 57]

Table 1 (Continued)

Molecular effector	Effect on lymphatic vasculature	Possible role(s) in lymphangiogenesis and nodal metastasis in NSCLC	References relevant to lymphangiogenesis in lung cancer
Neuropilin-2	– Co-receptor for VEGFR-3 – Direct receptor stimulation by VEGF-C and VEGF-D	– Receptor stimulation on lymphatic vasculature (Expression on NSCLC lymphatic vessels unknown.) – Cooperation with neuropilin-1 may contribute to blood angiogenesis (and possible lymphangiogenesis) in NSCLC	[58–60]
FGF-2	Soluble effector of both angiogenesis and lymphangiogenesis	– Paracrine lymphatic vessel growth stimulus released by tumor cells – Angiogenic stimulus (possible contribution to hematogenous lymph node metastasis)	[45, 49, 61]
FGFR-3	– Receptor for FGF on lymphatic endothelium	– Possible major lymphatic FGF receptor for FGF-dependent lymphangiogenesis – Cooperation with FGFR-1 in NSCLC (?)	[50]

Combining the body of animal studies showing strong genetic evidence for tumor lymphangiogenesis as an effector of lymph node metastasis with a growing body of mostly correlative evidence from the lung cancer literature to date, it appears likely that targeting some (or many) of the molecular pathways highlighted in Table 1 may limit lymphatic tumor progression and possibly improve outcomes in lung cancer. Considerations on how to practically apply such measurements in the clinical arena are outside the scope of this discussion. Nevertheless, it is clear from the evidence thus far that significant progress has been made in understanding the molecular control of tumor lymphangiogenesis, and that activation of several major pathways is a problem in lung cancer that is strongly associated with lymph node metastasis and poor outcomes. More work is needed to eventually translate the inhibition of these pathways toward blockade of clinical tumor lymphangiogenesis in lung cancer (e.g., as a dedicated form of secondary prevention or in combination with surgery and/or chemo/radiotherapy). Moreover, further research will be necessary to identify the patterns of lymphangiogenesis-associated biomarkers that may best predict (e.g., when applied to biopsy material) which lung cancer patients would respond with inhibition of lymphatic metastasis to interventions that may alter any combination of these molecular events.

Invasion of Lymphatic Vasculature in Lung Cancer

While lymphangiogenesis contributes to lymphatic invasion (and eventual lymph node metastasis) in the microenvironment of lung carcinomas, little is known about the molecular mechanisms that specifically effect *tumor migration* into the local tumor lymphatic vasculature. The mechanisms that promote tumor lymphangiogenesis discussed thus far are critical for establishing a level of lymphatic endothelial surface area that serves as the first lymphatic entry point for invading tumor cells that may subsequently seed sentinel or downstream hilar/mediastinal lymph nodes. It should be realized, however, that even the existing lymphatic vasculature around a developing lung carcinoma can provide sufficient conduit for the entry/uptake of invasive tumor cells, even in the absence of lymphangiogenesis [62]. Moreover, biophysical forces such as intra-tumoral hydrostatic pressure and pressure gradients directed outward from the tumor center in the face of an especially leaky lymphatic vascular surface area can greatly facilitate a "downstream" movement of motile or invasive tumor cells into larger collecting lymphatic vessels at the tumor periphery, with subsequent seeding of the nearest nodal regions [63].

In addition to lymphangiogenesis and biophysical (fluid-mechanical) forces that promote tumor cell entry into lymphatic vessels within the tumor microenvironment, certain lymphatic endothelial chemokines appear to promote attraction and/or adhesion of invading tumor cells that express cognate chemokine receptors [64, 65]. In particular, recent work shows that such chemokines may work in concert with biophysical factors involved in the establishment of chemokine gradients across peri-lymphatic extracellular matrix in tumors [66] to promote the movement of tumor toward and into local lymphatic vessels. Two important lymphatic endothelial chemokines that may mediate such migration include secondary lymphoid tissue chemokine (SLC)/CCL21 [67–69] and stromal cell-derived factor-1 alpha (SDF-1α)/CXCL12 [69–71]. The cited references describe the importance of these chemokines in promoting lymphatic metastasis in several carcinomas, including breast, squamous head and neck, melanoma, and cervical carcinomas. For lung carcinoma, there has also been some recent investigation on this topic, although most of the work describes critical roles for such chemokines acting in concert with their cognate receptors on lung cancer cells in the promotion of lymphatic metastasis using animal models [72]. Among clinical lung cancer specimens, both small and non-small cell lung carcinomas, among several other types of carcinomas, have been reported to strongly upregulate CCR7 and CXCR4, the cognate receptors for CCL21 and CXCL12, respectively [69, 73–77]. Moreover, Takanami [73] has shown that overexpression of CCR7 mRNA in NSCLC correlates with lymph node metastasis. Together, these findings indicate that CCL21/CCR7 and CXCL12/CXCR4 interactions may represent some of the most important chemokine/receptor interactions that drive tumor–lymphatic invasion and eventual lymph node metastasis in both lung cancer and several other carcinomas.

It is important to balance this discussion with the knowledge that tumor cells are not the only cells in the tumor microenvironment that express receptors for lymphatic endothelial chemokines. For example, the chemokines CCL21 and CXCL12, as well as the EBV-induced molecule 1 ligand chemokine CCL19, have been well characterized for their ability to affect lymphatic trafficking of dendritic cells as well as T cells in normal as well as neoplastic tissues [78–80]. In the tumor microenvironment, trafficking of such cells across lymphatic vasculature may mediate immunologic *antitumor* responses. Thus, combining these observations with the previous discussion, it appears that the release of such chemokines by tumor lymphatic vasculature may variably stimulate events that either promote lymph node metastasis (i.e., lymphatic vessel invasion by chemokine-responsive tumor cells) or limit lymphatic metastasis (i.e., lymphatic antitumor immune responses). Interestingly, the antitumor effects of CCL21-responsive immune cells have been exploited in novel immunotherapy lung cancer models, wherein dendritic cells transduced with a CCL21 expressing adenoviral vector delivered to the tumor environment have been used to drive immune-mediated tumor eradication following further tumor infiltration by responsive host dendritic cells and activated T cells [81]. However, in the absence of experimental or therapeutic augmentation of antitumor immune responses by such chemokines, the degree to which host tumor-infiltrating dendritic cells (or T cells) may counter the invasive effects of tumor cells responsive to the same chemokines remains to be determined. In this regard, it is worth noting that the maturation of dendritic cells that infiltrate human non-small cell lung carcinomas is often blocked at an immature stage [82]. Further work may lead to insightful methods to inhibit lymphatic vascular invasiveness by chemokine-responsive tumor cells while maintaining or even enhancing approaches that promote tumor immunization.

Modulation of Tumor Lymphangiogenesis and Lymphatic Invasion by Integrins and Proteoglycans

Several classes of molecules in the tumor environment may function as critical modulators that act either in concert with or directly facilitate the processes of lymphangiogenesis and the trafficking of both tumor cells and immune cells across tumor lymphatic vessels. Some of these molecules may function in a "broad" manner during lymphatic tumor progression, wherein their ability to simultaneously modulate the action of several pro-lymphangiogenic factors or multiple lymphatic vessel chemokines makes them important targets for future study and possibly therapeutic intervention. The discovery of molecular species that broadly control discrete steps in lymphatic tumor progression in lung cancer also introduces a rationale for overcoming redundancy in a system where the "magic-bullet" targeting of one major growth factor or chemokine, for example, might result in upregulation of other (non-targeted) factors that ultimately might contribute to completion, or even acceleration, of a given pathophysiologic step (e.g., lymphangiogenesis, controlled by multiple growth factors). Important species of molecules associated with lymphatic endothelium that may fall into this class include certain subclasses of integrins as well as proteoglycans. Herein, we highlight a few examples that apply to lung cancer; however, we also illustrate how growing experimental evidence might be applied to improve our understanding of how these molecules more generally affect lymphatic pathophysiology in cancer.

Lymphatic endothelium in the tumor environment may interact with both tumor cells and important matrix elements through the action of select members of the integrin family. Integrins are heterodimeric membrane glycoproteins that facilitate cell–cell interactions and migration of cells across extracellular matrix (ECM) through their ability to bind to both important ECM proteins such as fibronectin and immunoglobulin superfamily adhesion molecules such as vascular cell adhesion molecule-1 (VCAM-1) and intercellular adhesion molecule-1 (ICAM-1). Upon binding to such ligands, integrins co-cluster intracellular kinases and focal adhesion complex adaptor proteins, resulting in activation of signaling pathways that mediate cell migration and proliferation [83].

As a class, it appears likely that integrins expressed by lymphatic endothelium play important roles in modulating some of the critical pathophysiologic steps in lymph node metastasis that have been discussed, including tumor lymphangiogenesis and tumor attachment and migration across lymphatic vasculature. The roles of specific integrins in each of these processes have not been fully realized, and we currently have little clinical understanding of their specific function(s) in lung cancer lymphatic metastasis. However, several pieces of a puzzle that involves the action of both vascular (blood and lymphatic) and tumor-cell integrins are beginning to come together for cancer. For example, it is now evident that the integrin $\alpha 9\beta 1$ plays an important role in developmental lymphangiogenesis through both its upregulation by the major lymphatic transcription factor Prox-1 following growth factor stimulation and its ability to promote VEGF-C- and VEGF-D-mediated endothelial cell motility in vivo through direct binding to such factors [84, 85]. The latter may directly stimulate tumor lymphangiogenesis, although the specific role this integrin plays in cancer progression is not known. Other integrin members expressed on lymphatic endothelium appear to play important roles in pathologic lymphangiogenesis, including wound lymphangiogenesis ($\alpha 1\beta 1$, $\alpha 2\beta 1$) [86], corneal inflammatory lymphangiogenesis ($\alpha 5\beta 1$) [87], and tumor lymphangiogenesis ($\alpha 4\beta 1$) [88]. The latter appears to be strongly upregulated in lymphatic endothelium of experimental Lewis lung carcinoma tumor systems, and blockade of this integrin with antibodies is sufficient to inhibit tumor lymphangiogenesis and metastasis in the same in vivo models (J.A. Varner, unpublished data). In order to study the expression of certain integrins in clinical tumor-associated *lymphatic* vasculature, it may be useful to increase our use of high-sensitivity methodology such as laser capture microdissection (coupled with lymphatic-specific immuno-labeling) in clinical cancer specimens.

In lung cancer, a limited amount of clinical data has revealed that tumor expression of certain integrins correlates with nodal tumor spread. An example of this is the correlation between expression of $\alpha 5$ and $\beta 1$ integrins in NSCLC and lymph node metastasis [89]. It is possible that this might occur as a result of cross talk between the integrin-expressing tumor cell and cognate ligands expressed by the tumor lymphatic endothelium; however, the mechanisms that may mediate such interactions need further study. In squamous cell lung carcinoma, tumor expression of the integrins $\alpha 1\beta 1$ and $\alpha 2\beta 1$ directly correlates with metastatic progression [90], although the mechanism(s) whereby such integrins may promote *lymphatic* metastasis needs further study. While further clinical data are gathered for lung cancer, an important role for antagonists of specific integrins may also be realized, and experimental as well as clinical translational research may reveal the ability of such agents to block lymphatic tumor progression. More work is needed to further map the importance of specific integrins, including those associated with lymphatic endothelium, during nodal metastasis in lung cancer.

Another class of molecules that may modulate the action of several effectors that promote lymphatic tumor progression in lung cancer is proteoglycans. Members of this broad and ubiquitous class of glycan molecules are found at the cell surface and secreted from several mammalian cell types and consist of a core protein that bears one or more covalently attached glycosaminoglycan chains [91]. These include heparan sulfate proteoglycans (HSPGs), chondroitin sulfate proteoglycans (CSPGs), and other subclasses named after the nature of the repeating disaccharide unit that makes up the major part of their respective glyco-saminoglycan chains. A particularly unique feature of HSPGs is the presence of unique domains along the heparan sulfate chains that bear sulfate-modified motifs in clustered regions that confer binding capacity for several growth factors as well as chemokines that are known to play important roles in cell growth and migration, including vascular growth [92–94]. In cancer, it is possible that these properties of HSPGs may mediate not only blood-vascular progression (i.e., angiogenesis and tumor vascular invasion) but similar processes in lymphatic vasculature that promote lymph node metastasis, such as tumor lymphangiogenesis and lymphatic vessel tumor invasion.

Insights from the laboratory as well as in vivo gene-targeted experimental models have provided key insights on how HSPGs might facilitate important endothelial functions in carcinoma. This includes a consideration of tumor lymphatic endothelium as well. It is now well recognized that the interactions of some of the most important endothelial growth factors with their cognate receptors on vascular endothelium during developmental as well as pathologic angiogenesis are modulated by the co-receptor functions of HSPGs [95–97]. In tumor blood vasculature, endothelial cell surface and secreted HSPGs appear to serve as co-receptors as well as matrix scaffolds for a variety of soluble growth factors released by tumor cells, including VEGF-A, FGF-2, PDGF, HGF, heparin-binding epidermal growth factor (HB-EGF), and several other pro-angiogenic molecules [97–100]. Recent work shows that the major *angiogenic* effectors VEGF-A and FGF-2, for which HS may facilitate binding and signaling via endothelial VEGFR-2 and FGFR-1 receptors, may also stimulate lymphangiogenesis via the same receptors on lymphatic endothelium [43, 51, 65, 101–103]. The importance of HSPGs as co-receptors during that process remains to be examined. Moreover, the role of lymphatic endothelial HSPGs in mediating signaling by VEGF-C or VEGF-D during interactions with the cognate receptors VEGFR-3 (or VEGFR-2/3 heterodimers) has yet to be examined [104]. Preliminary data show that lymphatic endothelial cells that bear mutations in key HSPG biosynthetic enzymes show alterations in binding to such growth factors, and their ability to signal in response to specific growth factor stimulation also appears to be altered (M.M. Fuster, unpublished data). Beyond tumor lymphangiogenesis, the function of HSPGs in mediating any of the lymphatic chemokine interactions that have been discussed remains to be determined. For example, the chemokines CXCL12 and CCL21, which are associated with lymph node metastasis in several carcinomas, may be associated with lymphatic heparan sulfate during the establishment of chemokine gradients along lymphatic endothelium [105–107]. Since the cognate receptors for these chemokines are frequently overexpressed in both small cell and non-small cell lung carcinoma [73–75], it is possible that lymphatic endothelial HSPGs may serve critical functions in facilitating chemokine-mediated tumor invasion of lymphatic vasculature in lung cancer.

Little is known regarding tissue-specific expression of specific proteoglycans in lung carcinoma, and those specific families of HSPGs that most promote (blood or lymphatic) vascular progression have yet to be discovered. Some data suggest that the *stroma* of human lung cancer specimens shows elevated levels of certain cell-surface HSPGs that are distinct from those of tumor cells themselves and that differential regulation of unique families of HSPGs among different cell types within the tumor may result in the promotion of tumor metastasis. For example, while tumor-cell-associated HSPGs often facilitate growth factor signaling by a variety of tumor growth factors, distinct HSPGs may play unique roles in tumor differentiation; and in some cases, *down*regulated expression of a given HSPG (e.g., syndecan-1) by lung tumor cells appears to be associated with tumor *invasiveness*, as that particular HSPG may contribute to maintenance of a differentiated epithelial morphology [108]. On the other hand, recent work using microdissection-based tissue expression analyses has demonstrated that a distinct *up*regulation of syndecan-1 that occurs in *stroma*-associated cells of lung carcinomas (as well as other clinical tumors) may positively contribute to metastasis [109]. While much of this expression may be associated with myofibroblastic cells in the stroma, specific analyses on endothelial (including lymphatic endothelial) expression are lacking. It is also interesting to note that increased stromal expression of the CSPG versican in lung adenocarcinomas correlates with lymphatic metastasis as well as tumor recurrence [110]. More work is necessary to identify unique lymphatic endothelial proteoglycans that may contribute to tumor lymphatic progression in lung cancer.

Validation of specific integrins or heparan sulfate proteoglycans as molecular targets in the lymphatic vascular progression of lung cancer may be especially appealing since these classes of molecules may simultaneously mediate several lymphatic pathophysiologic processes. Targeting these pathways may thus alter the functions of multiple lymphatic growth factors, interfere with adhesion of blood-vascular and/or lymphatic endothelium with tumor cells, monocytes, or extracellular matrix, and possibly impair the trafficking of tumor cells across lymphatic endothelium during lymph node metastasis. Figure 1 highlights what appear to be the most important molecular mechanisms that promote tumor lymphangiogenesis and tumor lymphatic vascular invasion in lung cancer. As a final point with therapeutic implications, since much of our discussion has been centered on the lymphatic endothelium of the host, it should be mentioned that an advantage of targeting tumor endothelium in general is that it possesses greater genetic stability than tumor cells, resulting in a lower potential for induction of drug resistance [111]. As we expand our understanding of lymphatic molecular pathophysiology at the genetic and experimental level, it is hoped that translation to clinical lung cancer (either alone or in combination with

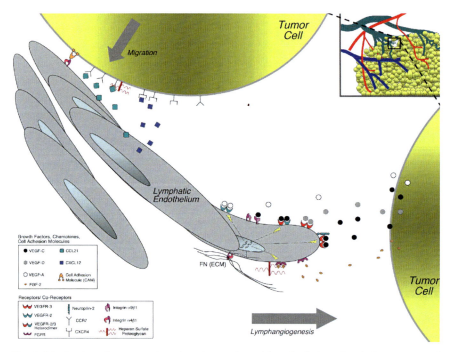

Fig. 1 Mechanisms for tumor lymphangiogenesis and lymphatic invasion in lung cancer: A proliferating primary lung carcinoma requires a blood vasculature, derived from surrounding host vessels through the process of angiogenesis (*red* and *blue* vessels in *upper right, inset*). Lymphatic vasculature (*green*) sprouts from host lymphatic vessels adjacent to the growing tumor and the molecular interactions between proliferating lymphatic endothelium and tumor cells (boxed area within the *inset*) are illustrated in the expanded figure. Tumor lymphangiogenesis (expanded view, *lower right*) is driven by a variety of potent lymphatic endothelial mitogens produced by tumor cells, including VEGF-C, VEGF-D, and the blood-endothelial growth factors VEGF-A and FGF-2. The ability of tumor-associated lymphatic vasculature to respond to these factors depends on the relative expression of the lymphatic receptors VEGFR-3 (that binds VEGF-C and VEGF-D), VEGFR-2 (that binds VEGF-A in addition to post-proteoly-tically processed variants of VEGF-C and VEGF-D), FGFR (binding to FGF-2), and even VEGFR-2/3 heterodimers. Receptor tyrosine kinase activation by these factors allows for activation of major endothelial proliferative signaling pathways (lymphatic nuclear activation, center). Lymphatic endothelial co-receptors that may play important roles in facilitating these interactions include neuropilin-2 (for VEGFR activation) and heparan sulfate proteoglycans (for FGF-2 and VEGFR activation). Integrins may play critical roles through their ability to both modulate growth factor interactions during lymphangiogenesis (e.g., integrin 91) and mediate interactions with extracellular matrix (ECM) components such as fibronectin (FN), allowing for concomitant lymphatic endothelial cytoskeletal changes that facilitate motility through matrix. Invasion of lymphatic vasculature by tumor cells in the tumor microenvironment (expanded view, *upper left*) involves both migration of tumor cells toward lymphatic vessels and attachment to the lymphatic endothelium. These processes are facilitated by a number of chemokine interactions, with some of the most important events being chemotaxis of CCR7-overexpressing carcinoma cells toward CCL21-producing lymphatic endothelial cells or chemotaxis of CXCR4-overexpressing tumor cells toward CXCL12 released from lymphatic endothelium. Heparan sulfate proteoglycans may play roles in stabilizing chemokine–receptor interactions. Following migration, such processes may also facilitate tumor-lymphatic adhesion, with additional stabilization by interactions between integrins and tumor cell adhesion molecules (CAMs). Legend is shown at the *lower left*

current therapy) will lead to promising targeted therapies that may prevent or inhibit lymphatic tumor progression and lymph node metastasis and improve patient outcomes.

Acknowledgments The authors acknowledge grant support from the American Cancer Society (RSG#116111 to MMF), the U.S. Department of Veterans Affairs (CDTA award to MMF), and NIH/NCI (RO1 CA126820-01A1 to JAV).

References

1. Alitalo, K., T. Tammela, and T.V. Petrova, *Lymphangiogenesis in development and human disease.* Nature, 2005. **438**(7070): 946–53.
2. Ji, R.C., *Lymphatic endothelial cells, tumor lymphangiogenesis and metastasis: New insights into intratumoral and peritumoral lymphatics.* Cancer Metastasis Rev, 2006. **25**(4): 677–94.
3. Makinen, T., C. Norrmen, and T.V. Petrova, *Molecular mechanisms of lymphatic vascular development.* Cell Mol Life Sci, 2007.
4. Liersch, R. and M. Detmar, *Lymphangiogenesis in development and disease.* Thromb Haemost, 2007. **98**(2): 304–10.
5. Mountain, C.F., *Revisions in the international system for staging lung cancer.* Chest, 1997. **111**(6): 1710–7.
6. Silvestri, G.A. et al., *Noninvasive staging of non-small cell lung cancer: ACCP evidenced-based clinical practice guidelines* (2nd edition). Chest, 2007. 132(3 Suppl): 178S–201S.
7. Scott, W.J. et al., *Treatment of non-small cell lung cancer stage I and stage II: ACCP evidence-based clinical practice guidelines* (2nd edition). Chest, 2007. 132(3 Suppl): 234S–242S.
8. Alitalo, K. and P. Carmeliet, *Molecular mechanisms of lymphangiogenesis in health and disease.* Cancer Cell, 2002. **1**(3): 219–27.
9. Nathanson, S.D., *Insights into the mechanisms of lymph node metastasis.* Cancer, 2003. **98**(2): 413–23.
10. Fidler, I.J., Molecular biology of cancer invasion and metastasis. In Cancer: Principles and Practice of Oncology, Fifth Edition, DeVita V.T., Hellman S., and Rosenberg S.A., Editor. 1997, Lippincott-Raven Publishers: Philadelphia, pp. 135–152.
11. He, Y. et al., *Preexisting lymphatic endothelium but not endothelial progenitor cells are essential for tumor lymphangiogenesis and lymphatic metastasis.* Cancer Res, 2004. **64**(11): 3737–40.
12. Oliver, G. and M. Detmar, *The rediscovery of the lymphatic system: old and new insights into the development and biological function of the lymphatic vasculature.* Genes Dev, 2002. **16**(7): 773–83.
13. Renyi-Vamos, F. et al., *Lymphangiogenesis correlates with lymph node metastasis, prognosis, and angiogenic phenotype in human non-small cell lung cancer.* Clin Cancer Res, 2005. **11**(20): 7344–53.
14. He, Y. et al., *Suppression of tumor lymphangiogenesis and lymph node metastasis by blocking vascular endothelial growth factor receptor 3 signaling.* J Natl Cancer Inst, 2002. **94**(11): 819–25.
15. Adams, R.H. and K. Alitalo, *Molecular regulation of angiogenesis and lymphangiogenesis.* Nat Rev Mol Cell Biol, 2007. **8**(6): 464–78.
16. Dadras, S.S. et al., *Tumor lymphangiogenesis predicts melanoma metastasis to sentinel lymph nodes.* Mod Pathol, 2005. **18**(9): 1232–42.
17. Joukov, V. et al., *A novel vascular endothelial growth factor, VEGF-C, is a ligand for the Flt4 (VEGFR-3) and KDR (VEGFR-2) receptor tyrosine kinases.* Embo J, 1996. **15**(7): 1751.

18. Makinen, T. et al., *Isolated lymphatic endothelial cells transduce growth, survival and migratory signals via the VEGF-C/D receptor VEGFR-3*. Embo J, 2001. **20**(17): 4762–73.
19. Joukov, V. et al., *Proteolytic processing regulates receptor specificity and activity of VEGF-C*. Embo J, 1997. **16**(13): 3898–911.
20. Achen, M.G. et al., *Vascular endothelial growth factor D (VEGF-D) is a ligand for the tyrosine kinases VEGF receptor 2 (Flk1) and VEGF receptor 3 (Flt4)*. Proc Natl Acad Sci U S A, 1998. **95**(2): 548–53.
21. Karkkainen, M.J. et al., *A model for gene therapy of human hereditary lymphedema*. Proc Natl Acad Sci U S A, 2001. **98**(22): 12677–82.
22. Olsson, A.K. et al., *VEGF receptor signalling – in control of vascular function*. Nat Rev Mol Cell Biol, 2006. **7**(5): 359–71.
23. Skobe, M. et al., *Induction of tumor lymphangiogenesis by VEGF-C promotes breast cancer metastasis*. Nat Med, 2001. **7**(2): 192–8.
24. Stacker, S.A. et al., *VEGF-D promotes the metastatic spread of tumor cells via the lymphatics*. Nat Med, 2001. **7**(2): 186–91.
25. Mandriota, S.J. et al., *Vascular endothelial growth factor-C-mediated lymphangiogenesis promotes tumour metastasis*. Embo J, 2001. **20**(4): 672–82.
26. Hirakawa, S. et al., *VEGF-C-induced lymphangiogenesis in sentinel lymph nodes promotes tumor metastasis to distant sites*. Blood, 2007. **109**(3): 1010–7.
27. Schmid, M.C. and J.A. Varner, *Myeloid cell trafficking and tumor angiogenesis*. Cancer Lett, 2007. **250**(1): 1–8.
28. Lin, E.Y. and J.W. Pollard, *Tumor-associated macrophages press the angiogenic switch in breast cancer*. Cancer Res, 2007. **67**(11): 5064–6.
29. Wigle, J.T. et al., *An essential role for Prox1 in the induction of the lymphatic endothelial cell phenotype*. Embo J, 2002. **21**(7): 1505–13.
30. Banerji, S. et al., *LYVE-1, a new homologue of the CD44 glycoprotein, is a lymph-specific receptor for hyaluronan*. J Cell Biol, 1999. **144**(4): 789–801.
31. Jain, R.K. and B.T. Fenton, Intratumoral lymphatic vessels: a case of mistaken identity or malfunction? J Natl Cancer Inst, 2002. **94**(6): 417–21.
32. Su, J.L. et al., *The VEGF-C/Flt-4 axis promotes invasion and metastasis of cancer cells*. Cancer Cell, 2006. **9**(3): 209–23.
33. Kajita, T. et al., *The expression of vascular endothelial growth factor C and its receptors in non-small cell lung cancer*. Br J Cancer, 2001. **85**(2): 255–60.
34. Nakashima, T. et al., *Expression of vascular endothelial growth factor-A and vascular endothelial growth factor-C as prognostic factors for non-small cell lung cancer*. Med Sci Monit, 2004. 10(6): BR157-65.
35. Li, Q. et al., *Clinical significance of co-expression of VEGF-C and VEGFR-3 in non-small cell lung cancer*. Chin Med J (Engl), 2003. **116**(5): 727–30.
36. Achen, M.G. et al., *The angiogenic and lymphangiogenic factor vascular endothelial growth factor-D exhibits a paracrine mode of action in cancer*. Growth Factors, 2002. **20**(2): 99–107.
37. Huang, C. et al., *Clinical application of biological markers for treatments of resectable non-small-cell lung cancers*. Br J Cancer, 2005. **92**(7): 1231–9.
38. Adachi, Y. et al., *Lymphatic vessel density in pulmonary adenocarcinoma immunohisto-chemically evaluated with anti-podoplanin or anti-D2-40 antibody is correlated with lymphatic invasion or lymph node metastases*. Pathol Int, 2007. **57**(4): 171–7.
39. Kojima, H. et al., *Clinical significance of vascular endothelial growth factor-C and vascular endothelial growth factor receptor 3 in patients with T1 lung adenocarcinoma*. Cancer, 2005. **104**(8): 1668–77.
40. Chen, F. et al., *Flt-4-positive endothelial cell density and its clinical significance in non-small cell lung cancer*. Clin Cancer Res, 2004. **10**(24): 8548–53.
41. Takizawa, H. et al., *The balance of VEGF-C and VEGFR-3 mRNA is a predictor of lymph node metastasis in non-small cell lung cancer*. Br J Cancer, 2006. **95**(1): 75–9.

42. Saintigny, P. et al., *Vascular endothelial growth factor-C and its receptor VEGFR-3 in non-small-cell lung cancer: concurrent expression in cancer cells from primary tumour and metastatic lymph node.* Lung Cancer, 2007. **58**(2): 205–13.

43. Nagy, J.A. et al., *Vascular permeability factor/vascular endothelial growth factor induces lymphangiogenesis as well as angiogenesis.* J Exp Med, 2002. **196**(11): 1497–506.

44. Tobler, N.E. and M. Detmar, *Tumor and lymph node lymphangiogenesis – impact on cancer metastasis.* J Leukoc Biol, 2006. **80**(4): 691–6.

45. Bremnes, R.M., C. Camps, and R. Sirera, *Angiogenesis in non-small cell lung cancer: the prognostic impact of neoangiogenesis and the cytokines VEGF and bFGF in tumours and blood.* Lung Cancer, 2006. **51**(2): 143–58.

46. O'Byrne, K.J. et al., *Vascular endothelial growth factor, platelet-derived endothelial cell growth factor and angiogenesis in non-small-cell lung cancer.* Br J Cancer, 2000. **82**(8): 1427–32.

47. Hirakawa, S. et al., *VEGF-A induces tumor and sentinel lymph node lymphangiogenesis and promotes lymphatic metastasis.* J Exp Med, 2005. **201**(7): 1089–99.

48. Baldwin, M.E. et al., *Multiple forms of mouse vascular endothelial growth factor-D are generated by RNA splicing and proteolysis.* J Biol Chem, 2001. **276**(47): 44307–14.

49. Takanami, I. et al., *Tumor angiogenesis in pulmonary adenocarcinomas: relationship with basic fibroblast growth factor, its receptor, and survival.* Neoplasma, 1997. **44**(5): 295–8.

50. Shin, J.W. et al., *Prox1 promotes lineage-specific expression of fibroblast growth factor (FGF) receptor-3 in lymphatic endothelium: a role for FGF signaling in lymphangiogenesis.* Mol Biol Cell, 2006. **17**(2): 576–84.

51. Chang, L.K. et al., *Dose-dependent response of FGF-2 for lymphangiogenesis.* Proc Natl Acad Sci U S A, 2004. **101**(32): 11658–63.

52. Tan, Y., *Basic fibroblast growth factor-mediated lymphangiogenesis of lymphatic endothelial cells isolated from dog thoracic ducts: effects of heparin.* Jpn J Physiol, 1998. **48**(2): 133–41.

53. Cao, Y., *Direct role of PDGF-BB in lymphangiogenesis and lymphatic metastasis.* Cell Cycle, 2005. **4**(2): 228–30.

54. Cao, R. et al., *Hepatocyte growth factor is a lymphangiogenic factor with an indirect mechanism of action.* Blood, 2006. **107**(9): 3531–6.

55. Achen, M.G., B.K. McColl, and S.A. Stacker, *Focus on lymphangiogenesis in tumor metastasis.* Cancer Cell, 2005. **7**(2): 121–7.

56. Seto, T. et al., *Prognostic value of expression of vascular endothelial growth factor and its flt-1 and KDR receptors in stage I non-small-cell lung cancer.* Lung Cancer, 2006. **53**(1): 91–6.

57. Cao, Y., *Opinion: emerging mechanisms of tumour lymphangiogenesis and lymphatic metastasis.* Nat Rev Cancer, 2005. **5**(9): 735–43.

58. Kawakami, T. et al., *Neuropilin 1 and neuropilin 2 co-expression is significantly correlated with increased vascularity and poor prognosis in nonsmall cell lung carcinoma.* Cancer, 2002. **95**(10): 2196–201.

59. Lantuejoul, S. et al., *Expression of VEGF, semaphorin SEMA3F, and their common receptors neuropilins NP1 and NP2 in preinvasive bronchial lesions, lung tumours, and cell lines.* J Pathol, 2003. **200**(3): 336–47.

60. Karpanen, T. et al., *Functional interaction of VEGF-C and VEGF-D with neuropilin receptors.* Faseb J, 2006. **20**(9): 1462–72.

61. Iwasaki, A. et al., *Basic fibroblast growth factor (bFGF) and vascular endothelial growth factor (VEGF) levels, as prognostic indicators in NSCLC.* Eur J Cardiothorac Surg, 2004. **25**(3): 443–8.

62. Pepper, M.S., *Lymphangiogenesis and tumor metastasis: myth or reality?* Clin Cancer Res, 2001. **7**(3): 462–8.

63. Padera, T.P. et al., *Lymphatic metastasis in the absence of functional intratumor lymphatics.* Science, 2002. **296**(5574): 1883–6.

64. Shields, J.D. et al., *Chemokine-mediated migration of melanoma cells towards lymphatics – a mechanism contributing to metastasis.* Oncogene, 2006.
65. Saharinen, P. et al., *Lymphatic vasculature: development, molecular regulation and role in tumor metastasis and inflammation.* Trends Immunol, 2004. **25**(7): 387–95.
66. Fleury, M.E., K.C. Boardman, and M.A. Swartz, *Autologous morphogen gradients by subtle interstitial flow and matrix interactions.* Biophys J, 2006. **91**(1): 113–21.
67. Kriehuber, E. et al., *Isolation and characterization of dermal lymphatic and blood endothelial cells reveal stable and functionally specialized cell lineages.* J Exp Med, 2001. **194**(6): 797–808.
68. Takeuchi, H. et al., *CCL21 chemokine regulates chemokine receptor CCR7 bearing malignant melanoma cells.* Clin Cancer Res, 2004. **10**(7): 2351–8.
69. Muller, A. et al., *Involvement of chemokine receptors in breast cancer metastasis.* Nature, 2001. **410**(6824): 50–6.
70. Uchida, D. et al., *Acquisition of lymph node, but not distant metastatic potentials, by the overexpression of CXCR4 in human oral squamous cell carcinoma.* Lab Invest, 2004. **84**(12): 1538–46.
71. Zhang, J.P. et al., *Study on CXCR4/SDF-1alpha axis in lymph node metastasis of cervical squamous cell carcinoma.* Int J Gynecol Cancer, 2007. **17**(2): 478–83.
72. Koizumi, K. et al., *CCL21 promotes the migration and adhesion of highly lymph node metastatic human non-small cell lung cancer Lu-99 in vitro.* Oncol Rep, 2007. **17**(6): 1511–6.
73. Takanami, I., Overexpression of CCR7 mRNA in nonsmall cell lung cancer: correlation with lymph node metastasis. Int J Cancer, 2003. **105**(2): 186–9.
74. Phillips, R.J. et al., *The stromal derived factor-1/CXCL12-CXC chemokine receptor 4 biological axis in non-small cell lung cancer metastases.* Am J Respir Crit Care Med, 2003. **167**(12): 1676–86.
75. Burger, M. et al., *Functional expression of CXCR4 (CD184) on small-cell lung cancer cells mediates migration, integrin activation, and adhesion to stromal cells.* Oncogene, 2003. **22**(50): 8093–101.
76. Mashino, K. et al., *Expression of chemokine receptor CCR7 is associated with lymph node metastasis of gastric carcinoma.* Cancer Res, 2002. **62**(10): 2937–41.
77. Almofti, A. et al., *The clinicopathological significance of the expression of CXCR4 protein in oral squamous cell carcinoma.* Int J Oncol, 2004. **25**(1): 65–71.
78. Luther, S.A. et al., *Differing activities of homeostatic chemokines CCL19, CCL21, and CXCL12 in lymphocyte and dendritic cell recruitment and lymphoid neogenesis.* J Immunol, 2002. **169**(1): 424–33.
79. Kabashima, K. et al., *CXCL12-CXCR4 engagement is required for migration of cutaneous dendritic cells.* Am J Pathol, 2007. **171**(4): 1249–57.
80. Ben-Baruch, A., *The multifaceted roles of chemokines in malignancy.* Cancer Metastasis Rev, 2006. **25**(3): 357–71.
81. Yang, S.C. et al., *Intratumoral administration of dendritic cells overexpressing CCL21 generates systemic antitumor responses and confers tumor immunity.* Clin Cancer Res, 2004. **10**(8): 2891–901.
82. Perrot, I. et al., *Dendritic cells infiltrating human non-small cell lung cancer are blocked at immature stage.* J Immunol, 2007. **178**(5): 2763–9.
83. Mitra, S.K., D.A. Hanson, and D.D. Schlaepfer, *Focal adhesion kinase: in command and control of cell motility.* Nat Rev Mol Cell Biol, 2005. **6**(1): 56–68.
84. Mishima, K. et al., *Prox1 induces lymphatic endothelial differentiation via integrin alpha9 and other signaling cascades.* Mol Biol Cell, 2007. **18**(4): 1421–9.
85. Vlahakis, N.E. et al., *The lymphangiogenic vascular endothelial growth factors VEGF-C and -D are ligands for the integrin alpha9beta1.* J Biol Chem, 2005. **280**(6): 4544–52.
86. Hong, Y.K. et al., *VEGF-A promotes tissue repair-associated lymphatic vessel formation via VEGFR-2 and the alpha1beta1 and alpha2beta1 integrins.* Faseb J, 2004. **18**(10): 1111–3.

87. Dietrich, T. et al., *Inhibition of inflammatory lymphangiogenesis by integrin {Alpha}5 blockade.* Am J Pathol, 2007. **171**(1): 361–72.
88. Garmy-Susini, B. et al., *Methods to study lymphatic vessel integrins.* Methods Enzymol, 2007. **426**: 415–38.
89. Han, J.Y. et al., *Immunohistochemical expression of integrins and extracellular matrix proteins in non-small cell lung cancer: correlation with lymph node metastasis.* Lung Cancer, 2003. **41**(1): 65–70.
90. Gogali, A., K. Charalabopoulos, and S. Constantopoulos, *Integrin receptors in primary lung cancer.* Exp Oncol, 2004. **26**(2): 106–10.
91. Bishop, J.R., M. Schuksz, and J.D. Esko, *Heparan sulphate proteoglycans fine-tune mammalian physiology.* Nature, 2007. **446**(7139): 1030–7.
92. Esko, J.D. and S.B. Selleck, *Order out of chaos: assembly of ligand binding sites in heparan sulfate.* Annu Rev Biochem, 2002. **71**: 435–71.
93. Fuster, M.M. and J.D. Esko, *The sweet and sour of cancer: glycans as novel therapeutic targets.* Nat Rev Cancer, 2005. **5**(7): 526–42.
94. Handel, T.M. et al., *Regulation of protein function by glycosaminoglycans – as exemplified by chemokines.* Annu Rev Biochem, 2005. **74**: 385–410.
95. Jakobsson, L. et al., *Heparan sulfate in trans potentiates VEGFR-mediated angiogenesis.* Dev Cell, 2006. **10**(5): 625–34.
96. Vlodavsky, I. and Y. Friedmann, *Molecular properties and involvement of heparanase in cancer metastasis and angiogenesis.* J Clin Invest, 2001. **108**(3): 341–7.
97. Fuster, M.M. et al., *Genetic alteration of endothelial heparan sulfate selectively inhibits tumor angiogenesis.* J Cell Biol, 2007. **177**(3): 539–49.
98. Sharma, B. et al., *Antisense targeting of perlecan blocks tumor growth and angiogenesis in vivo.* J Clin Invest, 1998. **102**(8): 1599–608.
99. Jiang, X. and J.R. Couchman, *Perlecan and tumor angiogenesis.* J Histochem Cytochem, 2003. **51**(11): 1393–410.
100. Iozzo, R.V. and J.D. San Antonio, *Heparan sulfate proteoglycans: heavy hitters in the angiogenesis arena.* J Clin Invest, 2001. **108**(3): 349–55.
101. Kubo, H. et al., *Blockade of vascular endothelial growth factor receptor-3 signaling inhibits fibroblast growth factor-2-induced lymphangiogenesis in mouse cornea.* Proc Natl Acad Sci U S A, 2002. **99**(13): 8868–73.
102. Veikkola, T. et al., *Intrinsic versus microenvironmental regulation of lymphatic endothelial cell phenotype and function.* Faseb J, 2003. **17**(14): 2006–13.
103. Scavelli, C. et al., *Crosstalk between angiogenesis and lymphangiogenesis in tumor progression.* Leukemia, 2004. **18**(6): 1054–8.
104. Yamazaki, Y. and T. Morita, *Molecular and functional diversity of vascular endothelial growth factors.* Mol Divers, 2006. **10**(4): 515–27.
105. Kuroshima, S. et al., *Expression of cys-cys chemokine ligand 21 on human gingival lymphatic vessels.* Tissue Cell, 2004. **36**(2): 121–7.
106. Amara, A. et al., *Stromal cell-derived factor-1alpha associates with heparan sulfates through the first beta-strand of the chemokine.* J Biol Chem, 1999. **274**(34): 23916–25.
107. Sadir, R. et al., *Characterization of the stromal cell-derived factor-1alpha-heparin complex.* J Biol Chem, 2001. **276**(11): 8288–96.
108. Shah, L. et al., *Expression of syndecan-1 and expression of epidermal growth factor receptor are associated with survival in patients with nonsmall cell lung carcinoma.* Cancer, 2004. **101**(7): 1632–8.
109. Mennerich, D. et al., *Shift of syndecan-1 expression from epithelial to stromal cells during progression of solid tumours.* Eur J Cancer, 2004. **40**(9): 1373–82.
110. Pirinen, R. et al., *Versican in nonsmall cell lung cancer: relation to hyaluronan, clinicopathologic factors, and prognosis.* Hum Pathol, 2005. **36**(1): 44–50.
111. Boehm, T. et al., *Antiangiogenic therapy of experimental cancer does not induce acquired drug resistance.* Nature, 1997. **390**(6658): 404–7.

Carcinoma-Associated Fibroblasts in Lung Cancer

Roya Navab, Bizhan Bandarchi, and Ming-Sound Tsao

Abstract There is growing evidence that carcinogenesis is influenced and controlled by the cellular interactions between tumor stroma, ECM, and neoplastic cells. Therefore, the stromal cells surrounding cancer epithelial cells, rather than being passive bystanders, appear to have an important role in modifying tumor development and progression. Clinical evidence also supports the significant contribution of stroma to the development of a wide variety of tumors. There is a higher incidence of tumor formation in tissues exhibiting a chronically inflamed stroma as well as those undergoing wound healing, in which the stroma plays a central role. The stromal microenvironment of human cancers is also different from that of the corresponding normal tissue. Studies have revealed reactive stroma that is characterized by modified ECM composition, increased microvasculature, inflammatory cells, and fibroblasts with "activated" phenotype. These modified fibroblasts are often referred to as activated fibroblasts, myofibroblasts, tumor-associated fibroblasts, or carcinoma-associated fibroblasts (CAFs). This chapter will focus its discussion on the characterization of CAFs, their role in human lung carcinogenesis and malignant progression, and as potential novel therapeutic targets.

Introduction

Fibroblasts are the predominant stromal cells in connective tissues, particularly fibrous connective tissue. Fibroblasts in normal tissue are responsible for the intracellular assembly of various extracellular fibrillary and nonfibrillary structural proteins such as procollagen and glycosaminoglycans, which form the ground substance of stromal tissue (1). The main product of fibroblasts is collagen, predominantly collagen type I, which is the major constituent of extracellular matrix (ECM). Cancer cells grow in a biologically complex stroma composed of various types of stromal and inflammatory cells and ECM, creating a tumor microenvironment [1, 2].

M.-S. Tsao (✉)
Ontario Cancer Institute and Princess Margaret Hospital, University Health Network and University of Toronto, University Avenue, Toronto, Ontario M5G 2M9, Canada
e-mail: ming.tsao@uhn.on.ca

V. Keshamouni et al. (eds.), *Lung Cancer Metastasis*,
DOI 10.1007/978-1-4419-0772-1_10, © Springer Science+Business Media, LLC 2009

There is growing evidence that carcinogenesis is influenced and controlled by the cellular interactions between tumor stroma, ECM, and neoplastic cells. Therefore, the stromal cells surrounding cancer epithelial cells, rather than being passive bystanders, appear to have an important role in modifying tumor development and progression. Clinical evidence also supports the significant contribution of stroma to the development of a wide variety of tumors. There is a higher incidence of tumor formation in tissues exhibiting a chronically inflamed stroma as well as those undergoing wound healing, in which the stroma plays a central role [3, 4]. The mouse models of tumorigenesis have also revealed that stromal cells, notably fibroblasts, endothelial cells, and inflammatory cells [5–8], actively support tumor growth by producing growth factors, cytokines, and chemokines, activating the surrounding ECM and inducing the selection and gene expression of the neoplastic cells [9, 10]. Earlier studies have demonstrated that inoculation of dissociated tumor cells might not be tumorigenic, whereas implantation of fragments of solid tumors containing stroma led to tumor growth [11].

The stromal microenvironment of human cancers is also different from that of the corresponding normal tissue. Studies have revealed reactive stroma that is characterized by modified ECM composition, increased microvasculature, inflammatory cells, and fibroblasts with "activated" phenotype [12]. These modified fibroblasts are often referred to as activated fibroblasts, myofibroblasts, tumor-associated fibroblasts, or carcinoma-associated fibroblasts (CAFs). These modified fibroblasts are characterized histologically as large spindle-shaped cells with indented nuclei [13–15]. They possess contractile filaments, prominent rough endoplasmic reticulum, intercellular gap junctions, and well-developed fibronexi (transmembrane complex with intracellular actin, integrins, and extracellular fibronectin). In contrast, the endoplasmic reticulum in quiescent adult fibroblasts is less abundant and the nucleus is flattened and heterochromatic [16]. Other studies have also implicated CAFs as important "coconspirators" in the development of the common carcinomas, such as those of the colon, lung, breast and prostate. These tumors originate from the epithelial cells lining the mucosa of intestines and lungs and the ductwork of mammary and prostate glands. Cunha et al. [7] showed that nonmalignant prostate epithelial cells cocultured with prostate CAFs acquired the ability to form tumors when transplanted into mice. They concluded that CAFs had undergone changes, which resulted in the production of growth factors or other substances that could transform epithelial cells.

Lung cancer is a highly metastatic tumor. Metastasis represents the final step of complex biological sequences that include invasion (loss of cell–cell adhesion, increased cell motility, and basement membrane degradation), vascular intravasation and extravasation, establishment of metastatic niche and angiogenesis. The role of the tumor microenvironment in human lung cancers has not been studied extensively. This chapter will focus its discussion on the characterization of CAFs, their role in human lung carcinogenesis and malignant progression, and as potential novel therapeutic targets.

Cancer Stroma

During the early stages of carcinogenesis, the proliferation of neoplastic epithelial cells is contained within the boundary of a basement membrane and separated from the surrounding stromal tissue [17]. This growth that is confined by the basement membrane is called carcinoma in situ (CIS). During CIS progression to invasive carcinoma, the tumor cells invade through the basement membrane [18, 19] into the stroma and induce its "reactive" appearances [18, 20]. This is associated with the expansion of the tumor stroma by increased proliferation of activated fibroblasts and deposition of ECM [21], a histological observation referred as desmoplasia [22]. In fact, activated fibroblasts appear as one of the key features not only in cancer stroma but also in a variety of inflammatory conditions including wound healing [13]. The histological term for activated fibroblasts is myofibroblast, which indicates an intermediate phenotype between smooth muscle cells and fibroblasts [14, 23]. Myofibroblasts are widely distributed and easy to culture in vitro. Although pathologists have identified the presence of myofibroblasts in cancer decades ago, the scientific interest in evaluating them remains preliminary. Consequently, our knowledge on myofibroblasts and CAFs remains fragmented. It should be noted that myofibroblasts are not per se a pathological cell type and are present in various tissues under normal conditions (e.g., lung, brain, prostate, breast, heart) [24].

Markers of Fibroblasts and CAFs

Fibroblast remains poorly defined in molecular terms. A lack of reliable and specific molecular fibroblast marker(s) is a limiting factor in studying fibroblasts in vivo. Among all the well-established markers of fibroblasts, fibroblast-specific protein-1 (FSP-1) appears to provide the best specificity in vivo (see Table 1). In addition, several other proteins can be considered as site-specific markers. CAFs are normally defined by the expression of α-smooth muscle actin (α-SMA) [18, 23, 25].

Chung et al. [26] showed that fibroblasts in mammals are highly heterogeneous, and those isolated from different sites show diversity (Table 1). They compared the genome-wide expression patterns of 50 human cultured fibroblasts isolated from 16 different organs and showed that gene expression patterns from different anatomical sites are as divergent as the gene expression patterns observed among distinct lineages of white blood cells [26]. This diversity is evident from the secretion of specific extracellular matrix (ECM) constituents, growth factors, or differentiation factors. For example, fetal skin fibroblasts express high levels of collagen types I and V, whereas fetal lung fibroblasts do not but express exclusively the lung-specific forkhead family transcription factors FOXF1 and FOXP1 [26].

Heterogeneity in human lung CAFs has also been observed. Nazaret et al. [27] established human lung TAFs which are characterized by the expression of human FSP-1, Thy-1, α-smooth muscle actin, and fibroblast activation protein (FAP)

Table 1 Putative fibroblast markers

Marker	Function	Types of fibroblast	Other cell types	References
Vimentin	Intermediate-filament-associated protein	Assorted	Endothelial cells, myoepithelial cells, and neurons	[92]
Cytoskeletal/Contractile filament protein	Another action isoform	Activated or resting fibroblast, myofibroblast	Vascular smooth muscle cells, pericytes, and myoepithelial cells	[18, 93]
Thy-1	Endothelial cell receptor, adhesion and transmigration of neutrophils	Liver fibroblasts, TAF from human colorectal liver metastases	Endothelial cells	[94]
Fibroblast-specific protein-1 (FSP1)/S100A4/MTS1	Intermediate-filament-associated protein	Assorted	Invasive carcinoma cells	[95]
Discoidin-domain receptor 2	Collagen receptor	Cardiac fibroblasts	Endothelial cells	[96, 97]
Fibroblast activation protein (FAP)	Serine protease	Activated fibroblasts	Activated melanocytes, human non-small cell lung cancer (NSCLC)	[98, 99]
Integrin $\alpha 11$	Collagen type 1 receptor	Activated fibroblasts	Human fetal myoblasts cells, mouse odontoblasts	[67, 100, 101]

Table 1 (Continued)

Marker	Function	Types of fibroblast	Other cell types	References
α1β1 integrin	Collagen receptor	Assorted	Monocytes and endothelial cells	[102, 103]
Prolyl 4-hydroxylase	Collagen biosynthesis	Assorted	Endothelial cells, cancer cells, and epithelial cells	[104, 105]
Procollagen α2	Collagen-1 biosynthesis	Assorted, lung fibroblasts	Osteoblasts and chondroblasts	[106]
Hyaluronan (hyaluronic acid or hyaluronate)	ECM component, cell proliferation, cell surface receptor interaction		Chondrocyte, skin	[107]
PDGFR-β	Tumor growth	Activated fibroblasts	Pericytes	[81]
Chondroitin sulfate proteoglycan (NG2)	Mediation of cellular interactions with the extracellular matrix	Assorted	Pericytes and vascular smooth muscle cells	[108]
Tenascin-C	Cell adhesion	Activated fibroblasts	Osteoblasts, perichondrial cells, and glial cells	[109]
Fibronectin-EDA	Cell adhesion and cell spreading	Activated fibroblasts	Endothelial cells and epithelial cells	[110]

(Table 1) but did not express CD45 and CD11b. These cells produce both soluble factors [e.g., TGF-β1, IFN-γ, IFN-γ-inducible protein-10, and monokine induced by IFN-γ (MIG)] and membrane-associated molecules (e.g., B7H1 and B7DC), which have been reported to exert immunomodulatory effects upon lymphocytes. A coculture experiment using TAFs and tumor-associated T cells (TATs) demonstrated that in some NSCLC tumors, TAFs enhanced TAT activation even in the presence of a TGF-β1-mediated suppressive effect. In other NSCLC tumors, TAFs suppressed TAT activation, possibly by hyporesponsiveness of TAT in the microenvironment to TGF-β1 produced by TAF [27]. Therefore, TAF in human NSCLC are functionally and phenotypically heterogeneous and may provide multiple complex regulatory signals in the tumor microenvironment.

Gene Expression Changes in Carcinoma or Senescent-Associated Fibroblasts

There is an increasing recognition of the importance of defining molecular mechanisms by which CAFs and stromal factors influence the development of epithelial cancers. These include cell surface molecules, secreted soluble factors, and ECM proteins. The identification of individual or combinations of secreted factors might suggest biomarkers for early detection of cancers or more importantly, those cancers with the propensity for metastasis.

Micke and Ostman [28] used laser capture microdissection and cDNA microarray to derive a comprehensive characterization of differences between CAFs and normal fibroblasts in basal cell carcinoma and normal skin from the same patients. The analysis revealed 415 upregulated and 458 downregulated genes. Among these were genes involved in growth regulation (amphiregulin, SDF-1, IGF-1, TGF-β3), angiogenesis (angiopoietin-2), and matrix remodeling (kallikrein-6, -10, -11, MMP-5, -11, TIMP-4). Nakamura et al. [29] used a cDNA filter array to identify five genes that were upregulated in CAFs from pulmonary adenocarcinoma compared to fibroblasts isolated from normal bronchus of the same patients. These upregulated genes were *E2F2* (regulatory transcription factors), *MLH1* (tumor suppressor gene), *Talin* (cell adhesion protein), *TGFβRI* (membrane receptors), and *TPA* (signaling intermediates).

Coculture models of lung fibroblasts and NSCLC cells mimicked the observation in other cancer types. NSCLC cells induce the secretion of angiogenic factors (e.g., FGF-2, IL-8) [30] as well as matrix proteases (e.g., MMP-11) in lung fibroblasts [31]. Gene expression profiling of normal human lung fibroblasts following coculture with NSCLC cells revealed alteration in gene expression profiles [32]. In this coculture model, Fromigue et al. [32] used magnetic cell sorting to separate fibroblasts from tumor cells. Using the DNA filter assay and cDNA microarray, a set of approximately 30 modulated genes coding for growth and survival factors, angiogenic factors, proteases and protease inhibitors, transmembrane receptors, kinases, and transcription regulators were identified (Table 2). These genes can

Table 2 Gene expression changes in fibroblasts cocultured with non-small cell lung cancer cells and isolated subsequently using magnetic cell sorting (MACS)

Category	Gene	Function	Up or down in coculture	References
Growth and survival factors	IGFBP (3,5)	Growth and survival	Down	[111, 112]
	LTBP2	Regulation of TGF-β	Down	[113]
	CTGF	Growth	Down	[114]
	Inhibin beta A (INHBA)	Proliferation	Up	[115]
Angiogenesis	FGF-2	Angiogenesis	Up	[31]
	IL-8	Angiogenesis	Up	[30]
	VEGF	Angiogenesis	Up	[116]
	Thrombospondin (THSB1)	Inhibition of angiogenesis	Down	[117]
Proteases/protease inhibitors	uPA, tPA	Migration, angiogenesis, metastasis, growth, and survival	Up	[118]
	TFPI-1, -2	Invasion and metastasis	Up	[119, 120]
	MMP-11	Migration, angiogenesis, metastasis, growth, and survival	Up	[121]
	MMP-9	Migration, angiogenesis, metastasis, growth, and survival	Up	[122]
	PAI-1, TIMP-3	Inhibition of invasion and metastasis	Down	[123, 124]

Abbreviations: IGFBP, insulin-like growth factor-binding protein; LTBP2, latent transforming growth factor β-binding protein; CTGF, connective tissue growth factor; INHBA, inhibin beta A; bFGF, basic fibroblast growth factor; IL-8, interleukin-8; VEGF, vascular endothelial growth factor; THSB1, thrombospondin-1; uPA, urokinase plasminogen activator; tPA, tissue plasminogen activator; TFPI-1, tissue factor pathway inhibitor; PAI-1, plasminogen activator inhibitor-1; TIMP-3, tissue inhibitor of metalloproteinase-3.

potentially affect the regulation of matrix degradation, angiogenesis, invasion, cell growth, and survival. A large number of these modulatory genes were secreted proteins. These findings could be of use to identify new potential markers and activated signaling pathways. As an example, the upregulation of Notch-3 in tumor-infiltrating fibroblasts is regulated by epithelial–mesenchymal interactions during development [33]. It is interesting to compare the consequences of such interactions in a coculture model using carcinoma-associated fibroblasts.

There is increasing evidence to suggest the contribution of senescent human fibroblasts to tumor growth by secreting factors such as VEGF that promote cancer progression [34, 35], a phenomenon that resembles carcinoma-associated fibroblasts. The ability of senescent fibroblasts to profoundly alter the growth characteristics of epithelial cells has led to further efforts in the identification of senescence- or aging-associated changes in gene expression using microarray-based global mRNA profiling strategies [36]. Table 3 summarizes the gene expression changes that have been reported in association with prostate fibroblast senescence program. These genes encode proteins that play important roles in autocrine/paracrine cell communication, immune and inflammatory responses, extracellular matrix structural components, and extracellular

Table 3 Putative senescence-associated markers in prostatic fibroblasts identified by gene-profiling studies

Marker	Functional category	Up or down in senescent fibroblasts	References
Amphiregulin, hepatoctye growth factor, bone morphogenic protein-1, macrophage-inhibitory cytokine 1, connective tissue growth factor, VEGF	Autocrine/paracrine growth factors	Up	[125]
IGFBP2, IGFBP3, IGFBP5, IGFBP6	Insulin-like growth factor-binding proteins	Up	[126]
CXCL12[1], CXCL1, CCL1, CCL13, CCL20, C17, IL6, IL8	Chemokines and cytokines	Up	[127]
Collagen 1α2, collagen III α1, collagen IV α5, collagen VI α1, collagen VI α2, collagen VII α1, collagen XV α1, laminin α4, laminin α2, integrin α5, integrin β1, integrin β4, osteonectin (SPARC), osteocalcin, osteopontin, syndecan-2, fibronectin-1	Extracellular matrix proteins	Up	[39, 128]
ADAMTS1, MMP2, MMP3, MMP9, cathepsin D, cathepsin O, cystatin S, cystatin B, cystatin C, TIMP1, TIMP2	Extracellular matrix proteases and protease inhibitors	Up	[128]

[1]SDF-1/CXCL12 is the most highly upregulated secreted protein.

proteases. Among the overexpressed cytokines, CXCL12 (SDF-1), CXCL1, IL-6, and IL-8 have been shown to enhance epithelial cell proliferation [36], while IL-8 and C17 as well as vascular endothelial growth factor (VEGF) are angiogenic factors [37]. Senescent fibroblasts also secrete amphiregulin that may stimulate the proliferation of prostate epithelial cells [38]. Among the extracellular matrix proteins, the high expression of osteopontin and osteocalcin was associated with increased metastasis of prostate carcinoma cell lines [39]. Matrix metalloproteinases may influence the availability of certain factors in the microenvironment. Matrix metalloproteinases are also involved in the processing of growth factors and their receptors, cytokines, chemokines, and other precursor proteins.

The invasiveness and metastatic features of prostate cancers appear to be dependent on the ratios of MMP-2 and MMP-9 to TIMP-1 [39]. The large number of changes in the expression of microenvironment constituents that associate with the senescence gene expression program provides challenges in determining which alteration represents the dominant influence on adjacent cell types. Nevertheless, the potential benefits of meeting this challenge are great as well, as identifying the key stromal effects on tumor cell characteristics would serve to prioritize methods to interfere with the detrimental signals.

CAFs Contribution to Carcinogenesis

CAFs are commonly observed in the stroma of a majority of invasive human cancers [40]. However, the specific contribution of these cells to tumor progression remains incompletely understood. CAFs possess greatly increased contractile ability, promote angiogenesis, and stimulate epithelial cell growth through the production of ECM and the secretion of growth factors and cytokines (Fig. 1). Activated fibroblasts secrete increased levels of ECM-degrading proteases such as matrix metalloproteinase-2 (MMP-2), MMP-3, and MMP-9, facilitating increased ECM turnover and altered ECM composition [41]. They often secrete increased amounts of growth factors such as hepatocyte growth factor (HGF), insulin-like growth factor (IGF), nerve growth factor (NGF), WNT1, EGF, and FGF-2, which may induce proliferative signals in adjacent epithelial cells [5]. Activated fibroblasts also have an important role as modulators of the immune response following tissue injury.

Several studies demonstrated a direct involvement of resident fibroblasts in the initiation of cancer (Table 4). A link between growth factors and CAFs in tumor initiation was indicated in a series of studies comparing the effect of normal fibroblasts and of CAFs isolated from the primary tumor site [7, 42]. Kuperwasser et al. [43] demonstrated that overexpression of TGF-β1 and/or hepatocyte growth factor (HGF) in mouse fibroblasts induced the initiation of breast cancer within the normal human epithelium. In addition to secreting growth factors that directly affect cell motility, activated fibroblasts are a source of ECM-degrading proteases such as the MMPs [44–46]. MMPs can

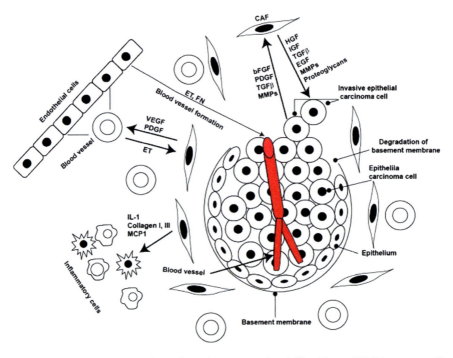

Fig. 1 Schematic representation of carcinoma-associated fibroblasts (CAFs)–cancer cell interaction in tumor stroma. CAFs interact with tumor cell, endothelial cells, and inflammatory cells through the secretion of growth factors and chemokines. CAFs increase deposition of collagen types I and III, which induce an altered extracellular matrix microenvironment leading to cancer progression. CAFs interact with the microvasculature by secreting matrix metalloproteinases (MMPs) and vascular endothelial growth factor (VEGF). CAFs regulate the inflammatory response by secreting chemokines such as monocyte chemotactic protein-1 (MCP-1) and interleukin-1 (IL-1). CAFs also secrete growth factors such as TGF-β and hepatocyte growth factor (HGF) to stimulate cancer cell proliferation and invasion. *Abbreviations*: TGF-β, transforming growth factor-β; PDGF, platelet-derived growth factor; bFGF, basic fibroblast growth factor; HGF, hepatocyte growth factor; VEGF, vascular endothelial growth factor; MMP, matrix metalloproteinase; ET, endothelin; FN, fibronectin; IGF, insulin-like growth factor; EGF, epidermal growth factor; MCP-1, monocyte chemotactic protein-1; IL-1, interleukin-1

directly affect the motility and invasiveness of cancer cells [44, 47] and allow the latter to cross the tumor–normal tissue boundaries during invasion.

While normal fibroblasts are required to maintain epithelial homeostasis, CAFs could play an important role in neoplastic initiation and promotion of epithelial cells. To investigate the importance of stroma during carcinogenesis, mammary epithelial cells and cleared fat pads of rats were exposed in vitro to the chemical carcinogen *N*-nitrosomethylurea (NMU) or vehicle and cross-implantation was performed. Neoplastic transformation of these mammary epithelial cells occurred only when vehicle-treated mammary epithelial cells or NMU-treated mammary epithelial cells were inoculated into the NMU-

Table 4 Selected functional/clinical studies of tumor–stroma interaction

Type of cancer	Type of study	Postulated mechanism	Prognosis	References
Prostate	Cocultures of prostate epithelium with senescent fibroblasts *or* Application of conditioned media from senescent fibroblasts	Paracrine-acting factors (especially amphiregulin) comprise majority of growth-promoting effect	Higher tumor cell proliferation	[38]
Non-small cell lung cancer	53 human clinical samples	TGF-β-1 / Hyaluronin	Negative impact on prognosis / Negative impact on prognosis	[60] / [62]
Small cell lung cancer	Comparison of laminin/matrigel impact upon SCLC cell injection into nude mice / Chemotherapy-induced apoptosis assay	Increased ECM proteins / Laminin, tenascin, fibronectin / Higher MMP expression	Tumor growth / Shorter survival / Negative impact on survival	[129] / [130] / [63]
Breast	Normal fibroblast/CAF comparison / Rat N-nitrosomethylurea exposure	TGF-β, HGF / Stroma as carcinogen – target	Identification of condition for tumor initiation / Identification of condition for neoplastic transformation	[43] / [48]
Ovary	Implantation into ovarian carcinoma spheroids	Angiopoietin-1, angiopoietin-2	Identification of condition for tumor initiation	[49, 50]
Pancreas	Effect of conditioned media from human pancreatic stellate cells *or* Coinjection of stellate cells in orthotopic model	Unknown soluble factors from stroma affect survival of pancreatic cancer patients	Identification of condition for tumor cell proliferation, migration, invasion, and anchorage-independent growth / Identification of condition for tumor incidence, increased growth, and metastasis	[131] / [131]

exposed fat pads. This finding suggests the importance of carcinogen exposure of stroma during carcinogenesis [48].

Myofibroblast infiltration into implanted ovarian carcinoma spheroids led the exit of tumors from dormancy and their contribution to vascular stabilization in ovarian tumors by expression of angiopoietin-1 and angiopoietin-2 [49, 50]. Orimo et al. [42] used RAS-transformed human MCF-7 breast cancer cells and coinjected these cells subcutaneously into nude mice in suspension with CAFs or normal fibroblasts. Their results showed that xenografts containing CAFs grew larger than xenografts containing normal fibroblasts. Such enhanced growth was associated with increased cancer cell proliferation (but not increased fibroblast proliferation) and angiogenesis. This finding indicates that CAFs might have both proliferative and angiogenic effects during tumorigenesis [42]. This study also demonstrated that CAFs-derived, stromal cell-derived factor-1 (SDF-1) mediates the recruitment of bone-marrow-derived endothelial cells and directly increases the proliferation of breast cancer cells (MCF-7-RAS). It remains unclear which aspect of this SDF-1 activity is the rate-determining step for tumor growth.

Contributions of CAFs in Metastasis

The presence of activated fibroblasts can promote the proliferation of cancer cells at the metastatic sites, similar to the effect of CAFs on tumor growth in the primary sites [51]. These metastasis-associated fibroblasts could represent a variant of CAFs [52]. Using a new model of human cancer-associated stellate cells, conditioned medium from human pancreatic stellate cells (HPSCs) stimulated pancreatic tumor cell proliferation, migration, invasion, and anchorage-independent growth in a dose-dependent manner. Coinjection of stellate cells increased tumor incidence, growth, and metastasis in an orthotopic model of pancreatic cancer. Moreover, conditioned media from HPSCs inhibited the response of tumor cells to chemotherapy and radiation. These observations indicate that soluble factors are produced by stellate cells and could stimulate the proliferation and survival of pancreatic cancer cells. Taken together, these studies indicate that the abundant stroma of pancreatic cancer plays an important role in the aggressiveness of this disease. The finding demonstrates that activated stellate cells might be important in creating a niche for the cancer cells and initiation of angiogenesis [53].

One of the important communication molecules in tumor–stroma interaction is transforming growth factor-β (TGF-β), a protein best known as a suppressor of tumor growth. There is evidence that TGF-β does not have to act directly on cancer cells to inhibit their growth. In a TGF-β receptor knockout mouse model in which fibroblasts lack the expression of TGF-β receptor, the animals developed early signs of prostate cancer and also more advanced invasive carcinomas of the stomach [54]. In a separate model, mammary carcinoma cells and fibroblasts lacking or normal in TGF-β receptor expression were cotransplanted into the mice. Animals implanted with the TGF-β receptor-deficient fibroblasts and tumor cells developed more aggressive cancers with greater number of metastases than when normal fibroblasts were used. The altered fibroblasts appear to stimulate cancer growth by producing transforming growth factor-α (TGF-α) and hepatocyte growth factor (HGF), which are mitogenic factors regulated normally by TGF-β1. Loss of the ability to respond to TGF-β1 might therefore be one of the changes that cause fibroblasts to stimulate cancer growth [55].

In contrast, other studies have reported that tumor-associated stromal cells are negative regulators of metastasis [56]. Immunohistochemical studies on non-small cell lung cancer (NSCLC) from 84 patients, including 51 squamous cell carcinomas and 33 nonsquamous cell carcinomas, revealed that basic fibroblast growth factor (FGF-2) and FGFR-1 were present in tumor and in tumor-associated stromal cells and vessels [56]. While FGFR-1 expression of tumor cells was directly correlated with tumor stage ($p = 0.03$), bFGF expression in tumor-associated stromal cells and vessels was inversely correlated with lymph node metastasis and advanced pathological stage. These findings suggested that FGF-2 expression might have an inhibitory role in NSCLC progression. These findings also suggest that tumor-associated stromal cells are functionally heterogeneous and provide several complex regulatory signals that have the potential to enhance or suppress tumor progression and metastasis in the tumor microenvironment.

Factors Expressed by CAF in Lung Cancer

Studies of the role of CAFs in lung carcinogenesis and malignant progression remain preliminary. However, similar to findings in other solid tumors, there is evidence that CAFs have similar tumorigenic potential in lung cancer. In non-small cell lung cancer (NSCLC), the expression of PDGF-α, -β, and TGF-β1 in tumor epithelial cells suggests their paracrine activities in the tumor microenvironment [57]. The PDGF-β receptor was expressed by CAFs in NSCLC but not in tumors that express the ligand PDGF-β [58, 59]. Overexpression of PDGF-β was associated with decreased survival [59], while TGF-β1 levels correlated with angiogenesis, tumor progression, and prognosis [60]. In NSCLC, the extensive amount of stroma alone has been reported to be an independent prognostic factor [61]. In the stroma of NSCLC, the level of hyaluronan, a polysaccharide synthesized by lung fibroblasts and an important ECM component, was negatively correlated with patient prognosis [62]. Increased MMP expression has also been identified as an independent negative predictor of survival in SCLC [63]. The growth factor receptor c-Met and its ligand HGF were reported as overexpressed in myofibroblasts of adenocarcinomas, suggesting an autocrine growth loop in the stromal compartment [64].

Integrin α11 as a Stromal Factor in NSCLC

Wang et al. [65] used the representational differences analysis technique to discover genes that were differentially expressed in lung adenocarcinoma compared to corresponding normal lung tissue. They identified six genes, the overexpression of which was validated subsequently by reverse transcriptase-quantitative polymerase chain reaction (RT-QPCR). Two of these, hyaluronan binding protein 2 (HABP2) and ceruloplasmin (CP), were secreted proteins. Three others were putatively stromal proteins: crystalline-mu (CRYM), collagen type XI alpha 1 (COL11A1), and integrin α11 (ITGA11). Interestingly, HABP2 and CRYM appear to be overexpressed mainly in adenocarcinoma, while the other three genes are overexpressed in both adenocarcinoma and squamous cell carcinoma. One gene is novel and remains to be cloned. The overexpression of these five known genes in high percentages of NSCLC was confirmed independently by another group of investigators [66].

Zhu et al. [67] confirmed subsequently that the protein product of ITGA11, referred to as α11, was expressed mainly in the stroma of primary NSCLC. Integrin α11β1 is one of the receptors for fibrillar collagens [68]. To investigate the biological role of α11 in the growth of NSCLC cells, immortalized mouse embryonic fibroblasts (MEF) that were normal or deficient in α11 expression were coimplanted with three different NSCLC cells. In all instances, fibroblasts enhanced the growth of these tumor cells, but enhancement was attenuated when the fibroblasts were deficient in α11 expression. It was subsequently shown that this growth-enhancing activity of α11 was mediated by IGF2, whose expression in fibroblasts was regulated by α11. The results of this study generate a novel paradigm whereby carcinoma–stromal interaction is mediated indirectly through interaction between matrix collagen and stromal fibroblasts to stimulate cancer cell growth.

Clinical Implication of CAFs in Targeted Therapy

Tumor stromal factors are potentially attractive targets for therapeutic intervention in cancer and possibly other diseases. The advantage of CAFs/stroma-targeted therapy has been emphasized on several recent reviews [28, 69, 70].

Stromal cells, in contrast to carcinoma cells, are diploid, exhibit limited proliferative capacity, and therefore stimulating immune responses against products of stromal cells could substantially reduce the incidence of immune evasion [71]. The facts that the stromal cells are genetically stable in contrast to carcinoma cells and expression of many stromal cell products is ubiquitous (i.e., present in almost all organ tissues) suggest that they could be targeted in most, if not all, cancer patients [72]. Based on mechanisms involved in tumor–stroma interaction, several strategies are possible for CAFs-targeted therapy [28].

The first strategy may focus on targeting signals from CAFs such as HGF, IGF, and MMPs that are responsible for tumor initiation and promotion, invasion, and metastasis [28]. ECM proteins (laminin, tenascin, fibronectin) protect from chemotherapy-induced apoptosis in small cell lung cancer [28]. The role of MMPs in lung cancer and their ability to degrade basement membrane and ECM have been investigated extensively [73, 74, 75]. Synthetic MMP inhibitors have been used in a variety of malignancies [73, 76]. However, in spite of promising preclinical studies with these inhibitors, large randomized trials in small cell lung carcinoma revealed no clinical benefit for these inhibitors [76]. The fact that MMPs act mainly during early stages of tumor progression was one of the explanations offered for the failure of these clinical trials [76]. Tumor-associated macrophages and fibroblasts also synthesize proteins such as VEGF, TGF-β, and IL-10 that contribute to local immunosuppressive environment and rendered tumor cells more chemoresistant [77–80].

The second strategy may focus on targeting (blocking) cancer cell signals that are responsible for recruitment of CAFs and their myofibroblastic differentiation or angiogenesis, such as TGF-β1, PDGF-BB, PDGF-C, and GM-CSF. Inhibitors against TGF-β1 and PDGF have been developed. Imatinib, a bcr-abl kinase inhibitor, was initially used on chronic myelogenous leukemia (CML) as a "magic bullet" [81] and later on for treatment of gastrointestinal tumor (GIST) through its activity against c-kit and PDGF receptor-α [82]. Targeting PDGF signaling was designed based on the presence of PDGF receptors (PDGFR) on pericytes and endothelial cells of tumor stroma [81]. Targeting PDGFR on tumor pericytes putatively would destabilize tumor blood vessels leading to vulnerability of these blood vessels to anti-VEGF therapies [83]. Pietras et al. [81, 84] offered evidence that targeting PDGF signaling in TAFs (PDGFR-α and -β) played a central role in tumor response to PDGFR blockade. Jain et al. [81] have also proposed that blocking PDGFR-α and -β by imatinib or monoclonal antibody against these two receptors can repress expression of FGF-2 and controls cervical cancer in a mouse model.

The last strategy is based on CAFs eradication, hence eliminating signals in both directions. One of the promising candidates for specifically targeting CAFs is a serine protease known as fibroblast activation protein (FAP), which is a 97-kDa cell surface glycoprotein with gelatinase and dipeptidyl peptidase activity expressed selectively on tumor stromal fibroblasts [85, 86]. Although normal fibroblasts do not express FAP, it is present transiently in healing wound tissue [87] or chronic inflammatory conditions such as cirrhosis [88]. These characteristics make FAP a potential therapeutic target [89]. FAP can function as a tumor rejection antigen [72]. Using melanoma, carcinoma, and lymphoma models, Lee et al. [72] have shown tumor growth inhibition in mice vaccinated against FAP that was similar in magnitude to that seen in mice vaccinated against tumor cell-expressed antigens. In their study, both subcutaneous implanted tumor and lung metastases were susceptible to anti-FAP immunotherapy. This antitumor response was further enhanced by the CD4 + T-cell arm of the anti-FAP immune response, achieved by using a lysosomal targeting sequence to redirect the translated FAP product into the class II presentation pathway [90] or by covaccination against FAP and a tumor cell-expressed antigen (tyrosine-related protein-2) [72]. CAFs are also the primary source of collagen type I, which contributes to decreased chemotherapeutic drug uptake in tumors [91]. Loeffler et al. [91] studied tumor tissue of FAP-vaccinated mice and showed markedly decreased collagen type I expression and up to 70% greater uptake of chemotherapeutic drugs, which led to a threefold prolongation of life span and a marked suppression of tumor growth.

Most of the therapeutic strategies mentioned have been investigated on cancers of different organs such as breast and colon, while studies in lung cancer remain very limited.

Conclusion

There is increasing evidence that CAFs play critical roles in carcinogenesis, tumor progression, and metastasis. Understanding the complex molecular interaction and signaling networks among various stromal host cells and tumor cells would provide important insights into developing novel diagnostic and therapeutic targets in human cancers.

Acknowledgments Supported by the Canadian Institutes of Health Research (CIHR) grant MOP-64345 and Princess Margaret Hospital "Investment in Research" grant. Dr. Tsao is the M. Qasim Choksi Chair in Lung Cancer Translational Research at the Princess Margaret Hospital and University of Toronto. Dr. Bandarchi is a Fellow of the CIHR Training Program in Molecular Pathology of Cancer (STP-53912).

We thank Dr. D. Gullberg (University of Bergen) for reviewing this chapter.

References

1. Bissell, M.J. and D. Radisky. Putting tumours in context. Nat Rev Cancer *1*: 46–54, 2001.
2. Mueller, M.M. and N.E. Fusenig. Friends or foes – bipolar effects of the tumour stroma in cancer. Nat Rev Cancer *4*: 839–49, 2004.
3. Coussens, L.M. and Z. Werb. Inflammation and cancer. Nature *420*: 860–7, 2002.
4. Jacobs, T.W., C. Byrne, G. Colditz, J.L. Connolly, and S.J. Schnitt. Radial scars in benign breast-biopsy specimens and the risk of breast cancer. N Engl J Med *340*: 430–6, 1999.
5. Bhowmick, N.A., E.G. Neilson, and H.L. Moses. Stromal fibroblasts in cancer initiation and progression. Nature *432*: 332–7, 2004.
6. Cunha, G.R., S.W. Hayward, Y.Z. Wang, and W.A. Ricke. Role of the stromal microenvironment in carcinogenesis of the prostate. Int J Cancer *107*: 1–10, 2003.
7. Olumi, A.F., G.D. Grossfeld, S.W. Hayward, P.R. Carroll, T.D. Tlsty, and G.R. Cunha. Carcinoma-associated fibroblasts direct tumor progression of initiated human prostatic epithelium. Cancer Res *59*: 5002–11, 1999.
8. Tlsty, T.D. Stromal cells can contribute oncogenic signals. Semin Cancer Biol *11*: 97–104, 2001.
9. Liotta, L.A. and E.C. Kohn. The microenvironment of the tumour–host interface. Nature *411*: 375–9, 2001.

10. Pupa, S.M., S. Menard, S. Forti, and E. Tagliabue. New insights into the role of extra-cellular matrix during tumor onset and progression. J Cell Physiol *192*: 259–67, 2002.
11. Singh, S., S.R. Ross, M. Acena, D.A. Rowley, and H. Schreiber. Stroma is critical for preventing or permitting immunological destruction of antigenic cancer cells. J Exp Med *175*: 139–46, 1992.
12. De Wever, O. and M. Mareel. Role of tissue stroma in cancer cell invasion. J Pathol *200*: 429–47, 2003.
13. Powell, D.W., R.C. Mifflin, J.D. Valentich, S.E. Crowe, J.I. Saada, and A.B. West. Myofibroblasts. I. Paracrine. cells important in health and disease. Am J Physiol *277*: C1-9, 1999.
14. Gabbiani, G., G.B. Ryan, and G. Majne. Presence of modified fibroblasts in granulation tissue and their possible role in wound contraction. Experientia *27*: 549–50, 1971.
15. Ronnov-Jessen, L., O.W. Petersen, V.E. Koteliansky, and M.J. Bissell. The origin of the myofibroblasts in breast cancer. Recapitulation of tumor environment in culture unravels diversity and implicates converted fibroblasts and recruited smooth muscle cells. J Clin Invest *95*: 859–73, 1995.
16. Tarin, D. and C.B. Croft. Ultrastructural features of wound healing in mouse skin. J Anat *105*: 189–90, 1969.
17. Hanahan, D. and R.A. Weinberg. The hallmarks of cancer. Cell *100*: 57–70, 2000.
18. Ronnov-Jessen, L., O.W. Petersen, and M.J. Bissell. Cellular changes involved in con-version of normal to malignant breast: importance of the stromal reaction. Physiol Rev *76*: 69–125, 1996.
19. Dvorak, H.F. Tumors: wounds that do not heal. Similarities between tumor stroma generation and wound healing. N Engl J Med *315*: 1650–9, 1986.
20. Dvorak, H.F., D.M. Form, E.J. Manseau, and B.D. Smith. Pathogenesis of desmoplasia. I. Immunofluorescence identification and localization of some structural proteins of line 1 and line 10 guinea pig tumors and of healing wounds. J Natl Cancer Inst *73*: 1195–205, 1984.
21. Shekhar, M.P., R. Pauley, and G. Heppner. Host microenvironment in breast cancer development: extracellular matrix-stromal cell contribution to neoplastic phenotype of epithelial cells in the breast. Breast Cancer Res *5*: 130–5, 2003.
22. Willis, R. Pathology of tumors. 4th edition. London: Butterworth and Company, 1967.
23. De Wever, O. and M. Mareel. Role of myofibroblasts at the invasion front. Biol Chem *383*: 55–67, 2002.
24. Hofer, S.O., G. Molema, R.A. Hermens, H.J. Wanebo, J.S. Reichner, and H.J. Hoekstra. The effect of surgical wounding on tumour development. Eur J Surg Oncol *25*: 231–43, 1999.
25. Arora, P.D. and C.A. McCulloch. The deletion of transforming growth factor-beta-induced myofibroblasts depends on growth conditions and actin organization. Am J Pathol *155*: 2087–99, 1999.
26. Chang, H.Y., J.T. Chi, S. Dudoit, C. Bondre, M. van de Rijn, D. Botstein, and P.O. Brown. Diversity, topographic differentiation, and positional memory in human fibro-blasts. Proc Natl Acad Sci USA *99*: 12877–82, 2002.
27. Nazareth, M.R., L. Broderick, M.R. Simpson-Abelson, R.J. Kelleher, Jr., S.J. Yokota, and R.B. Bankert. Characterization of human lung tumor-associated fibroblasts and their ability to modulate the activation of tumor-associated T cells. J Immunol *178*: 5552–62, 2007.
28. Micke, P. and A. Ostman. Tumour–stroma interaction: cancer-associated fibroblasts as novel targets in anti-cancer therapy? Lung Cancer *45(Suppl 2)*: S163–75, 2004.
29. Nakamura, N., T. Iijima, K. Mase, S. Furuya, J. Kano, Y. Morishita, and M. Noguchi. Phenotypic differences of proliferating fibroblasts in the stroma of lung adenocarcinoma and normal bronchus tissue. Cancer Sci *95*: 226–32, 2004.
30. Anderson, I.C., S.E. Mari, R.J. Broderick, B.P. Mari, and M.A. Shipp. The angiogenic factor interleukin 8 is induced in non-small cell lung cancer/pulmonary fibroblast cocul-tures. Cancer Res *60*: 269–72, 2000.

31. Mari, B.P., I.C. Anderson, S.E. Mari, Y. Ning, Y. Lutz, L. Kobzik, and M.A. Shipp. Stromelysin-3 is induced in tumor/stroma cocultures and inactivated via a tumor-specific and basic fibroblast growth factor-dependent mechanism. J Biol Chem *273*: 618–26, 1998.

32. Fromigue, O., K. Louis, M. Dayem, J. Milanini, G. Pages, S. Tartare-Deckert, G. Ponzio, P. Hofman, P. Barbry, P. Auberger, and B. Mari. Gene expression profiling of normal human pulmonary fibroblasts following coculture with non-small-cell lung cancer cells reveals alterations related to matrix degradation, angiogenesis, cell growth and survival. Oncogene *22*: 8487–97, 2003.

33. Mitsiadis, T.A., M. Lardelli, U. Lendahl, and I. Thesleff. Expression of Notch 1, 2 and 3 is regulated by epithelial–mesenchymal interactions and retinoic acid in the developing mouse tooth and associated with determination of ameloblast cell fate. J Cell Biol *130*: 407–18, 1995.

34. Coppe, J.P., K. Kauser, J. Campisi, and C.M. Beausejour. Secretion of vascular endothelial growth factor by primary human fibroblasts at senescence. J Biol Chem *281*: 29568–74, 2006.

35. Parrinello, S., J.P. Coppe, A. Krtolica, and J. Campisi. Stromal–epithelial interactions in aging and cancer: senescent fibroblasts alter epithelial cell differentiation. J Cell Sci *118*: 485–96, 2005.

36. Begley, L., C. Monteleon, R.B. Shah, J.W. Macdonald, and J.A. Macoska. CXCL12 overexpression and secretion by aging fibroblasts enhance human prostate epithelial proliferation in vitro. Aging Cell *4*: 291–8, 2005.

37. Lewis, C.E. and J.W. Pollard. Distinct role of macrophages in different tumor microenvironments. Cancer Res *66*: 605–12, 2006.

38. Bavik, C., I. Coleman, J.P. Dean, B. Knudsen, S. Plymate, and P.S. Nelson. The gene expression program of prostate fibroblast senescence modulates neoplastic epithelial cell proliferation through paracrine mechanisms. Cancer Res *66*: 794–802, 2006.

39. Stewart, D.A., C.R. Cooper, and R.A. Sikes. Changes in extracellular matrix (ECM) and ECM-associated proteins in the metastatic progression of prostate cancer. Reprod Biol Endocrinol *2*: 2, 2004.

40. Sappino, A.P., O. Skalli, B. Jackson, W. Schurch, and G. Gabbiani. Smooth-muscle differentiation in stromal cells of malignant and non-malignant breast tissues. Int J Cancer *41*: 707–12, 1988.

41. Rodemann, H.P. and G.A. Muller. Characterization of human renal fibroblasts in health and disease: II. In vitro growth, differentiation, and collagen synthesis of fibroblasts from kidneys with interstitial fibrosis. Am J Kidney Dis *17*: 684–6, 1991.

42. Orimo, A., P.B. Gupta, D.C. Sgroi, F. Arenzana-Seisdedos, T. Delaunay, R. Naeem, V.J. Carey, A.L. Richardson, and R.A. Weinberg. Stromal fibroblasts present in invasive human breast carcinomas promote tumor growth and angiogenesis through elevated SDF-1/CXCL12 secretion. Cell *121*: 335–48, 2005.

43. Kuperwasser, C., T. Chavarria, M. Wu, G. Magrane, J.W. Gray, L. Carey, A. Richardson, and R.A. Weinberg. Reconstruction of functionally normal and malignant human breast tissues in mice. Proc Natl Acad Sci USA *101*: 4966–71, 2004.

44. Boire, A., L. Covic, A. Agarwal, S. Jacques, S. Sherifi, and A. Kuliopulos. PAR1 is a matrix metalloprotease-1 receptor that promotes invasion and tumorigenesis of breast cancer cells. Cell *120*: 303–13, 2005.

45. Stetler-Stevenson, W.G., S. Aznavoorian, and L.A. Liotta. Tumor cell interactions with the extracellular matrix during invasion and metastasis. Annu Rev Cell Biol *9*: 541–73, 1993.

46. Sternlicht, M.D., A. Lochter, C.J. Sympson, B. Huey, J.P. Rougier, J.W. Gray, D. Pinkel, M.J. Bissell, and Z. Werb. The stromal proteinase MMP3/stromelysin-1 promotes mammary carcinogenesis. Cell *98*: 137–46, 1999.

47. Lochter, A., S. Galosy, J. Muschler, N. Freedman, Z. Werb, and M.J. Bissell. Matrix metalloproteinase stromelysin-1 triggers a cascade of molecular alterations that leads to

stable epithelial-to-mesenchymal conversion and a premalignant phenotype in mammary epithelial cells. J Cell Biol *139*: 1861–72, 1997.

48. Maffini, M.V., A.M. Soto, J.M. Calabro, A.A. Ucci, and C. Sonnenschein. The stroma as a crucial target in rat mammary gland carcinogenesis. J Cell Sci *117*: 1495–502, 2004.

49. Gilead, A., G. Meir, and M. Neeman. The role of angiogenesis, vascular maturation, regression and stroma infiltration in dormancy and growth of implanted MLS ovarian carcinoma spheroids. Int J Cancer *108*: 524–31, 2004.

50. Gilad, A.A., T. Israely, H. Dafni, G. Meir, B. Cohen, and M. Neeman. Functional and molecular mapping of uncoupling between vascular permeability and loss of vascular maturation in ovarian carcinoma xenografts: the role of stroma cells in tumor angiogenesis. Int J Cancer *117*: 202–11, 2005.

51. Olaso, E., A. Santisteban, J. Bidaurrazaga, A.M. Gressner, J. Rosenbaum, and F. Vidal-Vanaclocha. Tumor-dependent activation of rodent hepatic stellate cells during experimental melanoma metastasis. Hepatology *26*: 634–42, 1997.

52. Grum-Schwensen, B., J. Klingelhofer, C.H. Berg, C. El-Naaman, M. Grigorian, E. Lukanidin, and N. Ambartsumian. Suppression of tumor development and metastasis formation in mice lacking the S100A4(mts1) gene. Cancer Res *65*: 3772–80, 2005.

53. Olaso, E., C. Salado, E. Egilegor, V. Gutierrez, A. Santisteban, P. Sancho-Bru, S.L. Friedman, and F. Vidal-Vanaclocha. Proangiogenic role of tumor-activated hepatic stellate cells in experimental melanoma metastasis. Hepatology *37*: 674–85, 2003.

54. Bhowmick, N.A., A. Chytil, D. Plieth, A.E. Gorska, N. Dumont, S. Shappell, M.K. Washington, E.G. Neilson, and H.L. Moses. TGF-beta signaling in fibroblasts modulates the oncogenic potential of adjacent epithelia. Science *303*: 848–51, 2004.

55. Cheng, N., N.A. Bhowmick, A. Chytil, A.E. Gorksa, K.A. Brown, R. Muraoka, C.L. Arteaga, E.G. Neilson, S.W. Hayward, and H.L. Moses. Loss of TGF-beta type II receptor in fibroblasts promotes mammary carcinoma growth and invasion through upregulation of TGF-alpha-, MSP- and HGF-mediated signaling networks. Oncogene *24*: 5053–68, 2005.

56. Guddo, F., G. Fontanini, C. Reina, A.M. Vignola, A. Angeletti, and G. Bonsignore. The expression of basic fibroblast growth factor (bFGF) in tumor-associated stromal cells and vessels is inversely correlated with non-small cell lung cancer progression. Hum Pathol *30*: 788–94, 1999.

57. Soderdahl, G., C. Betsholtz, A. Johansson, K. Nilsson, and J. Bergh. Differential expression of platelet-derived growth factor and transforming growth factor genes in small- and non-small-cell human lung carcinoma lines. Int J Cancer *41*: 636–41, 1988.

58. Betsholtz, C., J. Bergh, M. Bywater, M. Pettersson, A. Johnsson, C.H. Heldin, R. Ohlsson, T.J. Knott, J. Scott, G.I. Bell et al. Expression of multiple growth factors in a human lung cancer cell line. Int J Cancer *39*: 502–7, 1987.

59. Kawai, T., S. Hiroi, and C. Torikata. Expression in lung carcinomas of platelet-derived growth factor and its receptors. Lab Invest *77*: 431–6, 1997.

60. Hasegawa, Y., S. Takanashi, Y. Kanehira, T. Tsushima, T. Imai, and K. Okumura. Transforming growth factor-beta1 level correlates with angiogenesis, tumor progression, and prognosis in patients with nonsmall cell lung carcinoma. Cancer *91*: 964–71, 2001.

61. Demarchi, L.M., M.M. Reis, S.A. Palomino, C. Farhat, T.Y. Takagaki, R. Beyruti, P.H. Saldiva, and V.L. Capelozzi. Prognostic values of stromal proportion and PCNA, Ki-67, and p53 proteins in patients with resected adenocarcinoma of the lung. Mod Pathol *13*: 511–20, 2000.

62. Pirinen, R., R. Tammi, M. Tammi, P. Hirvikoski, J.J. Parkkinen, R. Johansson, J. Bohm, S. Hollmen, and V.M. Kosma. Prognostic value of hyaluronan expression in non-small-cell lung cancer: Increased stromal expression indicates unfavorable outcome in patients with adenocarcinoma. Int J Cancer *95*: 12–7, 2001.

63. Michael, M., B. Babic, R. Khokha, M. Tsao, J. Ho, M. Pintilie, K. Leco, D. Chamberlain, and F.A. Shepherd. Expression and prognostic significance of metalloproteinases and their tissue inhibitors in patients with small-cell lung cancer. J Clin Oncol *17*: 1802–8, 1999.

64. Tokunou, M., T. Niki, K. Eguchi, S. Iba, H. Tsuda, T. Yamada, Y. Matsuno, H. Kondo, Y. Saitoh, H. Imamura, and S. Hirohashi. c-MET expression in myofibroblasts: role in autocrine activation and prognostic significance in lung adenocarcinoma. Am J Pathol *158*: 1451–63, 2001.
65. Wang, K.K., N. Liu, N. Radulovich, D.A. Wigle, M.R. Johnston, F.A. Shepherd, M.D. Minden, and M.S. Tsao. Novel candidate tumor marker genes for lung adenocarcinoma. Oncogene *21*: 7598–604, 2002.
66. Chong, I.W., M.Y. Chang, H.C. Chang, Y.P. Yu, C.C. Sheu, J.R. Tsai, J.Y. Hung, S.H. Chou, M.S. Tsai, J.J. Hwang, and S.R. Lin. Great potential of a panel of multiple hMTH1, SPD, ITGA11 and COL11A1 markers for diagnosis of patients with non-small cell lung cancer. Oncol Rep *16*: 981–8, 2006.
67. Zhu, C.Q., S.N. Popova, E.R. Brown, D. Barsyte-Lovejoy, R. Navab, W. Shih, M. Li, M. Lu, I. Jurisica, L.Z. Penn, D. Gullberg, and M.S. Tsao. Integrin alpha 11 regulates IGF2 expression in fibroblasts to enhance tumorigenicity of human non-small-cell lung cancer cells. Proc Natl Acad Sci USA *104*: 11754–9, 2007.
68. Tiger, C.F., F. Fougerousse, G. Grundstrom, T. Velling, and D. Gullberg. alpha11beta1 integrin is a receptor for interstitial collagens involved in cell migration and collagen reorganization on mesenchymal nonmuscle cells. Dev Biol *237*: 116–29, 2001.
69. Joyce, J.A. Therapeutic targeting of the tumor microenvironment. Cancer Cell *7*: 513–20, 2005.
70. Jain, R.K. Normalization of tumor vasculature: an emerging concept in antiangiogenic therapy. Science *307*: 58–62, 2005.
71. Gilboa, E. The promise of cancer vaccines. Nat Rev Cancer *4*: 401–11, 2004.
72. Lee, J., M. Fassnacht, S. Nair, D. Boczkowski, and E. Gilboa. Tumor immunotherapy targeting fibroblast activation protein, a product expressed in tumor-associated fibroblasts. Cancer Res *65*: 11156–63, 2005.
73. Chambers, A.F. and L.M. Matrisian. Changing views of the role of matrix metalloproteinases in metastasis. J Natl Cancer Inst *89*: 1260–70, 1997.
74. Thomas, P., R. Khokha, F.A. Shepherd, R. Feld, and M.S. Tsao. Differential expression of matrix metalloproteinases and their inhibitors in non-small cell lung cancer. J Pathol *190*: 150–6, 2000.
75. Kodate, M., T. Kasai, H. Hashimoto, K. Yasumoto, Y. Iwata, and H. Manabe. Expression of matrix metalloproteinase (gelatinase) in T1 adenocarcinoma of the lung. Pathol Int *47*: 461–9, 1997.
76. Shepherd, F.A., G. Giaccone, L. Seymour, C. Debruyne, A. Bezjak, V. Hirsh, M. Smylie, S. Rubin, H. Martins, A. Lamont, M. Krzakowski, A. Sadura, and B. Zee. Prospective, randomized, double-blind, placebo-controlled trial of marimastat after response to first-line chemotherapy in patients with small-cell lung cancer: a trial of the National Cancer Institute of Canada-Clinical Trials Group and the European Organization for Research and Treatment of Cancer. J Clin Oncol *20*: 4434–9, 2002.
77. Gabrilovich, D.I., H.L. Chen, K.R. Girgis, H.T. Cunningham, G.M. Meny, S. Nadaf, D. Kavanaugh, and D.P. Carbone. Production of vascular endothelial growth factor by human tumors inhibits the functional maturation of dendritic cells. Nat Med *2*: 1096–103, 1996.
78. O'Connor, D.S., J.S. Schechner, C. Adida, M. Mesri, A.L. Rothermel, F. Li, A.K. Nath, J.S. Pober, and D.C. Altieri. Control of apoptosis during angiogenesis by survivin expression in endothelial cells. Am J Pathol *156*: 393–8, 2000.
79. Muraoka, R.S., N. Dumont, C.A. Ritter, T.C. Dugger, D.M. Brantley, J. Chen, E. Easterly, L.R. Roebuck, S. Ryan, P.J. Gotwals, V. Koteliansky, and C.L. Arteaga. Blockade of TGF-beta inhibits mammary tumor cell viability, migration, and metastases. J Clin Invest *109*: 1551–9, 2002.
80. Yang, Y.A., O. Dukhanina, B. Tang, M. Mamura, J.J. Letterio, J. MacGregor, S.C. Patel, S. Khozin, Z.Y. Liu, J. Green, M.R. Anver, G. Merlino, and L.M. Wakefield.

Lifetime exposure to a soluble TGF-beta antagonist protects mice against metastasis without adverse side effects. J Clin Invest *109*: 1607–15, 2002.

81. Jain, R.K., J. Lahdenranta, and D. Fukumura. Targeting PDGF signaling in carcinoma-associated fibroblasts controls cervical cancer in mouse model. PLoS Med 5: e24, 2008.

82. Demetri, G.D., M. von Mehren, C.D. Blanke, A.D. Van den Abbeele, B. Eisenberg, P.J. Roberts, M.C. Heinrich, D.A. Tuveson, S. Singer, M. Janicek, J.A. Fletcher, S.G. Silverman, S.L. Silberman, R. Capdeville, B. Kiese, B. Peng, S. Dimitrijevic, B.J. Druker, C. Corless, C.D. Fletcher, and H. Joensuu. Efficacy and safety of imatinib mesylate in advanced gastrointestinal stromal tumors. N Engl J Med *347*: 472–80, 2002.

83. Bergers, G., S. Song, N. Meyer-Morse, E. Bergsland, and D. Hanahan. Benefits of targeting both pericytes and endothelial cells in the tumor vasculature with kinase inhibitors. J Clin Invest *111*: 1287–95, 2003.

84. Pietras, K., J. Pahler, G. Bergers, and D. Hanahan. Functions of paracrine PDGF signaling in the proangiogenic tumor stroma revealed by pharmacological targeting. PLoS Med 5: e19, 2008.

85. Park, J.E., M.C. Lenter, R.N. Zimmermann, P. Garin-Chesa, L.J. Old, and W.J. Rettig. Fibroblast activation protein, a dual specificity serine protease expressed in reactive human tumor stromal fibroblasts. J Biol Chem *274*: 36505–12, 1999.

86. Pineiro-Sanchez, M.L., L.A. Goldstein, J. Dodt, L. Howard, Y. Yeh, H. Tran, W.S. Argraves, and W.T. Chen. Identification of the 170-kDa melanoma membrane-bound gelatinase (seprase) as a serine integral membrane protease. J Biol Chem *272*: 7595–601, 1997.

87. Ghersi, G., H. Dong, L.A. Goldstein, Y. Yeh, L. Hakkinen, H.S. Larjava, and W.T. Chen. Regulation of fibroblast migration on collagenous matrix by a cell surface peptidase complex. J Biol Chem *277*: 29231–41, 2002.

88. Levy, M.T., G.W. McCaughan, G. Marinos, and M.D. Gorrell. Intrahepatic expression of the hepatic stellate cell marker fibroblast activation protein correlates with the degree of fibrosis in hepatitis C virus infection. Liver *22*: 93–101, 2002.

89. Henry, L.R., H.O. Lee, J.S. Lee, A. Klein-Szanto, P. Watts, E.A. Ross, W.T. Chen, and J. D. Cheng. Clinical implications of fibroblast activation protein in patients with colon cancer. Clin Cancer Res *13*: 1736–41, 2007.

90. Lin, K.Y., F.G. Guarnieri, K.F. Staveley-O'Carroll, H.I. Levitsky, J.T. August, D.M. Pardoll, and T.C. Wu. Treatment of established tumors with a novel vaccine that enhances major histocompatibility class II presentation of tumor antigen. Cancer Res *56*: 21–6, 1996.

91. Loeffler, M., J.A. Kruger, A.G. Niethammer, and R.A. Reisfeld. Targeting tumor-associated fibroblasts improves cancer chemotherapy by increasing intratumoral drug uptake. J Clin Invest *116*: 1955–62, 2006.

92. Mork, C., B. van Deurs, and O.W. Petersen. Regulation of vimentin expression in cultured human mammary epithelial cells. Differentiation *43*: 146–56, 1990.

93. Tomasek, J.J., G. Gabbiani, B. Hinz, C. Chaponnier, and R.A. Brown. Myofibroblasts and mechano-regulation of connective tissue remodelling. Nat Rev Mol Cell Biol *3*: 349–63, 2002.

94. Mueller, L., F.A. Goumas, M. Affeldt, S. Sandtner, U.M. Gehling, S. Brilloff, J. Walter, N. Karnatz, K. Lamszus, X. Rogiers, and D.C. Broering. Stromal fibroblasts in colorectal liver metastases originate from resident fibroblasts and generate an inflammatory microenvironment. Am J Pathol *171*: 1608–18, 2007.

95. Strutz, F., H. Okada, C.W. Lo, T. Danoff, R.L. Carone, J.E. Tomaszewski, and E.G. Neilson. Identification and characterization of a fibroblast marker: FSP1. J Cell Biol *130*: 393–405, 1995.

96. Vogel, W., G.D. Gish, F. Alves, and T. Pawson. The discoidin domain receptor tyrosine kinases are activated by collagen. Mol Cell *1*: 13–23, 1997.

97. Goldsmith, E.C., A. Hoffman, M.O. Morales, J.D. Potts, R.L. Price, A. McFadden, M. Rice, and T.K. Borg. Organization of fibroblasts in the heart. Dev Dyn *230*: 787–94, 2004.

98. Rettig, W.J., P. Garin-Chesa, J.H. Healey, S.L. Su, H.L. Ozer, M. Schwab, A.P. Albino, and L.J. Old. Regulation and heteromeric structure of the fibroblast activation protein in normal and transformed cells of mesenchymal and neuroectodermal origin. Cancer Res *53*: 3327–35, 1993.

99. Ramirez-Montagut, T., N.E. Blachere, E.V. Sviderskaya, D.C. Bennett, W.J. Rettig, P. Garin-Chesa, and A.N. Houghton. FAPalpha, a surface peptidase expressed during wound healing, is a tumor suppressor. Oncogene *23*: 5435–46, 2004.

100. Gullberg, D., G. Sjoberg, T. Velling, and T. Sejersen. Analysis of fibronectin and vitronectin receptors on human fetal skeletal muscle cells upon differentiation. Exp Cell Res *220*: 112–23, 1995.

101. Popova, S.N., Rodriguez-Sanchez, B., Liden, A., Betsholtz, C., Van Den Bos, T., and D. Gullberg. The mesenchymal alpha11beta1 integrin attenuates PDGF-BB-stimulated chemotaxis of embryonic fibroblasts on collagens. Dev Biol *270*: 427–42, 2004.

102. Gardner, H., J. Kreidberg, V. Koteliansky, and R. Jaenisch. Deletion of integrin alpha 1 by homologous recombination permits normal murine development but gives rise to a specific deficit in cell adhesion. Dev Biol *175*: 301–13, 1996.

103. Sudhakar, A., P. Nyberg, V.G. Keshamouni, A.P. Mannam, J. Li, H. Sugimoto, D. Cosgrove, and R. Kalluri. Human alpha1 type IV collagen NC1 domain exhibits distinct antiangiogenic activity mediated by alpha1beta1 integrin. J Clin Invest *115*: 2801–10, 2005.

104. Mussini, E., J.J. Hutton, Jr., and S. Udenfriend. Collagen proline hydroxylase in wound healing, granuloma formation, scurvy, and growth. Science *157*: 927–9, 1967.

105. Langness, U. and S. Udenfriend. Collagen biosynthesis in nonfibroblastic cell lines. Proc Natl Acad Sci USA *71*: 50–1, 1974.

106. Florin, L., H. Alter, H.J. Grone, A. Szabowski, G. Schutz, and P. Angel. Cre recombinase-mediated gene targeting of mesenchymal cells. Genesis *38*: 139–44, 2004.

107. Jenkins, R.H., G.J. Thomas, J.D. Williams, and R. Steadman. Myofibroblastic differentiation leads to hyaluronan accumulation through reduced hyaluronan turnover. J Biol Chem *279*: 41453–60, 2004.

108. Sugimoto, H., T.M. Mundel, M.W. Kieran, and R. Kalluri. Identification of fibroblast heterogeneity in the tumor microenvironment. Cancer Biol Ther *5*: 1640–6, 2006.

109. Chiquet-Ehrismann, R., P. Kalla, and C.A. Pearson. Participation of tenascin and transforming growth factor-beta in reciprocal epithelial–mesenchymal interactions of MCF7 cells and fibroblasts. Cancer Res *49*: 4322–5, 1989.

110. Serini, G., M.L. Bochaton-Piallat, P. Ropraz, A. Geinoz, L. Borsi, L. Zardi, and G. Gabbiani. The fibronectin domain ED-A is crucial for myofibroblastic phenotype induction by transforming growth factor-beta1. J Cell Biol *142*: 873–81, 1998.

111. Jaques, G., K. Noll, B. Wegmann, S. Witten, E. Kogan, R.T. Radulescu, and K. Havemann. Nuclear localization of insulin-like growth factor binding protein 3 in a lung cancer cell line. Endocrinology *138*: 1767–70, 1997.

112. Lee, H.Y., K.H. Chun, B. Liu, S.A. Wiehle, R.J. Cristiano, W.K. Hong, P. Cohen, and J.M. Kurie. Insulin-like growth factor binding protein-3 inhibits the growth of non-small cell lung cancer. Cancer Res *62*: 3530–7, 2002.

113. Taipale, J., J. Saharinen, and J. Keski-Oja. Extracellular matrix-associated transforming growth factor-beta: role in cancer cell growth and invasion. Adv Cancer Res *75*: 87–134, 1998.

114. Blom, I.E., R. Goldschmeding, and A. Leask. Gene regulation of connective tissue growth factor: new targets for antifibrotic therapy? Matrix Biol *21*: 473–82, 2002.

115. Robertson, D.M., E. Pruysers, H.G. Burger, T. Jobling, J. McNeilage, and D. Healy. Inhibins and ovarian cancer. Mol Cell Endocrinol *225*: 65–71, 2004.

116. Fukumura, D., R. Xavier, T. Sugiura, Y. Chen, E.C. Park, N. Lu, M. Selig, G. Nielsen, T. Taksir, R.K. Jain, and B. Seed. Tumor induction of VEGF promoter activity in stromal cells. Cell *94*: 715–25, 1998.

117. Mascaux, C., B. Martin, M. Paesmans, J.M. Verdebout, A. Verhest, P. Vermylen, T. Bosschaerts, V. Ninane, and J.P. Sculier. Expression of thrombospondin in non-small cell lung cancer. Anticancer Res *22*: 1273–7, 2002.

118. Ohtani, H. Stromal reaction in cancer tissue: pathophysiologic significance of the expression of matrix-degrading enzymes in relation to matrix turnover and immune/ inflammatory reactions. Pathol Int *48*: 1–9, 1998.

119. Wojtukiewicz, M.Z., L.R. Zacharski, M. Rucinska, L. Zimnoch, J. Jaromin, M. Rozanska-Kudelska, W. Kisiel, and B.J. Kudryk. Expression of tissue factor and tissue factor pathway inhibitor in situ in laryngeal carcinoma. Thromb Haemost *82*: 1659–62, 1999.

120. Lakka, S.S., S.D. Konduri, S. Mohanam, G.L. Nicolson, and J.S. Rao. In vitro modulation of human lung cancer cell line invasiveness by antisense cDNA of tissue factor pathway inhibitor-2. Clin Exp Metastasis *18*: 239–44, 2000.

121. Rabbani, S.A. Metalloproteases and urokinase in angiogenesis and tumor progression. In Vivo *12*: 135–42, 1998.

122. Lynch, C.C. and L.M. Matrisian. Matrix metalloproteinases in tumor-host cell communication. Differentiation *70*: 561–73, 2002.

123. Umeda, T., Y. Eguchi, K. Okino, M. Kodama, and T. Hattori. Cellular localization of urokinase-type plasminogen activator, its inhibitors, and their mRNAs in breast cancer tissues. J Pathol *183*: 388–97, 1997.

124. Kang, K.H., S.Y. Park, S.B. Rho, and J.H. Lee. Tissue inhibitor of metalloproteinases-3 interacts with angiotensin II type 2 receptor and additively inhibits angiogenesis. Cardiovasc Res, 2008.

125. Culig, Z., A. Hobisch, M.V. Cronauer, C. Radmayr, J. Trapman, A. Hittmair, G. Bartsch, and H. Klocker. Androgen receptor activation in prostatic tumor cell lines by insulin-like growth factor-I, keratinocyte growth factor, and epidermal growth factor. Cancer Res *54*: 5474–8, 1994.

126. Hrouda, D., D.L. Nicol, and R.A. Gardiner. The role of angiogenesis in prostate development and the pathogenesis of prostate cancer. Urol Res *30*: 347–55, 2003.

127. Engl, T., B. Relja, C. Blumenberg, I. Muller, E.M. Ringel, W.D. Beecken, D. Jonas, and R.A. Blaheta. Prostate tumor CXC-chemokine profile correlates with cell adhesion to endothelium and extracellular matrix. Life Sci *78*: 1784–93, 2006.

128. Dean, J.P. and P.S. Nelson. Profiling influences of senescent and aged fibroblasts on prostate carcinogenesis. Br J Cancer *98*: 245–9, 2008.

129. Fridman, R., G. Giaccone, T. Kanemoto, G.R. Martin, A.F. Gazdar, and J.L. Mulshine. Reconstituted basement membrane (matrigel) and laminin can enhance the tumorigenicity and the drug resistance of small cell lung cancer cell lines. Proc Natl Acad Sci USA *87*: 6698–702, 1990.

130. Sethi, T., R.C. Rintoul, S.M. Moore, A.C. MacKinnon, D. Salter, C. Choo, E.R. Chilvers, I. Dransfield, S.C. Donnelly, R. Strieter, and C. Haslett. Extracellular matrix proteins protect small cell lung cancer cells against apoptosis: a mechanism for small cell lung cancer growth and drug resistance in vivo. Nat Med *5*: 662–8, 1999.

131. Hwang, R.F., T. Moore, T. Arumugam, V. Ramachandran, K.D. Amos, A. Rivera, B. Ji, D.B. Evans, and C.D. Logsdon. Cancer-associated stromal fibroblasts promote pancreatic tumor progression. Cancer Res *68*: 918–26, 2008.

The Role of Tumor-Associated Macrophages and Other Innate Immune Cells in Metastatic Progression of Lung Cancer

Zvi G. Fridlender, M. Cecilia Crisanti, and Steven M. Albelda

Abstract There is increasing evidence that the immune cells within the tumor microenvironment play a key role in the ability of tumor cells to proliferate and spread. Given that macrophages are the most frequent hematopoietic cells found in the tumor microenvironment, they play an especially important part in tumor biology. There are numerous mechanisms by which tumor-associated innate immune cells can influence most aspects of the metastatic process. They play a role in the epithelial to mesenchymal transformation occurring in the original tumor cells and enhance basement membrane breakdown by the cancer cells invading neighboring tissue, lymph nodes, and blood vessels. Tumor-associated innate immune cells have been shown to have a crucial role in angiogenesis, in immunosuppression, and eventually in priming distant sites for the development of metastases. Unfortunately, we still know relatively little about the roles of these cells in lung cancer. Further work in animal models and using patient lung cancer samples is very much needed. With this knowledge, a better understanding of the role that these cells play in the metastatic process may facilitate development of new therapeutics, as well as the recognition of new diagnostic and prognostic markers. Modulation of the metastatic phenotype through intervention in the host innate immune response remains a promising future area of cancer therapy.

Introduction

For a cancer to metastasize, a subpopulation of tumor cells must breech normal tissue barriers (basement membranes), invade the vasculature, survive in the circulation, bind to and traverse the vascular endothelium and basement membrane, and grow in a secondary and foreign location [1]. Traditionally, research in metastasis has focused almost exclusively on the properties of the tumor cells

Z.G. Fridlender (✉)
Thoracic Oncology Research Laboratory, Pulmonary and Critical Care Division,
University of Pennsylvania Medical Center, Philadelphia, PA 19104-6160, USA
e-mail: gfrid@mail.med.upenn.edu

V. Keshamouni et al. (eds.), *Lung Cancer Metastasis*,   217
DOI 10.1007/978-1-4419-0772-1_11, © Springer Science+Business Media, LLC 2009

in this process. Although the intrinsic properties of tumor cells are certainly important, it has become increasingly well recognized that the other cells within the tumor microenvironment (i.e., leukocytes, mast cells, endothelial cells, and stromal cells) play a key role in the ability of tumor cells to proliferate and spread.

Leukocytes were first described to reside in tumors by Virchow [2]. It is now recognized that white blood cells are a major population of tumor-associated cells and can markedly affect the growth and metastasis of the tumor. Both innate immune cells (i.e., macrophages, neutrophils, natural killer cells, and mast cells) and those of the acquired immune system (T cells and B cells) have the potential to affect cancer growth and spread. In this chapter, we will focus on the role of tumor-associated innate immune cells in the development of lung metastasis.

Tumor-Associated Innate Immune Cells

Macrophages

It is well established that most of the hematopoietic cells found in the tumor microenvironment are macrophages [3]. These macrophages are known as tumor-infiltrating macrophages (TIMs) or tumor-associated macrophages (TAMs). Lung cancers are highly infiltrated by TAMs (Fig. 1).

Macrophages are derived from immature monocytes released from the bone marrow that circulate in the bloodstream and eventually migrate into tissues where they differentiate into specific macrophage phenotypes (i.e., alveolar macrophages). Several cytokines have been suggested to have a role in the recruitment of macrophages into tumors, including macrophage colony-stimulating factor (M-CSF) and vascular endothelial growth factor (VEGF) [4].

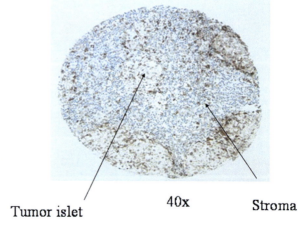

Fig. 1 A human lung cancer specimen stained with an antibody to CD68 shows intense infiltration with macrophages

Tumor islet   40x   Stroma

Monocyte-chemotactic protein-1 (MCP-1) and CCL-5 (RANTES) have been the most heavily implicated chemokines in monocyte recruitment to human tumors, and their expression has been shown to positively correlate with TAM numbers in some types of tumors [5, 6]. However, other CC chemokines may also be involved in monocyte recruitment to tumors. For example, CCL3, CCL4, CCL8 (monocyte-chemotactic protein-2), and CCL22 (macrophage-derived chemokine), all well-known monocyte attractants, have been detected in ovarian tumors [7]. Some CXC chemokines, particularly CXCL8, are highly expressed in human tumors and cell lines, but their role in directing the uptake of monocytes by tumors is not well defined [8]. CXCL12 (stromal-derived factor-1, SDF-1) is usually identified as a lymphocyte chemoattractant but has also been implicated in the metastasis of tumor cells expressing CXCR4, the receptor for this chemokine, to specific organs that have elevated CXCL12 levels, including the lungs [9]. Macrophages also express CXCR4 [10]; however, NSCLC do not express significant levels of CXCL12 [11], suggesting that this chemokine is unlikely to play a role in the attraction of macrophages into lung tumors [4].

The effects of macrophages seem dependent on the stage of tumor development. Early in the tumor process, TAMs appear to have an inflammatory, tumoricidal (so-called M1 or "classically activated") phenotype [12]. These macrophages, which have been studied in vitro by activation with bacterial products, endotoxin, TH1 cytokines, or other inducers of inflammation, are generally phagocytic, present antigens well, produce TH1-type inflammatory cytokines (like TNF-α), and are cytotoxic. Cytotoxicity is due to direct secretion of toxic substances such as reactive oxygen and nitrogen intermediates [13, 14]. Other agents secreted by TAMs with potential direct antitumoricidal properties include granulocyte/macrophage colony-stimulating factor (GM-CSF) [15], TNF-α [13], macrophage migration-inhibitory factor (MIF) [16], and IL-12. They may also indirectly promote cytotoxicity by activating other cells of the immune system, such as NK cells and T cells [17], via secretion of factors such as interferon-γ or IL-18 [18]. In addition, it is thought that these early TAMs, by production of mutagens (such as reactive oxygen species) and cytokines (such as MIF, TNF-α, and IL-6), can cause direct tissue damage and DNA mutations and support cell survival and tumorigenesis [19, 20].

However, as the tumor becomes established, macrophages begin to take on a phenotype called "alternative" or "M2 activation." In vitro, the M2 phenotype can be induced by exposure to IL-4, IL-13, IL-10, or immune complexes [21, 22]. It is not yet entirely clear what factors in the tumor microenvironment drive incoming monocytes toward the M2-like TAM phenotype, but in addition to these aforementioned factors, transforming growth factor-beta (TGF-β)has been implicated in many in vitro studies [22, 23]. This hypothesis is supported by our own observations showing that TGF-β inhibitors suppress the M2 phenotype.

Polarized M2 macrophages differ from M1 macrophages in receptor expression, antigen-presenting ability, function, and cytokine production [21]. Another key feature is the difference in arginine metabolism between the two phenotypes. Arginine metabolism is dominated by the enzyme arginase in M2 cells, resulting in the production of ornithine (which may help tumor growth) and urea. In contrast, M1 macrophages are characterized by high levels of inducible nitric oxide synthase (iNOS), catalyzing the production of nitric oxide (NO) from arginine [24]. The differences in cytokine production are probably another central feature in understanding the protumor effects of alternatively activated macrophages. Whereas M1 macrophages produce IL-12 and TNF-α, M2 macrophages produce immunoinhibitory cytokines and chemokines such as IL-10, TGF-β, IL-1 receptor antagonist (IL-1ra), CCL17, and CCL22 [21]. These different profiles of cytokines and chemokines appear to help regulate the generation of Th1 versus Th2 lymphocytes [24, 25]. M1 macrophages skew the microenvironment toward a Th1 milieu, while M2 macrophages, tend to promote a more protumor Th2 microenvironment [21, 23, 24]. M2 TAMs also appear to promote angiogenesis by the production of vascular endothelial growth factor (VEGF) [26]. As discussed below, these characteristics tend to favor tumor expansion and metastases.

Neutrophils (PMNs)

PMNs are the predominant circulating leukocyte population in humans, accounting for 50–70% of circulating leukocytes. They have been seen in vivo in close association with metastatic tumor cells, at the primary tumor, and within the vasculature [27]. However, the exact role of PMNs in the tumor cell microenvironment is a subject of controversy.

Neutrophils play a well-established role in host defense, where they extravasate from the circulation and enter tissues [28]. There, they phagocytose and kill invading microorganisms such as bacteria and fungi by release of activating cytokines (i.e., TNF-α, Interferons-, IL-1, IL-8 and others.), defensins, and through release of toxic substances such as hypochlorous acid and reactive oxygen species. There is some evidence showing that this same cytotoxic machinery can be used to kill tumor cells [29]. For example, in animal models, Ishihara et al. [30, 31] reported that neutrophils from bronchoalveolar lavage (BAL) and peripheral blood from tumor-bearing animals showed an enhanced cytotoxicity profile (measured by superoxide anion generation and phagocytosis) and induced a marked decrease in the size and number of metastatic foci in the lung. Another mechanism of neutrophil-mediated tumor cell killing is antibody-dependent, cell-mediated toxicity [29]. Finally, neutrophils have been shown as important adaptive immune cells that augment acquired antitumor immune responses [32]. Thus, under some circumstances, tumor-associated neutrophils (TANs) may be important antitumor effectors.

On the other hand, there are studies suggesting that tumor-associated neutrophils might augment the ability of tumor cells to grow, extravasate, and to metastasize. Proposed mechanisms (discussed in more detail below) include the ability to augment the capability of tumor cells to extravasate through endothelium (EC) [33], the induction of EC damage allowing enhanced adherence of tumor cells in the lung [34, 35], the secretion of basement membrane-degrading enzymes [36], the stimulation of motility and invasiveness [27, 37], the activation of an angiogenic switch [38], and the induction of immunosuppression [39, 40].

It is interesting that many patients with advanced cancer show high levels of neutrophilia [41]. The mechanisms by which neutrophilia is induced by tumors is still uncertain, although GM-CSF production has been implicated in some tumor systems, such as lung, melanoma, pancreas, and breast [42]. IL-8 secreted by the tumor cells may play an important role in attracting neutrophils to the tumor microenvironment. Importantly, once attracted into a tumor, TANs could help remodel the extracellular matrix, favoring neovascularization. Neutrophils have been implicated in some studies where passive immunization against IL-8 attenuated tumor growth and angiogenic response in mice with lung tumors [43, 44]. Neutrophilia is associated with poorer prognosis in bronchoalveolar carcinoma, metastatic melanoma, and renal carcinoma although in some tumors (i.e. gastric cancer), a high neutrophil count has been associated with a favorable prognosis [41, 45].

Natural Killer (NK) Cells

NK cells are lymphocytes of the innate immune system that can induce the death of allogeneic cells and autologous cells undergoing various forms of stress, such as upon microbial infection and malignant transformation. In humans, lymph node NK cells outnumber blood NK cells at a ratio of 10:1. NK cells express an array of activation and inhibitory receptors, whose engagement allows them to discriminate between target and nontarget cells. The repertoire of receptors includes scavenger, toll-like (TLR), and nucleotide oligomerization domain (NOD) receptors. NK cells thus broaden the strategies for the detection of pathogenic situations where "danger signals" are missing in vivo, such as in the case of poorly immunogenic tumors [46]. The cytotoxic properties of these cells have a critical role in suppressing the outgrowth and metastasis of tumor cells. Mice treated with inhibitors of NK cells reactivity (anti-NK MoAb, corticosteroids, cyclophosphamide, cigarette smoke) show a slower cancer cell clearance from the lungs and an increased metastatic rate [47, 48]. High numbers of intratumoral NK cells have been proposed as a prognostic indicator and correlate with early-stage tumors, less lymphatic invasion and lymph node metastasis, in colon, gastric, lung, and esophageal cancers [47].

Mast Cells

Mast cells (MCs) are important mediators of angiogenesis and invasiveness via release of a variety of mediators that do not involve VEGF [49, 50]. Heparin and histamine have angiogenic properties and can also increase the permeability of newly formed microvessels, increasing the leak of plasma proteins and deposition of fibrin, which is angiogenic. As shown by Azizkhan et al. [51], MCs secrete heparin which stimulates capillary endothelial cell migration. Enzymes, such as metalloproteinases MMP-2 and -9, contribute to the degradation of collagens IV, V, VII, X, and fibronectin, adding to invasiveness of the tumor. Tryptase (MCP-6) and chymase (MCP-4) degrade extracellular matrix components or release matrix-associated growth factors, as well as activate MMP and plasminogen activators. MCs also secrete polypeptide growth factors, cytokines, and chemokines such as FGF-2, VEGF, TGF-β, TNF-α, and IL-8 [49, 52]. All of these agents have been implicated in normal as well as in tumor-associated angiogenesis. Accumulation of MCs appears to be related to the release of factors from the neoplastic cells themselves [49]. Also, MCs seem to accumulate toward the border region of the tumor, where angiogenesis plays an active role in tumor progression [53].

MCs have been described in association with several solid tumors, such as breast cancer, hemangioma and hemangioblastoma, colorectal, uterine, laryngeal, small cell lung cancer, and melanoma [49].

How Could Tumor-Associated Innate Immune Cells Affect the Metastatic Process?

There are a number of steps along the pathway to metastasis that could be affected by the tumor-associated innate immune cells described above (Fig. 2).

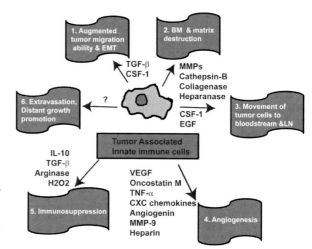

Fig. 2 The different actions and mediators of tumor-associated innate immune cells in the complex process of metastases formation

Epithelial to Mesenchymal Transformation-Augmented Migratory Ability

One of the first steps in the metastatic process in lung cancer is the conversion of cells from highly differentiated, contact-inhibited epithelial cells to a more invasive, motile cell, a process called epithelial to mesenchymal transformation [1]. Although this process can involve intrinsic or epigenetic changes, a number of secreted factors, most notably hepatocyte growth factor and TGF-β, can induce this process, at least in vitro [54]. TGF-β is actually growth inhibitory to normal epithelial cells, but as tumorigenesis progresses, cancer cells lose this response. At this point, TAMs, as well as the tumor cells themselves, often increase their production of TGF-β [55]. Thus, the high level of TGF-β secretion by TAMs can function to augment the invasiveness of tumor cells and enhance their ability to move into the stroma and vasculature [56, 57].

In a model of coculture of macrophages with breast or ovarian tumor cells, Hagemann et al. also showed that the macrophage's effect on the tumor is mediated via activation of NF-κB and JNK, leading to increased invasive capacity of the tumor cells [58]. Wycoff et al. [59] showed the existence of a paracrine loop between tumor cells and macrophages (involving CSF-1 and epidermal growth factor) that was required for tumor cell migration in mammary tumors.

Disruption of Basement Membranes and Matrix

An important early step in metastasis is the ability of tumor cell to cross basement membranes and matrix in order to enter blood vessels or lymphatics. The necessary remodeling of tissue structures is primarily achieved by proteases. Although tumor cells can make and activate proteases, tumor-associated macrophages, neutrophils, and mast cells are now recognized as a major source of MMPs and other proteases that have the ability to breakdown the basement membrane around areas of proliferating tumor cells, thereby prompting their escape into the surrounding healthy stroma for further growth [19]. Several proteolytic enzymes have been implicated. Cathepsin B was found in macrophages present at areas of BM breakdown [60]. TANs secrete high levels of basement membrane degrading enzymes such as type IV collagenase and heparanase, as well as elastase [29, 36]. Mast cells make tryptase (MCP-6) and chymase (MCP-4). TAMs, TANs, and MCs also make MMPs. In addition, coculturing macrophages with tumor cells enhances their ability to make their own matrix metalloproteinases [61]. MMP-2 and -9 contribute to the degradation of collagens IV, V, VII, X, and fibronectin, allowing the disruption of normal tissue architecture and breakdown of basement membranes, enabling metastatic spread [61]. MMP9, expressed in lung macrophages and endothelial cells in response to secretion of VEGF from the primary tumors, was shown to promote invasion of lung tissues by tumor cells, promoting metastases preferably to the lungs [62–64]. Although most of the actions of MMPs are protumorigenic, it is important to mention that MMP-12 was shown in a non-small cell lung cancer line to induce generation of the angiogenesis inhibitor angiostatin [65].

Movement of Tumor Cells to the Bloodstream and Lymph Nodes (Intravasation)

The ability of innate immune cells to enhance the migratory ability of tumor cells and break down vascular basement membranes (see above), as well as augment angiogenesis and lymphangiogenesis (see below), could theoretically increase the movement of tumor cells into the bloodstream and lymph nodes. TAMs were shown to have a role both in the shedding of cells from the primary tumor and in the establishment of distant metastases [19]. The specific role of macrophages in the intravasation of tumor cells to the bloodstream has also clearly been demonstrated in murine models of breast cancer. Neutrophils have also been shown to augment the ability of tumor cells to move through endothelium (EC) [33].

Angiogenesis

It is thought that angiogenesis and/or lymphangiogenesis are important features of tumors that allow metastatic spread [1]. Although tumor cells, themselves, can make angiogenic factors, it is becoming apparent that other tumor-associated innate immune cells also produce angiogenic factors. A number of investigators have shown correlations between increased TAM numbers and tumor vascularity in esophagus cancer [66] and in lung cancer [67, 68].

VEGF, the key factor of angiogenesis, has an autocrine loop with TAMs. VEGF is expressed by TAMs, but also acts as a chemotactic factor to macrophages, directing them to avascular parts of the tumor [69]. It was recently shown in a model of ovarian carcinoma that depletion of macrophages significantly decreases the level of peritoneal VEGF and reduces tumor invasiveness and metastases [70]. Another TAN-released molecule, oncostatin M, is involved in VEGF production in breast cancer, resulting in cell detachment and increased invasiveness [71]. In addition to directly producing VEGF, it has been shown in animal models that neutrophils can be a major source of MMP-9 that functionally activates VEGF, leading to activation of an "angiogenic switch" [38].

Other proangiogenic factors released by tumor-associated innate immune cells include TNF-α, angiogenin, and cyclooxygenase 2 (COX-2) [19].

Interleukin-8 (IL-8), also known as CXCL-8, and other CXC chemokines such as GRO-α (CXCL-1) and ENA-78 (CXCL-5) have been shown to play an important role in angiogenesis and metastasis, by directly enhancing endothelial cell proliferation, survival, and MMP expression [72]. Both TAMs and TANs make relatively large amounts of such chemokines [29, 32]. It has been shown that macrophages can be induced to secrete higher levels of angiogenic CXC chemokines by coculture with NSCLC cells [73]. This action was found to be dependent on the secretion of macrophage migration-inhibitory factor (MIF) by the tumor cells [73]. High levels of tumor-associated CXC chemokines and MIF are associated with the risk of recurrence after resection of lung cancer [74].

Interestingly, TAMs were also found to express VEGF-C, the lymphatic endothelial growth factor, suggesting a role in lymphangiogenesis as a potential way of tumor dissemination [75].

It has been demonstrated in different tumors that TAMs tend to migrate to the hypoxic areas formed around the tumor from the rapid disorganized blood vessel formation and the rapid tumor growth [76]. This migration occurs following hypoxic induction of several chemoattractants such as VEGF and endothelin [4, 77]. The macrophages appear to accumulate in these hypoxic areas, promote angiogenesis and tumor progression, and eventually increase lymph node involvement and confer poor prognosis [76].

Immunosuppression

Although local immunosuppression does not directly lead to metastasis, it is certainly a critical factor in allowing tumors to reach sufficient size and aggressiveness to ultimately spread. Although T-regulatory cells play an important role in immune suppression, a number of tumor-associated innate immune cells also contribute to this process.

As discussed above, several studies have shown that the TAMs, mainly in well-established tumors, predominately have the M2-type phenotype. These cells have immunosuppressive and anti-inflammatory activities and have been shown to promote angiogenesis and tumor metastatic spread through a variety of mechanisms [12, 21]. These macrophages no longer effectively lyse tumor cells themselves [78], nor do they efficiently present tumor-associated antigens and stimulate cytotoxic T cells [21]. The hallmark of that change from immunostimulation to immunosuppression is seen in reduced production of IL-12 and high production of the suppressive cytokines IL-10 and TGF-β [79].

In addition to its effect on tumor invasiveness, TGF-β is extremely immunosuppressive and potently inhibits any endogenous immune response that is generated against the tumor. As mentioned above, TGF-β has been shown to modulate tumor-associated macrophages and shift them from a more cytotoxic M1 phenotype to a more tumor-supportive M2 phenotype [80, 81]. An especially important consequence of this change may be the ability of TGF-β to stimulate the production of arginase by M2 macrophages [23, 24]. Arginase production in the tumor microenvironment by myeloid cells inhibits T-cell receptor expression and antigen-specific T-cell responses [82]. TGF-β also serves to inhibit leukocyte migration into tumors [83]. In addition, there are a number of direct effects on T cells. TGF-β affects the expression of key transcription factors and cytokines involved in T-cell development, differentiation, and activation (reviewed in Ref [80]). TGF-β also inhibits antigen presentation [84], shifts the T-cell repertoire to a primarily TH2 phenotype, and exerts inhibitory effects on T-cell proliferation by modulating the expression and signaling function of IL-2 and IL-2R [80]. Suppression of the transcription factors Tbet and GATA-3 levels by TGF-β hinders CD4 and CD8 T-cell differentiation. Additionally, TGF-β supports the maintenance of FOXP3 expression and supports the generation of peripheral CD4 + CD25 + regulatory T cells, including those found in the tumor microenvironment [85, 86]. TGF-β induces apoptosis in activated T cells, attenuates the acquisition and expression of T-cell effector function and directly acts on cytotoxic T cells to inhibit the expression of cytolytic gene targets (such as perforin granzymes and interferon-γ) [87–89].

The immunosuppressive role of neutrophils is being increasingly recognized. Granulocytes obtained from cancer patients are able to inhibit cytotoxic T cells due to the production of high levels of arginase [40] and/or hydrogen peroxide [39].

Killing of Circulating Metastatic Cells

After entry into the bloodstream, tumor cells must be able to survive several stresses, including physical damage from shear stresses and immune-mediated killing [1]. NK cells have shown effective antimetastatic activity with ability to eliminate circulating tumor cells in animal models and in humans as well. Several studies have shown that with reduced NK cell function, there is a higher risk of development of regional and distant metastases, and increased risk of recurrence after surgery with increased mortality [90]. These data suggest that NK cells are effective in killing circulating tumor cells on their way to becoming metastases [47, 90, 91].

Extravasation

Having survived the circulation, metastatic cells must exit at some point, traverse endothelial cells and migrate into target tissues. In addition to tumor cell factors (i.e., the expression of chemokine receptors, such as CXCR4), innate immune cells may also play a role. A study by Wu et al. [33] showed that in a series of in vitro experiments in breast cancer, PMNs exposed to tumor-conditioned media had an increased ability to adhere to tumor cells and to migrate through the endothelial barrier. Organ localization and metastasis of circulating cancer cells can be promoted by neutrophil-mediated microvascular injury.

Orr et al. [34, 35] have shown that the experimental induction of inflammation in the lung parenchyma was associated with endothelial lining disruption and increased lung metastatic foci. The specific extravasation of cells in distant sites was related to $CD11b^+$ myeloid cells. Primary tumors were shown to influence lung macrophages prior to the induction of metastases [62, 92]. Chemoattractants induced by distant primary tumors attract these myeloid cells to the premetastatic lung via VEGF-A, TNF-α, and TGF-β [93]. These changes in the distant sites for metastasis could assist specific migration of the tumor cells to them [93].

Distant Growth

Clinical studies showed that increased numbers of macrophages in lymph node metastases adjacent to the original tumor correlate with poor prognosis [94], suggesting that macrophages at the metastatic sites are as important for the distant growth of tumors as those within the original tumor.

Association Between Tumor-Associated Leukocytes and Lung Cancer Metastasis

As outlined in detail above, it seems likely that tumor-associated leukocytes could have major effects on the ability of lung cancer to metastasize. Most of the published work on the role of macrophages in the metastatic process describes mammary, colon, or melanoma tumors that metastasize to the lung. Only a few studies have addressed the specific question of the role of TAMs and TANs in the development of metastases originating from a lung tumor in animal models and human lung cancer patients. The data derived in these lung cancer studies are summarized below (see Table 1).

Animal Studies

Animal models with macrophage depletion have shown reduced tumor invasiveness. Convincing evidence for the important role of macrophages in the metastatic process was given by Lin et al. showing that depletion of macrophages in CSF-1 knockout mice significantly reduced the formation of lung metastases [95]. This was recently supported in a model of ovarian cancer, where local depletion of macrophages significantly reduced metastases [70].

Although a suitable animal model of metastasis of human lung cancer is required for an understanding of the cellular and molecular mechanisms of lung cancer metastasis, metastatic lung cancer models are not well developed. Most of the work has been done using metastatic clones of murine Lewis lung

Table 1 Studies examining the link between TAMs and clinical prognosis in lung cancer

	Year	Number of tumors evaluated	Methods	Findings	Reference
Takeo S	1986	77	Evaluation of the number of TAMs recovered by plastic adherence	TAMs changed by stage (I < II > III), N (N1 > N0/N2). No relation to T. No correlation between number of TAMs and recurrence, but significant correlation between their cytotoxicity and prognosis	[109]
Koukourakis MI	1998	141 Stage I–II	Evaluation of thymidine phosphorylase (TP) reactivity and its relation to macrophages density	Intense macrophage infiltration was associated with TP activity, which correlated with poor prognosis. However, in a subgroup of low vascularity, a group of better prognosis was defined	[68]
Kerr KM	1998	28	LC with histological features characteristic of regression in melanoma (found to have increased survival)	Increased CD68+ macrophages in the "regressing type" compared to 67 controls.	[116]
Takanami, T	1999	113	Evaluation of TAM density by IHC	Significant relation between TAM density and microvessel density. TAM density was negatively related to survival	[67]
Johnson SK	1999	95	Staining with CD68	Intratumoral infiltration of macrophages had no effect on survival	[110]
Arenberg DA	2000	15	Immunohistochemistry	Patients with recurrence of disease had higher levels of TAMs in their initial tumors	[117]

Table 1 (Continued)

	Year	Number of tumors evaluated	Methods	Findings	Reference
Toomey D	2003	113	Evaluation of TAM density by IHC Follow-up for 3 years	TAM density was not found to be correlated with prognosis	[111]
Chen JJ	2003	35	TAM density correlated with IHC and its relation to IL-8 mRNA and intratumoral microvessels	TAM density correlated significantly and positively with tumor IL-8 mRNA and intratumor microvessels, and significantly and negatively with patient survival	[102]
Tataroglu C	2004	63	IHC with CD68 staining	No correlation between TAMs and tumor stage	[118]
Welsh TJ	2005	175	IHC with CD68 staining accessing separately in tumor islets and stroma	Increased tumor islets macrophage density was found to be a positive prognostic factor, while increased stromal macrophage density was a strong independent predictor of reduced survival	[112]
Chen JJ	2005	41	Count of macrophage density in IHC and correlation with outcome	Significant negative correlation between macrophage density and disease-free survival	[108]
Fridlender ZG	2008	104	IHC with CD68 staining	No correlation between TAM density and lymph node invasion or stage	Not published

carcinoma (LLC) cells. Although these tumors metastasize, they produce only a small number of metastases and not to all the sites to which human lung cancer is known to metastasize. Another model used has been human xenografts grown in SCID/NK-depleted mice. Although these are human tumors, the requirement for immunodeficient mice prevents the study of the role of the acquired immune system [96].

Some of the early studies demonstrating the role of macrophages and macrophage-secreted cytokines on the metastatic process were done during the 1980s using the LLC model. Tumor-associated macrophages were shown to be suppressive to the immune reaction to cancer [97]. Coculture of tumor cells induced TAMs to secrete collagenase and other proteases causing BM degradation [98]. In another study, metastatic formation was augmented by inoculation of thioglycollate-elicited macrophages, now described as alternatively activated macrophages similar to TAMs [99]. The tumoricidal activity of alveolar macrophages (AMs) has also been evaluated, showing a change during tumor growth. Although AMs from LLC-bearing mice were cytotoxic, their activity was suppressed late in tumor growth, in a pattern similar to what has now been described in M2-like TAMs [100].

A partial validation of the important role of TAMs in NSCLC (and breast cancer) metastases has been recently done by Luo et al. [101]. This group showed that a specific reduction of TAMs in the tumor stroma using a vaccine against legumain, a specific M2 marker, reduced tumor cell proliferation, vascularization, and metastasis. This was shown to be related to a reduction in macrophage-released cytokines including VEGF, TNF-α, and TGF-β.

Macrophage-induced angiogenesis was also studied in the LLC lung cancer model. As previously mentioned, the role of the proangiogenic chemokine IL-8 (CXCL-8) was shown in NSCLC. The interaction between tumor cells and TAMs was shown to upregulate IL-8, as well as VEGF expression, in a paracrine manner [102]. On the other hand, a positive role of macrophages in preventing angiogenesis was also shown in the LLC model; macrophage-derived MMPs were shown to be an important factor in the secretion of angiostatin, a potent antiangiogenesis factor [103, 104].

Data about the role of TAMs in other tumors need to be validated in the lungs. Furthermore, specific questions related to the lung should be addressed. One example of these questions is the role of alveolar macrophages (AMs) in the development of lung tumor and metastases. Do the TAMs found in lung tumors originate from these local AM cells with a changed phenotype or are the TAM monocyte-derived cells recruited from the circulation [105]?

Specific animal studies examining the role of tumor-associated neutrophils in lung cancer are even more sparse. Protease activity was studied in lung and breast cancer cells, revealing that the presence of neutrophil elastase activity is related to a worsening of the prognosis with reduced survival and increased metastatic foci [106].

Human Studies

The connection between tumor-associated leukocytes and metastasis has also been examined in patients. More than 80% of the published studies found evidence for an association between the number and/or density of TAMs and the emergence of metastasis leading to reduced survival. This association has been reported in many types of tumors, including breast, prostate, ovary, and stomach [107].

Several studies have assessed the association between tumor macrophage infiltration and invasiveness or prognosis in NSCLC (Table 1); however, no clear conclusions can be reached. In the evaluation reported by Koukourakis et al., 141 cases of early-stage NSCLC that were treated with surgery alone were analyzed. Intense macrophage infiltration was found to be associated with bad prognosis [68]. Similar results were found in another three studies, which evaluated 330 patients [67, 102, 108]. In contrast, three other studies, evaluating 285 patients in total, found no clear correlation between intratumoral infiltration of macrophages and prognosis [109–111]. We have conducted a small study in 102 early-stage NSCLC patients who had surgery. Our data are similar to these latter studies in that we found no correlation between the numbers of TAMs (as defined by positive CD68 staining) and the stage of disease or lymph node metastases.

However, the location of the TAMs may be more important than their numbers. Welsh et al. found in a study of 175 patients that increased tumor islet macrophage density was a strong favorable independent prognostic factor, while tumor stromal macrophage density was an independent predictor of reduced survival [112]. Due to the diverse and multifaceted roles of macrophages within tumors, it seems reasonable to assume that the number of macrophages per se is not a sensitive enough tool to evaluate their influence on prognosis. It is probable that studying other factors, such as activation and maturation markers, will be needed in order to fully appreciate the role of TAM in tumor progression and metastases. Studies linking the presence of TAMs and prognosis in lung cancer are summarized in Table 1.

Rather than looking at macrophage numbers, several studies have linked specific macrophage products with NSCLC progression, development of metastasis, and prognosis. A clue for the importance of TAMs in the metastatic process, and specifically M2 phenotypes, arises from a study demonstrating that the expression of IL-10 by tumor macrophages is a negative prognostic factor in NSCLC and is associated with lymph node invasiveness, advanced stage, and lower survival [113]. In a study of 35 patients with NSCLC, the number of TAMs correlated with IL-8 mRNA and microvessel count and increases in these factors were inversely correlated with survival, suggesting that TAMs secrete angiogenic chemokines that have adverse effects [102]. Interestingly, YKL-40, a newly discovered growth factor with possible involvement in tumor cell proliferation and angiogenesis, was found to be secreted from TAMs and levels of YKL-40 were found to correlate with metastatic disease and poor prognosis [114].

Although little data exists related to tumor-associated neutrophils, neutrophilia is associated with poorer prognosis in bronchoalveolar carcinoma, metastatic melanoma, and renal carcinoma [41, 45, 115].

Despite their potential ability to augment angiogenesis, MCs have been implicated in conferring survival advantages in patients with NSCLC. More specifically, the presence of tumor cell islet MCs was associated with an improved prognosis, suggesting that they may have a protective effect on tumor progression [112]. In addition, a study on mediastinal lymph nodes showed that tumor-free mediastinal lymph nodes carried with them a higher MC count than did metastatic nodes. MC in the metastatic node were primarily located in T-cell areas, suggesting a positive relationship between MC and the T-cell system [52].

Conclusions

There is increasing evidence that the immune cells within the tumor microenvironment play a key role in the ability of tumor cells to proliferate and spread. Given that macrophages are the most frequent hematopoietic cells found in the tumor microenvironment, they play an especially important part in tumor biology. As discussed above, there are numerous mechanisms by which tumor-associated innate immune cells can influence most aspects of the metastatic process (Fig. 2). They play a role in the epithelial to mesenchymal transformation occurring in the original tumor cells and enhance basement membrane breakdown by the cancer cells invading neighboring tissue, lymph nodes, and blood vessels. Tumor-associated innate immune cells have been shown to have a crucial role in angiogenesis, in immunosuppression, and eventually in priming distant sites for the development of metastases. Unfortunately, we still know relatively little about the roles of these cells in lung cancer. Further work in animal models and using patient lung cancer samples is very much needed.

With this knowledge, a better understanding of the role that these cells play in the metastatic process may facilitate development of new therapeutics, as well as the recognition of new diagnostic and prognostic markers. Modulation of the metastatic phenotype through intervention in the host innate immune response remains a promising future area of cancer therapy.

References

1. Gupta, G.P. and Massague, J. 2006. Cancer metastasis: Building a framework. Cell 127: 679–695.
2. Virchow, R. 1863. Aetologie der neoplastichen geschwulste/pathogenie der neoplastichen geschwulste In Die krankhaften geschwulste (Berlin: Verlag von August Hirschwald; reprint).

 3. Pollard, J. 2004. Tumour-educated macrophages promote tumour progression and metastasis. Nat. Rev. Cancer 4: 71–78.
 4. Murdoch, C., Giannoudis, A., and Lewis, C.E. 2004. Mechanisms regulating the recruitment of macrophages into hypoxic areas of tumors and other ischemic tissues. Blood 104: 2224–2234.
 5. Luboshits, G., Shina, S., Kaplan, O., Engelberg, S., Nass, D., Lifshitz-Mercer, B., Chaitchik, S., Keydar, I., and Ben-Baruch, A. 1999. Elevated expression of the CC chemokine regulated on activation, normal T cell expressed and secreted (RANTES) in advanced breast carcinoma. Cancer Res. 59: 4681–4687.
 6. Ueno, T., Toi, M., Saji, H., Muta, M., Bando, H., Kuroi, K., Koike, M., Inadera, H., and Matsushima, K. 2000. Significance of macrophage chemoattractant protein-1 in macrophage recruitment, angiogenesis, and survival in human breast cancer. Clin. Cancer Res. 6: 3282–3289.
 7. Scotton, C., Milliken, D., Wilson, J., Raju, S., and Balkwill, F. 2001. Analysis of CC chemokine and chemokine receptor expression in solid ovarian tumours. Brit. J. Cancer 85: 891.
 8. Balkwill, F. 2003. Chemokine biology in cancer. Semin. Immunol. 15: 49–55.
 9. Muller, A., Homey, B., Soto, H., Ge, N., Catron, D., Buchanan, M.E., Mcclanahan, T., Murphy, E., Yuan, W., Wagner, S.N., Barrera, J.L., Mohar, A., Verastegui, E., and Zlotnik, A. 2001. Involvement of chemokine receptors in breast cancer metastasis. Nature 410: 50–56.
10. Scotton, C.J., Wilson, J.L., Scott, K., Stamp, G., Wilbanks, G.D., Fricker, S., Bridger, G., and Balkwill, F.R. 2002. Multiple actions of the chemokine CXCL2 on epithelial tumor cells in human ovarian cancer. Cancer Res. 62: 5930–5938.
11. Phillips, R.J., Burdick, M.D., Lutz, M., Belperio, J.A., Keane, M.P., and Strieter, R.M. 2003. The stromal derived factor-1/CXCL12-CXC chemokine receptor 4 biological axis in non-small cell lung cancer metastases. Am. J. Respir. Crit. Care Med. 167: 1676–1686.
12. Biswas, S.K., Sica, A., and Lewis, C.E. 2008. Plasticity of macrophage function during tumor progression: Regulation by distinct molecular mechanisms. J. Immunol. 180: 2011–2017.
13. Keller, R, K.R., Keist, R., Wechsler, A., Leist, T.P., and van der Meide, P.H. 1990. Mechanisms of macrophage-mediated tumor cell killing: A comparative analysis of the roles of reactive nitrogen intermediates and tumor necrosis factor. Int. J. Cancer 46: 682–686.
14. Martin, J.H. and Edwards, S.W. 1993. Changes in mechanisms of monocyte/macrophage-mediated cytotoxicity during culture. Reactive oxygen intermediates are involved in monocyte- mediated cytotoxicity, whereas reactive nitrogen intermediates are employed by macrophages in tumor cell killing. J. Immunol. 150: 3478–3486.
15. Grabstein, K.H., Urdal, D.L., Tushinski, R.J., Mochizuki, D.Y, Price, V.L., Cantrell, M. A., Gillis, S., and Conlon, P.J. 1986. Induction of macrophage tumoricidal activity by granulocyte-macrophage colony-stimulating factor. Science 232: 506–508.
16. Kamimura, A., Kamachi, M., Nishihira, J., Ogura, S., Isobe, H., Dosaka-Akita, H., Ogata, A., Shindoh, M., Ohbuchi, T., and Kawakami, Y. 2000. Intracellular distribution of macrophage migration inhibitory factor predicts the prognosis of patients with adenocarcinoma of the lung. Cancer 89: 334–341.
17. Janat-Amsbury, M.M., Yockman, J.W., Lee, M., Kern, S., Furgeson, D.Y., Bikram, M., and Kim, S.W. 2004. Combination of local, nonviral IL-12 gene therapy and systemic paclitaxel treatment in a metastatic breast cancer model. Mol. Ther. 9: 829–836.
18. Li, Q., Carr, A.L., Donald, E.J., Skitzki, J.J., Okuyama, R., Stoolman, L.M., and Chang, A.E. 2005. Synergistic effects of IL-12 and IL-18 in skewing tumor-reactive T-cell responses towards a type 1 pattern. Cancer Res. 65: 1063–1070.
19. Lewis, C.E. and Pollard, J.W. 2006. Distinct role of macrophages in different tumor microenvironments. Cancer Res. 66: 605–612.

20. Coussens, L.M. and Werb, Z. 2002. Inflammation and cancer. Nature 420: 860–867.
21. Mantovani, A., Sozzani, S., Locati M., Allavena, P., and Sica, A. 2002. Macrophage polarization: Tumor associated macrophages as a paradigm for polarized M2 mononuclear phagocytes. Trends Immunol. 23: 549–555.
22. Stout, R.D., Jiang, C., Matta, B., Tietzel, I., Watkins, S.K., and Suttles, J. 2005. Macrophages sequentially change their functional phenotype in response to changes in microenvironmental influences. J. Immunol. 175: 342–349.
23. Mills, C.D., Kincaid, K., Alt, J.M., Heilman, M.J., and Hill, A.M. 2000. M-1/m-2 macrophages and the TH1/TH2 paradigm. J. Immunol. 164: 6166–6173.
24. Munder, M., Eichmann, K., and Modolell, M. 1998. Alternative metabolic states in murine macrophages reflected by the nitric oxide synthase/arginase balance: Competitive regulation by CD4+ t cells correlates with TH1/TH2 phenotype. J. Immunol. 160: 5347–5354.
25. Bonecchi, R., Sozzani, S., Stine, J.T., Luini, W., D'amico, G., Allavena, P., Chantry, D., and Mantovani, A. 1998. Divergent effects of interleukin-4 and interferon-gamma on macrophage-derived chemokine production: An amplification circuit of polarized T helper 2 responses. Blood 92: 2668–2671.
26. Lewis, J.S., Landers, R.J., Underwood, J.C.E., Harris, A.L., and Lewis, C.E. 2000. Expression of vascular endothelial growth factor by macrophages is up-regulated in poorly vascularized areas of breast carcinomas. J. Pathol. 192: 150–158.
27. Welch, D.R., Schissel, D.J., Howrey, R.P., and Aeed, P.A. 1989. Tumor-elicited polymorphonuclear cells, in contrast to normal" circulating polymorphonuclear cells, stimulate invasive and metastatic potentials of rat mammary adenocarcinoma cells. Proc. Natl. Acad. Sci. 86: 5859–5863.
28. Heifets, L. 1982. Centennial of Metchnikoff's discovery. J. Reticuloendothel Soc. 31: 381–391.
29. Di Carlo, E., Forni, G., Lollini, P., Colombo, M.P., Modesti, A., and Musiani, P. 2001. The intriguing role of polymorphonuclear neutrophils in antitumor reactions. Blood 97: 339–345.
30. Ishihara, Y.F.T., Iijima, H., Saito, K., Matsunaga, K. 1998. The role of neutrophils as cytotoxic cells in lung metastasis: Suppression of tumor cell metastasis by a biological response modifier (psk). In Vivo 12: 175–182.
31. Ishihara, Y.I.H. and Matsunaga, K. 1998. Contribution of cytokines on the suppression of lung metastasis. Biotherapy 11: 267–275.
32. Scapini, P., Lapinet-Vera, J.A., Gasperini, S., Calzetti, F., Bazzoni, F., and Cassatella, M.A. 2000. The neutrophil as a cellular source of chemokines. Immunol. Rev. 177: 195–203.
33. Wu, Q.D., Wang, J.H., Condron, C., Bouchier-Hayes, D., and Redmond, H.P. 2001. Human neutrophils facilitate tumor cell transendothelial migration. Am. J. Physiol. Cell Physiol. 280: C814–822.
34. Orr, F.W. and Warner, D.J.A. 1990. Effects of systemic complement activation and neutrophil-mediated pulmonary injury on the retention and metastasis of circulating cancer cells in mouse lungs. Lab. Invest. 62: 331–338.
35. Orr, F.W. and Warner, D.J.A. 2001. Tumor cell interactions with the microvasculature: A rate-limiting step in metastasis. Surg. Oncol. Clin. N. Am. 10: 357–381.
36. Doi, K., Horiuchi, T., Uchinami, M., Tabo, T., Kimura, N., Yokomachi, J., Yoshida, M., and Tanaka, K. 2002. Neutrophil elastase inhibitor reduces hepatic metastases induced by ischaemia-reprefusion in rats. Eur. J. Surg. 168: 507.
37. Aeed, P.A., Nakajima, M., and Welch, D.R. 1988. The role of polymorphonuclear leukocytes (PMN) on the growth and metastatic potential of 13762nf mammary adenocarcinoma cells. Int. J. Cancer 42: 748–759.
38. Nozawa, H., Chiu, C., and Hanahan, D. 2006. Infiltrating neutrophils mediate the initial angiogenic switch in a mouse model of multistage carcinogenesis. Proc. Natl. Acad. Sci. 103: 12493–12498.

39. Schmielau, J. and Finn, O.J. 2001. Activated granulocytes and granulocyte-derived hydrogen peroxide are the underlying mechanism of suppression of T-cell function in advanced cancer patients. Cancer Res. 61: 4756–4760.
40. Zea, A.H., Rodriguez, P.C., Atkins, M.B., Hernandez, C., Signoretti, S., Zabaleta, J., McDermott, D., Quiceno, D., Youmans, A., O'neill, A., Mier, J., and Ochoa, A.C. 2005. Arginase-producing myeloid suppressor cells in renal cell carcinoma patients: A mechanism of tumor evasion. Cancer Res. 65: 3044–3048.
41. Schmidt, H., Bastholt, L., Geertsen, P., Christensen, I.J., Larsen, S., Gehl, J., and Von Der Maase, H. 2005. Elevated neutrophil and monocyte counts in peripheral blood are associated with poor survival in patients with metastatic melanoma: A prognostic model. Brit. J. Cancer 93: 273–278.
42. McGary, C.T., Miele, M.F., and Welch, D.R. 1995. Highly metastatic 13762NF rat mammary adenocarcinoma cell clones stimulate bone marrow by secretion of granulocyte-macrophage colony-stimulating factor/interleukin-3 activity. Am. J. Pathol. 147: 1668–1681.
43. De Larco, J.E., Wuertz, B.R.K., and Furcht, L.T. 2004. The potential role of neutrophils in promoting the metastatic phenotype of tumors releasing interleukin-8. Clin. Cancer Res. 10: 4895–4900.
44. De Larco, J.E., Wuertz, B.R.K., Yee, D., Rickert, B.L., and Furcht, L.T. 2003. Atypical methylation of the interleukin-8 gene correlates strongly with the metastatic potential of breast carcinoma cells. Proc. Natl. Acad. Sci. 100: 13988–13993.
45. Caruso, R.A., Bellocco, R., Pagano, M., Bertoli, G., Rigoli, L., and Inferrera, C. 2002. Prognostic value of intratumoral neutrophils in advanced gastric carcinoma in a high-risk area in northern Italy. Mod. Pathol. 15: 831–837.
46. Gregoire, C., Chasson, L., Luci, C., Tomasello, E., Geissmann, F., Vivier, E., and Walzer, T. 2007. The trafficking of natural killer cells. Immunol. Rev. 220: 169–182.
47. Yang, Q., Goding, S., Hokland, M., and Basse, P. 2006. Antitumor activity of NK cells. Immunol. Res. 36: 13–25.
48. Lu, L.-M., Zavitz, C.C.J., Chen, B., Kianpour, S., Wan, Y., and Stampfli, M.R. 2007. Cigarette smoke impairs NK cell-dependent tumor immune surveillance. J. Immunol. 178: 936–943.
49. Ribatti, D., Crivellato, E., Roccaro, A.M., Ria, R., and Vacca, A. 2004. Mast cell contribution to angiogenesis related to tumour progression. Clin. Exper. Allergy 34: 1660–1664.
50. Tomita, M., Matsuzaki, Y., and Onitsuka, T. 2000. Effect of mast cells on tumor angiogenesis in lung cancer. Ann. Thorac. Surg. 69: 1686–1690.
51. Azizkhan, R.G., Azizkhan, J.C., Zetter, B.R., and Folkman, J. 1980. Mast cell heparin stimulates migration of capillary endothelial cells in vitro. J. Exp. Med. 152: 931–944.
52. Tomita, M., Matsuzaki, Y., Edagawa, M., Shimizu, T., Hara, M., and Onitsuka, T. 2003. Distribution of mast cells in mediastinal lymph nodes from lung cancer patients. World J. Surg. Oncol. 1: 25.
53. Ibaraki, T., Muramatsu, M., Takai, S., Jin, D., Maruyama, H., Orino, T., Katsumata, T., and Miyazaki, M. 2005. The relationship of tryptase- and chymase-positive mast cells to angiogenesis in stage 1 non-small cell lung cancer. Eur. J. Cardio-Thorac. Surg. 28: 617–621.
54. Akhurst, R.J. and Derynck, R. 2001. TGF-β signaling in cancer – a double-edged sword. Trends Cell Biol. 11: S44–S51.
55. Ashley, D.M., Kong, F.M., Bigner, D.D., and Hale, L.P. 1998. Endogenous expression of transforming growth factor beta-1 inhibits growth and tumorigenicity and enhances fas-mediated apoptosis in a murine high-grade glioma model. Cancer Res. 58: 302–309.
56. Wrzesinski, S.H., Wan, Y.Y., and Flavell, R.A. 2007. Transforming growth factor-β and the immune response: Implications for anticancer therapy. Clin Cancer Res. 13: 5262–5270.
57. Bacman, D., Merkel, S., Croner, R., Papadopoulos, T., Brueckl, W., and Dimmler, A. 2007. TGF-beta receptor 2 downregulation in tumour-associated stroma worsens

prognosis and high-grade tumours show more tumour-associated macrophages and lower TGF-beta1 expression in colon carcinoma: A retrospective study. BMC Cancer 7: 156.

58. Hagemann, T., Wilson, J., Kulbe, H., Li, N.F., Leinster, D.A., Charles, K., Klemm, F., Pukrop, T., Binder, C., and Balkwill, F.R. 2005. Macrophages induce invasiveness of epithelial cancer cells via NFκB and JNK. J. Immunol. 175: 1197–1205.

59. Wyckoff, J., Wang, W., Lin, E.Y., Wang, Y., Pixley, F., Stanley, E.R., Graf, T., Pollard, J.W., Segall, J., and Condeelis, J. 2004. A paracrine loop between tumor cells and macrophages is required for tumor cell migration in mammary tumors. Cancer Res. 64: 7022–7029.

60. Domagala, W.S.G., Szadowska, A., Dukowicz, A., Weber, K., and Osborn, M. 1992. Cathepsin B in invasive ductal nos breast carcinoma as defined by immunohistochemistry. No correlation with survival at 5 years. Am. J. Pathol. 141: 1003–1012.

61. Hagemann, T., Robinson, S.C., Schulz, M., Trumper, L., Balkwill, F.R., and Binder, C. 2004. Enhanced invasiveness of breast cancer cell lines upon co-cultivation with macrophages is due to TNF-α dependent up-regulation of matrix metalloproteases. Carcinogenesis 25: 1543–1549.

62. Hiratsuka, S., Nakamura, K., Iwai, S., Murakami, M., Itoh, T., Kijima, H., Shipley, J.M., Senior, R.M., and Shibuya, M. 2002. Mmp9 induction by vascular endothelial growth factor receptor-1 is involved in lung-specific metastasis. Cancer Cell 2: 289–300.

63. Chen, X., Su, Y., Fingleton, B., Acuff, H., Matrisian, L.M., Zent, R., and Pozzi, A. 2005. Increased plasma MMP9 in integrin α1-null mice enhances lung metastasis of colon carcinoma cells. Int. J. Cancer 116: 52–61.

64. Williams, T.M., Medina, F., Badano, I., Hazan, R.B., Hutchinson, J., Muller, W.J., Chopra, N.G., Scherer, P.E., Pestell, R.G., and Lisanti, M.P. 2004. Caveolin-1 gene disruption promotes mammary tumorigenesis and dramatically enhances lung metastasis in vivo: Role of cav-1 in cell invasiveness and matrix metalloproteinase (MMP-2/9) secretion. J. Biol. Chem. 279: 51630–51646.

65. Zhongyun Dong, R.K., Xiulan, Y., and Fidler, I.J. 1997. Macrophage-derived metalloelastase is responsible for the generation of angiostatin in Lewis lung carcinoma. Cell 88: 801–810.

66. Koide, N., Nishio, A., Sato, T., Sugiyama, A., and Miyagawa, S. 2004. Significance of macrophage infiltration in squamous cell carcinoma of the esophagus. Am. J. Gastroenterol. 99: 1667–1674.

67. Takanami, T., Takeuchi, K., and Kodaira, S. 1999. Tumor-associated macrophage infiltration in pulmonary adenocarcinoma: Association with angiogenesis and poor prognosis. Oncology 57: 138–142.

68. Koukourakis Mi, G.A., Kakolyris, S., O'Byrne, K.J., Apostolikas, N., Skarlatos, J., Gatter, K.C., andHarris A.L. 1998. Different patterns of stromal and cancer cell thymidine phosphorylase reactivity in non-small-cell lung cancer: Impact on tumour neoangiogenesis and survival. Brit. J. Cancer. 77: 1696–1703.

69. Barleon, B., Sozzani, S., Zhou, D., Weich, H.A., Mantovani, A., and Marme, D. 1996. Migration of human monocytes in response to vascular endothelial growth factor (VEGF) is mediated via the VEGF receptor flt-1. Blood 87: 3336–3343.

70. Robinson-Smith, T.M., Isaacsohn, I., Mercer, C.A., Zhou, M., Van Rooijen, N., Husseinzadeh, N., Mcfarland-Mancini, M.M., and Drew, A.F. 2007. Macrophages mediate inflammation-enhanced metastasis of ovarian tumors in mice. Cancer Res. 67: 5708–5716.

71. Queen, M.M., Ryan, R.E., Holzer, R.G., Keller-Peck, C.R., and Jorcyk, C.L. 2005. Breast cancer cells stimulate neutrophils to produce oncostatin M: Potential implications for tumor progression. Cancer Res. 65: 8896–8904.

72. Li, A., Dubey, S., Varney, M.L., Dave, B.J., and Singh, R.K. 2003. IL-8 directly enhanced endothelial cell survival, proliferation, and matrix metalloproteinases production and regulated angiogenesis. J. Immunol. 170: 3369–3376.

73. White, E.S., Strom, S.R.B., Wys, N.L., and Arenberg, D.A. 2001. Non-small cell lung cancer cells induce monocytes to increase expression of angiogenic activity. J. Immunol. 166: 7549–7555.
74. White, E.S., Flaherty, K.R., Carskadon, S., Brant, A., Iannettoni, M.D., Yee, J., Orringer, M.B., and Arenberg, D.A. 2003. Macrophage migration inhibitory factor and cxc chemokine expression in non-small cell lung cancer: Role in angiogenesis and prognosis. Clin. Cancer Res. 9: 853–860.
75. Schoppmann, S.F., Birner, P., Stockl, J., Kalt, R., Ullrich, R., Caucig, C., Kriehuber, E., Nagy, K., Alitalo, K., and Kerjaschki, D. 2002. Tumor-associated macrophages express lymphatic endothelial growth factors and are related to peritumoral lymphangiogenesis. Am. J. Pathol. 161: 947–956.
76. Leek, R.D. and Lewis, C.L. 1999. Necrosis correlates with high vascular density and focal macrophage infiltration in invasive carcinoma of the breast. Brit. J. Cancer 79: 991–995.
77. Leek, R.D., Hunt, N.C., Landers, R.J., Lewis, C.E., Royds, J.A., and Harris, A.L. 2000. Macrophage infiltration is associated with VEGF and EGFR expression in breast cancer. J. Pathol. 190: 430–436.
78. Dinapoli, M.R., Calderon, C.L., and Lopez, D.M. 1996. The altered tumoricidal capacity of macrophages isolated from tumor- bearing mice is related to reduce expression of the inducible nitric oxide synthase gene. J. Exp. Med. 183: 1323–1329.
79. Sica, A., Saccani, A., Bottazzi, B., Polentarutti, N., Vecchi, A., Damme, J.V., and Mantovani, A. 2000. Autocrine production of il-10 mediates defective IL-12 production and NFκB activation in tumor-associated macrophages. J. Immunol. 164: 762–767.
80. Li, M.O., Wan, Y.Y., Sanjabi, S., Robertson, A.-K.L., and Flavell, R.A. 2006. Transforming growth factor-β; regulation of immune responses. Ann. Rev. Immunol. 24: 99–146.
81. Teicher, B.A. 2007. Transforming growth factor-β and the immune response to malignant disease. Clin. Cancer Res. 13: 6247–6251.
82. Rodriguez, P.C., Quiceno, D.G., Zabaleta, J., Ortiz, B., Zea, A.H., Piazuelo, M.B., Delgado, A., Correa, P., Brayer, J., Sotomayor, E.M., Antonia, S., Ochoa, J.B., and Ochoa, A.C. 2004. Arginase 1 production in the tumor microenvironment by mature myeloid cells inhibits T-cell receptor expression and antigen-specific T-cell responses. Cancer Res. 64: 5839–5849.
83. Mrass, P. and Weninger, W. 2006. Immune cell migration as a means to control immune privilege: Lessons from the CNS and tumors. Immunol. Rev. 213: 195–212.
84. Kobie, J.J., Wu, R.S., Kurt, R.A., Lou, S., Adelman, M.K., Whitesell, L.J., Ramanathapuram, L.V., Arteaga, C.L., and Akporiaye, E.T. 2003. Transforming growth factor-β inhibits the antigen-presenting functions and antitumor activity of dendritic cell vaccines. Cancer Res. 63: 1860–1864.
85. Marie, J.C., Letterio, J.J., Gavin, M., and Rudensky, A.Y. 2005. TGF-^{2}1 maintains suppressor function and foxp3 expression in CD4 + CD25 + regulatory T cells. J. Exp. Med. 201: 1061–1067.
86. Liu, V.C., Wong, L.Y., Jang, T., Shah, A.H., Park, I., Yang, X., Zhang, Q., Lonning, S., Teicher, B.A., and Lee, C. 2007. Tumor evasion of the immune system by converting CD4 + CD25– T-cells into CD4 + CD25 + T regulatory cells: Role of tumor-derived TGF-β. J. Immunol. 178: 2883–2892.
87. Chang, C.-J., Liao, C.-H., Wang, F.-H., and Lin, C.-M. 2003. Transforming growth factor-β^2 induces apoptosis in antigen-specific CD4 + T cells prepared for adoptive immunotherapy. Immunol. Lett. 86: 37–43.
88. Thomas, D.A. and Massague, J. 2005. TGF-β directly targets cytotoxic T cell functions during tumor evasion of immune surveillance. Cancer Cell 8: 369–380.
89. Ahmadzadeh, M. and Rosenberg, S.A. 2005. TGF-β1 attenuates the acquisition and expression of effector function by tumor antigen-specific human memory CD8 T cells. J. Immunol. 174: 5215–5223.

90. Jakobisiak, M., Lasek, W., and Golab, J. 2003. Natural mechanisms protecting against cancer. Immunol. Lett. 90: 103–122.

91. Hanna, N. 1982. Role of natural killer cells in control of cancer metastasis. Cancer Metastasis Rev. 1: 45–64.

92. Kaplan, R.N., Riba, R.D., Zacharoulis, S., Bramley, A.H., Vincent, L., Costa, C., Macdonald, D.D., Jin, D.K., Shido, K., Kerns, S.A., Zhu, Z., Hicklin, D., Wu, Y., Port, J.L., Altorki, N., Port, E.R., Ruggero, D., Shmelkov, S.V., Jensen, K.K., Rafii, S., and Lyden, D. 2005. VEGFR1-positive haematopoietic bone marrow progenitors initiate the pre-metastatic niche. Nature 438: 820–827.

93. Hiratsuka, S., Watanabe, A., Aburatani, H., and Maru, Y. 2006. Tumour-mediated upregulation of chemoattractants and recruitment of myeloid cells predetermines lung metastasis. Nat. Cell Biol. 8: 1369–1375.

94. Oberg, A., Samii, S., Stenling, R., and Lindmark, G. 2002. Different occurrence of cd8 +, CD45R0 +, and CD68 + immune cells in regional lymph node metastases from colorectal cancer as potential prognostic predictors. Int. J. Colorectal Dis. 17: 25–29.

95. Lin, E.Y., Nguven, A.V., Russell, R.G., and Pollard J.W. 2001. Colony stimulating factor 1 promotes progression of mammary tumors to malignancy. J. Exp. Med. 193: 727–740.

96. Yano, S., Nishioka, Y., Izumi, K., Tsuruo, T., Tanaka, T., Miyasaka, M., and Sone, S. 1996. Novel metastasis model of human lung cancer in SCID mice depleted of NK cells. Int. J. Cancer 67: 211–217.

97. Young, M.R. and Newby, M. 1986. Differential induction of suppressor macrophages by cloned lewis lung carcinoma variants in mice. J. Natl. Cancer Inst. 77: 1255–1260.

98. Henry, N., Van Lamsweerde, A.-L., and Vaes, G. 1983. Collagen degradation by metastatic variants of lewis lung carcinoma: Cooperation between tumor cells and macrophages. Cancer Res. 43: 5321–5327.

99. Gorelik, E., Wiltrout, R.H., Brunda, M.J., Holden, H.T., andHerberman, R.B. 1982. Augmentation of metastasis formation by thioglycollate-elicited macrophages. Int. J. Cancer 29: 575–581.

100. Duffie, G.P. and Young, M.R. 1991. Tumoricidal activity of alveolar and peritoneal macrophages of C57bl/6 mice bearing metastatic or nonmetastatic variants of lewis lung carcinoma. J. Leukoc. Biol. 49: 8–14.

101. Luo, Y., Zhou H., Krueger, J., Kaplan, C., Lee, S., Dolman, C., Markowitz, D., Wu, W., Liu, C., Reisfeld, R.A., Xiang, R. 2006. Targeting tumor-associated macrophages as a novel strategy against breast cancer. J. Clin. Invest. 116: 2132–2141.

102. Chen, J.J.W., Yao, P.-L., Yuan, A., Hong, T.-M., Shun, C.-T., Kuo, M.-L., Lee, Y.-C., and Yang, P.-C. 2003. Up-regulation of tumor interleukin-8 expression by infiltrating macrophages: Its correlation with tumor angiogenesis and patient survival in non-small cell lung cancer. Clin. Cancer Res. 9: 729–737.

103. Cornelius, L.A., Nehring, L.C., Harding, E., Bolanowski, M., Welgus, H.G., Kobayashi, D.K., Pierce, R.A., and Shapiro, S.D. 1998. Matrix metalloproteinases generate angiostatin: Effects on neovascularization. J. Immunol. 161: 6845–6852.

104. Dong, Z., Kumar, R., Yang, X., and Fidler, I.J. 1997. Macrophage-derived metalloelastase is responsible for the generation of angiostatin in lewis lung carcinoma. Cell 88: 801–810.

105. Montuenga, L.M. and Pio, R. 2007. Tumour-associated macrophages in nonsmall cell lung cancer: The role of interleukin-10. Eur. Respir. J. 30: 608–610.

106. Sato, T., Takahashi, S., Mizumoto, T., Harao, M., Akizuki, M., Takasugi, M., Fukutomi, T., and Yamashita, J.-I. 2006. Neutrophil elastase and cancer. Surg. Oncol. 15: 217–222.

107. Bingle, L., Brown, N., and Lewis, C.E. 2002. The role of tumor-associated macrophages in tumor progression: Implications for new anticancer therapies. J. Pathol. 196: 254–265.

108. Chen, J.J., Lin, Y.C., Yao, P.L., Yuan, A., Chen, H.Y., Shun, C.T., Tsai, M.F., Chen, C. H., and Yang, P.C. 2005. Tumor-associated macrophages: The double-edged sword in cancer progression. J. Clin. Oncol. 23: 953–964.

109. Takeo, S., Yasumoto, K., Nagashima, A., Nakahashi, H., Sugimachi, K., and Nomoto, K. 1986. Role of tumor-associated macrophages in lung cancer. Cancer Res. 46: 3179–3182.

110. Johnson, S.K., Kerr, K.M., Chapman, A.D., Kennedy, M.M., King, G., Cockburn, J.S., and Jeffrey, R.R. 1999. Immune cell infiltrates and prognosis in primary carcinoma of the lung. Lung Cancer 27: 27–35.

111. Toomey, D., Symthe, G., Condron, C., Kelly, J., Byrne, A.M., Kay, E., Conroy, R.M., Broe, P., and Bouchier-Hayes, D. 2003. Infiltrating immune cells, but not tumour cells, express fasl in non-small cell lung cancer: No association with prognosis identified in 3-year follow-up. Intl. J. Cancer 103: 408–412.

112. Welsh, T.J., Green, R.H., Richardson, D., Waller, D.A., O'byrne, K.J., and Bradding, P. 2005. Macrophage and mast-cell invasion of tumor cell islets confers a marked survival advantage in non-small-cell lung cancer. J. Clin. Oncol. 23: 8959–8967.

113. Zeni, E., Mazzetti, L., Miotto, D., Lo Cascio, N., Maestrelli, P., Querzoli, P., Pedriali, M., De Rosa, E., Fabbri, L.M., Mapp, C.E., and Boschetto, P. 2007. Macrophage expression of interleukin-10 is a prognostic factor in nonsmall cell lung cancer. Eur. Respir. J. 30: 627–632.

114. Junker, N., Johansen, J.S., Andersen, C.B., and Kristjansen, P.E.G. 2005. Expression of YKL-40 by peritumoral macrophages in human small cell lung cancer. Lung Cancer 48: 223–231.

115. Ferrigno, D.B.G. 2003. Hematologic counts and clinical correlates in 1201 newly diagnosed lung cancer patients. Monaldi Arch. Chest Dis. 59: 193–198.

116. Kerr, K.M., Johnson, S.K., King, G., Kennedy, M.M., Weir, J. and Jeffrey, R. 1998. Partial regression in primary carcinoma of the lung: Does it occur? Histopathology 33:55–63.

117. Arenberg, D.A., Keane, M.P. Digiovine, B., Kunkle, S.L., Strom, S.R, Burdick, M.D., Iannettoni, M.D., and Strieter, R.M. 2000. Macrophage infiltration in human non-small-cell lung cancer: The role of cc chemokines. Cancer Immunol. Immunother 49:63–70.

118. Tataroglu, C., Kargi, A., Ozkal, S., Esrefoglu, N., and Akkoclu, A. 2004. Association of macrophages, mast cells and eosinophil leukocytes with angiogenesis and tumor stage in non-small cell lung carcinomas (nsclc). Lung Cancer 43: 47–54.

Experimental Animal Models for Studying Lung Cancer

Jiang Liu and Michael R. Johnston

Abstract Lung cancer is the leading cause of cancer-related mortality for both men and women worldwide. The use of animal models of lung cancer is necessary to improve our understanding of lung tumor biology and facilitate novel therapies and diagnostics. To this end, animal models should mimic both the genetic alterations found in human lung tumors and their histological characteristics. Currently, several types of animal models are widely used for experimental lung cancer research. These include chemically induced lung tumors, transgenic mouse models, and human tumor xenografts. A single model system that faithfully recaptures the entire spectrum of lung cancer biology is unlikely to exist. Different models that accurately reflect the various aspects of the disease are necessary to properly investigate such a complex disease. Tumorigenesis, proliferation, invasion, angiogenesis, metastasis, prevention, and therapy are all areas where specific models are required to ensure proper experimental design.

The purpose of this chapter is to summarize the various lung cancer model systems in use today and define both their utility and limitations. We will briefly describe all of these models and provide a more detailed description of the orthotopic lung cancer xenograft models.

Introduction

Lung cancer is the leading cause of cancer-related mortality for both men and women worldwide. It presents a challenge to basic research to provide new steps toward therapeutic advances. Most patients die of progressive metastatic disease despite aggressive local and systemic therapies. The pathogenesis of lung cancer remains highly elusive due to its aggressive biologic nature and considerable heterogeneity, as compared to other cancers [1]. These circumstances

J. Liu (✉)

Division of Applied Molecular Oncology, Princess Margaret Hospital, University Health Network, Toronto, Ontario M5G 2M9, Canada

e-mail: jiang.liu@utoronto.ca

V. Keshamouni et al. (eds.), *Lung Cancer Metastasis*,
DOI 10.1007/978-1-4419-0772-1_12, © Springer Science+Business Media, LLC 2009

substantially impede the study of the disease in humans and necessitate the use of experimental models that can be used under more uniform, controlled conditions than that achievable in clinical settings. The development of animal models of lung cancer may aid in our understanding of lung tumor biology and facilitate the development and testing of novel therapeutic approaches and methods for early diagnosis. To this end, animal models should mimic both the genetic alterations found in human lung tumors and their histological characteristics.

The laboratory murine model has been used extensively in lung cancer research. Currently, several types of animal models are widely used for experimental lung cancer research. These include chemically induced lung tumors, transgenic mouse models, and human tumor xenografts.

A single model system that faithfully reflects the whole process of lung cancer carcinogenesis and progression is unlikely to be developed. Lung cancer models that accurately reflect the different aspects of the disease are necessary to properly investigate its myriad complexities. Tumorigenesis, proliferation, invasion, angiogenesis, metastasis, prevention, and therapy are all areas where specific models are required to ensure proper experimental design. To reflect the anticipated biological process being studied, model systems may require certain deviations from the human disease. Thus, we should interpret results of studies utilizing model systems with caution and with an appropriate understanding of their limitations. The purpose of this chapter is to summarize the various lung cancer model systems in use today and define both their utility and limitations. As Siemann stated [2], it is best to "... choose the model to address the question rather than force the question on the tumor model."

General Principles

Tumor–host interactions, including immunologic effects, vascular and stromal effects, and host-related pharmacologic and pharmacokinetic effects, are poorly modeled in vitro. Animal models to study these areas can be broadly divided into spontaneous or induced tumors and transplanted tumors. The former group consists of those induced by some extrinsic chemical or carcinogen and animals genetically modified to express genes that lead to lung tumor development. The latter group includes the widely used heterograft and xenograft models. We will briefly describe all of these models and provide a more detailed description of the orthotopic lung cancer xenograft models.

In general the spontaneous or chemical-induced tumor models most closely mimic the clinical situation [3]. The advantage offered by these models is that they mimic natural events, leading to the development of lung cancer. Several studies have shown that lung tumors developed in mice or rats are quite similar in histology, molecular characteristics, and histogenesis to human lung cancer [4, 5]. Unfortunately, these tumors are usually measurable only late in their course, their metastatic pattern is not uniform, and their response to therapy is generally poor. Because of these limitations, spontaneous and chemical-induced model systems are usually reserved for studies of carcinogenesis and cancer prevention [6].

The advent of transgenic technology has significantly improved the ability to define the role of specific genes in the process of transformation and disease progression. The mouse is a promising model system, as complex human genetic traits causal to lung cancer, from inherited polymorphisms to somatic mutations, can be recapitulated in its genome via genetic manipulation. The conventional transgenic mouse models for lung cancer constitutively expressed regulatory genes in the pulmonary epithelium. Subsequent generations of transgenic mouse models further enhanced the ability to clarify the specific molecular mechanisms by allowing for cell-specific-regulated expression or ablation of genes in the lung. These genetically engineered models can be exploited to define the molecular events that contribute to the pathogenesis and progression of this disease.

Transplanted animal tumor models and the human tumor xenografts are widely used in experimental therapeutics. Since malignant cells or tissues are directly inoculated into the host animal, effects on early events, such as initiation and carcinogenesis, are not well suited for study. Because tumor development uniformly follows inoculation with predictable growth and metastatic pattern, areas amenable for investigation include tumor growth, invasion, and metastasis. Testing of new therapeutic approaches and screening strategies is also particularly well suited for these models.

Chemical-Induced Lung Cancer Models

In our daily lives we are constantly exposed to potentially harmful mixtures of chemical and physical agents. The laboratory environment allows controlled administration of environmental and other toxins to animals. Chemical or carcinogen-induced lung tumors have been described in a variety of species, including dogs, cats, hamsters, mice, and ferrets; however, the mouse is most widely used. Specific inbred strains of mice susceptible to the development of spontaneous lung tumors, such as A/J and SWR, are also sensitive to chemically induced lung tumors [7]. This observation has led to the development of quantitative carcinogenicity bioassays [8] and screening systems for the efficacy of chemopreventive agents [9, 10]. If a newborn inbred A/J mouse is given a single intraperitoneal injection of ethyl carbamate (urethane), it will develop dozens of benign lung adenomas within a few months [8]. Some of these induced tumors eventually progress to adenocarcinomas that are histopathologically indistinguishable from human adenocarcinomas [11].

Strain A mice are also used extensively as a murine lung tumor bioassay to assess carcinogenic activity of chemicals and environmental agents, including urethane, benzopyrene, metals, aflatoxin, and constituents of tobacco smoke such as polyaromatic hydrocarbons and nitrosamines [8,12]. These agents can act as initiators and/or promoters of pulmonary tumorigenesis by accelerating tumor onset and increasing tumor multiplicity. The most common environmental exposure contributing to human lung cancer is tobacco smoke, which contains over 4,000 chemicals, gases, and volatiles. Developing an animal model for tobacco-induced cancer has generally relied on carcinogenicity studies of single components such as nitrosamine 4-(methylnitrosamino)-1-(3-pyridyl)-1-butanone (NNK). If male Balb/c and SWR mice are exposed to tobacco smoke for 5 months (6 h/day, 5 days/week; average concentration, 122 mg/m^3 of total suspended particulates followed by a recovery period of 4 months), there is an increase in incidence and number of lung tumors in both strains [13]. Second-hand or "environmental" tobacco smoke (ETS) exposure also induced lung tumors in a series of studies in which strain A/J mice were exposed to a well-defined ETS atmosphere. These studies provide convincing evidence that ETS is a potent mouse carcinogen [14]. Studying the mechanisms underlying lung tumor development in these tobacco-induced models may provide valuable clues to sorting out the initiation of smoking-related lung cancer in humans. In addition to chemicals, both radiation and viruses induce lung tumors in mice [15]. Although induction of lung tumors is highly reproducible [16], all chemical-induced lung tumors exhibit low metastatic potential. Table 1 summarizes data on some carcinogen-induced lung cancer models.

Table 1 Carcinogen-induced lung cancer models

Carcinogen	Route of administration	Phenotype	References
3-Methylcholanthrene	Transplacenta	Pulmonary adenomas	[17]
N-Nitrosobis-(2-chloroethyl) ureas	Topical	Squamous cell and adenosquamous carcinomas	[18]
Urethane	Intraperitoneal	Pulmonary adenomas	[19]
Benzo(a)pyrene Diethylnitrosamine Ethylnitrosourea Dimethylhydrazine	Intraperitoneal	Pulmonary adenomas	[20]

During tumor initiation and promotion, carcinogenesis is usually a result of changes in gene expression, rather than structural alteration. The carcinogenic process is therefore still reversible and a good opportunity for chemoprevention is potentially available. In addition to carcinogen detection, the strain A model has also been used to assess the ability of potential chemopreventive agents to protect against the development of carcinogen-induced lung tumors. A number of chemopreventive agents, including β-naphthoflavone [21], butylated hydroxyanisole [22], ellagic acid [23], phenethyl isothiocyanate [24], α-difluoromethylornithine combined with green tea, dexamethasone, and piroxicam [25], green tea, and black tea [26], were shown to inhibit chemical-induced lung tumors in strain A mice. In most instances, inhibition of lung tumorigenesis was correlated with effects of the chemopreventive agents on metabolic activation and/or detoxification of carcinogens.

Various anti-inflammatory drugs inhibit mouse lung tumorigenesis. These include nonsteroidal anti-inflammatory drugs, such as indomethacin, sulindac, and aspirin [27, 28]. Those that induce regression of benign colonic polyps in humans are modestly effective at lowering lung tumor incidence and multiplicity in mice [28]. The density of apoptotic cell bodies increased 2.9-fold in lung adenomas in A/J mice treated with indomethacin [29]. Studies have also shown that selective inhibition of COX-2 can reduce lung and regional lymph node metastasis in an in vivo lung cancer model [5, 30]. However, in some murine lung tumor models, celecoxib, a selective COX-2 inhibitor, was ineffective in suppressing tumor development [31]. In a recent study, prostacyclin synthase overexpression significantly decreased both the lung tumor incidence and the multiplicity in a tobacco-induced lung cancer model, providing additional evidence that manipulation of prostaglandin production distal to COX may be an attractive lung cancer chemopreventive strategy [32].

Because tumorigenesis in chemical-induced lung cancer is initiated by the investigator, each stage of neoplasia, such as hyperplasia, benign tumor formation, and the benign-to-malignant transition, can be studied independently. Thus, the molecular changes that precede the onset of hyperplastic foci and those during the evolution to malignancy can be distinguished from frank malignancy and phenotypes identified that might be useful for early diagnosis.

Despite the usefulness of chemical- or carcinogen-induced lung cancer models, there are major disadvantages of these models: a heterogenous response to the carcinogen with variable natural histories; a long incubation time; strain-dependent tumor development; and a very low rate of spontaneous metastasis. Mice develop primary lung tumors quite similar in structure, molecular characteristics, and histogenesis to human adenocarcinomas (ACs) and to the bronchioloalveolar carcinoma (BAC) subset of AC in particular. Small cell lung cancer and squamous cell carcinoma rarely occur in murine models. The major histological type induced by carcinogen exposure is BAC and by chemical exposure is adenocarcinoma, whereas squamous cell carcinoma is more common in animals exposed to high doses of radiation [33]. Finally, administration of chemicals or carcinogens can produce a variety of different tumor cell types, many of which might not be directly relevant to human lung cancer.

Transgenic Lung Cancer Models

Multiple genetic changes are involved in the development and progression of lung cancer. The cell-type-specific responses to oncogenic mutations that initiate and regulate lung cancer remain poorly defined. A better understanding of the relevant signaling pathways and mechanisms that control therapeutic outcome could also provide new insight. The generation of transgenic mouse strains able to develop lung cancer similar to the human situation enabled the identification of the genes that drive lung cancer development and progression. The ability to integrate a gene of interest into the genome of an animal provides a novel approach for cancer investigation. Transgenic mouse technology has proved useful in creating models of tumor development, in cloning immortalized cellular subpopulations, and in testing experimental therapeutic approaches [34, 35]. Gene transfection can be achieved with microinjection [36, 37], retroviral infection, or embryonic stem cell transfer [38, 39]. Transgenic mice are excellent models for studying the consequences of oncogene expression in animals, the effect of oncogenes on growth and differentiation, and their potential for cellular transformation. Conventionally, the transgene DNA construct is generated by the fusion of a cell-specific promoter to direct transcription of the gene of interest. This transgene DNA is subsequently microinjected into fertilized oocytes. The transgene is integrated into the host genome and then undergoes random integration into the mouse genome. The viable oocytes are then transferred into pseudopregnant mothers, and the DNA obtained from progeny is assessed for integration of the transgene into the mouse genome [40, 41]. Using this technology, gene expression has been directed in a cell-specific fashion to the lung. The first oncogene targeted specifically to the lung was the Simian virus large T antigen (Tag). Tag was targeted with both the surfactant protein C (*SP-C*) [42] and the Clara cell secretory protein (*CCSP*) [43] promoters. Both models resulted in adenocarcinoma of the lung.

When mutated H-*ras*, *p53*, or SV40 T antigen is used as a transgene and integrated into the host genome, lung tumors develop in mice soon after birth, resulting in early death of the animal. These genes may be nonspecifically expressed throughout the body or linked to lung-specific promoters so that their expression is selective for Clara cells or alveolar type II pneumocytes [44, 45]. Animals such as these are used to investigate molecular events in the progression of lung cancer. However, the rapid progression and early onset of cancer makes investigation of early events difficult [46]. When a new genetic material either is added to the genome or genes, such as tumor suppressor genes, or is removed from the genome (knockout), the effects can occur immediately and continue throughout the life span of the animal. Thus, mice develop tumors early in life and usually have a shortened life span. Human lung cancers often have mutations of both the retinoblastoma (*Rb*) and *p53* suppressor genes. When transgenic mice are created with the same mutations, they develop bronchial hyperplasia, but die of other neoplasms, including islet cell carcinoma, before progression to lung cancer can occur [47]. A limitation of using these approaches to generate transgenic models for lung cancer is the timing of the initiation of expression of these genes under the control of these promoters.

Currently, the most effective regulatory systems for conditional transgenic mice are the ligand-inducible binary transgenic systems that confer regulated expression of the desired gene [48, 49]. These systems consist of using at least two transgene constructs, a regulator transgene and a target transgene. The target transgene is silent until the regulator transgene is activated by the administration of an exogenous compound. An example is a bitransgenic model, such as the tetracycline transactivator-inducible system [50] in which mice are produced with two separate mutations that are activated or deactivated by tetracycline. This system has two major advantages over conventional transgenic mice. First, the transgene can be turned on at any time by administering tetracycline and thus resembles a somatic mutation. Second, regulated loss of expression (turning off the transgene by withdrawing tetracycline) can be used to determine whether the transgene is required to maintain growth and proliferation of the tumor.

A transgenic mouse model of lung adenocarcinoma with expression of a mutant active K-ras transgene was developed using this regulatory transgenic technology [51]. Tumors rapidly regress as a result of apoptosis when doxycycline, a tetracycline analog, is withdrawn. This is a clear demonstration of the role of K-ras in lung tumorigenesis. Several other lung cancer mouse models with conditional activation of oncogenic K-ras are also described [52]. The use of regulatory transgenic systems such as this provides a valuable tool for identifying targets for future drug development strategies.

An animal model of small cell lung cancer (SCLC) has been particularly difficult to develop. Recently, Meuwissen et al. established an animal model of SCLC with remarkable similarity to the human disease [53]. This model utilizes mice carrying Cre–LoxP-based conditional alleles of the Rb and p53 tumor suppressor genes. Deletion of these genes in the lung cells was achieved through intrabronchial injection of a recombinant adenovirus expressing the Cre recombinase (Ad-Cre). This method reproducibly resulted in the development of lung tumors with the histology, immunohistochemistry, and metastatic behavior of human SCLC. Most of these tumors spread diffusely through the lung and gave rise to extrapulmonary metastases at multiple sites, including bone, brain, adrenal gland, ovary, and liver. This model system exhibits several other important similarities to human SCLC. First, the coexistence of SCLC and NSCLC imitates a common clinical occurrence of both histologies present within the same tumor. Second, immunostaining revealed that most lesions are positive for the neuroendocrine marker synaptophysin (Syp) and the neural cell adhesion molecule Ncam1 (CD 56), indicating neuroendocrine differentiation. If the model exhibits an autocrine growth signal similar to human SCLC, it may be of value in developing therapies directed at blocking this signal. Improved conditional mouse models are now available as tools to improve the understanding of the cellular and molecular origins of adenocarcinoma. These models have already proven their utility in proof-of-principle experiments with new technologies including genomics and imaging [54]. Presently, there is no genetic mouse model of squamous cell carcinoma of the lung. A better understanding of the cell of origin that gives rise to lung squamous cell carcinoma might help the squamous cell carcinoma mouse model development. Tables 2 and 3 summarize some useful information concerning conventional and conditional transgenic lung cancer models, respectively.

Table 2 Conventional transgenic lung cancer models

Model design	Transgene/gene knockout/knock-in	Promoter	Phenotype	References
Viral oncogene	Tag	CCSP	Multifocal early onset bronchioloalveolar hyperplasias progressing to adenocarcinomas	[55]
	TAg	SP-C	Adenocarcinomas including papillary, solid, and bronchioloalveolar subtypes	[56]
	TAg	CaBP9K	Lung adenocarcinomas	[57]
Signaling/kinase	Myc	SP-C	Pulmonary tumors ranging from bronchioloalveolar adenomas to adenocarcinomas. Phenotype shows incomplete penetrance	[58]
	c-Raf-1	SP-C	Lung adenomas	[59]
	c-Raf-1-BxB	SP-C	Lung adenomas	[59]
	H-Ras	CGRP	Pulmonary neuroendocrine (NE) hyperplasia and non-NE adenocarcinomas	[60]
Growth factor receptor	RON	SP-C	Adenomas and adenocarcinomas	[61]
Growth factor	IgEGF	SP-C	Alveolar hyperplasia	[58]
	IgEGF × Myc	SP-C	Accelerated tumor progression	[58]
Transcription factor	hASH1	CC10	Airway hyperplasia and bronchioloalveolar metaplasia	[62]
	hASH1 × TAg	CC10	Adenocarcinoma with neuroendocrine features	[62]

Table 3 Conditional transgenic lung cancer models

Model design	Transgene	Promoter	Phenotype	References
Tumor suppressors	Rb, p53	Knock-in	Small cell lung carcinoma	Meuwissen et al. [53]
	p53	Knock-in	Adenocarcinoma	Meuwissen et al. [53]
Signaling/kinases	LSL-K-ras G12D	Knock-in	Adenocarcinoma and epithelial hyperplasia of the bronchioles	Jackson et al. [24]
	K-ras4b G12D	Tet-O	Adenocarcinomas that regress upon removal of doxycycline	Fisher et al. [51]
	rTA	CCSP		
	K-ras V12	B-actin	Adenocarcinomas	Meuwissen et al. [52]
Growth factor	FGF-3	UASG	Alveolar macrophage infiltration and alveolar type II cell hyperplasia	Zhao et al. [46]
	GLp65	SP-C		

Human Lung Tumor Xenografts

Cancer research started with transplanted tumors in animals, which provided the first reproducible and controllable materials for investigations. Transplanting human tumor into rodents and maintaining the histological and biological identity of tumor cells through successive passages in vivo revolutionized cancer research, in particular, drug development [63]. Since human neoplasms are rejected when implanted into another species, the host animal must be immunosuppressed. Irradiation, thymectomy, splenectomy, and corticosteroids were initially used to blunt acquired immunity. With the successful breeding of hairless nude mouse mutants (nu/nu homozygotes), severe combined immunodeficient (SCID) mice, and Rowett nude rats, laboratory animals are now readily available for the transplantation of human tumors.

Subcutaneous implantation in nude mice is the most common method of transplanting human tumor material. The procedure is straightforward and the site, usually the dorsal lateral flank, is easily accessible. Studies have shown that subcutaneous xenograft models can emulate clinical behavior [64], although recently some authors have questioned the accuracy of these data when applied to human drug trials [65]. These models, however, have major disadvantages including (1) a low tumor take rate for fresh clinical specimens [66]; (2) tumor growth in an unusual tissue compartment (the subcutis), the microenvironment of which might influence study results; and (3) the lack of consistent invasion and metastasis [67], properties that are closely linked to clinical outcome in humans.

In orthotopic models, human tumors are implanted in the laboratory animal directly into the appropriate organ or tissue of origin. Advantages include improved tumor take rates, along with enhanced invasive and metastatic properties [67, 68]. The metastatic phenotype of many tumors is expressed after orthotopic implantation; for example, colon carcinoma cells grown in the cecal wall, bladder carcinoma in the bladder, renal cell carcinoma cells under the renal capsule, and melanomas implanted subdermally all yield metastases at much higher frequency than when grown subcutaneously [69]. An organ-specific site presumably provides tumor cells with the most appropriate milieu for local growth and metastasis, thereby supporting Paget's hypothesis that metastasis is not a random phenomenon. Rather, he concluded that malignant cells have special affinity for growth in the environment of their origin, the familiar seed, and soil theory [70]. Although orthotopic tumors are more virulent and animal survival is shortened, the models in general are more complex and more costly than subcutaneous models.

Orthotopic Lung Cancer Models

Orthotopic lung cancer models are described using endobronchial, intrathoracic, or intravenous injection of tumor cell suspensions [71–73] and by surgical implantation of fresh tumor tissue [74, 75]. McLemore et al. [73] developed the first orthotopic lung cancer model by implanting lung cancer cell lines and disaggregated lung tumors into the lung of nude mice by endobronchial injection. The tumors grew more extensively within the lung than the same tumors implanted subcutaneously. However, most of the tumors stayed within the lung, resulting in only 3% metastasis to lymph nodes, liver, or spleen. A second model was developed by McLemore [76] by percutaneously injecting lung tumor cells into the pleural space. This model gave high tumor take rates, reproducible growth, and a mortality endpoint as a result of local disease progression; however, few metastases were seen. Since cancer cells are seeded into the pleural space rather than within the pulmonary parenchyma or bronchi, its relevance to human lung cancer is doubtful.

Our laboratory also used endobronchial implantation to grow non-small cell (A549, NCI-H460, and NCI-H125) and small cell (NCI-H345) lung tumors, but in nude rats rather than mice [71]. In these models, metastasis to mediastinal lymph nodes is frequently seen, but systemic metastases are rare. Subsequently, we described a systemic metastatic model by endobronchial implantation of tumor fragments derived from orthotopic lung tumors grown from the H460 cell line. This H460 nude rat model has a 100% primary tumor take rate in the lung with a rapid and reproducible growth rate of about 4 g over a 32–35-day period. It also metastasizes at a consistent rate to both regional mediastinal lymph nodes and distant systemic sites, including bone, brain, kidney, and contralateral lung. This is the first human lung cancer model to show extensive systemic metastasis from a primary lung site [72].

Several other intrathoracic human lung cancer models are described, all using immunocompromised mice. One is the traditional intravenous model in which the lung is colonized with tumor cells after tail vein injection [77, 78]. In another, tumor grows in a subpleural location from either tumor cell inoculation or fragments sewn onto the surface of the left lung [79, 611]. Recently, a SCID lung cancer model that develops lymphatic metastasis following percutaneous injection of cancer cells into the mouse lung was described [80]. None of these models grows from a primary endobronchial site and none develops a consistent metastatic pattern in extrathoracic locations.

The H460 orthotopic rat model has several advantages over the mouse models: (1) primary tumors originate within the bronchial tree, similar to most human lung cancers. (2) Primary tumors are confined to the right caudal lobe. This makes it unlikely that metastases arise from mechanical spread of the implanted tumor material. (3) A 10-fold larger size of the rat facilitates surgical manipulations, such as cannulation, and allows implantation of tumor fragments that are too large for the mouse bronchus.

Fresh human lung tumor tissues or tissues from metastatic lesions are also implanted orthotopically [81]. Such models putatively maintain intact critical stromal epithelial relationships, even though the source of most stromal tissue is probably from the host, rather than the xenograft [82]. Wang et al. [83] implanted human small cell lung cancer tissue into the mouse lung. Metastases were found in contralateral lung and mediastinal lymph nodes. Two tumor lines

Table 4 Orthotopic lung cancer models

Author	Animal	Tumor Material	Inoculation Method	Take rate	Regional	Distant	Average growth time
McLemore et al. [73]	Nude mice	H125, H358, H460, A549	Endobronchial	90%	Trachea 2%, peritracheal 6%, lymph node 90%	Left lung, liver, spleen 3%	9–61 days
Howard et al. [71]	Nude rats	H125, H460, A549, H345	Endobronchial	100%, 83%, 90%	Regional lymph nodes	H-125, A549 to contralateral lung	H460 (3 weeks) A549 (5 weeks) H125 (10 wks)
Howard et al. [72]	Nude rats	Tumor fragment derived from H460 lung tumors	Endobronchial	100%	Lymph node 100%	Bone, brain, kidney, left lung, soft tissue	32–35 days
Wang et al. [74]	SCID mice Nude mice	Tumor fragment from A549 subcut. tumor	Thoracotomy	3/5	Chest wall	Contralateral lung	N/A
Wang et al. [83]	SCID mice Nude mice	Human SCLC tumor fragment	Thoracotomy	100%	Mediastinum, chest wall lymph nodes	Contralateral lung	18.5–62 days

(Continued)

Table 4 (Continued)

Author	Animal	Tumor Material	Inoculation Method	Take rate	Regional	Distant	Average growth time
Nagamachi et al. [79]	Nude mice	A549, H23, H441, H157, Lu65, Lu99A PC9, PC14	Intrapleural	100% except H23	Mediastinum, lymph nodes	Contralateral lung	Depends on specific cell line PC14 within 30 days
Miyoshi et al. [80]	SCID mice	Ma-44	Percutaneous intrapulmonary	N/A	Lymph node 52%	Contralateral lung 52%	17.5 ± 6.0 days
Cuenca et al. [81]	SCID mice	Human NSCLC biopsy specimens	Anterior thoracotomy	31%	N/A	Metastasis rate 50%; contralateral lung 37.5%	4–6 months
Vertrees et al. (2000) [84]	Athymic nude mice	BZR-T33	Endobronchial intubation	100%	Lymph node	Axillary lymph node, liver, kidney	Approximately 5 weeks
Liu et al. [93]	Nude rats	H460SM	Endobronchial	100%	Lymph node	Bone, brain, kidney, left lung, soft tissue	32–35 days

derived from fresh human non-small cell lung cancer were established in our laboratory by endobronchial implantation in nude rats (unpublished data). Interestingly, one tumor line developed contralateral lung metastasis which was very similar in appearance to metastases in the patient from whom the tumor line originated. Table 4 provides a summary of orthotopic lung cancer models.

Useful Models for the Study of Lung Cancer Metastasis

Over 85% of lung cancer patients harbor overt or subclinical metastases at diagnosis, thus accounting for the poor prognosis in this disease. Unfortunately, little is known about the molecular pathways responsible for tumor progression to metastasis. Appropriate animal models to study these sequences may help us understand these complex pathways.

Entry of tumor cells into the circulation is a critical first step in the metastatic cascade, and although assayed in various ways [85], it has not been observed directly. Novel approaches to specifically "mark" the tumor cell hold promise. For example, one can engineer tumor cells to express the green fluorescence protein (GFP) for in vivo fluorescence imaging. In order to understand the metastatic pattern of non-small cell lung cancer (NSCLC), Yang M et al. developed a high-expression GFP transductant of human lung cancer cell line H460 (H460-GFP), which visualized widespread skeletal metastases when implanted orthotopically in nude mice [86]. This makes possible the direct study of tumor growth and metastasis as well as tumor angiogenesis and gene expression. It can reveal the microscopic stages of tumor growth and metastatic seeding as real-time visualization of micrometastases, even down to the single-cell level.

Neoplasms are biologically heterogeneous and contain genotypically and phenotypically diverse subpopulations of tumor cells, each of which has the potential to complete some but not all of the steps in the metastatic process [87, 88]. Recent studies using in situ hybridization and immunohistochemical staining show that the expression of genes and proteins associated with proliferation, angiogenesis, cohesion, motility, and invasion varies among different regions of a neoplasm [89]. Studies have also shown that tissue obtained from metastatic sites grows more readily than ablated primary tumors [90]. This is consistent with the ability of metastatic cells to grow at a foreign site and suggests that these metastatic adaptations are also applicable to growth at xenotransplantation sites. In general, metastasis favors the survival and growth of a few subpopulations of cells that preexist within the parent neoplasm. In addition, metastases may have a clonal origin, with different metastases originating from the proliferation of different single cells. Therefore, the search for those metastasis-associated genes and proteins cannot be conducted by an indiscriminate and nonselective processing of tumor tissues. Isolating these clones from other cell populations in the parent neoplasm provides a powerful tool to study those properties that distinguish metastatic from nonmetastatic cells [91, 92]. One method to separate these cell populations is to develop cell variants through in vivo propagation and selection. By selectively harvesting tumor cells from mediastinal lymph nodes in our H460 orthotopic lung cancer model and subjecting them to several cycles of in vitro and in vivo orthotopic passage, we have established a clonal H460SM variant cell line that spontaneously produces widespread systemic metastases following orthotopic implantation [93]. In contrast to the two-step NCI-H460 metastatic model mentioned previously [72], the one-step metastatic model with the H460SM cell line provides a simpler system to characterize molecular mechanisms leading to nodal and systemic metastases. To our knowledge, the H460SM orthotopic model represents the first lung cancer rodent model derived from a human lung cancer cell line that closely mimics the spectrum of common metastatic sites observed in NSCLC patients.

Kozaki et al. [94] also used the NCI-H460 cell line as a basis to establish a lymphatic metastasis model of NSCLC. In their model, the H460-LNM35 cell line was established following serial in vivo selection steps that included two rounds of implantation into the abdominal wall of nude mice and culturing of cells from the lung metastatic nodules. Cells were then passaged through the subcutaneous tissue and the LNM35 cell line was established from metastatic tumor cells in the axillary lymph node. When implanted subcutaneously, the LNM35 cell line gave rise to axillary lymph node metastases in 100% of animals. Following endobronchial (orthotopic) implantation of LNM35 cells into the lungs of nude mice, mediastinal lymph node metastases were also noted in 100% of the animals. In contrast to the H460SM model, neither subcutaneous nor orthotopic implantation of the LNM35 cell line resulted in systemic metastases.

The H460SM and H460-LNM35 variant cell lines show a higher incidence of metastasis when implanted in immunocompromised rodents compared to the parent cell line. Such paired parent and variant cell lines constitute a useful model for the discovery of genes involved in lung cancer metastasis. By comparing microarray data from each cell line, parent, and variant, genes suspected of expressing the metastatic phenotype can be identified and further investigated [93].

Lung Cancer Models in Preclinical Cancer Drug Development

Despite advances in basic cancer biology, animal models, especially human tumor xenografts, will remain pivotal to preclinical cancer drug discovery and development. The value of such models depends upon their validity, selectivity, predictability, reproducibility, and cost. Initially, lung tumor xenografts were intended to facilitate patient-specific chemotherapy. In this scenario, a patient's tumor is implanted as a xenograft in nude mice and the animals treated with various chemotherapy agents. By learning the drug responsiveness of the xeno-graft, treatment of the patient can then be individualized. Unfortunately, variations in take rate, the time required for the xenografts to grow, and the expense incurred make this strategy untenable.

In general, xenografts derived directly from patient biopsies, in contrast to those derived from continuous cell lines, appear to better retain the morphological properties and molecular markers reminiscent of the source tumors in man. In contrast, xenografts derived from cell lines generally show a more homogeneous, undifferentiated histology, probably indicative of the higher selection pressure in vitro during extensive culturing. Once a xenograph is established from a patient biopsy, however, it is difficult to subsequently develop cell lines. Therefore, establishing parallel in vitro cell lines (valuable as a continued source of pure human tumor cells for biochemical and molecular studies) and corresponding xenograft lines (valuable for pharmacological and pharmacodynamic studies) is quite difficult. In general it does appear that both xenografts derived from cell lines and those derived directly from patient biopsies provide some predictive power for selecting cytotoxics with clinical activity.

Early drug screening systems utilized the L1210 mouse lymphoma or P388 mouse leukemia models. Anticancer agents had to prove themselves in these murine models before passing on to further in vivo animal model testing. However, only 2% of drugs active in the L1210 or P388 models were subsequently shown to have in vivo activity in Lewis lung or colon 38 adenocarcinoma models [6]. This persuaded the US National Cancer Institute (NCI) to shift from a compound-oriented to a disease-oriented screening system. A high-throughput in vitro screening method capable of screening 20,000 compounds per year was developed using a panel of 60 cell lines representing all of the major human solid tumors (http://dtp.nci.nih.gov/branches/btb/ivclsp.html). Drugs found to have a favorable activity profile to a particular tumor histology or site are further tested in appropriate xenografts. The xeno-grafts are used as a secondary screening system to judge efficacy prior to considering a drug for early phase human studies [95].

Subcutaneous xenograft models have a long history in the pharmaceutical industry because of their utility, ease of use, and economy. Models are selected to demonstrate a specific cytotoxic effect of a drug or a biological agent, such as xenografts that reflect the chemosensitivities of their tumors of origin. For instance, the growth of small cell lung cancer xenografts is inhibited by cisplatin, etoposide, cyclophosphamide, doxorubicin, and vincristine, whereas non-small cell grafts are much less responsive to those same agents [96].

Although the subcutaneous xenograft model is widely employed as an in vivo drug screen, the more complicated orthotopic models may be better suited for preclinical studies. Since orthotopic rodent tumors mimic biological aspects of clinical cancer (e.g., disease progression and metastasis), they are likely to provide more relevant pharmacokinetic and pharmacodynamic information than subcutaneous tumors [97]. Carcinogen-induced and genetically modified murine lung cancer models that have been shown to mimic the human disease, either histologically or in terms of gene expression, may also provide predictive models for performing preclinical testing of therapeutic efficacy. Genetically modified murine cancer models are used to examine the efficacy of some targeted therapeutics. For example, farnesyltransferase inhibitors (FTIs) that act to inhibit *Ras* signaling have been tested in several models where upregulation of *ras* signaling results in tumor development. These studies demonstrated that FTIs are often effective in causing regression or preventing progression of tumor growth [98].

A range of methods are used to evaluate drug effect on tumors in animal models. Tumor size and tumor weight or volume changes are simple and easily reproducible parameters in subcutaneous xenograft models, but are more difficult, except at necropsy, in most orthotopic models. We used a mammographic imaging technique to assess both primary tumor growth and metastases in our orthotopic model [99]. Miniaturized human imaging methods, such as computed tomography, magnetic resonance imaging, and positron emission tomography, are now available for laboratory use. Morphologic changes and alterations in tumor immunogenicity or invasiveness are other markers of response. Survival, perhaps the ultimate parameter, is a valid endpoint only if clinically relevant tumor progression, such as systemic metastasis, is responsible for the animal's demise, a parameter better assessed in orthotopic than subcutaneous models.

To accurately evaluate anticancer activity in an animal model system, validation of the model is critical. This entails the design of studies aimed at assessing tumor response to drugs or other agents known to have efficacy in patients with the particular type of cancer represented by the model. We validated our H460 orthotopic lung cancer model [100] by treating tumor-bearing nude rats with one of four chemotherapy agents: doxorubicin, mitomycin, cisplatin, and the novel matrix metalloproteinase inhibitor batimastat. The model showed consistent responses in the form of tumor weight, metastatic pattern, and longevity to cisplatin and mitomycin treatment. The other two agents, for the most part, were ineffective, which accurately reflects drug sensitivity patterns in NSCLC and the H460 cell line. The model also detected cisplatin toxicity, as assessed by body weight changes and kidney damage. A similar study was performed using two human lung cancers implanted in the pleural cavity of nude mice [101]. Both studies show that selective cytotoxic agents may reduce primary tumor burden and prolong the survival of tumor-bearing animals. However, none of these agents was capable of completely eradicating tumor, reflecting the resistance of this disease to standard chemotherapy.

The orthotopic site may be crucial to a clinically relevant drug response. An orthotopic model of human small cell lung carcinoma (SCLC) demonstrates sensitivity to cisplatin and resistance to mitomycin C, reflecting the clinical situation [78]. However, the same tumor xenograft implanted subcutaneously responded to mitomycin and not to cisplatin, thus failing to match clinical behavior for SCLC. Similar phenomena that underscore the effect of the microenvironment on drug sensitivity have been observed [102].

A number of orthotopic models were developed as in vivo preclinical screens for novel therapies that target invasion, metastasis, and angiogenesis [103–106]. Our own studies in the H460 orthotopic lung cancer model include the matrix metalloproteinase inhibitors prinomastat (AG3340) and the integrin-linked kinase (ILK) inhibitor KP-392 [107, 108]. Assessment of multiple endpoints, such as tumor weight, metastatic pattern, and survival, appears to improve the sensitivity of the model system to demonstrate a treatment effect. By describing patterns of response in a model system, the results may also suggest mechanisms of action or biological properties of a particular agent. For instance, prinomastat was found to significantly increase the length of survival despite the fact that it showed no consistent effect on tumor size or on the incidence of metastases. Thus, the drug may be slowing, but not eradicating, the metastatic process.

In preclinical drug development, the orthotopic model also takes into account the role of the microenvironment, which is biologically unique for each organ system. For instance, endothelial cells in the vasculature of various organs express different cell-surface receptors [109] and growth factors that may influence the phenotype of primary tumors or metastases developing in these organs. Therapeutic efficacy can depend on multiple interactions of tumor cells with its microenvironment. Therefore, therapy should be targeted not only against the cancer cells themselves but also against the specific homeostatic factors that promote tumor cell growth, survival, angiogenesis, invasion, and metastasis.

A concern in testing anticancer agents with animal models derived from human cell lines is the potential loss of tumor heterogeneity [110]. In other words, does serial passage of cell lines over months and years select out and propagate only certain specific clonal elements of a tumor? Studies have shown that the molecular characteristics of both breast and lung cancer cell lines closely match their original human tumor [111]. From a phenotypic perspective, the H460 cell line used in our studies continues to exhibit consistent invasive and metastatic properties and has maintained its drug sensitivity profile for over 10 years and in thousands of experimental animals. However, other important characteristics, such as cytokine production or still unknown gene expressions, may be lost or muted through serial passaging. And so, as mentioned at the outset, it behooves the investigator to understand both the strengths and limitations of the tumor model chosen for lung cancer studies.

Hence, one needs to interpret xenograft studies with caution and bearing in mind the many variables that exist. Major variables include the origin of the tumor (i.e., cell line versus patient biopsy), the target/receptor status of the tumor, the site of tumor implantation (e.g., s.c., i.p., orthotopic), the size of the tumor at the onset of agent treatment, growth rate and growth characteristics, agent dose, formulation, scheduling and route of administration, and experimental endpoints. In addition, one needs to bear in mind the fact that the stromal compartment of xenografts is largely of murine origin. Therefore, when studying antiangiogenic and antivascular strategies using humanized antibodies (immunotherapy), the effector function being targeted is that of mouse or rat.

Lung Cancer Model for Studying Adjuvant Modalities

Surgery is the mainstay for treatment of NSCLC. Adjuvant therapy, including chemotherapy and radiation, has limited but important therapeutic benefits in this disease [112]. Effective adjuvant modalities are needed to improve the survival of lung cancer patients. Ideally, these novel therapies need to be tested in suitable adjuvant lung cancer models prior to clinical development. Surgical extirpation of the lung tumor is necessary to construct such model systems which can simulate clinical lung cancer patients who receive surgical intervention. The anticipated therapeutic effect is to control regional and systemic micrometastasis, therefore reducing the incidence of tumor recurrence. By complete removal of an orthotopically growing tumor in the H460 lung cancer model soon after tumor implantation, we established an orthotopic lung cancer model with significant potential for tumor recurrence both locally and systemically [113]. We used this model system to investigate a novel lymphatic drug delivery system as an adjuvant modality [114]. By adjusting the time of tumor resection following tumor implantation and selecting different tumor cell lines, the model system can potentially be refined to reflect many facets of lung cancer in the adjuvant setting.

Summary

Although the available lung cancer animal models have been informative and further propel our understanding of human lung cancer, they still do not fully recapitulate the complexities of human lung cancer. Each has its own advantages and disadvantages that should be understood and evaluated before their use. In selecting the best model system, consideration should be given to the genetic stability and heterogeneity of the transplanted cell line, its immunogenicity within the host animal, and the appropriate biologic endpoints. There is increasing pressure on the research community to reduce or even eliminate the use of animals in research. However, relevant animal model systems provide an appropriate interface between the laboratory bench and a patient's bedside for continued progress in cancer research and drug development. As in many other diseases, even more sophisticated lung cancer models will be needed in the future, as the complexities of this devastating disease are slowly unravelled.

References

1. Liu J, Johnston MR (2002) Animal models for studying lung cancer and evaluating novel intervention strategies. Surg Oncol 11:217–27.
2. Siemann DW (1984) Modification of chemotherapy by nitroimidazoles. Int J Radiat Oncol Biol Phys 10: 1585–94.
3. Corbett TH, Roberts BJ, Leopold WR, Peckham JC, Wilkoff LJ, Griswold DP, Schabel FM (1984) Induction and chemotherapeutic response of two transplantable ductal adenocarcinomas of the pancreas in C57BL/6 mice. Cancer Res 44: 717–26.
4. Balmain A, Harris CC (2000) Carcinogenesis in mouse and human cells: parallels and paradoxes. Carcinogenesis 21: 371–7.
5. Malkinson AM (2001) Primary lung tumors in mice as an aid for understanding, preventing, and treating human adenocarcinoma of the lung. Lung Cancer 32: 265–79.
6. Curt GA (1994) The use of animal models in cancer drug discovery and development. Stem Cells 12: 23–9.
7. Tuveson DA, Jacks T (1999) Modeling human lung cancer in mice: similarities and shortcomings. Oncogene 18: 5318–24.
8. Shimkin MB, Stoner GD (1975) Lung tumors in mice: application to carcinogenesis bioassay. Adv Cancer Res 21: 1–58.
9. Stoner GD, Adam-Rodwell G, Morse MA (1993) Lung tumors in strain A mice: application for studies in cancer chemoprevention. J Cell Biochem Suppl. 17F: 95–103.
10. Wattenberg LW, Leong JL (1970) Inhibition of the carcinogenic action of benzo(a)pyrene by flavones. Cancer Res 30: 1922–5.
11. Malkinson AM (1992) Primary lung tumors in mice: an experimentally manipulable model of human adenocarcinoma. Cancer Res 52: 2670s–6s.
12. Kim SH, Lee CS (1996) Induction of benign and malignant pulmonary tumors in mice with benzo(a)pyrene. Anticancer Res 16: 465–70.
13. Witschi H, Espiritu I, Dance ST, Miller MS (2002) A mouse lung tumor model of tobacco smoke carcinogenesis. Toxicol Sci 68: 322–30.
14. Bogen KT et al. (2002) Lung tumors in A/J mice exposed to environmental tobacco smoke: estimated potency and implied human risk. Carcinogenesis 23: 511–9.
15. Rapp UR, Todaro GJ (1980) Generation of oncogenic mouse type C viruses: in vitro selection of carcinoma-inducing variants. Proc Natl Acad Sci USA 77: 624–8.
16. Malkinson AM (1989) The genetic basis of susceptibility to lung tumors in mice. Toxicology 54: 241–71.
17. Miller MS, Jones AB, Chauhan DP et al. (1990) Role of the maternal environment in determining susceptibility to transplacentally induced chemical carcinogenesis in mouse fetuses. Carcinogenesis 11:1979–84
18. Rehm S, Lijinsky W, Singh G et al. (1991) Mouse bronchiolar cell carcinogenesis. Histologic characterization and expression of Clara cell antigen in lesions induced by N-nitrosobis-(2-chloroethyl) ureas. Am J Pathol 139:413–22
19. White MR, Grendon A, Jones HB (1970) Tumor incidence and cellularity in lungs of mice given various dose schedules of urethan. Cancer Res 30:1030–6.
20. Stoner GD, Greisiger EA, Schut HA (1984) A comparison of the lung adenoma response in strain A/J mice after intraperitoneal and oral administration of carcinogens. Toxicol Appl Pharmacol 72:313–23.
21. Anderson LM, Priest LJ (1980) Reduction in the transplacental carcinogenic effect of methylcholanthrene in mice by prior treatment with beta-naphthoflavone. Res Commun Chem Pathol Pharmacol 30: 431–46.
22. Wattenberg LW (1973) Inhibition of chemical carcinogen-induced pulmonary neoplasia by butylated hydroxyanisole. J Natl Cancer Inst 50: 1541–4.
23. Lesca P (1983) Protective effects of ellagic acid and other plant phenols on benzo[a]pyrene-induced neoplasia in mice. Carcinogenesis 4: 1651–3.

24. Jackson EL, Willis N, Mercer K et al. (2001) Analysis of lung tumor initiation and progression using conditional expression of oncogenic K-ras. Genes Dev 15: 3243–48.
25. Gunning WT, Kramer PM, Lubet RA, Steele VE, Pereira MA (2000) Chemoprevention of vinyl carbamate-induced lung tumors in strain A mice. Exp Lung Res 26: 757–72.
26. Wang ZY, Hong JY, Huang MT, Reuhl KR, Conney AH, Yang CS (1992) Inhibition of N-nitrosodiethylamine- and 4-(methylnitrosamino)-1-(3-pyridyl)-1-butanone-induced tumorigenesis in A/J mice by green tea and black tea. Cancer Res 52(7):1943–7.
27. Jalbert G, Castonguay A (1992) Effects of NSAIDs on NNK-induced pulmonary and gastric tumorigenesis in A/J mice. Cancer Lett 66: 21–8.
28. Duperron C, Castonguay A (1997) Chemopreventive efficacies of aspirin and sulindac against lung tumorigenesis in A/J mice. Carcinogenesis 18: 1001–6.
29. Moody TW, Leyton J, Zakowicz H et al. (2001) Indomethacin reduces lung adenoma number in A/J mice. Anticancer Res 21: 1749–55.
30. Kozaki K, Koshikawa K, Tatematsu Y et al. (2001) Multi-faceted analyses of a highly metastatic human lung cancer cell line NCI-H460-LNM35 suggest mimicry of inflammatory cells in metastasis. Oncogene 20: 4228–34.
31. Kisley LR, Barrett BS, Dwyer-Nield LD, Bauer AK, Thompson DC, Malkinson AM (2002) Celecoxib reduces pulmonary inflammation but not lung tumorigenesis in mice. Carcinogenesis 23: 1653–60.
32. Keith RL, Miller YE, Hudish TM et al. (2004) Pulmonary Prostacyclin Synthase Overexpression Chemoprevents Tobacco Smoke Lung Carcinogenesis in Mice. Cancer Res 64: 5897–904.
33. Hahn FF, Lundgren DL (1992) Pulmonary neoplasms in rats that inhaled cerium-144 dioxide. Toxicol Pathol 20: 169–78.
34. Adams JM, Cory S (1991) Transgenic models of tumor development. Science 254: 1161–7.
35. Thomas H, Balkwill F (1995) Assessing new anti-tumour agents and strategies in oncogene transgenic mice. Cancer Metastasis Rev 14: 91–5.
36. Hogan B (1986) Manipulating the mouse embryo: a laboratory manual. In: Hanahan D (eds) Cold Spring Harbor Laboratory Manual. Cold Spring Harbor, New York.
37. Gordon JW, Ruddle FH (1983) Gene transfer into mouse embryos: production of transgenic mice by pronuclear injection. Methods Enzymol 101: 411–33.
38. Jaenisch R (1980) Retroviruses and embryogenesis: microinjection of Moloney leukemia virus into midgestation mouse embryos. Cell 19: 181–8.
39. Soriano P, Jaenisch R (1986) Retroviruses as probes for mammalian development: allocation of cells to the somatic and germ cell lineages. Cell 46: 19–29.
40. Dosaka-Akita H, Cagle PT, Hiroumi H et al. (2000) Differential retinoblastoma and p16(INK4A) protein expression in neuroendocrine tumors of the lung. Cancer 88: 550–6.
41. Ehrhardt A, Bartels T, Geick A, Klocke R, Paul D, Halter R (2001) Development of pulmonary bronchiolo-alveolar adenocarcinomas in transgenic mice overexpressing murine c-myc and epidermal growth factor in alveolar type II pneumocytes. Br J Cancer 84: 813–8.
42. Fijneman RJ, de Vries SS, Jansen RC, Demant P (1996) Complex interactions of new quantitative trait loci, Sluc1, Sluc2, Sluc3, and Sluc4, that influence the susceptibility to lung cancer in the mouse. Nat Genet 14: 465–7.
43. Fong KM, Sekido Y, Minna JD (1999) Molecular pathogenesis of lung cancer. J Thorac Cardiovasc Surg 118:1136–52.
44. Suda Y, Aizawa S, Hirai S, Inoue T, Furuta Y, Suzuki M, Hirohashi S, Ikawa Y (1987) Driven by the same Ig enhancer and SV40 T promoter ras induced lung adenomatous tumors, myc induced pre-B cell lymphomas and SV40 large T gene a variety of tumors in transgenic mice. EMBO J 6: 4055–65.
45. Sandmoller A, Halter R, Suske G, Paul D, Beato M (1995) A transgenic mouse model for lung adenocarcinoma. Cell Growth Differ 6: 97–103.

46. Zhao B, Magdaleno S, Chua S et al. (2000) Transgenic mouse models for lung cancer. Exp. Lung Res 26: 567–79.
47. Macleod KF, Jacks T (1999) Insights into cancer from transgenic mouse models. J Pathol 187: 43–60.
48. DeMayo FJ, Tsai SY (2001) Targeted gene regulation and gene ablation. Trends Endocrinol Metab 12: 348–53.
49. Lewandoski M (2001) Conditional control of gene expression in the mouse. Nat Rev Genet 2: 743–55.
50. Shockett PE, Schatz DG (1996) Diverse strategies for tetracycline-regulated inducible gene expression. Proc Natl Acad Sci USA 93: 5173–6.
51. Fisher GH, Wellen SL, Klimstra D et al. (2001) Induction and apoptotic regression of lung adenocarcinomas by regulation of a K-Ras transgene in the presence and absence of tumor suppressor genes. Genes Dev 15: 3249–62.
52. Meuwissen R, Linn SC, van der Valk M, Mooi WJ, Berns A (2001) Mouse model for lung tumorigenesis through Cre/lox controlled sporadic activation of the K-Ras oncogene. Oncogene 20: 6551–8.
53. Meuwissen R, Linn SC, Linnoila RI, Zevenhoven J, Mooi WJ, Berns A (2003) Induction of small cell lung cancer by somatic inactivation of both Trp53 and Rb1 in a conditional mouse model. Cancer Cell 4: 181–9.
54. Kim CF, Jackson EL, Kirsch DG, et al. (2005) Mouse models of human non-small-cell lung cancer: raising the bar. Cold Spring Harb Symp Quant Biol 70:241–50.
55. DeMayo FJ, Finegold MJ, Hansen TN et al. (1991) Expression of SV40 T antigen under control of rabbit uteroglobin promoter in transgenic mice. Am J Physiol 261: L70–6.
56. Wikenheiser KA, Clark JC, Linnoila RI et al. (1992) Simian virus 40 large T antigen directed by transcriptional elements of the human surfactant protein C gene produces pulmonary adenocarcinomas in transgenic mice. Cancer Res 52:5342–52.
57. Chailley-Heu B, Rambaud C, Barlier-Mur AM et al. (2001) A model of pulmonary adenocarcinoma in transgenic mice expressing the simian virus 40 T antigen driven by the rat Calbindin-D9K (CaBP9K) promoter. J Pathol 195:482–9.
58. Ehrhardt A, Bartels T, Geick A et al. (2001) Development of pulmonary bronchiolo-alveolar adenocarcinomas in transgenic mice overexpressing murine c-myc and epidermal growth factor in alveolar type II pneumocytes. Br J Cancer 84:813–8.
59. Kerkhoff E, Fedorov LM, Siefken R et al. (2000) Lung-targeted expression of the c-Raf-1 kinase in transgenic mice exposes a novel oncogenic character of the wild-type protein. Cell Growth Differ 11:185–90.
60. Sunday ME, Haley KJ, Sikorski K et al. (1999) Calcitonin driven v-Ha-ras induces multilineage pulmonary epithelial hyperplasias and neoplasms. Oncogene 18:4336–47.
61. Chen YQ, Zhou YQ, Fu LH et al. (2002) Multiple pulmonary adenomas in the lung of transgenic mice overexpressing the RON receptor tyrosine kinase. Recepteur d'origine nantais. Carcinogenesis 23:1811–9.
62. Linnoila RI, Sahu A, Miki M et al. (2000) Morphometric analysis of CC10-hASH1 transgenic mouse lung: a model for bronchiolization of alveoli and neuroendocrine carcinoma. Exp Lung Res 26:595–615.
63. Sharkey FE, Fogh J, Hajdu S et al. (1978) Experience in surgical pathology with human tumor growth in the nude mouse. In: Fogh J, Giovanella B, The nude mouse in experimental and clinical research. Academic Press, New York, p. 188.
64. Boven E, Winograd B, Berger DP, et al. (1992) Phase II preclinical drug screening in human tumor xenografts: a first European multicenter collaborative study. Cancer Res 52: 5940–7.
65. Takimoto CH (2001) Why drugs fail: of mice and men revisited. Clin Cancer Res 7: 229–30.
66. Fodstad O (1988) Representativity of xenografts for clinical cancer. Tumor and host characteristics as variables of tumor take rate. In Winograd B, Peckham MJ, Pinedo HM

(eds.), Human Tumor Xenografts in Anticancer Drug Development. Springer-Verlag, Berlin, pp. 15–21.

67. Fidler IJ (1986) Rationale and methods for the use of nude mice to study the biology and therapy of human cancer metastasis. Cancer Metastasis Rev 5: 29–49.

68. Fidler IJ (1991) Orthotopic implantation of human colon carcinomas into nude mice provides a valuable model for the biology and therapy of metastasis. Cancer Metastasis Rev 10: 229–43.

69. Kerbel RS, Cornil I, Theodorescu D (1991) Importance of orthotopic transplantation procedures in assessing the effects of transfected genes on human tumor growth and metastasis. Cancer Metastasis Rev 10: 201–15.

70. Paget S (1889) Secondary growths of cancer of breast. Lancet 1: 571–3.

71. Howard RB, Chu H, Zeligman BE (1991). Irradiated nude rat model for orthotopic human lung cancers. Cancer Res 51: 3274–80.

72. Howard RB, Mullen JB, Pagura ME, Johnston MR (1999) Characterization of a highly metastatic, orthotopic lung cancer model in the nude rat. Clin Exp Metastasis 17: 157–62.

73. McLemore TL, Liu MC, Blacker PC et al. (1987) Novel intrapulmonary model for orthotopic propagation of human lung cancers in athymic nude mice. Cancer Res 47: 5132–40.

74. Wang X., Fu X, Hoffman RM (1992) A new patient-like metastatic model of human lung cancer constructed orthotopically with intact tissue via thoracotomy in immunodeficient mice. Int J Cancer 51: 992–5.

75. Rashidi B, Yang M, Jiang P (2000) A highly metastatic Lewis lung carcinoma orthotopic green fluorescent protein model. Clin Exp Metastasis 18: 57–60.

76. McLemore TL, Eggleston JC, Shoemaker RH et al. (1988) Comparison of intrapulmonary, percutaneous intrathoracic, and subcutaneous models for the propagation of human pulmonary and nonpulmonary cancer cell lines in athymic nude mice. Cancer Res 48: 2880–6.

77. Kuo TH, Kubota T, Watanabe M et al. (1992) Orthotopic reconstitution of human small-cell lung carcinoma after intravenous transplantation in SCID mice. Anticancer Res 12: 1407–10.

78. Kuo TH, Kubota T, Watanabe M. (1993) Site-specific chemosensitivity of human small-cell lung carcinoma growing orthotopically compared to subcutaneously in SCID mice: the importance of orthotopic models to obtain relevant drug evaluation data. Anticancer Res 13: 627–30.

79. Nagamachi Y, Tani M, Shimizu K, Tsuda H, Niitsu Y, Yokota J (1998) Orthotopic growth and metastasis of human non-small cell lung carcinoma cell injected into the pleural cavity of nude mice. Cancer Lett 127: 203–9.

80. Miyoshi T, Kondo K, Ishikura H, Kinoshita H, Matsumori Y, Monden Y (2000) SCID Mouse Lymphogenous Metastatic Model of Human Lung Cancer Constructed Using Orthotopic Inoculation of Cancer Cells. Anticancer Res 20: 161–4.

81. Cuenca RE, Takita H, Bankert R (1996) Orthotopic engraftment of human lung tumours in SCID mice for the study of metastasis. Surg Oncol 5: 85–91.

82. Van Weerden WM, Romijn JC (2000) Use of nude mouse xenograft models in prostate cancer research. Prostate 43: 263–71.

83. Wang X, Fu X, Kubota T, Hoffman RM (1992) A new patient-like metastatic model of human small-cell lung cancer constructed orthotopically with intact tissue via thoracotomy in nude mice. Anticancer Res 12: 1403–6.

84. Vertrees RA, Deyo DJ, Quast M et al. (2000) Development of a human to murine orthotopic xenotransplanted lung cancer model. J Invest Surg 13:349–58.

85. Glaves D (1986) Detection of circulating metastatic cells. Prog Clin Biol Res 212: 151–67.

86. Yang M, Hasegawa S, Jiang P et al. (1998) Widespread skeletal metastatic potential of human lung cancer revealed by green fluorescent protein expression. Cancer Res 58: 4217–21.

87. Clark EA, Golub TR, Lander ES, Hynes RO (2000) Genomic analysis of metastasis reveals an essential role for RhoC. Nature 406: 532–5.
88. Fidler IJ, Poste G (1985) The cellular heterogeneity of malignant neoplasms: implications for adjuvant chemotherapy. Semin Oncol 12: 207–21.
89. Fidler IJ (2002) The organ microenvironment and cancer metastasis. Differentiation 70: 498–505.
90. Carmichael J and Smyth JF (1988) Chemotherapy studies in human non-small cell lung cancer xenografts transplanted in immune-deprived mice. In: Winograd B, Peckham MJ, Pinedo HM (eds.), Human Tumour Xenografts in Anticancer Drug Development, Springer, New York, pp. 51–56.
91. Dinney CP, Fishbeck R, Singh RK et al. (1995) Isolation and characterization of metastatic variants from human transitional cell carcinoma passaged by orthotopic implantation in athymic nude mice. J Urol 154: 1532–8.
92. Chu LW, Pettaway CA, Liang JC (2001) Genetic abnormalities specifically associated with varying metastatic potential of prostate cancer cell lines as detected by comparative genomic hybridization. Cancer Genet Cytogenet 127: 161–7.
93. Liu J, Blackhall F, Seiden-Long I et al. (2004) Modeling of lung cancer by an orthotopically growing H460SM variant cell line reveals novel candidate genes for systemic metastasis. Oncogene 23: 6316–24.
94. Kozaki K, Miyaishi O, Tsukamoto T, Tatematsu Y, Hida T, Takahashi T, Takahashi T (2000) Establishment and characterization of a human lung cancer cell line NCI- H460-LNM35 with consistent lymphogenous metastasis via both subcutaneous and orthotopic propagation. Cancer Res 60: 2535–40.
95. Khleif SN, Curt GA (1997) Animal models in drug development. In: Holland JF, Bast RC, Morton DL, Weichselbaum RR (eds.), Cancer Medicine. Williams & Wilkins, Baltimore, pp. 855–68.
96. Shoemaker RH, McLemore TL, Abbott BJ et al. (1988) Human tumor xenograft models for use with an in vitro-based, disease-oriented antitumor drug screening program. In: Winograd B, Peckham MJ, Pinedo HM (eds), Human Tumor xenografts in Anticancer Drug Development. Springer-Verlag, Berlin, pp. 115–20.
97. Mulvin DW, Howard RB, Mitchell DH et al. (1992) Secondary screening system for preclinical testing of human lung cancer therapies. J Natl Cancer Inst 84: 31–7.
98. Van Dyke T, Jacks T (2002) Cancer modeling in the modern era: progress and challenges. Cell 108: 135–44.
99. Zeligman BE, Howard RB, Marcell T, Chu H, Rossi RP, Mulvin D, Johnston MR (1992) Chest roentgenographic techniques for demonstrating human lung tumour xenografts in nude rats. Lab Anim 26: 100–106.
100. Johnston MR, Mullen JB, Pagura M, Howard RB (2001) Validation of an orthotopic model of human lung cancer with regional and systemic metastases. Ann Thorac Surg 71: 1120–5.
101. Kraus-Berthier L, Jan M, Guilbaud N, Naze M, Pierre A, Atassi G (2002) Histology and sensitivity to anticancer drugs of two human non-small lung cell lung carcinomas implanted in the pleural cavity of nude mice. Clin Cancer Res 6: 297–304.
102. Wilmanns C, Fan D, O'Brian CA, Bucana CD, Fidler IJ (1992) Orthotopic and ectopic organ environments differentially influence the sensitivity of murine colon carcinoma cells to doxorubicin and 5- fluorouracil. Int J Cancer 52: 98–104.
103. Davies B, Brown PD, East N, Crimmin MJ, Balkwill FR (1993) A synthetic matrix metalloproteinase inhibitor decreases tumor burden and prolongs survival of mice bearing human ovarian carcinoma xenografts. Cancer Res 53: 2087–91.
104. Marincola FM, Da Pozzo LF, Drucker BJ, Holder WD (1990) Adoptive immunotherapy of human pancreatic cancer with lymphokine- activated killer cells and interleukin-2 in a nude mouse model. Surgery 108: 919–29.

105. Russell PJ, Ho SI, Boniface GR, Izard ME, Philips J, Raghavan D, Walker KZ (1991) Growth and metastasis of human bladder cancer xenografts in the bladder of nude rats. A model for intravesical radioimmunotherapy. Urol Res 19: 207–13.
106. Schuster JM, Friedman HS, Archer GE, Fuchs HE, McLendon RE, Colvin OM, Bigner DD (1993) Intraarterial therapy of human glioma xenografts in athymic rats using 4-hydroperoxycyclophosphamide. Cancer Res 53: 2338–43.
107. Liu J, Tsao MS, Pagura M, Shalinsky DR, Khoka R, Fata J, Johnston MR (2003) Early combined treatment with carboplatin and the MMP inhibitor prolongs survival and reduces systemic metastasis in an aggressive orthotopic lung cancer model. Lung Cancer 42:335–44.
108. Liu J, Costello PC, Pham N, Pintillie M, Jabali M, Sanghera J, Tsao MS, Johnston MR (2006) Integrin linked kinase (ILK) inhibitor KP-392 inhibits tumor growth and metastasis in an orthotopic human non small lung cancer model. J Thorac Oncol 1:771–9.
109. Pasqualini R, Ruoslahti E (1996) Organ targeting in vivo using phage display peptide libraries. Nature 380: 364–6.
110. Price JE (1994) Analyzing the metastatic phenotype. J Cell Biochem 56: 16–22.
111. 97. Wistuba II, Bryant D, Behrens C, Milchgrub S, Virmani AK, Ashfaq R, Minna JD, Gazdar AF (1999) Comparison of features of human lung cancer cell lines and their corresponding tumors. Clin Cancer Res 5: 991–1000.
112. Winton T, Livingston R, Johnson D et al. (2005) Vinorelbine plus cisplatin vs. observation in resected non-small-cell lung cancer. N Engl J Med 352:2589–97.
113. Liu J, Li M, Tsao MS, Johnston MR (2003) An experimental lung cancer model for the assessment of adjuvant therapies following surgical resection. Proc Am Assoc Cancer Res Toronto, Canada.
114. Liu J, Wong H, Moselhy J, Bowen B, Wu XY, Johnston MR (2006) Targeting colloidal particulates to thoracic lymph nodes. Lung Cancer 51:377–86.

Molecular Imaging in Lung Cancer Metastases

Mahaveer Swaroop Bhojani, Shyam Nyati, Hyma R. Rao, Brian D. Ross, and Alnawaz Rehemtulla

Abstract Advances in gene profiling technology have led to the identification of novel gene expression signatures and individual biomarkers associated with the cancer and the spread of malignancy to distant organs. Molecular imaging is a very promising technology which provides the potential for utilizing these biomarkers for monitoring tumor progression and therapeutic response. This technology may allow real-time, dynamic, and quantifiable monitoring of biomarker activity. This chapter describes molecular imaging modalities that are currently available for monitoring clinical and experimental metastasis, their application and potential to monitor tumor progression and therapeutic outcome of a treatment regimen in real time, and in the discovery and development of novel drugs that target metastatic disease.

Introduction

To date, most clinically relevant cancers are staged by assessing gross structural features including the extent of local invasion, the presence of enlarged lymph nodes, and the detection of lesions in distant organs [1–3]. At the same time, significant progress in the field of molecular and cellular oncology has led to a better understanding of certain irregularities in signal transduction and gene alterations that occur during various stages of tumor initiation and metastases. Such insights, aided by sequencing of the genome of various organisms and advances in molecular profiling technologies such as microarrays and proteomics, have led to the identification of biomarkers and gene expression signatures for the prognosis and diagnosis of cancer [4–9]. Thus, there is a grievous disconnect between the identification of biomarkers in the research laboratories and their application in clinical oncology. This is partly due to the fact that technologies for the quantitation of these biomarkers and their signaling

M.S. Bhojani (✉)
Departments of Radiation Oncology, University of Michigan, Ann Arbor,
MI 48109, USA
e-mail: mahaveer@umich.edu

V. Keshamouni et al. (eds.), *Lung Cancer Metastasis*,
DOI 10.1007/978-1-4419-0772-1_13, © Springer Science+Business Media, LLC 2009

cascades are still in their infancy and have not kept pace with the identification of novel biomarkers. Additionally, molecular profiling strategies utilize tumor biopsies, which provide only a snapshot of the biomarker activity at the time of sample retrieval. Thus, it fails to provide any information about dynamic changes within the malignancy and its surrounding milieu. Therefore, for molecular characterization of cancer to have a clinical impact, innovative modalities are vital for noninvasive and real-time monitoring of activities of biomarkers and events regulated by them. The field of molecular imaging attempts to bridge this lacuna. It aims at developing suitable probes for non-invasive visualization of biological processes at the cellular and molecular level in an entire organism as well as producing the instrumentations and methodologies needed to make this type of visualization and measurement possible [10–16]. At present, molecular imaging is largely in the preclinical phase (animal studies) but has the potential to impact clinical care by using molecular characterization to (1) diagnose cancer at an earlier stage; (2) predict the risk of precancerous lesion progression; (3) quantify the activity of specific molecules that are involved in tumor growth, metastasis, and invasion; (4) select for rational molecular therapies; and (5) assess the efficiency of chemo- and radio-therapeutic agents in real time [14, 17–24].

A major technical challenge for molecular imaging of metastases is that this process involves multiple complex steps involving numerous alterations at different molecular levels. Intriguingly, some of the phenotypic changes that cells may undergo during metastases are strikingly distinct, such as epithelial–mesenchymal transition (EMT) and mesenchymal–epithelial transition (MET; refer Chapter 4). Therefore, the molecular profile of cells at these stages may also differ significantly. Since the procurement of samples at the stage of intravasation, circulation, and extravasation is difficult, majority of the molecular profiling investigations for metastasis are based on the gene expression comparisons from the primary and the corresponding metastatic tumor specimens.

Molecular Probes

Innovations in the field of molecular imaging are made possible from break-throughs achieved in developing novel molecular probes, which include injectible radiopharmaceuticals, novel contrast agents, and genetically encoded reporters such as luciferase, fluorescent proteins, and thymidine kinase. When utilizing a particular probe for imaging, factors including specificity, uptake, distribution, metabolism, excretion, and biodetectability are considered before establishing the usefulness of a probe [17, 20, 25–30]. Based on the above factors, molecular probes are classified into following three categories: (1) nonspecific probes; (2) targeted probes; and (3) "smart" probes. Nonspecific probes usually have a low molecular weight and have a differential distribution depending on the tissue architecture. Even though these probes do not measure precise pathological alterations at molecular level, they measure and help visualize gross changes in the physiological processes such as changes in blood volume, flow, and perfusion between normal tissue and tumors [31]. Targeted probes are designed to recognize specific biomarkers, which in cancer are typically upregulated proteins. Some common molecular interactions utilized in imaging are antigen–antibody, ligand–receptor, and inhibitor–receptor interactions [32, 33]. In contrast to nonspecific probes, targeted probes increase the signal-to-noise ratio [31], but signal from unbound probe remains a major hurdle [31]. In order to overcome this problem, there needs to be a clear understanding of the pharmacokinetics of each probe so that clearance of the unbound probe may be permitted while the probe–target interaction is imaged. In addition to this, the signal intensity strongly depends on the density or availability of target receptors, and it is limited by nonspecific cellular uptake [20]. The newer imaging agents, "smart" probes, also known as molecular beacons, participate in a specific molecular interaction and then change their physical properties [20]. An example of "smart" probes is fluorescent molecular beacons, which are based on the fluorescence quenching–dequenching strategy [20]. Here, probes in their native form are constructed in such a way that a fluorochrome and a quencher are juxtapositioned, leading to quenching of fluorescence. However, modification of the probe by a specific enzyme either alters the conformation or cleaves the probe such that the fluorescence and quencher are no longer in close apposition and fluorescence can then be detected [20]. This method increases the signal-to-noise ratio and also includes a signal amplification step wherein multiple quenched probes are cleaved by a single enzyme. Smart probes are being currently explored to dynamically monitor activities of enzymes that have a vital role in cancer such as matrix metalloproteinases, prostate-specific antigens, caspases, and cathepsins [34–38].

Simultaneous progress in the development of probes and instrumentation essential for real-time functional imaging presented researchers with powerful tools to perform noninvasive experiments on dynamic biological processes in intact cells as well as in whole organisms. Biological processes that are monitored by this technology include transcriptional and translational regulation, signal transduction, protein–protein interactions, oncogenic and viral transformation, cell migration and trafficking, monitoring tumor burden, and metastatic tumor progression [16, 39–47].

Imaging Modalities for Clinical Metastases

In addition to radiography-based detection modalities, new developments in the field of magnetic resonance imaging (MRI) and nuclear imaging have brought new hope to early and sensitive detection of lung nodules and metastases. In this section, the MRI and the nuclear imaging modality will be discussed.

Magnetic Resonance Imaging

MRI is a method of imaging in which information is gleaned from atomic nuclei (most commonly hydrogen) by using radio waves in the presence of a magnetic field [46, 48, 49]. Various endogenous tissue properties are used in MRI in order to assess gross tumor morphology and growth in a noninvasive way [21]. High spatial resolution for structural imaging (25–100 μm), the absence of reduced resolution quality due to changes in tissue depth, and the ability to use different frequency pulse sequences to measure multiple physiological parameters are a few of the major MRI advantages [46, 48, 49]. Such features make MRI preferable when imaging gene expression, localizing tumor margins, and tracking stem cells, lymphocytes, and oligodendrocyte progenitors. There are, however, a few concerns in reference to MRI as a molecular imaging tool; some of them are the following: (a) a relatively long data acquisition time, which could sometimes extend to several hours; (b) potential toxicity of injection of contrast agents such as gadolinium or superparamagnetic iron oxide with higher doses or repeated use; and (c) comparatively poor sensitivity [46].

Nuclear Imaging (SPECT and PET)

Of all the modalities available for molecular imaging, nuclear imaging is the most sensitive, tomographic, and quantitative [46]. PET is the current paradigm for sensitivity for in vivo detection of molecular probes which can be visualized and quantitated at the concentration of 10^{-10} to 10^{-12} M [30, 46, 50]. Therefore, genes that are delivered by vectors with weak promoters (e.g., tissue specific) or low transfection efficacy (e.g., plasmid) can still be detected by PET. In addition, the brief half-life of the radioactive substrates offers another advantage to PET imaging since short half-lives enable recurrent imaging of tracer in targeted tissues. Clinically, PET is now routinely utilized for detection of primary and metastatic tumor sites utilizing fluorodeoxyglucose (FDG), a glucose analog labeled with radioactive fluorine that emits positrons. As the positrons encounter electrons, they produce paired gamma rays that travel in opposite directions. These gamma rays are then detected by the PET scanner, which positions the FDG spatially within the patient's body. The idea behind the use of FDG for PET imaging is based on the finding of Nobel Prize winner Otto Heinrich Warburg, which suggests differential uptake of glucose by tumor cells and normal cells. Tumor cells overexpress genes that are involved in glucose transport since they utilize inefficient nonoxidative glycolysis pathway for generation of energy [51, 52]. PET is therefore a unique imaging modality in its ability to metabolically characterize biologic tissues according to their utilization of glucose and their likely malignant nature.

SPECT is more economical than PET, and it is a powerful technique used for imaging molecular processes. SPECT takes into account the rotation of a photon detector array around the body in order to detect γ-emitting radio-nuclides, thus obtaining numerous projections [46]. Sodium iodide or solid-state cadmium zinc telluride detectors are used to spot γ photons and when optimized, these detectors provide a spatial resolution of 1–2 mm. Common SPECT radionuclides are $^{99}Tc^m$ (6 h), ^{111}In (2.8 days), ^{123}I (13.2 h), and ^{125}I (59.5 days) [53]. Generally, SPECT is used to track cells and molecules such as during the radiolabeling of annexin V as an early marker of apoptosis [54, 55].

Molecular Imaging for Experimental Metastasis

The majority of developments that the field of molecular imaging has seen have not progressed beyond experimental animal systems. Bioluminescence- and fluorescence-based imaging are the two major optical imaging modalities used for monitoring experimental metastasis.

Bioluminescent Optical Imaging

Bioluminescence imaging has emerged as a useful and complementary experimental imaging technique for small animals. This imaging modality detects a scant number of photons generated by the expression of genetically encoded luciferase and provides a robust modality for high-throughput screening, monitoring in vivo drug–target interactions, and identifying combination therapies. For such assays, tumor cells or cancer-related genes are tagged with a reporter gene that encodes a light-generating enzyme, luciferase [11, 50, 56]. When this reporter oxidizes its substrate, luciferin, a blue to yellow-green light with an emission spectra peaking at a wavelength between 490 and 620 nm is produced [56]. An extremely sensitive, cooled, charge-coupled device (CCD) camera detects any low light that is emitted during the bioluminescence reaction. Due to its extreme sensitivity, broad dynamic range, and exceptionally large signal-to-noise ratio, this type of noninvasive imaging permits a real-time analysis of a number of biological events [11]. However, major disadvantages of biolumi-nescent imaging is that it provides two-dimensional datasets which lead to positional uncertainty of the signal and bioluminescence remains contingent upon on the pharmacokinetics of the substrate. Although there are more than 30 luciferase–luciferin systems, the most frequently used luciferase for in vivo molecular imaging is the ATP-dependent firefly (*Photinus pyralis*) luciferase [57]. The reason for this is that 30% of the light produced by firefly luciferase has an emission spectra above 600 nm, a region in which the signal attenuation by the absorption and scatter properties of live mammalian tissue is at a minimum [11, 57]. Even though in basic research, luciferases demonstrate a vital advantage in assessing many biological functions such as gene expression, promoter regulation, protein stability, protein–protein interaction, and enzyme activity, such genetically encoded reporters have a small chance of playing a major clinical role in the near future since their application is dependent upon the approval of gene therapy protocols for patients.

Fluorescent Optical Imaging

Fluorescence-based imaging is another powerful modality for molecular imaging. This area of optical imaging received a great impetus when the green fluorescent protein was discovered and recognition when the discoverers were awarded the Nobel Prize in chemistry for 2008 (for review see [50]). The key advantage of fluorescence imaging is that it is independent of the substrate and, therefore, disengages the signal readout from the pharmacokinetics of the substrate. However, the major drawback of this method is that the wavelength of light used for excitation of fluorochrome can also excite other naturally occurring fluorescent molecules in the body (for example, hemoglobin partially absorbs visible light). This may frequently produce higher levels of background autofluorescence in the blue-green spectral region, resulting in a decreased signal-to-noise ratio. Additionally, in fluorescence imaging, the signal is partially attenuated by water in the infrared region. This leads to photon scattering in the tissues and inaccuracies in the quantitation of photon output. To counteract such shortcomings, the last decade has seen intensive investigations targeted to identifying probes that emit in the region of the electromagnetic spectrum that imparts greater tissue penetration and minimal signal attenuation in live tissues. Near-infrared fluorescent (NIRF) probes and red-shifted fluorescent proteins are recent discoveries from these efforts [20, 58–62]. The development of sensitive photon-sensing detectors, in vivo optoelectronic, confocal, and multiphoton microscopy, and advances in mathematical modeling of photon propagation in tissues have led to new imaging techniques including fluorescence tomography, spectrally resolved whole animal imaging, and intravital multiphoton imaging [19, 26, 63–66]. Researchers are now able to detect the activity of matrix metalloproteinases, annexin V, cathepsins, caspases, and lymph node metastasis because of enhancements in imaging devices and noninvasive NIRF imaging using molecular beacons [29, 37, 38, 59, 65, 67–72]. Such advances are reforming the detection of biomarkers or molecular events specific to cancer. Research in the field of fluorescence imaging has the potential to have clinical applications due to the launch of extremely photostable NIRF semiconductor nanocrystals (quantum dots or qdots) and its application in confocal microscopy, total internal reflection microscopy, or basic wide-field epifluorescence microscopy [73–77].

Common parameters used for the selection of an individual modality for imaging include cost, spatial and temporal resolution, complexity of operation, motion artifacts, depth of signal detection, acquisition time, and clinical relevance. No single technique has the ability to provide the panacea for all the molecular imaging needs and each technique has its unique advantages and disadvantages when imaging certain events. Hence, a new area of multimodality imaging is emerging in which the beneficial qualities from each of these imaging modalities are merged together. The creation of such a system would enhance the ability to quantify, interpret, and locate molecular events and biological processes [13, 78, 79]. A vector that harbors a fusion protein consisting of a bioluminescent reporter (Renilla luciferase), a fluorescence reporter (red or green fluorescence protein), and a PET reporter (mutant herpes simplex virus thymidine kinase) retained most of the activity of each protein constituent when expressed. This fusion protein was utilized in investigating lymphocytic migration, gene therapy, and metastasis [80, 81]. In analyzing cervical carcinoma with bladder invasion, fusion imaging of Thallium-201 single-photon emission computed tomography (Tl-201 SPECT) and F-18 fluorodeoxyglucose positron emission tomography (FDG PET) was employed. The multimodality image system of registration and fusion applied here bypasses the inadequate image resolution of SPECT and the low sensitivity of PET, and therefore presents an effective procedure for recognizing bladder invasion in cervical cancer [82]. At present, multimodality imaging is becoming prevalent in molecular-genetic studies, but it also has great potential to become the conventional approach for reporter gene imaging studies [80, 81, 83, 84].

Applications of Bioluminescent and Fluorescent Optical Imaging

Recently, protein complementation assays have been in the limelight for their ability to allow noninvasive, near-real-time detection of changes in signaling pathways [85–88]. This strategy relies on unique splitting of a monomeric reporter enzyme into two distinct inactive components which when forced into juxtaposition reconstitute the original enzymatic activity [89]. Historically, the yeast two-hybrid system first described by Stanley Fields [88] is based on protein complementation of GAL4, a transcriptional activator protein. This system revolutionized the characterization of signaling cascades in eukaryotes by the ability to identify interaction partners of signaling components. Recently, a number of different proteins have been tested for complementation assays and these include dihydrofolate reductase, β-galactosidase, green fluorescent protein, yellow fluorescent protein, β-lactamase, and luciferases (firefly, Gaussia, and Renilla). Of the different complementation assays, the bioluminescence reporter is one of the most useful modalities for small animal imaging. Luker et al. optimized firefly luciferase protein complementation by screening incremental truncation libraries of N- and C-terminal fragments of luciferase

[115]. Since then, this system has been utilized to monitor near-real-time interaction between mTOR and FK506-binding protein, Cdc25c and 14-3-3ε, EGFR and shc, EGFR and Grb2, MyoD and Id [90], insulin and TGF-β (for complete list, see Table 1).

Table 1 Applications of split luciferase-based reporters for monitoring protein–protein interactions, kinase activity, and protease activity

Reporter	Protein interaction or activity	Luciferase source
Protein–protein interaction		
FRB-NFLuc CFLuc-FKBP	FRB (rapamycin-binding domain of mTOR) and FKBP (FK506-binding protein type 12) [116, 125]	Firefly
NFLuc-Id MyoD-CFLuc	MyoD (myogenic regulatory protein from skeletal muscle) and Id (inhibitor of DNA binding 1) [126]	Firefly
NFLuc-DnaEN-ID and MyoD-DnaEC-CFLuc	DnaE C/N (N-terminal or C-terminal of DNA polymerase III catalytic subunit) [126]	Firefly
CFLuc-CXCR4 CXCR7-NRLuc	CXCR4 chemokine (C–X–C motif) receptor 4 and 7 [127]	Firefly
EGFR-NLuc, Grb2-NLuc, EGFR-CLuc, Shc-CLuc	EGFR interaction with growth factor receptor-binding protein 2 (Grb2) and Src homology 2 domain containing (Shc2) [128]	Firefly
FRB-hGLuc(1) FKBP-hGLuc(2)	FRB (rapamycin-binding domain of mTOR) and FKBP (FK506-binding protein type 12) [118]	Gaussia
NhRLuc-MyoD Id-ChRluc	MyoD (myogenic regulatory protein from skeletal muscle) and Id (inhibitor of DNA binding 1) [90]	Renilla
NhRLuc-FRB FKBP12-ChRLuc	FRB (rapamycin-binding domain of mTOR) and FKBP (FK506-binding protein type 12) interaction [129]	Renilla
NRLuc-CaM-M13-CRLuc	CaM (calmodulin) and M13(CaM-binding domain of skeletal muscle MLCK) interaction [130]	Renilla
Kinase activity		
NLuc-FHA2-pepCLuc	Akt kinase activity [99, 131]	Firefly
EGFR-NLuc, Grb2-NLuc, EGFR-CLuc, and Shc-CLuc	Ligand-mediated EGFR activation and subsequent phosphorylation of its target proteins Grb2 and Shc2 [128]	Firefly
NLuc-SH2-SH3-CD-CLuc	Bcr-Abl kinase activity [101]	Firefly
Protease activity		
pepA-NLuc pepB-CLuc	Caspase 3 activity [113]	Firefly
Other		
Probe1-CRLuc Probe2-CRLuc	Oligonucleotide probe interaction [132]	Renilla

Imaging Kinases

Protein kinases are enzymes that post-translationally modify substrate proteins by catalyzing the covalent addition of a negatively charged phosphate group from *ATP* to a specific *amino acid* [91–96]. These enzymes are one of the principle regulators of signaling cascades influencing a plurality of cellular decisions. Phosphorylation of target residues in proteins results in changes in substrate activity, subcellular location, and/or interaction with other proteins which mediate a bulk of kinase signaling [93–98]. Years of intensive investigations have led to the identification of key kinase biomarkers in cancer initiation and progression. For example, in breast cancer, overexpression and/or amplification of Her-2 is observed in nearly 25% of the patients and is mostly associated with aggressive and metastatic breast cancer. Many such oncogenic kinases have been identified; however, a majority of these biomarkers remain undrugged partly due to the unavailability of simple and reproducible cell-based assays to monitor kinases.

We have recently developed a luciferase complementation-based kinase imaging platform that allows quantitative, real-time, noninvasive imaging of kinase activity and is easily amenable for high-throughput screening of new drugs [97, 99, 100]. As a prototype, we constructed an Akt reporter, which was a fusion of an Akt consensus substrate peptide and phosphoamino acid-binding domain (FHA2) flanked by the amino- (N-Luc) and carboxyl- (C-Luc) terminal domains of the firefly luciferase reporter molecule (Fig. 1). N-Luc and C-Luc are split luciferase components that are inactive when expressed individually but can reconstitute luciferase activity when juxtaposed. In the presence of Akt kinase activity, phosphorylation of the Akt consensus substrate sequences within the reporter results in its interaction with the FHA2 domain, thus stearically preventing reconstitution of a functional luciferase reporter molecule (see Fig. 1B and 2). In the absence of an Akt kinase activity, release of this stearic constraint allows reconstitution of the luciferase activity. When cells were transfected with this reporter and treated with Akt inhibitor, API2, or a PI-3K inhibitor, perifosine, an increase in bioluminescence activity in a time- and dose-dependent manner was observed. This indicated that the Akt reporter monitors Akt activity noninvasively, in near real time, and quantitatively [99, 100]. This finding was corroborated with conventional Western blotting using antibodies to phosphorylated Akt [99]. The Akt reporter was also used to probe upstream signaling event: stimulation of EGFR using EGF resulted in a decrease in reporter activity, while an increase in bioluminescence was observed when treated with erlotinib, an EGFR inhibitor. Additionally, the use of erlotinib in the erlotinib-sensitive and -resistant cell lines resulted in differential activation of the Akt reporter. Finally, activation of the reporter was also monitored in vivo in mice bearing tumors when treated with erlotinib, API-2, or perifosine, further substantiating the utility of this kinase reporter. In summary, the Akt reporter allows imaging of signaling events, leading to activation /inactivation of Akt in a quantitative, dynamic, and noninvasive

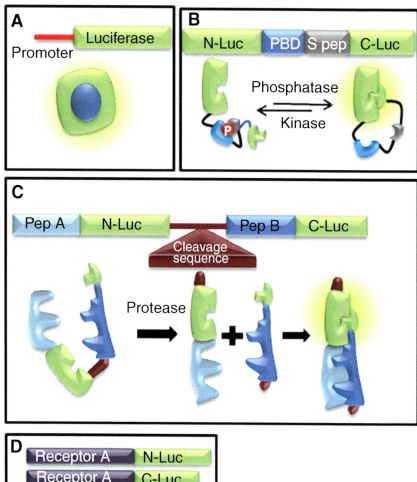

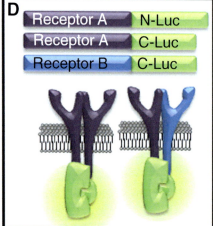

Fig. 1 Molecular imaging of signaling during metastases. Tumor metastases may be monitored using a promoter tagged reporter expressing cell line and following the fate of such cells

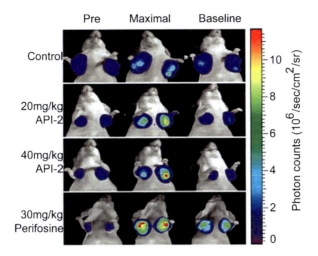

Fig. 2 Imaging of Akt activity in preclinical experimental model system. Mice transplanted with D54 cells stably expressing bioluminescent Akt reporter (BAR) were treated with vehicle control (20% DMSO in PBS), API-2 (20 mg/kg or 40 mg/kg), or perifosine (30 mg/kg). Images of representative mice are shown before treatment, during maximal luciferase signal upon treatment (Max), and after treatment

manner. Very recently, this imaging strategy was adapted for monitoring Abl kinase [101], suggesting that luciferase complementation-based kinase imaging platforms are versatile sensors for detecting kinase activity and should be exploited for monitoring metastatic kinases.

Fig. 1 (continued) in animals. (**a**) This allows tracking of cells during different stages of metastases and identification of new abode of the cancer cells (see I–V green cells). A number of receptor or nonreceptor tyrosine or serine/threonine kinases influence the metastatic behavior of cancer cells. (**b**) depicts a strategy to monitor kinase activity based on the luciferase complementation. The chimeric kinase reporter is a fusion of N-Luc and C-Luc components of luciferase complementation system (see text) separated by the kinase substrate peptide (S Pep) harboring a consensus phosphorylation site and phosphoamino acid-binding domain (PBD). Phosphorylation of the substrate peptide within the reporter results in inter-action with the PBD causing stearic constraints on the C-Luc and N-Luc. Inhibition of the kinase results in decreased binding of substrate peptide and PBD domain enabling the N-Luc and C-Luc interaction to restore bioluminescence. (**c**) Schematic representation of the biolu-minescent caspase-3 reporter, PepA-NLuc-DEVD-pepB-CLuc. Apoptosis imaging reporter constitutes the split luciferase (N-Luc and C-Luc) domains fused to strongly interacting peptide pair, pepA and pepB, with an intervening caspase-3 cleavage motif. Upon induction of apoptosis, the reporter molecule is proteolytically cleaved by caspase-3 at the DEVD motif. This cleavage enables interaction between pepA-NLuc and pepB-CLuc, thus reconstituting luciferase activity. Monitoring protein–protein interaction by the luciferase complementation involves creating of two distinct fusion proteins proteinA-NLuc and ProteinB-CLuc which when interacting generate light due to complementation. (**d**) is schematic representation of utilization of luciferase complementation assay to monitor homodimeric and heterodimeric receptor interactions. The reporter can be modified to sense any protein–protein interaction

Imaging Proteases

A crucial step during metastasis is the destruction of biological barriers such as the basement membrane, which requires activation of proteolytic enzymes [102–104]. A concerted effort of a number of proteases is needed for every step starting from the breakdown of the basal membrane of the primary tumor to the extended growth of established metastases. Among them, members of the plasminogen activator pathway and matrix metalloproteinase (MMP) family are well-documented contributors to tumor invasion, metastasis, and angiogenesis. Additionally, loss of caspase has been reported in the growth of metastatic tumors, presumably to evade apoptotic death [105]. This section is dedicated to the description of the molecular imaging strategies that were developed by our lab and others in order to noninvasively monitor protease activity in cells and animals. We suggest that similar strategies could be exploited in monitoring proteases involved in signaling during metastases.

Caspases, a family of cysteine-dependent aspartate-directed proteases, are key initiators and executors of both extrinsic and intrinsic apoptotic pathways [106–110]. We have recently constructed a caspase-3 activity sensor namely pepA-NLuc-DEVD-pepB-CLuc. In this reporter, pepA and pepB, a pair of peptides that have been reported to interact with each other with strong affinity [111, 112], are fused to N-Luc and C-Luc, respectively, with an intervening caspase-3 cleavage site. In a nonapoptotic cell, this chimeric luciferase reporter has reduced or no background luciferase activity as the N-Luc and the C-Luc are unable to complement when expressed as a fusion protein. However, in the presence of caspase-3 activity, the reporter is cleaved, and pepA and pepB associate through a high-affinity interaction and facilitate complementation of N-Luc and C-Luc domains, which reconstitutes luciferase. This apoptosis reporter system is a highly sensitive, dynamic, and quantitative reporter of caspase-3 activity both in vitro and in vivo [113] and may be adapted to monitor other cytosolic metastatic proteases. We have recently utilized this reporter system for in vivo optimization of dose, combination, and schedule of novel therapies in a dynamic and noninvasive manner [113]. These results highlight the power of molecular imaging in screening of novel combinations of therapies in experimental animal systems to derive therapies which can rein in aggressive and metastatic cancers.

Imaging Protein–Protein Interaction

Protein complementation assays have garnered a lot of attention for monitoring protein–protein interaction [85–88]. Ever since it was pioneered in 1989, yeast two hybrid screening, based on complementation of GAL4 and utilized for monitoring protein-protein interactions, has remarkably influenced our understanding of the signaling cascades. Recently, complementation of a number of different reporters has been developed; these include fluorescent proteins (GFP and YFP), bioluminescent enzymes (firefly luciferase, Renilla luciferase,

Gaussia luciferase), β-galactosidase, dihydrofolate reductase (DHFR), and TME1 b-lactamase [89, 114–119]. Of the different complementation assays, the bioluminescence reporter is one of the most useful modalities for small animal imaging. Using incremental truncation libraries of N and C-terminal fragments of firefly luciferase, a protein complementation assay for luciferase, was established by luker et al. [115]. They utilized the complementation assay for demonstrating an interaction between human Cdc25C and 14-3-3-e in real time noninvasively both in vitro and in vivo. Along similar lines, Paulmurugan and Gambhir [90] developed a Renilla luciferase complementation assay and monitored the interaction of MyoD and Id in real time. Similarly, Gaussia luciferase complementation assays were developed by Remy and Michnick [118], where they monitored cross talk of TGFb and insulin signaling. For a list of reporters constructed utilizing split luciferase complementation assays, see Table 1. In summary, protein–protein interactions can be monitored by luciferase complementation assays and thus can be exploited for monitoring such interactions specific for metastases.

Molecular Imaging Modality in Monitoring Therapeutic Response

The efficacy of a therapeutic regimen in clinic is assessed by anatomical measurements months after the end of treatment. Such assessments have had deleterious effect on the outcome of the patients, especially for those that have tumors that are resistant to the first line of therapy. Molecular imaging is extremely useful in preclinical determination of dose, schedule, combination, and efficacy of a therapeutic regimen. This allows clinicians to make informed clinical decisions on the efficacy of a particular therapy. This would also result in improved quality of life for patients by not subjecting them to a nonefficacious therapy and shifting them to alternate experimental or established therapy. Further, the capacity to prognosticate early in therapy will reduce the high cost associated with drug usage and utilization of resources. One such technique which has shown significant potential for determining, in real time, the efficacy of a therapy is diffusion MRI [21, 22, 120]. In this technique, the diffusion of water is used to evaluate the impact of a therapy and the main hypothesis asserts that though a tumor can be treated successfully with the aid of anticancer agents, there is still significant damage to cells and cell death that alters the integrity of the plasma membrane and the degree of cellularity. Thus, cell loss leads to the subsequent increase in the fractional volume of the interstitial space, which results in amplified levels of water diffusion within the tumor's damaged tissue. It is also interesting that the use of water diffusion as a substitute marker for probing tissue cellularity strongly impinges upon the molecular viscosity and membrane permeability between intra- and extracellular compartments, the active transport, and the flow and the directionality of tissue/cellular structures that impede water mobility [21, 120]. Accordingly, diffusion MRI has applications in detecting tumor regions with high cellular density, differentiating cystic masses from solid lesions in tumors and other modes of tumor characterizations [120, 121]. This method was corroborated to examine early events in the treatment of various tumor models and recently in patients with CNS tumor [121].

Other technology that is clinically relevant for very early measures of response is FDG-positron emission tomography (PET). Stroobants et al. showed, in soft tissue sarcoma treated with imatinib, a profound decline in FDG uptake within 48 hours of treatment and that the early response monitored by FDG uptake was able to predict progression-free survival [122]. Additionally, radionuclide imaging of apoptosis and cellular proliferation are also reported for monitoring response to therapy [123, 124].

Molecular Imaging in Drug Discovery and Development

Discovery and development of drugs for treating human diseases is a protracted and expensive process, requiring years of investigation and a budget close to $800 million for every drug that receives FDA approval. At an early stage of drug discovery, molecular imaging assists to support the proof-of-concept testing. Additionally, it aids not only in early detection of promising candidates but also in aborting research on candidates that are toxic and unlikely to pass the rigorous process of drug development. Further, it has the potential to hasten preclinical studies by noninvasively quantifying the biomarker activity and monitoring the drug–target interaction in vivo. Furthermore, cell-based molecular imaging assays monitor biomarker activity or its inhibition in the native environment of the target. Thus, this leads to identification of hits that usually possess the ideal solubility, ability to traverse membranes, and inhibit the biomarker in its innate milieu compartment (pH, concentrations of specific ions, etc.). Therefore, molecular imaging has the potential to reduce time and cost at various stages of drug development starting from developing surrogate assays for various biological processes that can be utilized in high-throughput drug discovery screens through assessing drug–target interactions, identification of patients, and finally in monitoring response of diseased tissue to therapeutic agents.

A significant advantage of complementation-based bioluminescent kinase or protease reporters described above is their adaptability to high-throughput screening. Bioluminescence generated in luciferase assays offers increased sensitivity compared to FRET-based systems due to amplification of the signal and shows higher robustness toward nonspecific interference by compounds. Luciferase complementation-based assays are a "gain of function assay" wherein the inhibition of kinase activity results in an increase in bioluminescence. Such assays are better suited for high-throughput screening when compared to promoter-driven luciferase, which are fraught with false positives. For example, compounds that kill cells (and thus result in a loss of signal) or those that inhibit luciferase activity may show up as false positives in typical luciferase/fluorescent/enzyme-based assays. However, specific inhibition of reporters like a kinase complementation reporter results in an increase in bioluminescence activity and thus nonspecific cytotoxic agents are eliminated. Such carefully designed screening methodology will enable narrowing the number of positive compounds to a smaller group of "true positives" and play an important role in hastening the drug discovery process.

Concluding Remarks

Molecular imaging provides a unique opportunity to integrate tumor molecular profiling information to preclinical and clinical utilization for monitoring tumor growth, metastasis, biomarker activity, therapeutic responsiveness, high-throughput screening for new drugs, drug–target interaction, and developing new schedules of therapies.

Acknowledgments We thank Terry Williams for critical reading of the manuscript. This work was supported by US National Institutes of Health grants P01CA85878, P50CA01014, R24CA83099, R01RCA129623A and a grant from the John and Suzanne Munn Endowed Research Fund of the University of Michigan Comprehensive Cancer Center (to MSB).

References

1. Cady, B. Regional lymph node metastases; a singular manifestation of the process of clinical metastases in cancer: contemporary animal research and clinical reports suggest unifying concepts. Ann Surg Oncol *14*: 1790–800, 2007.
2. Leong, S.P., B. Cady, D.M. Jablons, J. Garcia-Aguilar, D. Reintgen, J. Jakub, S. Pendas, L. Duhaime, R. Cassell, M. Gardner, R. Giuliano, V. Archie, D. Calvin, L. Mensha, S. Shivers, C. Cox, J.A. Werner, Y. Kitagawa, and M. Kitajima. Clinical patterns of metastasis. Cancer Metastasis Rev *25*: 221–32, 2006.
3. Leong, S.P., B. Cady, D.M. Jablons, J. Garcia-Aguilar, D. Reintgen, J.A. Werner, and Y. Kitagawa. Patterns of metastasis in human solid cancers. Cancer Treat Res *135*: 209–21, 2007.
4. Vicent, S., D. Luis-Ravelo, I. Anton, I. Garcia-Tunon, F. Borras-Cuesta, J. Dotor, J. De Las Rivas, and F. Lecanda. A novel lung cancer signature mediates metastatic bone colonization by a dual mechanism. Cancer Res *68*: 2275–85, 2008.
5. Inamura, K., T. Shimoji, H. Ninomiya, M. Hiramatsu, M. Okui, Y. Satoh, S. Okumura, K. Nakagawa, T. Noda, M. Fukayama, and Y. Ishikawa. A metastatic signature in entire lung adenocarcinomas irrespective of morphological heterogeneity. Hum Pathol *38*: 702–9, 2007.
6. Montel, V., T.Y. Huang, E. Mose, K. Pestonjamasp, and D. Tarin. Expression profiling of primary tumors and matched lymphatic and lung metastases in a xenogeneic breast cancer model. Am J Pathol *166*: 1565–79, 2005.
7. Hu, J., F. Bianchi, M. Ferguson, A. Cesario, S. Margaritora, P. Granone, P. Goldstraw, M. Tetlow, C. Ratcliffe, A.G. Nicholson, A. Harris, K. Gatter, and F. Pezzella. Gene expression signature for angiogenic and nonangiogenic non-small-cell lung cancer. Oncogene *24*: 1212–9, 2005.

8. Li, C., Z. Chen, Z. Xiao, X. Wu, X. Zhan, X. Zhang, M. Li, J. Li, X. Feng, S. Liang, P. Chen, and J.Y. Xie. Comparative proteomics analysis of human lung squamous carcinoma. Biochem Biophys Res Commun *309*: 253–60, 2003.
9. Yanagisawa, K., B.J. Xu, D.P. Carbone, and R.M. Caprioli. Molecular fingerprinting in human lung cancer. Clin Lung Cancer *5*: 113–8, 2003.
10. Sharma, V., G.D. Luker, and D. Piwnica-Worms. Molecular imaging of gene expression and protein function in vivo with PET and SPECT. J Magn Reson Imaging *16*: 336–51, 2002.
11. Contag, C.H. and M.H. Bachmann. Advances in in vivo bioluminescence imaging of gene expression. Annu Rev Biomed Eng *4*: 235–60, 2002.
12. Weissleder, R. Scaling down imaging: molecular mapping of cancer in mice. Nat Rev Cancer *2*: 11–8, 2002.
13. Blasberg, R.G. Molecular imaging and cancer. Mol Cancer Ther *2*: 335–43, 2003.
14. Gelovani Tjuvajev, J. and R.G. Blasberg. In vivo imaging of molecular-genetic targets for cancer therapy. Cancer Cell *3*: 327–32, 2003.
15. Herschman, H.R. Molecular imaging: looking at problems, seeing solutions. Science *302*: 605–8, 2003.
16. Gross, S. and D. Piwnica-Worms. Spying on cancer: molecular imaging in vivo with genetically encoded reporters. Cancer Cell *7*: 5–15, 2005.
17. Jaffer, F.A. and R. Weissleder. Molecular imaging in the clinical arena. Jama *293*: 855–62, 2005.
18. Weissleder, R. and U. Mahmood. Molecular imaging. Radiology *219*: 316–33, 2001.
19. Weissleder, R. and V. Ntziachristos. Shedding light onto live molecular targets. Nat Med *9*: 123–8, 2003.
20. Mahmood, U. and R. Weissleder. Near-infrared optical imaging of proteases in cancer. Mol Cancer Ther *2*: 489–96, 2003.
21. Chenevert, T.L., L.D. Stegman, J.M. Taylor, P.L. Robertson, H.S. Greenberg, A. Rehemtulla, and B.D. Ross. Diffusion magnetic resonance imaging: an early surrogate marker of therapeutic efficacy in brain tumors. J Natl Cancer Inst *92*: 2029–36, 2000.
22. Moffat, B.A., D.E. Hall, J. Stojanovska, P.J. McConville, J.B. Moody, T.L. Chenevert, A. Rehemtulla, and B.D. Ross. Diffusion imaging for evaluation of tumor therapies in preclinical animal models. Magma *17*: 249–59, 2004.
23. Guccione, S., K.C. Li, and M.D. Bednarski. Molecular imaging and therapy directed at the neovasculature in pathologies. How imaging can be incorporated into vascular-targeted delivery systems to generate active therapeutic agents. IEEE Eng Med Biol Mag *23*: 50–6, 2004.
24. Morgan, B., M.A. Horsfield, and W.P. Steward. The role of imaging in the clinical development of antiangiogenic agents. Hematol Oncol Clin North Am *18*: 1183–206, x, 2004.
25. Louie, A.Y., M.M. Huber, E.T. Ahrens, U. Rothbacher, R. Moats, R.E. Jacobs, S.E. Fraser, and T.J. Meade. In vivo visualization of gene expression using magnetic resonance imaging. Nat Biotechnol *18*: 321–5, 2000.
26. Ntziachristos, V., C. Bremer, E.E. Graves, J. Ripoll, and R. Weissleder. In vivo tomographic imaging of near-infrared fluorescent probes. Mol Imaging *1*: 82–8, 2002.
27. Bremer, C., V. Ntziachristos, and R. Weissleder. Optical-based molecular imaging: contrast agents and potential medical applications. Eur Radiol *13*: 231–43, 2003.
28. Funovics, M., R. Weissleder, and C.H. Tung. Protease sensors for bioimaging. Anal Bioanal Chem *377*: 956–63, 2003.
29. Ntziachristos, V., E.A. Schellenberger, J. Ripoll, D. Yessayan, E. Graves, A. Bogdanov, Jr., L. Josephson, and R. Weissleder. Visualization of antitumor treatment by means of fluorescence molecular tomography with an annexin V-Cy5.5 conjugate. Proc Natl Acad Sci USA *101*: 12294–9, 2004.
30. Dzik-Jurasz, A.S. Molecular imaging in vivo: an introduction. Br J Radiol *76 Spec No 2*: S98–109, 2003.

31. Bhojani, M.S., B. Laxman, B.D. Ross, and A. Rehemtulla. Molecular imaging in cancer. In *ApoptosisandCancerTherapy*, K.-M.DebatinandS.Fulda,eds.(Weinheim:Wiley-VCH,2006).

32. Buchsbaum, D., R. Lloyd, J. Juni, I. Wollner, P. Brubaker, D. Hanna, J. Spicker, F. Burns, Z. Steplewski, D. Colcher et al. Localization and imaging of radiolabeled monoclonal antibodies against colorectal carcinoma in tumor-bearing nude mice. Cancer Res *48*: 4324–33, 1988.

33. Buchsbaum, D.J. Imaging and therapy of tumors induced to express somatostatin receptor by gene transfer using radiolabeled peptides and single chain antibody constructs. Semin Nucl Med *34*: 32–46, 2004.

34. Figueiredo, J.L., H. Alencar, R. Weissleder, and U. Mahmood. Near infrared thoracoscopy of tumoral protease activity for improved detection of peripheral lung cancer. Int J Cancer *118*: 2672–7, 2006.

35. Blum, G., G. von Degenfeld, M.J. Merchant, H.M. Blau, and M. Bogyo. Noninvasive optical imaging of cysteine protease activity using fluorescently quenched activity-based probes. Nat Chem Biol *3*: 668–77, 2007.

36. Tung, C.H., U. Mahmood, S. Bredow, and R. Weissleder. In vivo imaging of proteolytic enzyme activity using a novel molecular reporter. Cancer Res *60*: 4953–8, 2000.

37. Bremer, C., S. Bredow, U. Mahmood, R. Weissleder, and C.H. Tung. Optical imaging of matrix metalloproteinase-2 activity in tumors: feasibility study in a mouse model. Radiology *221*: 523–9, 2001.

38. Tung, C.H., S. Bredow, U. Mahmood, and R. Weissleder. Preparation of a cathepsin D sensitive near-infrared fluorescence probe for imaging. Bioconjug Chem *10*: 892–6, 1999.

39. Rehemtulla, A., L.D. Stegman, S.J. Cardozo, S. Gupta, D.E. Hall, C.H. Contag, and B.D. Ross. Rapid and quantitative assessment of cancer treatment response using in vivo bioluminescence imaging. Neoplasia *2*: 491–5, 2000.

40. Ciana, P., M. Raviscioni, P. Mussi, E. Vegeto, I. Que, M.G. Parker, C. Lowik, and A. Maggi. In vivo imaging of transcriptionally active estrogen receptors. Nat Med *9*: 82–6, 2003.

41. Carlsen, H., J.O. Moskaug, S.H. Fromm, and R. Blomhoff. In vivo imaging of NF-kappa B activity. J Immunol *168*: 1441–6, 2002.

42. Doubrovin, M., V. Ponomarev, T. Beresten, J. Balatoni, W. Bornmann, R. Finn, J. Humm, S. Larson, M. Sadelain, R. Blasberg, and J. Gelovani. Tjuvajev Imaging transcriptional regulation of p53-dependent genes with positron emission tomography in vivo. Proc Natl Acad Sci USA *98*: 9300–5, 2001.

43. Rehemtulla, A., N. Taneja, and B.D. Ross. Bioluminescence detection of cells having stabilized p53 in response to a genotoxic event. Mol Imaging *3*: 63–8, 2004.

44. Laxman, B., D.E. Hall, M.S. Bhojani, D.A. Hamstra, T.L. Chenevert, B.D. Ross, and A. Rehemtulla. Noninvasive real-time imaging of apoptosis. Proc Natl Acad Sci USA *99*: 16551–5, 2002.

45. Luker, G.D., V. Sharma, C.M. Pica, J.L. Prior, W. Li, and D. Piwnica-Worms. Molecular imaging of protein–protein interactions: controlled expression of p53 and large T-antigen fusion proteins in vivo. Cancer Res *63*: 1780–8, 2003.

46. Massoud, T.F. and S.S. Gambhir. Molecular imaging in living subjects: seeing fundamental biological processes in a new light. Genes Dev *17*: 545–80, 2003.

47. Stell, A., S. Belcredito, B. Ramachandran, A. Biserni, G. Rando, P. Ciana, and A. Maggi. Multimodality imaging: novel pharmacological applications of reporter systems. Q J Nucl Med Mol Imaging *51*: 127–38, 2007.

48. Ross, B.D., T.L. Chenevert, and A. Rehemtulla. Magnetic resonance imaging in cancer research. Eur J Cancer *38*: 2147–56, 2002.

49. Rees, J. Advances in magnetic resonance imaging of brain tumours. Curr Opin Neurol *16*: 643–50, 2003.

50. Choy, G., P. Choyke, and S.K. Libutti. Current advances in molecular imaging: noninvasive in vivo bioluminescent and fluorescent optical imaging in cancer research. Mol Imaging *2*: 303–12, 2003.

51. Bartrons, R. and J. Caro. Hypoxia, glucose metabolism and the Warburg's effect. J Bioenerg Biomembr *39*: 223–9, 2007.
52. Wallace, D.C. Mitochondria and cancer: Warburg addressed. Cold Spring Harb Symp Quant Biol *70*: 363–74, 2005.
53. Massoud, T.F., R. Paulmurugan, and S.S. Gambhir. Molecular imaging of homodimeric protein–protein interactions in living subjects. Faseb J *18*: 1105–7, 2004.
54. Blasberg, R.G. and J. Gelovani. Molecular-genetic imaging: a nuclear medicine-based perspective. Mol Imaging *1*: 280–300, 2002.
55. Blankenberg, F.G., C. Mari, and H.W. Strauss. Development of radiocontrast agents for vascular imaging: progress to date. Am J Cardiovasc Drugs *2*: 357–65, 2002.
56. McCaffrey, A., M.A. Kay, and C.H. Contag. Advancing molecular therapies through in vivo bioluminescent imaging. Mol Imaging *2*: 75–86, 2003.
57. Greer, L.F., 3rd and A.A. Szalay. Imaging of light emission from the expression of luciferases in living cells and organisms: a review. Luminescence *17*: 43–74, 2002.
58. Mahmood, U. Near infrared optical applications in molecular imaging. Earlier, more accurate assessment of disease presence, disease course, and efficacy of disease treatment. IEEE Eng Med Biol Mag *23*: 58–66, 2004.
59. Weissleder, R., C.H. Tung, U. Mahmood, and A. Bogdanov, Jr. In vivo imaging of tumors with protease-activated near-infrared fluorescent probes. Nat Biotechnol *17*: 375–8, 1999.
60. Campbell, R.E., O. Tour, A.E. Palmer, P.A. Steinbach, G.S. Baird, D.A. Zacharias, and R.Y. Tsien. A monomeric red fluorescent protein. Proc Natl Acad Sci USA *99*: 7877–82, 2002.
61. Shaner, N.C., R.E. Campbell, P.A. Steinbach, B.N. Giepmans, A.E. Palmer, and R.Y. Tsien. Improved monomeric red, orange and yellow fluorescent proteins derived from Discosoma sp. red fluorescent protein. Nat Biotechnol *22*: 1567–72, 2004.
62. Zhang, H.G., J. Wang, X. Yang, H.C. Hsu, and J.D. Mountz. Regulation of apoptosis proteins in cancer cells by ubiquitin. Oncogene *23*: 2009–15, 2004.
63. Zipfel, W.R., R.M. Williams, R. Christie, A.Y. Nikitin, B.T. Hyman, and W.W. Webb. Live tissue intrinsic emission microscopy using multiphoton-excited native fluorescence and second harmonic generation. Proc Natl Acad Sci USA *100*: 7075–80, 2003.
64. Zipfel, W.R., R.M. Williams, and W.W. Webb. Nonlinear magic: multiphoton microscopy in the biosciences. Nat Biotechnol *21*: 1369–77, 2003.
65. Bhojani, M.S., G. Chen, B.D. Ross, D.G. Beer, and A. Rehemtulla. Nuclear localized phosphorylated FADD induces cell proliferation and is associated with aggressive lung cancer. Cell Cycle *4*: 1478–81, 2005.
66. Ntziachristos, V., C.H. Tung, C. Bremer, and R. Weissleder. Fluorescence molecular tomography resolves protease activity in vivo. Nat Med *8*: 757–60, 2002.
67. Messerli, S.M., S. Prabhakar, Y. Tang, K. Shah, M.L. Cortes, V. Murthy, R. Weissleder, X.O. Breakefield, and C.H. Tung. A novel method for imaging apoptosis using a caspase-1 near-infrared fluorescent probe. Neoplasia *6*: 95–105, 2004.
68. Mahmood, U., C.H. Tung, A. Bogdanov, Jr., and R. Weissleder. Near-infrared optical imaging of protease activity for tumor detection. Radiology *213*: 866–70, 1999.
69. Chen, J., C.H. Tung, U. Mahmood, V. Ntziachristos, R. Gyurko, M.C. Fishman, P.L. Huang, and R. Weissleder. In vivo imaging of proteolytic activity in atherosclerosis. Circulation *105*: 2766–71, 2002.
70. Parungo, C.P., S. Ohnishi, A.M. De Grand, R.G. Laurence, E.G. Soltesz, Y.L. Colson, P.M. Kang, T. Mihaljevic, L.H. Cohn, and J.V. Frangioni. In vivo optical imaging of pleural space drainage to lymph nodes of prognostic significance. Ann Surg Oncol *11*: 1085–92, 2004.
71. Parungo, C.P., S. Ohnishi, S.W. Kim, S. Kim, R.G. Laurence, E.G. Soltesz, F.Y. Chen, Y.L. Colson, L.H. Cohn, M.G. Bawendi, and J.V. Frangioni. Intraoperative identification of esophageal sentinel lymph nodes with near-infrared fluorescence imaging. J Thorac Cardiovasc Surg *129*: 844–50, 2005.

72. Josephson, L., U. Mahmood, P. Wunderbaldinger, Y. Tang, and R. Weissleder. Pan and sentinel lymph node visualization using a near-infrared fluorescent probe. Mol Imaging 2: 18–23, 2003.
73. Michalet, X., F.F. Pinaud, L.A. Bentolila, J.M. Tsay, S. Doose, J.J. Li, G. Sundaresan, A.M. Wu, S.S. Gambhir, and S. Weiss. Quantum dots for live cells, in vivo imaging, and diagnostics. Science 307: 538–44, 2005.
74. Gao, X., Y. Cui, R.M. Levenson, L.W. Chung, and S. Nie. In vivo cancer targeting and imaging with semiconductor quantum dots. Nat Biotechnol 22: 969–76, 2004.
75. Lacoste, T.D., X. Michalet, F. Pinaud, D.S. Chemla, A.P. Alivisatos, and S. Weiss. Ultrahigh-resolution multicolor colocalization of single fluorescent probes. Proc Natl Acad Sci USA 97: 9461–6, 2000.
76. Dahan, M., S. Levi, C. Luccardini, P. Rostaing, B. Riveau, and A. Triller. Diffusion dynamics of glycine receptors revealed by single-quantum dot tracking. Science 302: 442–5, 2003.
77. Hohng, S. and T. Ha. Near-complete suppression of quantum dot blinking in ambient conditions. J Am Chem Soc 126: 1324–5, 2004.
78. Ponomarev, V., M. Doubrovin, I. Serganova, J. Vider, A. Shavrin, T. Beresten, A. Ivanova, L. Ageyeva, V. Tourkova, J. Balatoni, W. Bornmann, R. Blasberg, and J. Gelovani. Tjuvajev A novel triple-modality reporter gene for whole-body fluorescent, bioluminescent, and nuclear noninvasive imaging. Eur J Nucl Med Mol Imaging 31: 740–51, 2004.
79. Doubrovin, M., I. Serganova, P. Mayer-Kuckuk, V. Ponomarev, and R.G. Blasberg. Multimodality in vivo molecular-genetic imaging. Bioconjug Chem 15: 1376–88, 2004.
80. Ray, P., A. De, J.J. Min, R.Y. Tsien, and S.S. Gambhir. Imaging tri-fusion multimodality reporter gene expression in living subjects. Cancer Res 64: 1323–30, 2004.
81. Kim, Y.J., P. Dubey, P. Ray, S.S. Gambhir, and O.N. Witte. Multimodality imaging of lymphocytic migration using lentiviral-based transduction of a tri-fusion reporter gene. Mol Imaging Biol 6: 331–40, 2004.
82. Yen, K.Y., J.A. Liang, A.C. Shiau, T.C. Hsieh, S.S. Sun, and C.H. Kao. Fusion images of Tl-201 SPECT and FDG PET with CT in detection of cervical carcinoma with bladder invasion. Clin Nucl Med 30: 278–80, 2005.
83. Blasberg, R.G. and J.G. Tjuvajev. Molecular-genetic imaging: current and future perspectives. J Clin Invest 111: 1620–9, 2003.
84. Schellenberger, E.A., D. Sosnovik, R. Weissleder, and L. Josephson. Magneto/optical annexin V, a multimodal protein. Bioconjug Chem 15: 1062–7, 2004.
85. Kerppola, T.K. Visualization of molecular interactions by fluorescence complementation. Nat Rev Mol Cell Biol 7: 449–56, 2006.
86. Michnick, S.W., M.L. MacDonald, and J.K. Westwick. Chemical genetic strategies to delineate MAP kinase signaling pathways using protein-fragment complementation assays (PCA). Methods 40: 287–93, 2006.
87. Shyu, Y.J. and C.D. Hu. Fluorescence complementation: an emerging tool for biological research. Trends Biotechnol 26: 622–30, 2008.
88. Fields, S. and O. Song. A novel genetic system to detect protein–protein interactions. Nature 340: 245–6, 1989.
89. Michnick, S.W., P.H. Ear, E.N. Manderson, I. Remy, and E. Stefan. Universal strategies in research and drug discovery based on protein-fragment complementation assays. Nat Rev Drug Discov 6: 569–82, 2007.
90. Paulmurugan, R. and S.S. Gambhir. Monitoring protein–protein interactions using split synthetic renilla luciferase protein-fragment-assisted complementation. Anal Chem 75: 1584–9, 2003.
91. Manning, G., G.D. Plowman, T. Hunter, and S. Sudarsanam. Evolution of protein kinase signaling from yeast to man. Trends Biochem Sci 27: 514–20, 2002.
92. Manning, G., D.B. Whyte, R. Martinez, T. Hunter, and S. Sudarsanam. The protein kinase complement of the human genome. Science 298: 1912–34, 2002.

93. Edelman, A.M., D.K. Blumenthal, and E.G. Krebs. Protein serine/threonine kinases. Annu Rev Biochem *56*: 567–613, 1987.
94. Hubbard, S.R. and J.H. Till. Protein tyrosine kinase structure and function. Annu Rev Biochem *69*: 373–98, 2000.
95. Hunter, T. and J.A. Cooper. Protein-tyrosine kinases. Annu Rev Biochem *54*: 897–930, 1985.
96. Tsygankov, A.Y. Non-receptor protein tyrosine kinases. Front Biosci *8*: s595–635, 2003.
97. Zhang, L., M.S. Bhojani, B.D. Ross, and A. Rehemtulla. Molecular imaging of protein kinases. Cell Cycle *7*: 314–7, 2008.
98. Blume-Jensen, P. and T. Hunter. Oncogenic kinase signalling. Nature *411*: 355–65, 2001.
99. Zhang, L., K.C. Lee, M.S. Bhojani, A.P. Khan, A. Shilman, E.C. Holland, B.D. Ross, and A. Rehemtulla. Molecular imaging of Akt kinase activity. Nat Med *13*: 1114–9, 2007.
100. Zhang, L., M.S. Bhojani, B.D. Ross, and A. Rehemtulla. Enhancing Akt imaging through targeted reporter expression. Mol Imaging *7*: 168–74, 2008.
101. Zhou, V., X. Gao, S. Han, A. Brinker, J.S. Caldwell, and X.J. Gu. An intracellular conformational sensor assay for Abl T315I. Anal Biochem *385*: 300–8, 2009.
102. Liotta, L.A., K. Tryggvason, S. Garbisa, I. Hart, C.M. Foltz, and S. Shafie. Metastatic potential correlates with enzymatic degradation of basement membrane collagen. Nature *284*: 67–8, 1980.
103. Liotta, L.A., P.S. Steeg, and W.G. Stetler-Stevenson. Cancer metastasis and angiogenesis: an imbalance of positive and negative regulation. Cell *64*: 327–36, 1991.
104. Coussens, L.M., B. Fingleton, and L.M. Matrisian. Matrix metalloproteinase inhibitors and cancer: trials and tribulations. Science *295*: 2387–92, 2002.
105. Stupack, D.G., T. Teitz, M.D. Potter, D. Mikolon, P.J. Houghton, V.J. Kidd, J.M. Lahti, and D.A. Cheresh. Potentiation of neuroblastoma metastasis by loss of caspase-8. Nature *439*: 95–9, 2006.
106. Shi, Y. Apoptosome: the cellular engine for the activation of caspase-9. Structure *10*: 285–8, 2002.
107. Nicholson, D.W. and N.A. Thornberry. Caspases: killer proteases. Trends Biochem Sci *22*: 299–306, 1997.
108. Nicholson, D.W. and N.A. Thornberry. Apoptosis. Life and death decisions. Science *299*: 214–5, 2003.
109. Bhojani, M.S., Ross, B.D., and A. Rehemtulla. TRAIL in Cancer Therapy. In Death Receptor in Cancer Therapy, El-Deiry, W.S., ed., Series Cancer Drug Discovery and Development (Totowa NJ: Humana, 2004).
110. Bhojani, M.S., B.D. Rossu, and A. Rehemtulla. TRAIL and anti-tumor responses. Cancer Biol Ther *2*: S71–8, 2003.
111. Thormeyer, D., O. Ammerpohl, O. Larsson, Y. Xu, A. Asinger, C. Wahlestedt, and Z. Liang. Characterization of lacZ complementation deletions using membrane receptor dimerization. Biotechniques *34*: 346–50, 352–5, 2003.
112. Zhang, G., X. Zhou, C. Wang, M. Yao, H. Yu, and Q. Xie. mRNA and protein expression of Fas associated death domain protein in apoptotic hepatocyte induced by tumor necrosis factor-alpha. Zhonghua Gan Zang Bing Za Zhi *9*: 10–2, 2001.
113. Coppola, J.M., B.D. Ross, and A. Rehemtulla. Noninvasive imaging of apoptosis and its application in cancer therapeutics. Clin Cancer Res *14*: 2492–501, 2008.
114. Hu, C.D., Y. Chinenov, and T.K. Kerppola. Visualization of interactions among bZIP and Rel family proteins in living cells using bimolecular fluorescence complementation. Mol Cell *9*: 789–98, 2002.
115. Luker, G.D., V. Sharma, C.M. Pica, J.L. Dahlheimer, W. Li, J. Ochesky, C.E. Ryan, H. Piwnica-Worms, and D. Piwnica.-Worms Noninvasive imaging of protein–protein interactions in living animals. Proc Natl Acad Sci USA *99*: 6961–6, 2002.
116. Luker, K.E. and D. Piwnica-Worms. Optimizing luciferase protein fragment complementation for bioluminescent imaging of protein–protein interactions in live cells and animals. Methods Enzymol *385*: 349–60, 2004.

117. Galarneau, A., M. Primeau, L.E. Trudeau, and S.W. Michnick. Beta-lactamase protein fragment complementation assays as in vivo and in vitro sensors of protein protein interactions. Nat Biotechnol *20*: 619–22, 2002.
118. Remy, I. and S.W. Michnick. A highly sensitive protein–protein interaction assay based on Gaussia luciferase. Nat Methods *3*: 977–9, 2006.
119. Remy, I. and S.W. Michnick. Application of protein-fragment complementation assays in cell biology. Biotechniques *42*: 137, 139, 141 passim, 2007.
120. Chenevert, T.L., C.R. Meyer, B.A. Moffat, A. Rehemtulla, S.K. Mukherji, S.S. Gebarski, D.J. Quint, P.L. Robertson, T.S. Lawrence, L. Junck, J.M. Taylor, T.D. Johnson, Q. Dong, K.M. Muraszko, J.A. Brunberg, and B.D. Ross. Diffusion MRI: a new strategy for assessment of cancer therapeutic efficacy. Mol Imaging *1*: 336–43, 2002.
121. Moffat, B.A., T.L. Chenevert, T.S. Lawrence, C.R. Meyer, T.D. Johnson, Q. Dong, C. Tsien, S. Mukherji, D.J. Quint, S.S. Gebarski, P.L. Robertson, L.R. Junck, A. Rehemtulla, and B.D. Ross. Functional diffusion map: a noninvasive MRI biomarker for early stratification of clinical brain tumor response. Proc Natl Acad Sci USA *102*: 5524–9, 2005.
122. Stroobants, S., J. Goeminne, M. Seegers, S. Dimitrijevic, P. Dupont, J. Nuyts, M. Martens, B. van den Borne, P. Cole, R. Sciot, H. Dumez, S. Silberman, L. Mortelmans, and A. van Oosterom. 18FDG-Positron emission tomography for the early prediction of response in advanced soft tissue sarcoma treated with imatinib mesylate (Glivec). Eur J Cancer *39*: 2012–20, 2003.
123. Mankoff, D.A., A.F. Shields, and K.A. Krohn. PET imaging of cellular proliferation. Radiol Clin North Am *43*: 153–67, 2005.
124. Blankenberg, F., K. Ohtsuki, and H.W. Strauss. Dying a thousand deaths. Radionuclide imaging of apoptosis. Q J Nucl Med *43*: 170–6, 1999.
125. Luker, K.E., M.C. Smith, G.D. Luker, S.T. Gammon, H. Piwnica-Worms, and D. Piwnica-Worms. Kinetics of regulated protein–protein interactions revealed with firefly luciferase complementation imaging in cells and living animals. Proc Natl Acad Sci USA *101*: 12288–93, 2004.
126. Paulmurugan, R., Y. Umezawa, and S.S. Gambhir. Noninvasive imaging of protein–protein interactions in living subjects by using reporter protein complementation and reconstitution strategies. Proc Natl Acad Sci USA *99*: 15608–13, 2002.
127. Luker, K.E., M. Gupta, and G.D. Luker. Imaging CXCR4 signaling with firefly luciferase complementation. Anal Chem *80*: 5565–73, 2008.
128. Li, W.R., F. Li, Q. Huang, B. Frederick, S.D. Bao, and C.Y. Li. Noninvasive imaging and quantification of epidermal growth factor receptor kinase activation in vivo. Cancer Res *68*: 4990–4997, 2008.
129. Paulmurugan, R., T.F. Massoud, J. Huang, and S.S. Gambhir. Molecular imaging of drug-modulated protein–protein interactions in living subjects. Cancer Res *64*: 2113–9, 2004.
130. Kaihara, A., Y. Umezawa, and T. Furukawa. Bioluminescent indicators for Ca2 + based on split renilla luciferase complementation in living cells. Analytical Sciences *24*: 1405–8, 2008.
131. Chan, C.T., R. Paulmurugan, O.S. Gheysens, J. Kim, G. Chiosis, and S.S. Gambhir. Molecular imaging of the efficacy of heat shock protein 90 inhibitors in living subjects. Cancer Res *68*: 216–226, 2008.
132. Cissell, K.A., Y. Rahimi, S. Shrestha, and S.K. Deo. Reassembly of a bioluminescent protein renilla luciferase directed through dna hybridization. Bioconjug Chem 2008.

Biomarker Discovery for Metastatic Disease

Gilbert S. Omenn and James D. Cavalcoli

Abstract Emerging knowledge about the many features of metastasis offers numerous possibilities for discovery and exploitation of diagnostic and prognostic biomarkers and targets for therapy. A systems biology approach that encompasses differential expression of mRNAs (gene expression), microRNAs (gene regulators), and proteins in primary and metastatic tumors, in proximal biofluids, and in the blood plasma generates potentially complementary molecular signatures. We illustrate the use of Oncomine and Molecular Concepts Maps and the biological amplification of tumor protein signals with immune *responses that produce autoantibodies in relation to lung cancers.*

Introduction

There are two complementary but very different needs for biomarkers of cancers. The first is to diagnose cancers at early stages, presumably much more treatable for cure, or even in preclinical stages when chemoprevention might be successful. The second is to gain information about the prognosis, both in response to particular therapies and in relation to likelihood of metastasis. Despite a voluminous literature about potential mRNA and protein biomarker profiles for various cancers and a compelling clinical need for diagnostic tests and prognostic tests, progress has been limited.

Currently, new methods and new instruments are being employed to try to accelerate the discovery phase. Biomarkers may be assayed directly in primary or metastatic tumor specimens, in biofluids proximal to the tumor (bronchial lavage, urine, CSF), or in the circulation (plasma, serum). Given the heterogeneity of tumor mechanisms and the limitations of specific analytical methods, it is likely that a variety of strategies will be needed and will be complementary

G.S. Omenn (✉)
Internal Medicine, Human Genetics, Public Health, and Center for Computational Medicine and Bioinformatics, University of Michigan, Ann Arbor, MI 48109-2218, USA
e-mail: gomenn@umich.edu

V. Keshamouni et al. (eds.), *Lung Cancer Metastasis*,
DOI 10.1007/978-1-4419-0772-1_14, © Springer Science+Business Media, LLC 2009

[1]. Molecular biomarkers for lung cancers would be particularly useful for screening and for differential diagnosis, since they could be combined with imaging modalities, such as spiral CT imaging of the lung [2, 3].

The vast majority of deaths from cancers, an estimated 90% [4, 5], are due to metastases from the primary tumor site. Understanding what mediates metastasis is the aim of this book. Molecular markers or signatures that could help predict which tumors have a propensity and the capability to metastasize would be useful clinically. Host genotypes and phenotypes, perhaps specific for particular organ sites or tissue types, might influence or even determine whether micrometastases take root and grow into harmful lesions. Starting from the metastatic lesion, molecular markers for response to therapy would be important, especially when there are alternative therapeutic regimens or new regimens need to be devised for nonresponders. In some cases, having molecular markers for a metastatic lesion that would reveal its likely source of origin would be valuable, especially in the absence of a known primary tumor and in the differentiation of primary and metastatic single lesions in the lung.

Different primary tumors have different propensities for sites of metastasis. Sometimes the reasons are obvious, like the dissemination of colorectal cancer cells via the portal vein to the liver and appearance of metastases in lymph nodes draining the breast, oral cavity, and other primary sites. Other times the propensity is less obvious, like the metastasis of lung cancer cells to the adrenal gland. We are in the infancy of such studies.

In *The Biology of Cancer* [6], Weinberg emphasizes that the reasons are still obscure why tumors arising in certain tissues have a high probability of metastasis, while those arising in other tissues rarely do so. Contrasting examples are melanomas and squamous cell carcinomas of the skin. The fundamental question is whether primary tumors with a high propensity to metastasize already have distinguishable characteristics that reveal that propensity – at one extreme for early metastasis (like lung and pancreatic cancers) or at the opposite extreme for emergence of late metastases long after successful treatment of the primary lesion (like breast). A tiny subpopulation of tumor cells, the cancer stem cells, may govern the risk of recurrence after successful therapy to markedly reduce tumor mass; perhaps different cells drive metastasis. The cellular and molecular processes involved in multistep tumor progression and metastasis facilitate migration and invasion, which are amply addressed in this book; survival without stroma and extracellular matrix in the lymphatics or circulating blood; and complex responses in distant sites that somehow determine the colonization, growth, and fate of micrometastases.

Most likely the results are a combination of the properties of the primary tumor and its heterogeneous cells and stroma and the properties of the microenvironment at distant sites in different individuals ("seed" and "soil"). The relatively large size of cancer cells released into the circulation or of cancer cells coated with platelets causes them to lodge in the first capillaries or small arterioles they encounter, commonly in the lungs, accounting for the high incidence of metastatic lesions in the lungs. How some of these circulating cells escape from the lungs to reach distant sites is much less clear, perhaps involving arteriovenous shunts. Also it is unclear how much of the lodging of cancer cells and subsequent extravasation through the vessel wall into the surrounding tissue is physical trapping and how much reflects a role for integrins and other specific cell surface receptors on endothelial cells. Specifically, cancer cells are thought to lack the complex capabilities of leukocytes that facilitate diapedesis, the process by which these cells escape from post-capillary venules to perform inflammatory functions in the tissue. Cancer cells release proteases into microthrombi that may facilitate extravasation. In addition, angiogenesis provides an increased density of immature, highly permeable blood vessels that have few intercellular junction complexes. Based on clinical, functional, and molecular evidence, Padua et al. [7] showed that the cytokine TGF-beta in the breast tumor microenvironment primes cancer cells for metastasis to the lungs by inducing angiopoietin-like 4 (Angptl4), via the Smad signaling pathway. Angptl4 in breast cancer cells that are about to enter the circulation enhances their subsequent retention in the lungs, but not in the bone. Tumor cell-derived Angptl4 disrupts vascular endothelial cell–cell junctions, increases the permeability of lung capillaries, and facilitates the transendothelial passage of tumor cells. Thus, a cytokine in the primary tumor microenvironment induces the expression of another cytokine in departing tumor cells, empowering these cells to disrupt lung capillary walls and seed pulmonary metastases [8].

It is feasible to identify and track micrometastases in experimental animals using antibodies against cytokeratins for the blood and against epithelial cell adhesion molecules (EpCAM) for the lymph, with sensitivity to detect even one cancer cell among 100,000 or more mesenchymal cells. A primary tumor of 1 g mass with 10(9) cells in the mouse may release a million cells per day into the circulation with few or no metastases resulting [6]. The rate-limiting step is colonization at the distant site. Dormant micrometastases have been demonstrated unequivocally in mouse experiments. Fluorescent dye-labeled cancer cells introduced via the portal circulation formed large numbers of single-cell micrometastases in the liver; 11 weeks later, viable cells were recovered with fluorescence undiluted by cell division. These cells still generated xenografts when injected s.c. into other host mice [9]. These single-cell micrometastases may be a greater threat for later activation than small colonies of cells in which the rate of proliferation has been balanced by apoptosis, perhaps due to failure to execute the angiogenic switch.

All of these different cellular phenotypes should have distinguishable molecular signatures and treatment targets revealed with mRNA gene expression, miRNA, or proteins. The vascular endothelium may be characterized with a combination of imaging and molecular signatures, as demonstrated by Schnitzer and colleagues [10]. Murphy et al. [11] targeted integrin $\alpha v \beta 3$, which is found on a subset of tumor blood vessels and is associated with angiogenesis and malignant tumor growth. They designed a nanoparticle encapsulating the cytotoxic drug doxorubicin (Dox) for targeted drug delivery to the $\alpha v \beta 3$-expressing tumor vasculature. They obtained selective apoptosis in regions of the αvβ3-expressing tumor vasculature. In clinically relevant pancreatic and renal cell orthotopic models of spontaneous metastasis, this treatment produced a 15-fold increase in anti-metastatic activity without producing drug-associated weight loss as observed with systemic administration of the free drug.

Biomarkers have been sought also for diagnosis and prognosis of skeletal metastases from lung cancers [12]. The incidence of skeletal metastases in patients with non-small cell lung cancers is between 8 and 34%, as detected by bone scans, and 24–30% as detected by PET imaging, with two-thirds of the patients found to have such metastases at the time of initial staging. Biomarkers assess the balance of osteoclastic and osteoblastic activity in the continuous remodeling of bone. Activated osteoclasts resorb bone by attaching to the mineral surface and secreting hydrolytic enzymes which acidify, dissolve, and release mineral and collagen breakdown products. Malignant cells secrete molecules that uncouple bone remodeling, at least in part through induction of receptor activator of nuclear factor kappa B (RANK) ligand (RANKL). The interaction between tumor cells and osteoclasts exacerbates resorption, leading to pain, pathologic fractures, hypercalcemia, and spinal cord compression, collectively termed "skeletal-related events" [12]. The best biomarkers of bone turnover are bone-specific alkaline phosphatase for bone formation and N-terminal telopeptide of collagen type I (NTx) for bone resorption. These biomarkers are highly correlated with incidence of SREs and with response to therapies, both bisphosphonates and Denosumab, a human monoclonal antibody that binds and neutralizes RANK ligand.

Analyses of Gene Expression in Primary Tumors and Metastases

By far the most exploited approach to molecular signatures of tumors involves microarray analysis for differences in gene expression. Klein et al. [13] used comparative genomic hybridization to show extensive heterogeneity among single-cell micrometastases in bone marrow biopsies of patients with surgically removed primary adenocarcinomas and, later, much less heterogeneity among larger metastases. Their interpretation is that certain cells undergo additional chromosomal rearrangements or mutations in their distant site and initiate a new wave of micrometastases that have greater capability to colonize and grow into clinically significant lesions. These metastases have a clonal origin and much less heterogeneity.

Wu et al. [14] compared primary and metastatic breast cancer gene expression profiles in 10 patients with metastatic breast cancers, after postmortem intervals of 1–4 hours. They constructed single-patient tissue microarrays from the patients' archived primary tumors and multiple different metastatic lesions harvested at autopsy. They performed immunohistochemical labeling for multiple biomarkers and analyzed methylation of multiple gene promoters. Extensive heterogeneity was observed between the primary tumors and their paired metastatic lesions, as well as among multiple metastatic lesions from the same patient. Estrogen and progesterone receptors tended to be uniformly down-regulated in metastases. E-cadherin was downregulated in a subset of the metastases of one case. Variable overexpression in metastatic compared with the primary tumor was observed for cyclooxygenase-2 (five cases), epidermal growth factor receptor (four cases), MET (four cases), and mesothelin (four cases). No case strongly overexpressed HER-2/neu by immunohistochemistry, but eight cases showed variable protein expression ranging from negative to equivocal (2 +) in different metastases. EGFR and MET overexpressions were restricted to the four basal-type cancers. EGFR protein overexpression did not correlate with EGFR gene amplification. Hypermethylation of promoters was reported earlier by the same group [15] for RASSF1A, HIN-1, cyclin D2, Twist, and RAR-beta in four breast cancer metastatic sites – lymph node, bone, lung, and brain.

Clearly, there are differences between primary and metastatic tumors in the same patient, with extensive heterogeneity across patients and within a single patient. Reactivation of genes silenced by hypermethylation of their promoters might be achieved with demethylating agents, histone deactylase inhibitors, and/or differentiation-enhancing (like retinoids) agents.

The Oncomine Resource for Microarray Gene Expression Data Sets

Thousands of large-scale DNA microarray experiments have been performed in the past decade, yielding global quantitative profiles for various cancers. Micro-array repositories such as GEO [16] and ArrayExpress [17] are now available, enhanced by requirements of journals to deposit data before publication. For example, Van't Veer et al. [18], from microarray results on specimens from 117 breast cancer patients, generated a classifier that would identify patients who needed adjuvant systemic therapy and patients who did not. The microarray results also yielded patterns for ER-positive tumors and for BRCA-1 (heredi-tary) breast cancers.

Oncomine 3.0 is a highly useful "meta-data" resource developed by Rhodes, Chinnaiyan, and colleagues at the University of Michigan. It presents and synthesizes the results of >18,000 cancer gene expression experiments and embedded statistical and informatics tools to explore differences between types of cancers, effects of various therapies, and differences between primary and metastatic tumors [19]. There is automated analysis of the genes, pathways, transcription factor binding sites, regulatory networks, and functional net-works activated or repressed in these cancers. Oncomine version 1.0 was released in 2003, version 2.0 in October 2004, and version 3.0 in 2007. Oncomine has three general layers: data input, with annotation, curation, and standardi-zation of the sample information; automated data analysis of cancer vs. normal, cancer vs. cancer, histologic subtype, grade, stage, molecular phenotypes and targets, co-expression of genes, and prognosis/survival; and data visualization, with heatmaps, boxplots, and other formats. Scalable vector graphics (SVG) were adopted for visualizing gene expression data and analysis. Additional methods now include molecular concepts mapping, interactome analysis, enrichment analysis, meta-analysis, and cancer outlier profile analysis [20, 21]. It is important to note, given the large number of cross-comparisons, that p values for statistical differences are corrected for multiple hypothesis testing. The Molecular Concepts Maps utilize multiple existing data resources (Gene Ontology, InterPro, Biocarta, KEGG, HPRD, Transfac) and the literature.

The usual first step with Oncomine is gene search, which yields a differential activity map for that selected gene(s), a visual summary of all the tissues and comparison of types of tumors in which that gene is differentially expressed, with statistical significance at a level chosen by the user. After intermediate analyses by tumor type, outliers due to heterogeneity, transcription factor binding sites, or protein–protein interactions, we commonly now move to sets of related genes captured as "molecular concepts," such as pathways, processes, and protein complexes.

Rhodes et al. [19] illustrated the utility of the cancer subtype profile method by searching for differential expression of known therapeutic targets in metastatic prostate cancer. Altogether 347 genes encoding proteins that have literature-defined inhibitors, antagonists, or blockers in the Therapeutic Target Database were put through this filter. Two striking targets are PRKCZ (protein kinase c, zeta), which is inhibited by bisindolylmaleimide I, and SHMT2 (serine hydroxymethyltransferase 2, mitochondrial), which is inhibited by a plant amino acid, mimosine (see [17], Fig. 3). Both show higher gene expression in two or three independent data sets, in the order of metastatic > localized > normal and benign prostate. This analysis generated suggestions of new classes of drugs to try on prostate cancer cells and tumors. Comparing multiple data sets in a meta-analysis reveals more robust findings, a way of overcoming the known problem of high false-positive results in microarray studies.

A meta-analysis of the original 40 data sets in Oncomine 1.0 identified potentially universal cancer signatures across cancer types relative to normal tissues and for genes activated in poorly differentiated cancers vs. well-differentiated cancers [22]. The strategy underlying such a meta-analysis with large numbers of differentially expressed genes is to search the intersection of observations across many data sets. The essential features should be enriched, while the epiphenomena, batch or sample factors, and system-specific or cancer type-specific features should be underrepresented. Such an analysis identified common transcriptional mechanisms of dedifferentiation. A complementary analysis could reveal genes different between similar tumors in different patients or metastases in different organs from the same tumor in the same patient (or animal). Meta-profiling of seven data sets for undifferentiated vs. differentiated signatures yielded 69 genes with significantly differential expression in at least four of the seven data sets (vs. one expected by chance). Three genes unique to the undifferentiated signature have a known role in chromatin remodeling and broad spectrum transcriptional regulation – the polycomb group protein EZH2 and histone variant proteins H2AFX and H2AFZ, which control euchromatin–heterochromatin transitions. EZH2 independently was found to be notably overexpressed in metastatic prostate cancer, compared with localized prostate cancer or benign tissue [23] and has been licensed as a biomarker candidate for prognosis.

EZH2 is a critical component of a multiprotein complex that methylates Lys27 of histone 3 (H3K27), leading to repression of target gene expression in embryonic stem cells and probably cancer stem cells. EZH2 (enhancer of zeste 2), SUZ12 (suppressor of zeste 12), and EED (embryonic ectoderm development) form the polycomb repressive complex 2 (PRC2), which specifically trimethylates H3K27 on target gene promoters [24]. Such repression is associated with poor prognosis [25]. Yu et al. [25] mapped genome-wide H3K27 methylation in aggressive, disseminated human prostate cancer tissues. They reported a signature of 14 gene targets for polycomb repression in metastatic tumors. Then, using the Oncomine and Molecular Concepts Maps, they found the same signature, represented by H3K27me3-occupied promoters in 87 genes with the most striking repression, in other metastatic solid tumors, including breast and lung (lung data set from Garber et al. [26]). For example, in metastatic prostate tumors, WNT2, CXCL12, and KRT17 were >100-fold downregulated.

Finally, high-grade Gleason-score prostate cancers, compared with low grade after laser microdissection of 101 cell populations, showed marked enrichment ($p < 10-16$) for an attenuated androgen signaling signature similar to that for metastatic prostate cancer. There is a concomitant decrease in protein synthesis [27]. The molecular concepts support a coherent model for hormone-naïve and hormone-refractory stages of metastatic prostate cancer. Similar analyses could be done for metastatic lung cancers.

Special Analysis for Metastatic Lung Cancer Phenotypes Using Oncomine

For this study, we utilized the Oncomine database resource (academic version: http://www.oncomine.org) to explore and attempt to identify common pathways or genes which are over- or underexpressed in metastatic lung cancers compared with the localized lung adenocarcinomas. These analyses are illustrative, not definitive, given our opportunistic use of data sets that were generated to ask other questions.

Oncomine utilizes the tumor and outcome data which are available from the various published microarray experiments, supplemented by primary data obtained directly from many of the investigators. For that reason, it is not always feasible to find the data in the original papers that are presented and reanalyzed in Oncomine. Oncomine generates evidence of differential expression of genes whose expression signatures or protein products might serve as potential biomarkers.

For demonstration purposes, we selected three studies which reported genes that are differentially expressed in lung tumor samples:

(1) The Garber study [26] includes lung adenocarcinomas from primary resection ($n = 40$, stage not identified in this paper) and lung adenocarcinoma metastases to the lymph nodes ($n = 6$). [The study also contained SCC ($n = 5$), large cell lung cancer ($n = 5$), and small cell lung cancer ($n = 5$), which were not used in the expression comparison presented here.]

(2) The Beer study [28] contains results for 86 lung adenocarcinomas, primarily comparing stage I with stage III. Oncomine obtained additional lymph node status data to compare N0 ($n = 69$) with N1 ($n = 2$) + N2 ($n = 15$). N0 has none, while N1–3 represent increasing involvement of lobar, hilar, and mediastinal lymph nodes, respectively.

(3) The Bhattacharjee study [29] similarly provided data in which lung adenocarcinomas could be divided into N0 ($n = 69$) vs. N1 ($n = 20$), N2 ($n = 7$), and N3 ($n = 1$).

When we performed a combined analysis on the Beer and Bhattacharjee studies, there were approximately 100 genes overexpressed in both studies ($p < 0.05$). Then we combined with the Garber signatures for node metastases vs. primary tumors and used a cutoff value of $p < 0.1$ for genes overexpressed in all three studies. The result is the list of 69 genes shown in Table 1.

To understand the mechanisms at a higher level rather than at a gene-by-gene level, we explored the pathways involved to see if there were common

Table 1 Genes overexpressed ($p < 0.1$) across the Beer and Bhattacharjee (lymph node status N1–N3 vs. N0) and Garber data sets (lymph node metastasis vs. primary lung adenocarcinoma). Genes were identified using the Oncomine meta-analysis feature to compare across different data sets

Gene symbol	Gene name
NKX3-1	NK3 homeobox 1
RPS6KB1	Ribosomal protein S6 kinase, 70 kDa, polypeptide 1
FEZ2	Fasciculation and elongation protein zeta 2 (zygin II)
IGF1R	Insulin-like growth factor 1 receptor
MTHFD2	Methylenetetrahydrofolate dehydrogenase (NADP-dependent) 2, methylenetetrahydrofolate cyclohydrolase
GIT2	G protein-coupled receptor kinase interactor 2
ETF1	Eukaryotic translation termination factor 1
PGK1	Phosphoglycerate kinase 1
NPC1	Niemann–Pick disease, type C1
NTRK2	Neurotrophic tyrosine kinase, receptor, type 2
SIAH1	Seven in absentia homolog 1 (*Drosophila*)
COX7B	Cytochrome *c* oxidase subunit VIIb

Table 1 (continued)

Gene symbol	Gene name
CASR	Calcium-sensing receptor (hypocalciuric hypercalcemia 1, severe neonatal hyperparathyroidism)
AUH	AU RNA-binding protein/enoyl-Coenzyme A hydratase
COX5A	Cytochrome *c* oxidase subunit Va
EPB42	Erythrocyte membrane protein band 4.2
APC	Adenomatosis polyposis coli
XPA	Xeroderma pigmentosum, complementation group A
CEBPG	CCAAT/enhancer-binding protein (C/EBP), gamma
S100A10	S100 calcium-binding protein A10
HSPE1	Heat shock 10 kDa protein 1 (chaperonin 10)
PAICS	Phosphoribosylaminoimidazole carboxylase, phosphoribosylaminoimidazole succinocarboxamide synthetase
USP14	Ubiquitin-specific peptidase 14 (tRNA-guanine transglycosylase)
AHDC1	AT hook, DNA-binding motif, containing 1
PARG	Poly (ADP-ribose) glycohydrolase
CCR6	Chemokine (C–C motif) receptor 6
EEF1B2	Eukaryotic translation elongation factor 1 beta 2
VRK2	Vaccinia-related kinase 2
MARCKS	Myristoylated alanine-rich protein kinase C substrate
CTRB1	Chymotrypsinogen B1
RRM1	Ribonucleotide reductase M1 polypeptide
FUBP3	Far upstream element (FUSE)-binding protein 3
EIF3A	Eukaryotic translation initiation factor 3, subunit A
HINT1	Histidine triad nucleotide-binding protein 1
SLBP	Stem-loop (histone)-binding protein
TNPO1	Transportin 1
SCAMP1	Secretory carrier membrane protein 1
KIAA0020	KIAA0020
CDKN3	Cyclin-dependent kinase inhibitor 3 (CDK2-associated dual specificity phosphatase)
RAB2A	RAB2A, member RAS oncogene family
HMGB1	High-mobility group box 1
NDUFB7	NADH dehydrogenase (ubiquinone) 1 beta subcomplex, 7, 18 kDa
TERF1	Telomeric repeat-binding factor (NIMA-interacting) 1
ATP5O	ATP synthase, H + transporting, mitochondrial F1 complex, O subunit (oligomycin sensitivity conferring protein)
PRDX2	Peroxiredoxin 2
NF1	Neurofibromin 1 (neurofibromatosis, von Recklinghausen disease, Watson disease)
CDK6	Cyclin-dependent kinase 6
CGREF1	Cell growth regulator with EF-hand domain 1
OSTF1	Osteoclast stimulating factor 1
RAD23B	RAD23 homolog B (*Saccharomyces cerevisiae*)
PSMB7	Proteasome (prosome, macropain) subunit, beta type, 7
NEK2	NIMA (never in mitosis gene a)-related kinase 2
TSN	Translin
DST	Dystonin

Table 1 (continued)

Gene symbol	Gene name
CYP2E1	Cytochrome P450, family 2, subfamily E, polypeptide 1
SRP54	Signal recognition particle 54 kDa
ATXN3	Ataxin 3
GLRX	Gglutaredoxin (thioltransferase)
ARL4A	ADP-ribosylation factor-like 4A
AMPH	Amphiphysin
BZW1	Basic leucine zipper and W2 domains 1
GAD1	Glutamate decarboxylase 1 (brain, 67 kDa)
PCCB	Propionyl Coenzyme A carboxylase, beta polypeptide
SNRPD3	Small nuclear ribonucleoprotein D3 polypeptide 18 kDa
MPHOSPH9	M-phase phosphoprotein 9
FARSA	Phenylalanyl-tRNA synthetase, alpha subunit
PSMA4	Proteasome (prosome, macropain) subunit, alpha type 4
SMS	Spermine synthase
EFNB2	Ephrin-B2

pathways. We took the gene list from Table 1 and extracted protein interaction data from the Michigan Molecular Interactions database (MiMI; http://www.mimi.ncibi.org) [30]. Several of the proteins of those genes have been shown to interact (Table 2); the pathways involved in these groups are clearly related to cell proliferation and tumorigenesis.

We then used the MiMI database, MiMI plug-in (http://mimi.ncibi.org/MimiWeb/MimiWebApplication.html), and Cytoscape visualization tool (www.cytoscape.org) to identify the protein–protein interaction nearest

Table 2 Protein–protein interactions among genes from Table 1. Extracted from MiMI using the MiMI plug-in for Cytoscape (with provenance indicated)

ATXN3, RAD23B, XPA	RAD23B and XPA are both involved in DNA excision/repair and are in an indirect complex together [prov: Reactome]; ATXN3 in a mutant form is found to bind RAD23B (affinity capture; [prov: BIND, HPRD, and others)
COX5A, COX7B, ATP50, NDUFB7, NTRK2, and PAICS	COX5A and 7B, ATP50, and NDUFB7 are primarily involved in the oxidative phosphorylation pathway (KEGG). NTRK2 and PAICS are both involved in ATP binding and are neighboring reactions
PSMA4 and PSMB7	Part of the proteasome complex (macropain); directly interact in that complex
APC and SIAH1	Wnt signaling pathway members involved in cell adhesion (APC) and cell morphogenesis (SIAH1): APC and Siah-1 mediate a novel beta-catenin degradation pathway linking p53 activation to cell cycle control [86], which may have particular relevance in lung cancers

neighbors for the 69 genes overexpressed in the Beer, Bhattacharjee, and Garber studies. This produces a complicated graph of interactions among 1,365 nearest neighbors, which is too complex to interpret visually. However, the MCODE module [31] in Cytoscape helps identify clusters of highly interacting proteins. The top subclusters of highly connected proteins were grouped into the following pathways: ribosomal structure/binding, oxidative phosphorylation, proteasome/protein catabolism, GTPase activation/glutathione transferase, purine metabolism, urea cycle metabolism, Wnt signaling/adhesion, ErbB signaling, ATP binding (cell cycle, differentiation, glycolysis), DNA excision/repair, cell division/kinase signaling, and nucleotide metabolism.

We examined the 69 signature genes using the same method as [20] and identified 1,192 protein-interacting nearest neighbors. We wanted to see if the pathways involved were the same or similar, even though the specific genes were different between the analyses. The top subclusters/pathways from the Rhodes signature gene list were ribosomal structure, threonine metabolism, NTP binding/ATPase activation, cell cycle control/apoptosis, basal transcription, purine/pyrimidine metabolism, urea cycle control, DNA excision/repair, MAPK signaling (also Toll/Wnt), and ECM receptor interactions. Many of the major pathways are in common, and these are groups of proteins/pathways which would be involved in cell proliferation (ribosomal proteins, cell cycle, cell division) and invasive properties, cell remodeling and adaptation to a new microenvironment (Wnt signaling, adhesion, proteasome, and protein catabolism).

These groups of pathways indicate that tumor progression may have a common trend or pattern based on the requirements for overall metastasis. In addition, specific signature subsets of genes may be unique to specific tumor types. Alternatively, there may be many signatures for metastases (both genes and overall pathways), reflecting the microenvironments at the site of metastasis, combined with the inherent features of the primary tumors. A study by Talbot et al. [32] showed that metastatic SCC tumors in the lung could be classified based on their origin (tongue SCC, in this case), based on unique gene expression from the site of origin. Initial comparison of the genes overexpressed in this data set did not identify a large number of overexpressed genes in common with our signature of 69 genes (data not shown).

These illustrative analyses may stimulate others to identify not only biomarkers but pathways important for diagnosis, stratification of patients, prognosis, and therapeutic choices. There are many additional lung cancer data sets in Oncomine for further analyses [32–48].

miRNAs as New Biomarkers for Lung Cancers

A whole additional layer of molecular expression has emerged with the discovery in multiple organisms and in cancer cells of important roles for small noncoding RNA molecules (microRNAs, miRNA), typically 22 nucleotides in length. Weiss et al. [49] examined EGFR regulation by microRNAs in lung cancer, correlating clinical response and survival after gefitinib therapy with EGFR expression in cell lines. Since allelic loss in chromosome 3p is one of the most frequent and earliest genetic events in lung carcinogenesis, they focused on microRNA-128b, which is located on chromosome 3p and is a putative regulator of epidermal growth factor receptor (EGFR). Loss of microRNA-128b would be equivalent to losing a tumor suppressor gene because it would allow increased expression of EGFR.

They tested microRNA-128b expression levels in non-small cell lung cancer (NSCLC) cell lines by quantitative RT–PCR, genomic copy number by quantitative PCR, and mutations in the mature microRNA-128b by sequencing. They determined whether microRNA-128b loss of heterozygosity (LOH) in 58 NSCLC patient samples correlated with response to gefitinib and evaluated EGFR expression and mutation status. The evidence supports the view that microRNA-128b directly regulates EGFR. MicroRNA-128b LOH was frequent in tumor samples and correlated significantly with clinical response and survival following gefitinib. However, EGFR expression and mutation status did not correlate with survival outcome unrelated to therapy.

Each known miRNA has a large number of predicted targets. For example, members of the let-7/miR-98 family are upregulated late in embryonic development and downregulated early in carcinogenesis, indicating that let-7-regulated oncofetal genes are reexpressed in cancer cells. Boyerinas et al. [50] identified 12 such genes, including HMGA2 and IMP-1/CRD-BP, which were confirmed with proteomics as major miRNA targets involved in cell growth and motility. IMP-1 is an RNA-binding protein that recognizes c-myc, IGF2, tau, FMR1, semaphorin, beta-TrCP1 mRNAs, and H19 RNA and shields them from degradation.

MicroRNA regulators of oncogenes could have far-reaching implications for lung cancer patients through improving patient selection for targeted agents, development of novel therapeutics, or as biomarkers of early or metastatic disease.

Discovery of Protein Biomarkers Using Proteomics

There are many approaches to protein biomarkers. One can study individual proteins or proteomic patterns in the tumor and in subcellular compartments, like cell surface membranes, secretory pathways, and the nucleus. Proteins can be analyzed in biofluids, ranging from bronchial lavage, sputum, and pleural effusions to urine and cerebrospinal fluid. Then all sources point to the circulation, where EDTA–plasma is the preferred sample [51] for proteomic analyses. The challenge with plasma is the huge dynamic range of concentrations from albumin at 40 mg/ml to cytokines and other molecules 1ng/ml (nanogram) or lower. The most abundant proteins dominate most analyses, with albumin accounting for

50% of the protein mass and the top 22 proteins accounting for 99% of protein mass. Investigators may wish to focus on modifications of traditional plasma proteins, like acute-phase reactants, or on proteins released from or secreted from cancer cells. Extensive fractionation of the plasma specimen, including antibody-based depletion of the most abundant proteins, enhances detection of proteins of moderate to low concentration.

Proteomic Analyses of Lung Cancers and Biofluids

In a companion study to the Beer et al. [28] study of transcriptional profiles that predict survival for patients with stage I lung adenocarcinoma, Chen et al. [52] used quantitative two-dimensional polyacrylamide gel electrophoresis and mass spectrometry to identify a total of 682 individual protein spots in 90 lung adenocarcinomas. A protein profile using the top 20 survival-associated proteins identified by Cox modeling predicted survival among stage I patients ($p<0.01$). Expression of 12 of the candidate proteins identified by mass spectrometry was confirmed with immunohistochemical analysis of tumor tissue microarrays. Combined analysis of protein and mRNA data revealed upregulation of 11 components of the glycolysis pathway associated with poor survival, which is compatible with the "Warburg effect" of shift from Krebs cycle to glycolysis [53]. Among these candidates, elevated levels of phosphoglycerate kinase 1 in the serum were significantly correlated with poor outcome in an independent validation set of 107 patients with lung adenocarcinomas using ELISA analysis. These studies help explain why even stage I patients (according to clinical, radiologic, and histologic criteria) have only moderate overall 5-year survival.

A similar study was reported by Yanagisawa et al. [54]. MALDI mass spectrometry was performed on 174 frozen-tissue specimens from resected non-small cell lung cancers (NSCLC) and 27 specimens from normal lung tissue, divided into a training set (116 cancers and 20 normals) and a test set (58 tumors and 7 normals). Protein signals differentially associated with specimens from patients who died within 5 years of surgery compared with those alive with no symptoms of relapse after a mean of 89 months of follow-up were selected with several statistical tests to yield a prognostic signature of 25 signals, which was validated with the test set. The hazard ratio for death was 61 (CI 9–419, $p<0.001$) and for relapse was 12 (CI 3.1–44.8, $p<0.001$). A variety of proteins identified with ion-trap mass spectrometry included ribosomal protein L26-like 1, acylphosphatase, and phosphoprotein enriched in astrocytes 15.

Malignant pleural effusions of advanced lung adenocarcinomas are a useful source of biomarkers of diagnosis and prognosis. Soltermann et al. [55] used a powerful method for capture and analysis of N-glycosylated proteins in routine cytology specimens, eliminating albumin and other non-glycosylated proteins. They compared five patients with adenocarcinoma of the lung and five nonmalignant controls with triplicate analysis. A total of 170 and 278 nonredundant proteins were detected, using threshold probabilities of $p \geq 0.9$ and $p \geq 0.5$, respectively, and reaching down into the range of mcg to ng/ml concentration. N-glycosylated proteins associated with tumor progression or metastasis included CA-125, CD44, CD166, lysosome-associated membrane glycoprotein 2 (LAMP-2), multimerin 2, and periostin. Validation with antibodies was performed on the effusion fluid and the tumor tissue. Lung-specific proteins such as tracheobronchial mucin 5B, surfactant protein A, and thyroid transcription factor 1 were also identified. These findings of the N-glycosylated protein subproteome partly overlap the proteins identified by Tyan et al. [56], using a global proteomic tandem MS/MS method.

A panel of immunohistochemical markers has been pursued to meet the need to differentiate primary vs. metastatic carcinoma in the lung [57]. The thyroid transcription factor 1 mentioned above is a tissue-specific nuclear protein with DNA-binding activity, a member of the 40 kDa NKx2 family of homeodomain transcription factors. In normal lung, it regulates expression of surfactant proteins and Clara cell secretory protein genes. It is highly specific for thyroid and lung. Napsin A is an aspartic proteinase expressed normally in lysosomes of type II pneumocytes and alveolar macrophages and also in proximal and convoluted tubules of the kidney. Napsin A has been strongly positive in up to 80% of primary lung adenocarcinomas but is negative in poorly differentiated cancers, as well as in squamous and small cell carcinomas of the lung. Not many other proteins show much promise at present. For example, surfactant proteins A and B turned out to be stained in only 63% of primary lung carcinomas and then in 46% of metastatic carcinomas, especially primary breast cancers. Enteric types of lung adenocarcinomas tend to aberrantly express colonic-type biomarkers, such as CDX-2, cytokeratin CK20, and MUC3, while losing expression of TTF-1, surfactant proteins, and napsin. Cytokeratin CK7 may be usefully positive, since it is negative in primary colon cancers.

Pleural mesotheliomas also have been analyzed for biomarkers of prognosis. Mesotheliomas often have complex chromosomal rearrangements, including losses of chromosome 10, which was a clue for analysis of PTEN, the tumor suppressor gene phosphatase and tensin homolog at 10p23. Opitz et al. [58] prepared tissue microarrays from 341 mesothelioma cases and performed immunohistochemistry with a monoclonal mouse anti-PTEN antibody, scoring expression semi-quantitatively as negative, weak, moderate, and strong. Survival time was correlated to PTEN expression in 126 cases with complete follow-up data. Comparing any PTEN expression with no expression, median survival time was significantly longer (log rank test $p = 0.0001$) in patients with PTEN (15.5 months vs. 9.7 months). Cox regression analysis demonstrated an association between PTEN expression and survival ($p = 0.003$) independent of histologic subtype ($p = -0.7$). Loss of PTEN implies activation of the PI3K-AKT/protein kinase B pathway, which thereby becomes a target for therapy.

Carbone, Caprioli, and colleagues at Vanderbilt University have pursued a unique path to biomarkers of lung cancers, using direct MALDI-TOF mass spectrometry (MS) on lung tumor specimens and sera [59–62]. For example, Rahman et al. [59] obtained MS profiles from 10-μm sections of fresh-frozen tissue samples: 25 normal lung, 29 normal bronchial epithelium, and 20 preinvasive and 36 invasive lung tumor tissue samples from 53 patients. They found a specific proteomic profile that allows an overall predictive accuracy of over 90% of normal, preinvasive, and invasive lung tissues. The proteomic profiles of these tissues were distinct from each other within a disease continuum. They trained their prediction model in a previously published data set and tested it in a new blinded test set to reach an overall 74% accuracy in classifying tumors vs. normal tissues. Amann et al. [60] developed a method compatible with MALDI-TOF MS to facilitate selective analysis of cancer cells in mixed clinical samples such as fine-needle aspirates. Taguchi et al. [61] developed and tested the ability of a predictive algorithm based on MALDI-MS analysis of pretreatment serum to identify patients who are likely to benefit from treatment with EGFR tyrosine kinase inhibitors. An algorithm developed from a training set of 139 patients from three cohorts was tested in two independent validation cohorts of 67 and 96 patients who were treated with gefitinib and erlotinib, respectively, and in three control cohorts of patients who were not treated with EGFR TKIs to analyze clinical outcomes of survival and time to progression. The algorithm based on just eight distinct m/z features identified patients who showed improved outcomes after EGFR TKI treatment. In one cohort, median survival of patients in the predicted "good" and "poor" groups was 207 and 92 days, respectively (hazard ratio [HR] of death in the good vs. poor groups = 0.50, 95% confidence interval [CI] = 0.24–0.78). In the other cohort, median survivals were 306 vs. 107 days (HR = 0.41, 95% CI = 0.17–0.63). The classifier did not predict outcomes in patients who did not receive EGFR TKI treatment. Such a method may assist in the stratification and selection of appropriate subgroups of NSCLC patients for treatment with EGFR TKIs. Finally, Yildiz et al. [62] used the MALDI-MS analysis of the most abundant peptides in unfractionated serum to distinguish lung cancer cases from matched controls. A serum proteomic signature of seven features in the training set reached an overall accuracy of 78%, sensitivity 67%, and specificity 89%. In the blinded test set, this signature gave overall accuracy of 73%, sensitivity just 58%, and specificity 86%. The serum signature was associated with the diagnosis of lung cancer independently of gender, smoking status, smoking pack-years, and C-reactive protein levels. Three discriminatory features were identified as members of a cluster of truncated forms of serum amyloid A (see also Gao et al. [63]).

Proteomics Analyses of Serum from Patients with Lung Cancers

Serum samples from lung cancer patients have been analyzed using a method of very limited power and reliability, called surface-enhanced laser desorption/ionization (SELDI) time-of-flight mass spectrometry [64]. Protein peak identification (mass/charge ratio) and clustering were performed on proteomic spectra for sera from 89 patients and 68 age- and sex-matched healthy controls as a training set and then for sera from 62 patients and 34 controls as a test set. The software identified only 48 mass speaks per spectrum; three peaks were used to construct a classification tree, which was reported to separate patients from controls with sensitivity of 91% and specificity of 97% and then 89% and 91% in the test set. The marker pattern outperformed immunoassays of Cyfra21-1 and carcinoembryonic antigen. This method based on patterns lacking protein identifications has lost standing as instrumentation for extensive identification of proteins in the proteome has become widely available.

A different glycoprotein capture method using multiple lectins to bind the proteins during affinity chromatography has been applied to sera from patients with lung adenocarcinoma. Heo et al. [65] isolated glycoproteins from three patients and three healthy individuals, treated with peptide-N-glycosidase F, digested in-gel with trypsin, and analyzed tryptic peptides with ESI-MS/MS and bioinformatics tools. A total of 148 glycoproteins were detected and identified among the 3 cancer patient sera and 132 glycoproteins in the normal sera. Of 99 proteins detected in all 3 cancer patients, they identified 38 with 1.5-fold higher peptide hit numbers in sera from patients; 6 were immunoglobulins, 1 hemoglobin, 8 high-abundance proteins such as haptoglobin, inter-alpha-trypsin inhibitor heavy chain 4, complement C3 precursor, and leucine-rich alpha-2 glycoprotein, and 23 (60%) previously reported as low abundance proteins in human sera. Plasma kallikrein (KLKB1) and inter-alpha-trypsin heavy chain 3 were increased in the cancer patient sera and confirmed by Western blot analysis. An 18 kDa plasma kallikrein protein fragment was detected at high levels in 25 of 28 patient sera vs. weakly detectable in only 1 of 8 normals. S100 A-8/calgranulin A was another promising cancer-associated protein. Relying on just three patients and three controls for the discovery phase reveals the laborious nature of discovery phase proteomics and the limitations of the conclusions. Several of the relatively abundant cancer-associated proteins had been reported previously using 2D gel electrophoresis and MALDI-TOF analyses [66, 67].

Serum Protein Profiles Associated with Lung Cancers Involving Detection of Abundant Proteins with Antibody Microarrays

As noted above, tissue- or tumor-derived proteins are often difficult to detect in the circulation, especially with direct mass spectrometric profiling, due the limited sensitivity, difficulty in proving the identification of the proteins, and very low throughput. A complementary, quite feasible approach is the quantitation of highly abundant serum or plasma proteins associated with the host response to disease, such as serum amyloid A, haptoglobin, alpha-1 anti-trypsin, and C-reactive protein. Gao et al. [63] used antibody microarrays with 84 antibodies specific for a wide range of serum proteins, spotted on nitrocellulose-coated microscope slides. The slides were exposed to serum from various groups of patients and controls, and immunoreactivity was quantified using two-color rolling-circle amplification. Among 24 newly diagnosed individuals with lung cancers, 24 healthy controls, and 32 patients with chronic obstructive pulmonary disease, 7 proteins gave a significant difference for the lung cancer patients as compared to either healthy controls or COPD patients. Higher abundances were found for C-reactive protein (CRP), increased 13-fold; serum amyloid A (SAA), increased 2.0-fold; and mucin 1 (MUC1) and alpha-1 anti-trypsin (AAT), each increased 1.4-fold. At a cutoff where all 56 of the nontumor samples were correctly classified, 15/24 lung cancer patients were correctly identified. There was no striking correlation with adenocarcinoma, squamous cell, or small cell histology. These patients were not subclassified into localized vs. metastatic, but such studies could readily be performed. With appropriate antibodies, much less abundant proteins could be assayed with the same approach.

The MUC1 protein is known to be aberrantly expressed on many solid tumor cancers. In contrast to its apical clustering on healthy epithelial cells, it is uniformly distributed over cancer cells. Mahanta et al. [68] reported that a membrane-bound MUC1 cleavage product, MUC1*, is the predominant form of the protein on cultured cancer cells and on cancerous tissues. Furthermore, transfection of a minimal fragment of MUC1, containing 45 amino acids of the extracellular domain, is sufficient to confer the full oncogenic activities of the full-length protein. Dimerization of the extracellular domain of MUC1* activates the MAP kinase signaling cascade and stimulates cell growth.

Using the Immune System's Production of Autoantibodies as a Form of Biological Amplification

Instead of searching for circulating tumor-associated proteins, an attractive option is to screen for autoantibodies against such tumor-associated proteins. Consider the remarkable impact of polymerase chain reaction (PCR) amplification of very low concentrations of DNA or RNA in nucleic acid studies. There is no in vitro counterpart for proteins. However, the body has its own biological amplification method for protein signals, namely the highly specific immune response with autoantibodies against one's own proteins. In general, these autoantibodies circulate at a concentration on the order of 1,000 times that of the protein antigen. Combining this approach with proteomic analyses permits detection of proteins with their native posttranslational modifications, which are often critical for their biological functions and their antigenicity [69, 70].

Hanash and colleagues [70] reported use of 2D polyacrylamide gel electrophoresis of A549 lung adenocarcinoma cell lysates, followed by Western blotting with serum specimens from patients and controls. Annexins I and II and UCHL3 (PGP9.5) (a ubiquitin lyase) were reported to have autoantibodies in the sera of lung cancer patients (one or more of these three) in about 60% of cases, with no such reactivity in healthy controls or patients with most other cancers (except esophageal CA) [71] [72]. Pereira-Faca et al. [73] extended this approach to 14-3-3-theta. Recently, Qiu et al. [74] tested pre-diagnostic sera from participants in the Beta-Carotene and Retinol Efficacy Trial [75] using extensively fractionated A549 lysates (1824 fractions). They found autoantibodies to annexin I, to 14-3-3 theta, and to LAMR1 in sera from patients up to 12 months before their diagnosis. PGP9.5 autoantibodies were not detected among these 85 patients and 85 controls.

Another method for detection of autoantibodies employs phage display. Tomlins et al. [21] published a 22-epitope panel for sera from prostate cancer patients with AUC characteristics far superior to prostate-specific antigen. Using the same approach, Chen et al. reported a (different) 22-epitope panel as highly discriminating for lung cancer from patient sera; the most interesting protein identified is ubiquilin-1 [76]. These epitope panels so far include only a few specifically identified proteins and are produced in batch methods, which introduce some challenges in reproducibility.

Proteomics Analysis of the Epithelial–Mesenchymal Transition (EMT) in Lung Adenocarcinoma Cells, an In Vitro Model for Metastasis

One path to understanding the nature and variability of metastases is to analyze the changes in gene and protein expression that occur during the epithelial–mesenchymal transition or invasion–metastasis cascade. Gene expression and protein expression changes in EMT are becoming well established, starting with distinctive loss of E-cadherin, which immobilizes cells in epithelial layers, gain of vimentin and N-cadherin, which favor cell motility, and release of matrix metalloproteinases by inflammatory cells, macrophages, and fibroblasts in the stroma. E-cadherin is particularly salient in this process, since advanced tumors in many sites have loss of E-cadherin activity, through a variety of different types of mutations, and restoration of E-cadherin activity with an expression vector can suppress the invasiveness and metastasis of these cancer cells [6]. Using iTRAQ labeling (isobaric tags for relative and absolute quantitation), tandem mass spectrometry, and MetaCore network analysis software for proteomics data, Keshamouni et al. [77,78] revealed a network of genes and proteins important to cytoskeletal function. The moesin–ezrin–radixin complex, integrin-beta1, Hsp27, tropomyosins, cofilin, filamins A,B,C, 14-3-3 zeta, and transglutaminase2 were all upregulated by TGF-beta-induced EMT in A549 human lung adenocarcinoma cells in vitro. Downregulated proteins were primarily enzymes involved in regulating nutrient or drug metabolism. This work has been extended with complementary methods, including iTRAQ time-course experiments (Keshamouni et al., 2009) and stable isotope labeling with amino acids in cultured cells (SILAC) and fluorescent differential in-gel electrophoresis (DIGE) (Keshamouni et al., unpublished), which readily show upregulation of vimentin, which was not detected for some reason with iTRAQ (see Chapter 6 by Moustakas and Keshamouni for details about EMT).

Tumor-associated stroma produces TGF-beta; maintenance of TGF-beta signaling through a positive-feedback loop appears to be important in many epithelial cancers, often in association with *ras* mutations. The molecular signature for EMT in these lung adenocarcinoma cells shows no overlap with the Oncomine molecular signatures for transcripts shown in Tables 1 and 2 (above), consistent with the interpretation that EMT is a transitional state before the establishment of a stable metastatic phenotype. EMT, meanwhile, is a reversible process, meaning that some or many of the features may disappear in the metastatic lesion. The high importance of the primary tumor microenvironment strongly suggests analogous critical roles for the microenvironments of micro-metastases. Clearly the malignant phenotypes of cancer cells are not specified solely by the genomes and proteomes of the neoplastic cells.

Use of Genetically Engineered Mouse Models of Specific Human Cancers

The National Cancer Institute has supported a major program to generate strains of mice with the precise primary molecular lesions of specific human cancers, such as Her2/neu amplification in breast cancer, Kras G12D activation and Ink4A/Arf deletion in pancreatic cancer, Kras activation and PTEN deletion in ovarian cancer, and Kras activation and p53 deletion in lung cancer [http://emice.nci.nih.gov/mouse_models/]. Plasma specimens from the tumor-prone and tumor-bearing mice were compared with plasma specimens from the wild-type mice, using extensive fractionation, labeling, and proteomic analyses with advanced instruments. The findings are beginning to appear, including breast [79] and pancreas [80]. In each case, numerous cancer-associated proteins were identified in plasma; these are a basis for searching for the homologous proteins in patients with the homologous cancers. For example, Faca et al. [80] identified 1,442 proteins distributed across 7 orders of magnitude of abundance in plasma and showed differences between pancreatic tumor-bearing mice and wild-type mice for 165 proteins, of which 45 were less abundant with human orthologs. A set of three proteins (PTTGF, TNFRSF1, and ALCAM) gave good discrimination on immunohistochemistry and a set of nine proteins (ALCAM, ICAM1, LCN2, TNFRSF1A, TIMP1, REG1A, REG3, WFDC2, and IGFBP4) gave good discrimination on ELISA between newly diagnosed patients with pancreatic cancer and healthy or pancreatitis controls. A panel of five proteins selected on the basis of their increased level at an early stage of tumor development in the mouse (LCN2, TIMP1, REG1A, REG3, and IGFBP4) was tested in a blinded study in 26 humans at high risk for lung cancer (long-time smokers and former smokers, plus asbestos-exposed workers) from the CARET (Carotene and Retinol Efficacy Trial) cohort [75]. The panel discriminated pancreatic cancer cases from matched controls in pre-diagnostic blood specimens obtained between 7 and 13 months prior to the development of symptoms and clinical diagnosis of pancreatic cancer. Corresponding studies are pending on the lung cancer models.

Finally, we have initiated a novel method to detect alternative splice isoforms of proteins [81]. MS/MS spectra are interrogated for novel splice isoforms using a nonredundant database containing an exhaustive three-frame translation of Ensembl transcripts and gene models from ECgene. The integrated analyses combining Trans Proteomic Pipeline (TPP) and Michigan Peptide to Protein Integration (MPPI) have identified both known isoforms and novel isoforms not previously noted in the gene and protein databases [82]. Work is in progress on the lung cancer data sets.

Conclusion

Emerging knowledge about the many features of metastasis offers numerous possibilities for discovery and exploitation of diagnostic and prognostic biomarkers and targets for therapy. A systems biology approach that encompasses differential expression of mRNAs (gene expression), microRNAs (gene regulators), and proteins and metabolites [83] in primary and metastatic tumors, in proximal biofluids, and in the blood plasma generates potentially complementary molecular signatures. We have illustrated the use of Oncomine and Molecular Concepts Maps and biological amplification of tumor protein signals with immune responses that produce autoantibodies in relation to lung cancers.

We have taken a systems biology approach to biomarker discovery, starting with mRNA transcripts in tumors and cultured cells to detect mRNA overexpression, some of which will be correlated with protein overexpression. Some of those proteins may be secreted or released into proximal biofluids and reach the circulation. Detection of low-abundance tumor proteins in the complex and dynamic mixture that is plasma requires combinations of increasingly powerful technologies. The biological amplification of protein signals through the immune system offers autoantibodies against tumor-associated proteins or protein fragments as potential biomarkers. Higher abundance proteins, including acute-phase reactants, may have practical value, especially if the proteins are structurally modified as part of the cancer processes, by protease action or glycosylation, for example. Promising biomarker candidates must be confirmed in the same lab and then in independent laboratories. Then they must be subjected to higher throughput methods, either multiplex ELISA or multiple reaction monitoring, a mass spectrometric method for identifying and quantifying unique peptides for targeted proteins [84]. These methods are practical for large-scale validation studies to establish sensitivity, specificity, and predictive value in both screening and prognostic scenarios. Standardized operating procedures for specimen handling, design and use of reference standards [85], care to avoid bias and confounding, and guidelines for reporting findings and contributing data sets should enhance the prospects for predictive profiling of people at risk for cancers and of patients at risk for metastasis.

Acknowledgments This work was supported by grants MEDC 687, NIH U54 DA02159, and SAIC/NCI 23X110A. We thank Denise Taylor-Moon for expert assistance with the manuscript.

References

1. Omenn, G.S. Strategies for plasma proteomic profiling of cancers. Proteomics 6: 5662–73, 2006.
2. Henschke, C.I., D.F. Yankelevitz, D.M. Libby, M.W. Pasmantier, J.P. Smith, and O.S. Miettinen. Survival of patients with stage I lung cancer detected on CT screening. N Engl J Med 355: 1763–71, 2006.
3. Omenn, G.S. Human lung cancer chemoprevention strategies: Parker B. Francis lecture. Chest 125: 123S–7S, 2004.
4. Sporn, M.B. The war on cancer. Lancet 347: 1377–81, 1996.
5. Hanahan, D. and R.A. Weinberg. The hallmarks of cancer. Cell 100: 57–70, 2000.
6. Weinberg, R.A. Moving out: invasion and metastasis, in The Biology of Cancer (New York: Garland Science, Taylor & Francis Group, 2006). Chapter 14, 587–654.
7. Padua, D., X.H. Zhang, Q. Wang, C. Nadal, W.L. Gerald, R.R. Gomis, and J. Massague. TGFbeta primes breast tumors for lung metastasis seeding through angiopoietin-like 4. Cell 133: 66–77, 2008.
8. Dvorak, H.F., M. Detmar, K.P. Claffey, J.A. Nagy, L. van de Water, and D.R. Senger. Vascular permeability factor/vascular endothelial growth factor: an important mediator of angiogenesis in malignancy and inflammation. Int Arch Allergy Immunol 107: 233–5, 1995.
9. Naumov, G.N., I.C. MacDonald, P.M. Weinmeister, N. Kerkvliet, K.V. Nadkarni, S.M. Wilson, V.L. Morris, A.C. Groom, and A.F. Chambers. Persistence of solitary mammary carcinoma cells in a secondary site: a possible contributor to dormancy. Cancer Res 62: 2162–8, 2002.
10. Simonson, A.B. and J.E. Schnitzer. Vascular proteomic mapping in vivo. J Thromb Haemost 5 Suppl 1: 183–7, 2007.
11. Murphy, E.A., B.K. Majeti, L.A. Barnes, M. Makale, S.M. Weis, K. Lutu-Fuga, W. Wrasidlo, and D.A. Cheresh. Nanoparticle-mediated drug delivery to tumor vasculature suppresses metastasis. Proc Natl Acad Sci USA 105: 9343–8, 2008.
12. Kosteva, J. and C. Langer. The changing landscape of the medical management of skeletal metastases in nonsmall cell lung cancer. Curr Opin Oncol 20: 155–61, 2008.
13. Klein, C.A., T.J. Blankenstein, O. Schmidt-Kittler, M. Petronio, B. Polzer, N.H. Stoecklein, and G. Riethmuller. Genetic heterogeneity of single disseminated tumour cells in minimal residual cancer. Lancet 360: 683–9, 2002.
14. Wu, J.M., M.J. Fackler, M.K. Halushka, D.W. Molavi, M.E. Taylor, W.W. Teo, C. Griffin, J. Fetting, N.E. Davidson, A.M. De Marzo, J.L. Hicks, D. Chitale, M. Ladanyi, S. Sukumar, and P. Argani. Heterogeneity of breast cancer metastases: comparison of therapeutic target expression and promoter methylation between primary tumors and their multifocal metastases. Clin Cancer Res 14: 1938–46, 2008.

15. Mehrotra, J., M. Vali, M. McVeigh, S.L. Kominsky, M.J. Fackler, J. Lahti-Domenici, K. Polyak, N. Sacchi, E. Garrett-Mayer, P. Argani, and S. Sukumar. Very high frequency of hypermethylated genes in breast cancer metastasis to the bone, brain, and lung. Clin Cancer Res *10*: 3104–9, 2004.

16. Barrett, T., T.O. Suzek, D.B. Troup, S.E. Wilhite, W.C. Ngau, P. Ledoux, D. Rudnev, A. E. Lash, W. Fujibuchi, and R. Edgar. NCBI GEO: mining millions of expression profiles – database and tools. Nucleic Acids Res *33*: D562–6, 2005.

17. Parkinson, H., U. Sarkans, M. Shojatalab, N. Abeygunawardena, S. Contrino, R. Coulson, A. Farne, G.G. Lara, E. Holloway, M. Kapushesky, P. Lilja, G. Mukherjee, A. Oezcimen, T. Rayner, P. Rocca-Serra, A. Sharma, S. Sansone, and A. Brazma. ArrayExpress – a public repository for microarray gene expression data at the EBI. Nucleic Acids Res *33*: D553–5, 2005.

18. van 't Veer, L.J., H. Dai, M.J. van de Vijver, Y.D. He, A.A. Hart, M. Mao, H.L. Peterse, K. van der Kooy, M.J. Marton, A.T. Witteveen, G.J. Schreiber, R.M. Kerkhoven, C. Roberts, P.S. Linsley, R. Bernards, and S.H. Friend. Gene expression profiling predicts clinical outcome of breast cancer. Nature *415*: 530–6, 2002.

19. Rhodes, D.R., S. Kalyana-Sundaram, V. Mahavisno, R. Varambally, J. Yu, B.B. Briggs, T.R. Barrette, M.J. Anstet, C. Kincead-Beal, P. Kulkarni, S. Varambally, D. Ghosh, and A.M. Chinnaiyan. Oncomine 3.0: genes, pathways, and networks in a collection of 18,000 cancer gene expression profiles. Neoplasia *9*: 166–80, 2007.

20. Rhodes, D.R. and A.M. Chinnaiyan. Integrative analysis of the cancer transcriptome. Nat Genet *37 Suppl*: S31–7, 2005.

21. Tomlins, S.A., D.R. Rhodes, S. Perner, S.M. Dhanasekaran, R. Mehra, X.W. Sun, S. Varambally, X. Cao, J. Tchinda, R. Kuefer, C. Lee, J.E. Montie, R.B. Shah, K.J. Pienta, M.A. Rubin, and A.M. Chinnaiyan. Recurrent fusion of TMPRSS2 and ETS transcription factor genes in prostate cancer. Science *310*: 644–8, 2005.

22. Rhodes, D.R., J. Yu, K. Shanker, N. Deshpande, R. Varambally, D. Ghosh, T. Barrette, A. Pandey, and A.M. Chinnaiyan. Large-scale meta-analysis of cancer microarray data identifies common transcriptional profiles of neoplastic transformation and progression. Proc Natl Acad Sci USA *101*: 9309–14, 2004.

23. Varambally, S., S.M. Dhanasekaran, M. Zhou, T.R. Barrette, C. Kumar-Sinha, M.G. Sanda, D. Ghosh, K.J. Pienta, R.G. Sewalt, A.P. Otte, M.A. Rubin, and A.M. Chinnaiyan. The polycomb group protein EZH2 is involved in progression of prostate cancer. Nature *419*: 624–9, 2002.

24. Kirmizis, A., S.M. Bartley, A. Kuzmichev, R. Margueron, D. Reinberg, R. Green, and P.J. Farnham. Silencing of human polycomb target genes is associated with methylation of histone H3 Lys 27. Genes Dev *18*: 1592–605, 2004.

25. Yu, J., D.R. Rhodes, S.A. Tomlins, X. Cao, G. Chen, R. Mehra, X. Wang, D. Ghosh, R. B. Shah, S. Varambally, K.J. Pienta, and A.M. Chinnaiyan. A polycomb repression signature in metastatic prostate cancer predicts cancer outcome. Cancer Res *67*: 10657–63, 2007.

26. Garber, M.E., O.G. Troyanskaya, K. Schluens, S. Petersen, Z. Thaesler, M. Pacyna-Gengelbach, M. van de Rijn, G.D. Rosen, C.M. Perou, R.I. Whyte, R.B. Altman, P.O. Brown, D. Botstein, and I. Petersen. Diversity of gene expression in adenocarcinoma of the lung. Proc Natl Acad Sci USA *98*: 13784–9, 2001.

27. Tomlins, S.A., R. Mehra, D.R. Rhodes, X. Cao, L. Wang, S.M. Dhanasekaran, S. Kalyana-Sundaram, J.T. Wei, M.A. Rubin, K.J. Pienta, R.B. Shah, and A.M. Chinnaiyan. Integrative molecular concept modeling of prostate cancer progression. Nat Genet *39*: 41–51, 2007.

28. Beer, D.G., S.L. Kardia, C.C. Huang, T.J. Giordano, A.M. Levin, D.E. Misek, L. Lin, G. Chen, T.G. Gharib, D.G. Thomas, M.L. Lizyness, R. Kuick, S. Hayasaka, J.M. Taylor, M.D. Iannettoni, M.B. Orringer, and S. Hanash. Gene-expression profiles predict survival of patients with lung adenocarcinoma. Nat Med *8*: 816–24, 2002.

29. Bhattacharjee, A., W.G. Richards, J. Staunton, C. Li, S. Monti, P. Vasa, C. Ladd, J. Beheshti, R. Bueno, M. Gillette, M. Loda, G. Weber, E.J. Mark, E.S. Lander, W. Wong, B.E. Johnson, T.R. Golub, D.J. Sugarbaker, and M. Meyerson. Classification of human lung carcinomas by mRNA expression profiling reveals distinct adenocarcinoma sub-classes. Proc Natl Acad Sci USA 98: 13790–5, 2001.

30. Jayapandian, M., A. Chapman, V.G. Tarcea, C. Yu, A. Elkiss, A. Ianni, B. Liu, A. Nandi, C. Santos, P. Andrews, B. Athey, D. States, and H.V. Jagadish. Michigan Molecular Interactions (MiMI): putting the jigsaw puzzle together. Nucleic Acids Res 35: D566–71, 2007.

31. Bader, G.D. and C.W. Hogue. An automated method for finding molecular complexes in large protein interaction networks. BMC Bioinformatics 4: 2, 2003.

32. Talbot, S.G., C. Estilo, E. Maghami, I.S. Sarkaria, D.K. Pham, P. Oc, N.D. Socci, I. Ngai, D. Carlson, R. Ghossein, A. Viale, B.J. Park, V.W. Rusch, and B. Singh. Gene expression profiling allows distinction between primary and metastatic squamous cell carcinomas in the lung. Cancer Res 65: 3063–71, 2005.

33. Bild, A.H., G. Yao, J.T. Chang, Q. Wang, A. Potti, D. Chasse, M.B. Joshi, D. Harpole, J. M. Lancaster, A. Berchuck, J.A. Olson, Jr., J.R. Marks, H.K. Dressman, M. West, and J. R. Nevins. Oncogenic pathway signatures in human cancers as a guide to targeted therapies. Nature 439: 353–7, 2006.

34. Bittner, M. A window on the dynamics of biological switches. Nat Biotechnol 23: 183–4, 2005.

35. Chen, H.Y., S.L. Yu, C.H. Chen, G.C. Chang, C.Y. Chen, A. Yuan, C.L. Cheng, C.H. Wang, H.J. Terng, S.F. Kao, W.K. Chan, H.N. Li, C.C. Liu, S. Singh, W.J. Chen, J.J. Chen, and P.C. Yang. A five-gene signature and clinical outcome in non-small-cell lung cancer. N Engl J Med 356: 11–20, 2007.

36. Gordon, G.J., R.V. Jensen, L.L. Hsiao, S.R. Gullans, J.E. Blumenstock, S. Ramaswamy, W.G. Richards, D.J. Sugarbaker, and R. Bueno. Translation of microarray data into clinically relevant cancer diagnostic tests using gene expression ratios in lung cancer and mesothelioma. Cancer Res 62: 4963–7, 2002.

37. Larsen, J.E., S.J. Pavey, L.H. Passmore, R. Bowman, B.E. Clarke, N.K. Hayward, and K.M. Fong. Expression profiling defines a recurrence signature in lung squamous cell carcinoma. Carcinogenesis 28: 760–6, 2007.

38. Minn, A.J., G.P. Gupta, P.M. Siegel, P.D. Bos, W. Shu, D.D. Giri, A. Viale, A.B. Olshen, W.L. Gerald, and J. Massague. Genes that mediate breast cancer metastasis to lung. Nature 436: 518–24, 2005.

39. Nielsen, T.O., R.B. West, S.C. Linn, O. Alter, M.A. Knowling, J.X. O'Connell, S. Zhu, M. Fero, G. Sherlock, J.R. Pollack, P.O. Brown, D. Botstein, and M. van de Rijn. Molecular characterisation of soft tissue tumours: a gene expression study. Lancet 359: 1301–7, 2002.

40. Powell, C.A., A. Spira, A. Derti, C. DeLisi, G. Liu, A. Borczuk, S. Busch, S. Sahasrabudhe, Y. Chen, D. Sugarbaker, R. Bueno, W.G. Richards, and J.S. Brody. Gene expression in lung adenocarcinomas of smokers and nonsmokers. Am J Respir Cell Mol Biol 29: 157–62, 2003.

41. Ramaswamy, S., P. Tamayo, R. Rifkin, S. Mukherjee, C.H. Yeang, M. Angelo, C. Ladd, M. Reich, E. Latulippe, J.P. Mesirov, T. Poggio, W. Gerald, M. Loda, E.S. Lander, and T.R. Golub. Multiclass cancer diagnosis using tumor gene expression signatures. Proc Natl Acad Sci USA 98: 15149–54, 2001.

42. Raponi, M., Y. Zhang, J. Yu, G. Chen, G. Lee, J.M. Taylor, J. Macdonald, D. Thomas, C. Moskaluk, Y. Wang, and D.G. Beer. Gene expression signatures for predicting prognosis of squamous cell and adenocarcinomas of the lung. Cancer Res 66: 7466–72, 2006.

43. Su, A.I., J.B. Welsh, L.M. Sapinoso, S.G. Kern, P. Dimitrov, H. Lapp, P.G. Schultz, S.M. Powell, C.A. Moskaluk, H.F. Frierson, Jr., and G.M. Hampton. Molecular classification of human carcinomas by use of gene expression signatures. Cancer Res 61: 7388–93, 2001.

44. Stearman, R.S., L. Dwyer-Nield, L. Zerbe, S.A. Blaine, Z. Chan, P.A. Bunn, Jr., G.L. Johnson, F.R. Hirsch, D.T. Merrick, W.A. Franklin, A.E. Baron, R.L. Keith, R.A. Nemenoff, A.M. Malkinson, and M.W. Geraci. Analysis of orthologous gene expression between human pulmonary adenocarcinoma and a carcinogen-induced murine model. Am J Pathol *167*: 1763–75, 2005.
45. Tomida, S., K. Koshikawa, Y. Yatabe, T. Harano, N. Ogura, T. Mitsudomi, M. Some, K. Yanagisawa, T. Takahashi, and H. Osada. Gene expression-based, individualized outcome prediction for surgically treated lung cancer patients. Oncogene *23*: 5360–70, 2004.
46. Wachi, S., K. Yoneda, and R. Wu. Interactome-transcriptome analysis reveals the high centrality of genes differentially expressed in lung cancer tissues. Bioinformatics *21*: 4205–8, 2005.
47. Wigle, D.A., I. Jurisica, N. Radulovich, M. Pintilie, J. Rossant, N. Liu, C. Lu, J. Woodgett, I. Seiden, M. Johnston, S. Keshavjee, G. Darling, T. Winton, B.J. Breitkreutz, P. Jorgenson, M. Tyers, F.A. Shepherd, and M.S. Tsao. Molecular profiling of non-small cell lung cancer and correlation with disease-free survival. Cancer Res *62*: 3005–8, 2002.
48. Yamagata, N., Y. Shyr, K. Yanagisawa, M. Edgerton, T.P. Dang, A. Gonzalez, S. Nadaf, P. Larsen, J.R. Roberts, J.C. Nesbitt, R. Jensen, S. Levy, J.H. Moore, J.D. Minna, and D. P. Carbone. A training-testing approach to the molecular classification of resected non-small cell lung cancer. Clin Cancer Res *9*: 4695–704, 2003.
49. Weiss, G.J., L.T. Bemis, E. Nakajima, M. Sugita, D.K. Birks, W.A. Robinson, M. Varella-Garcia, P.A. Bunn, Jr., J. Haney, B.A. Helfrich, H. Kato, F.R. Hirsch, and W.A. Franklin. EGFR regulation by microRNA in lung cancer: correlation with clinical response and survival to gefitinib and EGFR expression in cell lines. Ann Oncol *19*: 1053–9, 2008.
50. Boyerinas, B., S.M. Park, N. Shomron, M.M. Hedegaard, J. Vinther, J.S. Andersen, C. Feig, J. Xu, C.B. Burge, and M.E. Peter. Identification of let-7-regulated oncofetal genes. Cancer Res *68*: 2587–91, 2008.
51. Omenn, G.S., D.J. States, M. Adamski, T.W. Blackwell, R. Menon, H. Hermjakob, R. Apweiler, B.B. Haab, R.J. Simpson, J.S. Eddes, E.A. Kapp, R.L. Moritz, D.W. Chan, A. J. Rai, A. Admon, R. Aebersold, J. Eng, W.S. Hancock, S.A. Hefta, H. Meyer, Y.K. Paik, J.S. Yoo, P. Ping, J. Pounds, J. Adkins, X. Qian, R. Wang, V. Wasinger, C.Y. Wu, X. Zhao, R. Zeng, A. Archakov, A. Tsugita, I. Beer, A. Pandey, M. Pisano, P. Andrews, H. Tammen, D.W. Speicher, and S.M. Hanash. Overview of the HUPO Plasma Proteome Project: results from the pilot phase with 35 collaborating laboratories and multiple analytical groups, generating a core dataset of 3020 proteins and a publicly-available database. Proteomics *5*: 3226–45, 2005.
52. Chen, G., T.G. Gharib, H. Wang, C.C. Huang, R. Kuick, D.G. Thomas, K.A. Shedden, D.E. Misek, J.M. Taylor, T.J. Giordano, S.L. Kardia, M.D. Iannettoni, J. Yee, P.J. Hogg, M.B. Orringer, S.M. Hanash, and D.G. Beer. Protein profiles associated with survival in lung adenocarcinoma. Proc Natl Acad Sci USA *100*: 13537–42, 2003.
53. Warburg, O. The Chemical Constitution of Respiration Ferment. Science *68*: 437–43, 1928.
54. Yanagisawa, K., S. Tomida, Y. Shimada, Y. Yatabe, T. Mitsudomi, and T. Takahashi. A 25-signal proteomic signature and outcome for patients with resected non-small-cell lung cancer. J Natl Cancer Inst *99*: 858–67, 2007.
55. Soltermann, A., R. Ossola, S. Kilgus-Hawelski, A. von Eckardstein, T. Suter, R. Aebersold, and H. Moch. N-glycoprotein profiling of lung adenocarcinoma pleural effusions by shotgun proteomics. Cancer *114*: 124–33, 2008.
56. Tyan, Y.C., H.Y. Wu, W.C. Su, P.W. Chen, and P.C. Liao. Proteomic analysis of human pleural effusion. Proteomics *5*: 1062–74, 2005.
57. Jagirdar, J. Application of immunohistochemistry to the diagnosis of primary and metastatic carcinoma to the lung. Arch Pathol Lab Med *132*: 384–96, 2008.
58. Opitz, I., A. Soltermann, M. Abaecherli, M. Hinterberger, N. Probst-Hensch, R. Stahel, H. Moch, and W. Weder. PTEN expression is a strong predictor of survival in mesothelioma patients. Eur J Cardiothorac Surg *33*: 502–6, 2008.

59. Rahman, S.M., Y. Shyr, P.B. Yildiz, A.L. Gonzalez, H. Li, X. Zhang, P. Chaurand, K. Yanagisawa, B.S. Slovis, R.F. Miller, M. Ninan, Y.E. Miller, W.A. Franklin, R.M. Caprioli, D.P. Carbone, and P.P. Massion. Proteomic patterns of preinvasive bronchial lesions. Am J Respir Crit Care Med *172*: 1556–62, 2005.

60. Amann, J.M., P. Chaurand, A. Gonzalez, J.A. Mobley, P.P. Massion, D.P. Carbone, and R.M. Caprioli. Selective profiling of proteins in lung cancer cells from fine-needle aspirates by matrix-assisted laser desorption ionization time-of-flight mass spectrometry. Clin Cancer Res *12*: 5142–50, 2006.

61. Taguchi, F., B. Solomon, V. Gregorc, H. Roder, R. Gray, K. Kasahara, M. Nishio, J. Brahmer, A. Spreafico, V. Ludovini, P.P. Massion, R. Dziadziuszko, J. Schiller, J. Grigorieva, M. Tsypin, S.W. Hunsucker, R. Caprioli, M.W. Duncan, F.R. Hirsch, P.A. Bunn, Jr., and D.P. Carbone. Mass spectrometry to classify non-small-cell lung cancer patients for clinical outcome after treatment with epidermal growth factor receptor tyrosine kinase inhibitors: a multicohort cross-institutional study. J Natl Cancer Inst *99*: 838–46, 2007.

62. Yildiz, P.B., Y. Shyr, J.S. Rahman, N.R. Wardwell, L.J. Zimmerman, B. Shakhtour, W. H. Gray, S. Chen, M. Li, H. Roder, D.C. Liebler, W.L. Bigbee, J.M. Siegfried, J.L. Weissfeld, A.L. Gonzalez, M. Ninan, D.H. Johnson, D.P. Carbone, R.M. Caprioli, and P.P. Massion. Diagnostic accuracy of MALDI mass spectrometric analysis of unfractionated serum in lung cancer. J Thorac Oncol *2*: 893–901, 2007.

63. Gao, W.M., R. Kuick, R.P. Orchekowski, D.E. Misek, J. Qiu, A.K. Greenberg, W.N. Rom, D.E. Brenner, G.S. Omenn, B.B. Haab, and S.M. Hanash. Distinctive serum protein profiles involving abundant proteins in lung cancer patients based upon antibody microarray analysis. BMC Cancer *5*: 110, 2005.

64. Han, K.Q., G. Huang, C.F. Gao, X.L. Wang, B. Ma, L.Q. Sun, and Z.J. Wei. Identification of lung cancer patients by serum protein profiling using surface-enhanced laser desorption/ionization time-of-flight mass spectrometry. Am J Clin Oncol *31*: 133–9, 2008.

65. Heo, S.H., S.J. Lee, H.M. Ryoo, J.Y. Park, and J.Y. Cho. Identification of putative serum glycoprotein biomarkers for human lung adenocarcinoma by multilectin affinity chromatography and LC-MS/MS. Proteomics *7*: 4292–302, 2007.

66. Maciel, C.M., M. Junqueira, M.E. Paschoal, M.T. Kawamura, R.L. Duarte, G. Carvalho Mda, and G.B. Domont. Differential proteomic serum pattern of low molecular weight proteins expressed by adenocarcinoma lung cancer patients. J Exp Ther Oncol *5*: 31–8, 2005.

67. Okano, T., T. Kondo, T. Kakisaka, K. Fujii, M. Yamada, H. Kato, T. Nishimura, A. Gemma, S. Kudoh, and S. Hirohashi. Plasma proteomics of lung cancer by a linkage of multi-dimensional liquid chromatography and two-dimensional difference gel electrophoresis. Proteomics *6*: 3938–48, 2006.

68. Mahanta, S., S.P. Fessler, J. Park, and C. Bamdad. A minimal fragment of MUC1 mediates growth of cancer cells. PLoS ONE *3*: e2054, 2008.

69. Stockert, E., E. Jager, Y.T. Chen, M.J. Scanlan, I. Gout, J. Karbach, M. Arand, A. Knuth, and L.J. Old. A survey of the humoral immune response of cancer patients to a panel of human tumor antigens. J Exp Med *187*: 1349–54, 1998.

70. Hanash, S. Harnessing immunity for cancer marker discovery. Nat Biotechnol *21*: 37–8, 2003.

71. Brichory, F., D. Beer, F. Le Naour, T. Giordano, and S. Hanash. Proteomics-based identification of protein gene product 9.5 as a tumor antigen that induces a humoral immune response in lung cancer. Cancer Res *61*: 7908–12, 2001.

72. Brichory, F.M., D.E. Misek, A.M. Yim, M.C. Krause, T.J. Giordano, D.G. Beer, and S. M. Hanash. An immune response manifested by the common occurrence of annexins I and II autoantibodies and high circulating levels of IL-6 in lung cancer. Proc Natl Acad Sci USA *98*: 9824–9, 2001.

73. Pereira-Faca, S.R., R. Kuick, E. Puravs, Q. Zhang, A.L. Krasnoselsky, D. Phanstiel, J. Qiu, D.E. Misek, R. Hinderer, M. Tammemagi, M.T. Landi, N. Caporaso, R. Pfeiffer, C. Edelstein, G. Goodman, M. Barnett, M. Thornquist, D. Brenner, and S.M. Hanash. Identification of 14-3-3 theta as an antigen that induces a humoral response in lung cancer. Cancer Res 67: 12000–6, 2007.

74. Qiu, J., G. Choi, L. Lin, H. Wang, S.J. Pitteri, S.R. Pereira-Faca, A.L. Krasnoselsky, T.W. Randolph, C. Edelstein, M. Barnett, M. Thornquist, G. Goodman, G. S. Omenn, D. Brenner, Z. Feng, and S.M. Hanash. Occurrence of autoantibodies to annexin 1, 14-3-3 theta and LAMR1 in pre diagnostic lung cancer sera. J Clin Oncol 26: 5060–6, 2008.

75. Omenn, G.S., G.E. Goodman, M.D. Thornquist, J. Balmes, M.R. Cullen, A. Glass, J.P. Keogh, F.L. Meyskens, B. Valanis, J.H. Williams, S. Barnhart, and S. Hammar. Effects of a combination of beta carotene and vitamin A on lung cancer and cardiovascular disease. N Engl J Med 334: 1150–5, 1996.

76. Chen, G., X. Wang, J. Yu, S. Varambally, D.G. Thomas, M.Y. Lin, P. Vishnu, Z. Wang, R. Wang, J. Fielhauer, D. Ghosh, T.J. Giordano, D. Giacherio, A.C. Chang, M.B. Orringer, T. El-Hefnawy, W.L. Bigbee, D.G. Beer, and A.M. Chinnaiyan. Autoantibody profiles reveal ubiquilin 1 as a humoral immune response target in lung adenocarcinoma. Cancer Res 67: 3461–7, 2007.

77. Keshamouni, V.G., G. Michailidis, C.S. Grasso, S. Anthwal, J.R. Strahler, A. Walker, D. A. Arenberg, R.C. Reddy, S. Akulapalli, V.J. Thannickal, T.J. Standiford, P.C. Andrews, and G.S. Omenn. Differential protein expression profiling by iTRAQ-2DLC-MS/MS of lung cancer cells undergoing epithelial-mesenchymal transition reveals a migratory/invasive phenotype. J Proteome Res 5: 1143–54, 2006.

78. Keshamouni, V.G., Jagtap, P., Michailidi, G., Strahler, J.R., Kuick, R., Reka, A.K., Papoulias, P., Krishnapuram, R., Srirangam, A., Standiford, T.J., Andrews, P.C., Omenn, G.S. Temporal quantitative proteomics by iTRAQ 2D-LC-MS/MS and corresponding mRNA expression analysis identify post-transcriptional modulation of action-cytoskeleton regulators during TGF-beta-induced epithelial-mesenchymal transition. J Proteome Res 8: 35–47, 2009. PMID: 19118450.

79. Whiteaker, J.R., H. Zhang, L. Zhao, P. Wang, K.S. Kelly-Spratt, R.G. Ivey, B.D. Piening, L.C. Feng, E. Kasarda, K.E. Gurley, J.K. Eng, L.A. Chodosh, C.J. Kemp, M. W. McIntosh, and A.G. Paulovich. Integrated pipeline for mass spectrometry-based discovery and confirmation of biomarkers demonstrated in a mouse model of breast cancer. J Proteome Res 6: 3962–75, 2007.

80. Faca, V.M., K.S. Song, H. Wang, Q. Zhang, A.L. Krasnoselsky, L.F. Newcomb, R.R. Plentz, S. Gurumurthy, M.S. Redston, S.J. Pitteri, S.R. Pereira-Faca, R.C. Ireton, H. Katayama, V. Glukhova, D. Phanstiel, D.E. Brenner, M.A. Anderson, D. Misek, N. Scholler, N.D. Urban, M.J. Barnett, C. Edelstein, G.E. Goodman, M.D. Thornquist, M. W. McIntosh, R.A. DePinho, N. Bardeesy, and S.M. Hanash. A mouse to human search for plasma proteome changes associated with pancreatic tumor development. PLoS Med 5: e123, 2008.

81. Fermin, D., B.B. Allen, T.W. Blackwell, R. Menon, M. Adamski, Y. Xu, P. Ulintz, G.S. Omenn, and D.J. States. Novel gene and gene model detection using a whole genome open reading frame analysis in proteomics. Genome Biol 7: R35, 2006.

82. Menon, R., Zhang, Q., Zhang, Y., Fermin, D., Bardeesy, N., DePinho, R.A., Lu, C., Hanash, S.M., Omenn, G.S., States, D.J. Identification of novel alternative splice iso-forms of circulating proteins iin a mouse model of human pancreatic cancer. Cancer Res 69: 300–9, 2009. PMID: 19118015.

83. Sreekumar, A., Poisson, L.M., Rajendiran, T.M., Khan, A.P., Cao, Q., Yu, J., Laxman, B., Mehra, R., Loniga, R.J., Li., Y., Nyati, M.K., Ahsan, A., Kalyana-Sundaram, S., Han, B., Cao, X., Byun, J., Omenn, G.S., Ghosh, D., Pennathur, S., Alexander, D.C., Berger, A., Shuster, J.R., Wei, J.T., Varambally, S., Beecher, C., Chinnaiyan, A.M.

Metabolomic profiles delineate potential role for sarcosine in prostate cancer progression. Nature, *457*: 910–4, 2009. PMID: 19212411.

84. Anderson, L. and C.L. Hunter. Quantitative mass spectrometric multiple reaction monitoring assays for major plasma proteins. Mol Cell Proteomics 5: 573–88, 2006.

85. Barker, P.E., P.D. Wagner, S.E. Stein, D.M. Bunk, S. Srivastava, and G.S. Omenn. Standards for plasma and serum proteomics in early cancer detection: a needs assessment report from the national institute of standards and technology – National Cancer Institute Standards, Methods, Assays, Reagents and Technologies Workshop, August 18–19, 2005. Clin Chem *52*: 1669–74, 2006.

86. Liu, J., J. Stevens, C.A. Rote, H.J. Yost, Y. Hu, K.L. Neufeld, R.L. White, and N. Matsunami. Siah-1 mediates a novel beta-catenin degradation pathway linking p53 to the adenomatous polyposis coli protein. Mol Cell 7: 927–36, 2001.

Current Clinical Management of Metastatic Lung Cancer

Bryan J. Schneider and Suresh S. Ramalingam

Abstract Approximately 40% of patients with non-small cell lung cancer (NSCLC) and 70% of patients with small cell lung cancer (SCLC) present with advanced, hematogenously metastatic, incurable disease. Systemic chemotherapy is the mainstay of therapy in these patients with the primary goals of palliating symptoms, maintaining quality of life, and prolonging life. For patients with advanced NSCLC, standard treatment consists of two-drug, platinum-based chemotherapy with or without bevacizumab, a monoclonal antibody targeting the vascular endothelial growth factor which controls tumor angiogenesis. In NSCLC, second- and third-line therapy with chemotherapy or epidermal growth factor receptor inhibitors has also been shown to provide a survival benefit. Recent studies have begun to define specific clinical, histological, and molecular characteristics that can help identify subsets of patients with NSCLC who will or will not respond to particular chemotherapeutic or molecularly targeted agents. For patients with extensive-stage SCLC, initial platinum-based chemotherapy yields impressive response rates, but long-term survival remains extremely limited. Despite extensive knowledge of the biology of SCLC, studies of molecularly targeted therapies have yet to demonstrate any significant clinical benefits in this disease.

Introduction

More than 200,000 new cases of lung cancer are diagnosed each year in the United States, with non-small cell lung cancer (NSCLC) accounting for approximately 85% of all cases [1]. In the past two decades, the proportion of patients diagnosed with small cell lung cancer (SCLC) has decreased [2]. NSCLC comprises various histological subtypes including adenocarcinoma, squamous cell carcinoma, large cell carcinoma, and bronchioloalveolar

B.J. Schneider (✉)
Division of Hematology/Oncology Department of Internal Medicine, Presbyterian-Weill Cornell Medical Center, New York, NY 10065, USA
e-mail: bjs2004@med.cornell.edu

V. Keshamouni et al. (eds.), *Lung Cancer Metastasis*,
DOI 10.1007/978-1-4419-0772-1_15, © Springer Science+Business Media, LLC 2009

carcinoma. The incidence of adenocarcinoma has gradually increased in the past three decades, whereas that of squamous cell carcinoma has decreased.

Approximately 40% of patients with NSCLC are diagnosed with advanced or metastatic disease and are not candidates for definitive local therapy [1]. Similarly, two-thirds of patients with SCLC present with extensive-stage disease. Systemic therapy leads to improvements in both overall survival and quality of life for patients with advanced-stage SCLC and NSCLC [3]. In recent years, a number of newer chemotherapeutic agents and novel combination regimens have been added to the therapeutic armamentarium. In addition, improved understanding of the molecular mechanisms that underlie lung cancer progression and metastasis has now led to the development of novel targeted agents. Inhibitors of epidermal growth factor receptor (EGFR) and vascular endothelial growth factor (VEGF) are already in routine clinical use. Selection of therapy based on molecular characteristics of the tumor in individual patients has now become a major goal of clinical/translational investigations. This chapter will describe the current treatment of advanced-stage lung cancer and the role of emerging new agents.

Non-small Cell Lung Cancer

Patients with hematogenous metastases to distant organs or other lobes of the lungs (ipsilateral or contralateral) are categorized as having advanced-stage or stage IV disease. In addition, patients with malignant pleural or pericardial effusions (T4 disease, stage IIIB) have comparable survival outcomes to those with stage IV disease and are treated in a similar manner. Advanced-stage NSCLC is treated primarily with systemic therapy, which includes chemotherapeutic agents and molecularly targeted agents. Performance status is the main determinant of outcome in patients with advanced-stage NSCLC [4]. Those with a score of 0 or 1 on the Eastern Cooperative Oncology Group (ECOG) performance status scale have the most favorable outcome, whereas those with a score of 2 or worse have a poor survival [5]. Performance status is considered to be a composite measure that combines the impact of both lung cancer aggressiveness and comorbid illness. Since the majority of clinical trials include only patients with a good performance status, treatment guidelines are less defined for patients with a poor performance status.

Systemic Chemotherapy

Platinum-based combination chemotherapy is considered the standard therapy for patients with advanced NSCLC with a good performance status [6].

Although the anticancer activity of single-agent cisplatin or carboplatin is modest, their combination with a second chemotherapeutic agent such as paclitaxel, docetaxel, vinorelbine, gemcitabine, or pemetrexed results in improved efficacy [7–9]. Several randomized clinical trials have compared the efficacy of single-agent cisplatin to cisplatin-based two-drug combinations [9–11]. Overall, combination regimens result in superior response rates, time to disease progression, and overall survival, but also increase the incidence of adverse events. Carboplatin is associated with a more favorable nonhematological toxicity profile than cisplatin and has now become the more commonly used platinum compound for the treatment of patients with advanced NSCLC in the United States. Studies that compared cisplatin-based combinations to carboplatin-based regimens have demonstrated comparable survival in this setting [7, 12]. A recent meta-analysis of studies that compared cisplatin-based regimens with carboplatin-based regimens in patients with advanced NSCLC suggested slightly greater response rates with the former but no clinically significant difference in survival [13]. Since the intent of treatment in patients with advanced NSCLC is primarily palliation, the more favorable toxicity profile of carboplatin-based regimens has led to their adoption for routine clinical use. In curative settings such as adjuvant therapy for early stage, completely resected NSCLC, cisplatin is generally preferred over carboplatin.

A number of newer chemotherapeutic agents have been combined with platinum compounds and have demonstrated anticancer efficacy in the treatment of patients with advanced-stage NSCLC. Phase II studies of the combination of either cisplatin or carboplatin with paclitaxel, docetaxel, vinorelbine, gemcitabine, irinotecan, or pemetrexed in patients with advanced NSCLC have shown response rates of 30–50% and median survival times of 8–12 months. These encouraging data paved the way for randomized phase III studies that compared various platinum-based combination regimens (Table 1). The ECOG 1594 study compared three different combination regimens (cisplatin + docetaxel, cisplatin + gemcitabine, and carboplatin + paclitaxel) to the regimen of cisplatin + paclitaxel [7]. All four regimens demonstrated comparable efficacy in terms of response rate, time to progression, and overall survival with no clear advantage for one over another. The regimens differed only in regard to their toxicity profiles, with carboplatin + paclitaxel having the most favorable therapeutic index. Another study that compared carboplatin + paclitaxel to cisplatin + vinorelbine also yielded comparable efficacy results between the regimens [14]. The therapeutic equivalence of various platinum-based doublets has been confirmed in several large, randomized phase III studies [8, 15–17].

Substitution of platinum-based regimens with nonplatinum two-drug regimens has also undergone extensive investigation. Randomized studies have demonstrated comparable efficacy of various nonplatinum regimens to platinum-based chemotherapy combinations [18, 19]. However, there was no major advantage in the adverse event profile of nonplatinum regimens that would justify them supplanting the use of platinum-based combinations for first-line treatment of patients with advanced NSCLC. For selected patients who are unlikely to tolerate platinum-based therapy, the nonplatinum regimens are an acceptable therapeutic alternative. Although two-drug combinations are superior to single-agent therapy, the addition of a third cytotoxic drug does not result in improved efficacy [20]. However, three-drug combinations are associated with greater toxicity and are not recommended for the treatment of patients with advanced NSCLC.

Table 1 Selected phase III studies of platinum-based two-drug combinations for advanced NSCLC

Author	Regimen	Response rate (%)	Median survival (m)	1-Year survival (%)
Schiller	Cisplatin–paclitaxel	21	7.8	31
[7]	Cisplatin–docetaxel	17	7.4	31
	Cisplatin–gemcitabine	22	8.1	36
	Carboplatin–paclitaxel	17	8.1	34
Kelly [14]	Cisplatin–vinorelbine	28	8.0	36
	Carboplatin–paclitaxel	25	8.0	38
Ohe [145]	Cisplatin–irinotecan	31	13.9	59
	Cisplatin–gemcitabine	30	14.0	60
	Cisplatin–vinorelbine	33	11.8	44
	Carboplatin–paclitaxel	32	12.3	51
Fossella	Cisplatin–vinorelbine	25	10.1	41
[15]	Cisplatin–docetaxel	31	11.3	46
	Carboplatin–docetaxel	24	9.4	38
Scagliotti	Cisplatin–gemcitabine	28	10.3	Not reported
[8]	Cisplatin–pemetrexed	31	10.3	

Customized Chemotherapy Based on Tumor Characteristics

The efficacy of various combination chemotherapy regimens appears similar across the histological subtypes of NSCLC. However, a recently reported study demonstrated varying efficacy for the cisplatin + pemetrexed regimen based on histological subtype. Pemetrexed, a novel multitargeted antifolate compound, has demonstrated anticancer activity as a single-agent in patients with relapsed NSCLC [21]. A phase III study that compared the regimen of cisplatin + pemetrexed to cisplatin + gemcitabine in patients with advanced-stage NSCLC demonstrated noninferiority of the cisplatin + pemetrexed combination, which was also associated with a more favorable toxicity profile [8]. Intriguingly, a preplanned subset analysis demonstrated superior survival with cisplatin + pemetrexed for patients with adenocarcinoma. The biological basis for this may be the higher frequency of methylthioadenosine phosphorylase (MTAP) deletions in adenocarcinoma relative to other histological subtypes [22, 23]. MTAP plays an important role in the salvage pathway for the synthesis of adenosine and tumors with MTAP deletions appear to be associated with a heightened sensitivity to treatment with pemetrexed [24]. Tumor specimens from patients enrolled in this study are being evaluated for MTAP deletions to confirm this hypothesis. If proven to be true, the presence of an MTAP deletion could serve as a marker for preferential selection of the cisplatin + pemetrexed regimen.

Other strategies are also being evaluated to select the most appropriate chemotherapy regimen based on patient-specific tumor molecular characteristics. The excision repair cross-complementing (ERCC) gene is involved in DNA repair [25]. Since platinum compounds induce lethality by the formation of DNA adducts, an inherent impairment in cellular DNA repair capacity is associated with heightened sensitivity to platinum-based therapy [26]. Based on this premise, a randomized clinical trial was conducted to select therapy for individual patients based on the level of tumor ERCC1 expression. Patients with ERCC1 overexpressing tumors were treated with nonplatinum regimens, while those with low ERCC1-expressing tumors were treated with platinum-based therapy [27]. The response rate was higher in patients with low ERCC1-expressing tumors receiving platinum-based therapy than in a control group of unselected patients treated with cisplatin + docetaxel. A similar finding was observed in patients receiving adjuvant therapy for early-stage NSCLC, where those with tumors with low ERCC1 expression had significant benefit from cisplatin-based therapy, while those with high ERCC1 expression derived no survival benefit from such therapy.

The results of another phase II study in patients with advanced NSCLC also support the feasibility and promise of customizing therapy based on biomarkers. Simon et al. evaluated both ERCC1 for the prediction of cisplatin sensitivity and the ribonucleotide reductase subunit M1 (RRM1) enzyme, which catalyzes deoxynucleotide production and is inversely associated with sensitivity to gemcitabine [28]. An initial tumor biopsy was used to evaluate the expression of ERCC1 and RRM1 by reverse transcriptase-polymerase chain reaction and the treatment regimen was chosen based on the expression level of the two genes. Patients whose tumors had low ERCC1 and RRM1 were treated with the combination of carboplatin + gemcitabine, whereas those with high expression levels received docetaxel + vinorelbine. With customized therapy, a promising response rate of 44% and a median survival time of 13.3 months were noted in 85 patients with advanced NSCLC. The therapeutic advantage associated with this approach is now being tested in a phase III study conducted by the same investigators.

Salvage Chemotherapy for Progressive Disease

A number of therapeutic options have emerged in the past few years for the treatment of patients with advanced NSCLC who have disease progression following initial chemotherapy. Docetaxel, a tubulin-binding agent, was the first to receive FDA approval in the United States as salvage therapy for NSCLC. Two randomized studies established the efficacy of single-agent docetaxel in this setting [29, 30]. At a dose of 75 mg/m^2 every 3 weeks, docetaxel is associated with a response rate of 5–10% and a median survival time of approximately 8 months. Improvements in several qualitative parameters, such as performance status, global quality of life scores, and pain, were noted with docetaxel. Pemetrexed has also been approved by the FDA based on demonstrated efficacy as salvage therapy for patients with NSCLC. A phase III study that compared pemetrexed to docetaxel as salvage therapy reported comparable efficacy between the two agents, though pemetrexed had a more favorable toxicity profile. Several other agents have also demonstrated efficacy as salvage therapy, including oral topotecan, vinflunine (a vinca alkaloid), and polyglutamated paclitaxel (a novel macromolecular formulation), although they do not offer any clear advantage over docetaxel or pemetrexed [31, 32]. Erlotinib, an inhibitor of the epidermal growth factor receptor (EGFR), has also been approved by the FDA as salvage therapy for NSCLC and will be discussed below. Combination regimens do not have any survival advantage over single agents in the salvage setting, though response rates do appear to be slightly higher. The current wave of clinical investigations in the salvage setting involves the study of various combinations of a cytotoxic agent with a molecularly targeted agent.

EGFR Inhibitors

EGFR inhibitors are now in routine clinical use for the treatment of patients with advanced-stage NSCLC. Gefitinib was the first EGFR inhibitor to demonstrate anticancer activity in NSCLC (Table 2). Two doses of gefitinib (250 mg/day and 500 mg/day) were compared in patients with advanced-stage NSCLC following progression after standard therapy [33, 34]. The objective response rate was 10–19% with an additional 30–40% of patients experiencing disease stabilization. Improvements in quality of life and lung cancer symptom scores were also noted in many patients. No difference in efficacy was noted between the two doses, though the lower dose was associated with a more favorable toxicity profile. However, a subsequent phase III study that compared gefitinib to placebo failed to demonstrate a progression-free or overall survival advantage for gefitinib as salvage treatment for patients with advanced NSCLC [35]. This finding effectively halted the use of this agent in patients with advanced-stage NSCLC in the United States. However, selected subgroups of patients, including never-smokers and those of East Asian ethnicity, had superior survival with gefitinib over placebo, suggesting a possible role for this agent in clinically or molecularly selected subsets of patients with NSCLC.

Erlotinib, another EGFR tyrosine kinase inhibitor (TKI), is currently approved for the treatment of patients with advanced NSCLC. Following demonstration of its anticancer activity in a phase II study [36], erlotinib was compared to placebo in a randomized phase III study in patients with advanced NSCLC who had progressed after one or two prior chemotherapy

Table 2 EGFR inhibitors in clinical use for treatment of NSCLC

Author	Agent	Response rate (%)	Median survival (m)	1-Year survival (%)
Kris [34]	Gefitinib 250 mg	12	7.0	27
	Gefitinib 500 mg	9	6.0	24
Fukuoka [33]	Gefitinib 250 mg	18	7.6	35
	Gefitinib 500 mg	19	8.0	29
Thatcher [35]	Gefitinib 250 mg	8	5.6	27
	Placebo	1	5.1	22
Perez-Soler [36]	Erlotinib 150 mg	12	8.4	40
Shepherd [37]	Erlotinib 150 mg	9	6.7	31
	Placebo	<1	4.7	21

regimens [37]. The median survival time was superior with erlotinib (6.7 months vs. 4.7 months), and erlotinib yielded a response rate of 9% and a disease stabilization rate of 35%. Improvements were also noted in time to symptomatic deterioration in patients treated with erlotinib. The main side effects were skin rash in 75% of patients and diarrhea in 54%. This study led to the FDA approval of erlotinib as second- or third-line therapy for patients with advanced-stage NSCLC.

Cetuximab, a monoclonal antibody targeting EGFR, also has modest single-agent efficacy in patients with NSCLC. In a phase II study of patients with previously treated advanced NSCLC, cetuximab demonstrated a response rate of 5% and a disease stabilization rate of 30% [38]. The incidence of skin rash was high, but diarrhea was uncommon. Following the demonstration of efficacy of EGFR inhibitors as single agents, randomized clinical trials have been conducted to study them in combination with chemotherapy. This was supported by preclinical evidence that the coadministration of EGFR inhibitors and chemotherapeutic agents resulted in supraadditive effects in NSCLC cell lines [39]. However, the clinical trials have failed to demonstrate any improvement in overall survival or progression-free survival with combinations of an EGFR TKI plus standard platinum-based chemotherapy over chemotherapy alone in patients with advanced-stage NSCLC [40, 41]. Although the reasons behind the conflicting preclinical and clinical findings are not entirely clear, further development of combination regimens of EGFR TKIs plus chemotherapy has been discontinued.

In contrast, cetuximab, the anti-EGFR monoclonal antibody, was associated with promising response rates and survival duration when combined with chemotherapy in phase II studies for patients with advanced-stage NSCLC [42–44]. Subsequent phase III studies of chemotherapy with or without cetuximab in patients with chemotherapy-naïve advanced-stage NSCLC have yielded conflicting results, with one study that combined cetuximab with carboplatin plus a taxane showing no improvement in progression-free survival over chemotherapy alone, while another study that combined cetuximab with cisplatin + vinorelbine demonstrating improved survival in patients with EGFR-expressing tumors (Press release, Imclone Pharmaceuticals, Inc, September 2007). The detailed results of this trial are yet to be reported. Of note, the positive study with cetuximab was unique in that it selected patients for therapy based on EGFR expression status. Clinical development of panitumumab, a fully human anti-EGFR monoclonal antibody, was discontinued based on data from a randomized phase II study of carboplatin + paclitaxel with or without panitumumab that showed no improvement in any efficacy parameters with the addition of panitumumab to chemotherapy [45]. Appropriate patient selection using molecular and clinical factors is a key subject of ongoing research efforts evaluating the potential utility of EGFR inhibition in patients with NSCLC.

Molecular Predictive Markers for EGFR Inhibition

EGFR protein expression: Initial studies in NSCLC with EGFR inhibitors were conducted only in patients with EGFR-expressing tumors [36, 38]. However, subsequent studies have enrolled patients regardless of EGFR status due to the lack of clear correlation between EGFR expression and response. In the randomized BR.21 trial that led to FDA approval of erlotinib for patients with NSCLC, a retrospective evaluation of receptor expression in tumor tissues from one-third of the participating patients suggested a lack of benefit for erlotinib in patients with EGFR-negative tumors [37]. The utility of this marker for treatment selection remains unclear due to conflicting data on the correlation between EGFR expression and response to EGFR inhibitors noted in other tumor types, such as colon cancer. Potential challenges to the use of EGFR protein expression by immunohistochemistry (IHC) for patient selection include the low sensitivity of the IHC techniques, interobserver variability in scoring, and the variation in EGFR expression both within the same tumor and between metastatic sites [46].

EGFR gene copy number: The number of *EGFR* gene copies has been linked to treatment outcomes with EGFR inhibitors [47, 48]. Amplification of the *EGFR* gene is noted in tumors from 10 to 15% of patients with NSCLC, but there does not appear to be a clear correlation between *EGFR* gene amplification and protein expression [49]. In a predictive algorithm developed by Hirsch et al., a higher gene copy number, assessed by fluorescent in situ hybridization (FISH), was associated with improved outcome for patients treated with gefitinib or erlotinib for advanced NSCLC. FISH positivity was defined as the presence of more than four copies of the *EGFR* gene in at least 40% of tumor cells. Based on this definition, the investigators were able to identify patients who were likely to experience improved survival. In a retrospective analysis conducted on tumor specimens from patients who participated in the ISEL study of gefitinib vs. placebo, the hazard ratio for survival with gefitinib in FISH-positive patients was 0.61, compared to 1.16 in FISH-negative patients. This observation has also been noted in a retrospective analysis of the BR.21 study with erlotinib [50]. Prospective studies are now underway to evaluate the predictive potential of *EGFR* gene copy number for response to EGFR inhibitors in NSCLC. However, planned subset analyses of two recently reported studies have provided conflicting results. The randomized phase III INTEREST study that compared gefitinib to docetaxel as salvage therapy in unselected patients met its primary endpoint of noninferiority for gefitinib. However, a preplanned subset analysis in FISH-positive patients failed to demonstrate superiority for gefitinib over docetaxel [51]. Similarly, the randomized INVITE study that compared gefitinib to vinorelbine in elderly patients with NSCLC demonstrated a lack of improved outcome for FISH-positive patients treated with the EGFR inhibitor [52]. Therefore, until results from ongoing prospective studies are available, testing for *EGFR* gene amplification cannot be recommended for routine clinical practice.

EGFR mutation: The presence of specific mutations in the tyrosine kinase domain of the EGFR is associated with a higher likelihood of response to treatment with EGFR TKIs. Both in-frame deletions of four amino acids in exon 19 and point mutations resulting in the substitution of an amino acid in exon 21 of the *EGFR* gene have been noted in tumors of patients with NSCLC who had a robust response to EGFR TKIs [53]. These mutations have not been identified in other tumor types. The EGFR mutations do not confer constitutive activity but result in heightened responsiveness to receptor activation. The prevalence of these EGFR mutations in Caucasian patients is only 10–15%, but they are found in a higher proportion of patients of East Asian ethnicity [54]. Other clinical characteristics that are associated with a higher prevalence of EGFR mutations include female gender, never-smoking status, and adenocarcinoma histology, perhaps accounting for the higher response rates to EGFR inhibitors noted in these patient subsets. Contrary to this hypothesis, a retrospective analysis of the BR.21 study failed to demonstrate a survival advantage for erlotinib over placebo in patients with tumors harboring an EGFR mutation [50]. This study was limited, however, by the small number of patients whose tumors were available for analysis. Recently, the results from prospective studies have suggested very high response rates and prolonged time to progression with the use of EGFR TKIs in patients with EGFR mutations. In a study by the Spanish Lung Cancer Group, 38 patients with EGFR mutations treated with single-agent erlotinib as first-line therapy for advanced NSCLC had a response rate of 82% and a median progression-free survival of over 12 months [55]. Of note, the response rate was higher in patients with a mutation in exon 19 than in exon 21, suggesting differential biological effects of the two mutations. This observation has been confirmed further by other studies [56, 57]. Although the EGFR TKIs are more active in patients with EGFR mutations, the effect of mutations on the efficacy of anti-EGFR monoclonal antibodies is unclear. In preclinical studies, TKIs are more potent than monoclonal antibodies against mutant EGFR-bearing NSCLC cell lines [58]. Furthermore, the question remains as to whether EGFR mutations have a prognostic or predictive effect in patients with NSCLC, since an analysis of a phase III trial that compared chemotherapy with or without erlotinib noted that even patients in the chemotherapy-alone arm had a better outcome if their tumors harbored an EGFR mutation [59]. Therefore, the utility of EGFR mutations in patient selection for EGFR TKIs remains a subject of ongoing investigations.

Recently, a secondary mutation in exon 20 of the EGFR has been reported. This mutation confers structural changes in the tyrosine kinase domain and results in resistance to therapy with EGFR TKIs [60]. It is commonly found in the tumors of patients with exon 19 or 21 mutations after treatment with an EGFR TKI. Agents specific for patients with this secondary EGFR mutation are now under clinical evaluation. Alternative mechanisms of resistance to EGFR inhibition such as activation of the C-MET pathway have also been described in NSCLC [61].

Serum proteomic analysis: Mass spectroscopic analysis of serum samples has recently been shown to identify patients who are likely to derive a survival benefit from EGFR TKIs [62]. Eight specific protein peaks were noted to differentiate patients with a "good" outcome with EGFR TKIs from those with a "poor" outcome. The predictive potential of serum proteomic analysis to select patients for treatment with EGFR TKIs is now being tested in prospective clinical trials. If proven useful, this could be an inexpensive and non-invasive method for selecting appropriate patients for therapy with EGFR inhibitors.

Antiangiogenic Agents

The formation of new blood vessels is critical for the proliferation and metastasis of cancer cells [63]. Vascular endothelial growth factor (VEGF), the rate-limiting factor for neoangiogenesis under physiological conditions, also plays a major role in the tumor milieu [64]. Therefore, a number of agents that block VEGF or its receptors are under development as anticancer drugs (Table 3). Bevacizumab, a monoclonal antibody targeting VEGF, augments the anticancer effects of chemotherapy in multiple tumor types [65]. In NSCLC, the limited available evidence suggests that bevacizumab is not active as a single agent [66]. However, in a randomized phase II study conducted in patients with advanced NSCLC, the addition of bevacizumab to chemotherapy resulted in a higher response rate and improved overall survival. Subsequently, ECOG conducted a phase III study (ECOG 4599) to evaluate whether the addition of bevacizumab to the regimen of carboplatin plus paclitaxel improves overall survival in patients with advanced-stage NSCLC [67]. Patients with squamous

Table 3 VEGF inhibitors in treatment of advanced NSCLC

Author	Phase	Regimen	Response rate	Median PFS
Sandler* [67]	III	Carboplatin–paclitaxel–bevacizumab (15 mg/kg)	35%	6.2 m
		Carboplatin–paclitaxel	15%	4.8 m
Manegold* [68]	III	Cisplatin–gemcitabine–bevacizumab (7.5 mg/kg)	34%	6.7 m
		Cisplatin–gemcitabine–bevacizumab (15 mg/kg)	30%	6.5 m
		Cisplatin–gemcitabine–placebo	20%	6.1 m
Natale [69]	II	Vandetanib 300 mg	8%	11 wk
Socinski [70]	II	Sunitinib	10%	11.3 wk
Gatzemeier [71]	II	Sorafenib	0	11.9 wk
Schiller [146]	II	Axitinib	9%	25 wk
Gauler [147]	II	Vatalanib (BID dosing)	7%	12.1 wk

* Study conducted in patients with previously untreated advanced NSCLC

cell histology, prior hemoptysis, and brain metastasis were excluded. The higher incidence of life-threatening hemoptysis in the preceding phase II study in patients with squamous cell carcinoma prompted the exclusion of this histological subtype. The addition of bevacizumab to chemotherapy resulted in an improvement in response rate (35% vs. 15%) and overall survival (12.3 months vs. 10.3 months) compared to chemotherapy alone. Salient adverse events associated with the bevacizumab plus chemotherapy combination included neutropenia, hypertension, proteinuria, and bleeding events. The number of treatment-related deaths was also higher with the addition of bevacizumab.

The results of the ECOG study led to FDA approval of bevacizumab in combination with carboplatin and paclitaxel for patients with previously untreated, advanced nonsquamous NSCLC. A second randomized study that evaluated the addition of bevacizumab to chemotherapy (cisplatin + gemcitabine) demonstrated a modest improvement in progression-free survival, though overall survival results have not yet been reported [68].

In contrast to bevacizumab, a number of novel agents that inhibit the VEGF receptor tyrosine kinase have demonstrated single-agent activity in advanced NSCLC. Vandetanib, a dual inhibitor of EGF and VEGF receptors, resulted in a response rate of 8% when given as a single agent to patients with relapsed advanced NSCLC [69]. Sunitinib, another small-molecule inhibitor of VEGF receptors, was also associated with a response rate of approximately 10% [70]. Other agents of this class that are undergoing active investigation include sorafenib, axitinib, and vatalanib [71, 72]. In addition to the common adverse events associated with VEGF inhibition, such as hypertension and proteinuria, the VEGFR TKIs are associated with other toxicities such as hand–foot syndrome and fatigue. These agents are now being tested in combination with chemotherapy, but it remains to be seen if the small-molecule inhibitors will offer any therapeutic advantage over bevacizumab.

Efforts to identify predictive biomarkers for clinical benefit from VEGF inhibition are now underway. In the ECOG 4599 study, analysis of baseline and posttreatment serum samples showed no correlation between baseline VEGF expression levels and response to therapy with the bevacizumab plus chemotherapy regimen [73]. However, lower baseline levels of intracellular adhesion molecule (ICAM) were associated with improved outcome with bevacizumab-based therapy. This observation is yet to be validated in prospective studies. Phosphorylation of the VEGF receptor in circulating endothelial cells is also being studied as a potential surrogate biomarker of VEGF inhibition.

Proteosome Inhibition

The 26S proteosome is a multisubunit protein complex that is involved in the degradation of a variety of proteins with critical functions, such as regulation of the cell cycle, transcription, and apoptosis [74]. Bortezomib is a specific inhibitor of the 26S proteosome that has been shown in preclinical models to induce apoptosis and enhance the efficacy of chemotherapy against a variety of cancer cell lines. It is approved for the treatment of multiple myeloma in the United States. Based on promising preclinical studies, bortezomib has been evaluated for the treatment of patients with advanced NSCLC in multiple clinical trials. In a phase II study, patients with advanced NSCLC patients ($N = 155$) who progressed following one prior chemotherapy regimen were randomized to receive either bortezomib alone or in combination with docetaxel [75]. The response rate was 8% with single-agent bortezomib compared to 9% with the combination, but the median time to progression favored the combination (4 months vs. 1.5 months). In another phase II study by the Southwest Oncology Group (SWOG), bortezomib was combined with the regimen of carboplatin plus gemcitabine for first-line therapy in patients with advanced NSCLC ($N = 121$) [76]. The combination was well tolerated and was associated with a median survival of 11 months and a median time to progression of 5 months. The main toxicities associated with the combination included thrombocytopenia, neutropenia, and neuropathy. Bortezomib has also been evaluated in combination with other targeted agents, including EGFR inhibitors, in preclinical studies [77]. Favorable results have led to early-phase clinical trials with novel bortezomib-based combinations. Thus far, bortezomib appears to have some activity against NSCLC; however, large randomized clinical trials are necessary to determine whether the addition of bortezomib to chemotherapy will result in improved survival for patients with advanced NSCLC.

Histone Deacetylase (HDAC) Inhibitors

HDAC mediates the transcription of a number of genes relevant for cell cycle regulation and apoptosis. By altering the dynamic equilibrium between histone acetylation and deacetylation, HDAC inhibitors have been noted to exert anticancer effects against a variety of cancer cell lines [78]. The anticancer activity of HDAC inhibitors has also been attributed to their effects on non-histone targets, such as p53, heat-shock protein 90, and α-tubulin. A number of novel agents that inhibit HDAC are currently under development.

Vorinostat (SAHA) is an orally administered inhibitor of HDAC that has recently been approved by the FDA for the treatment of refractory cutaneous T-cell lymphoma. Early-phase clinical trials with vorinostat have demonstrated activity against mesothelioma and NSCLC [79]. Vorinostat also enhances the activity of other commonly used anticancer agents, such as the platinum compounds and taxanes [80, 81]. Therefore, a phase I study was designed to evaluate the combination of vorinostat with carboplatin plus paclitaxel in 19 patients with previously untreated NSCLC [82]. Vorinostat at a dose of 400 mg/day (2 weeks on, 1 week off) was combined safely with carboplatin (AUC = 6 mg/ml × min) and paclitaxel (200 mg/m^2). Ten patients had an objective response and four had disease stabilization.

These promising results have led to a phase II study that randomizes patients with advanced NSCLC to receive carboplatin plus paclitaxel in combination with either vorinostat or placebo. Vorinostat is also being evaluated in combination with a number of targeted agents, such as EGFR inhibitors. In particular, vorinostat has been shown to have synergistic interactions with EGFR TKI in resistant cell lines through its effects on E-cadherin [83]. Several other HDAC inhibitors, such as PXD101, MS275, and LBH589 are in early-phase clinical trials for advanced NSCLC.

mTOR Pathway Inhibitors

The mammalian target of rapamycin (mTOR) is a 289-kDa serine/threonine kinase that plays a central role in regulating cell growth, proliferation, and survival [84]. mTOR functions downstream of the PI3K/Akt pathway, which is a major cell survival pathway [85]. mTOR is dysregulated in several malignancies and has therefore become a target for the treatment of cancer. Agents such as CCI-779 (temsirolimus) and RAD 001 (everolimus) are in various stages of clinical evaluation. A phase III study in patients with advanced renal cell carcinoma demonstrated a survival advantage for high-risk patients treated with CCI-779 over therapy with interferon [86].

In lung cancer, mTOR inhibitors are under evaluation as single agents and in combination with proven agents. A phase I/II study of the combination of erlotinib and RAD 001 for patients with refractory NSCLC reported promising anticancer activity, though the optimal doses are yet to be established [87]. This approach involves combined inhibition of the postreceptor "survival" pathway (Akt-PI3K) and the proliferation pathway (Ras-Raf-MAPK) which is downstream of EGFR. In order to understand the effects of RAD 001 on the tumor, an ongoing study is evaluating RAD 001 as a preoperative therapy for a brief duration followed by surgical resection. Tumor tissue from the baseline biopsy and the surgical specimen will be evaluated for various downstream effects of mTOR inhibition. The results of such studies will provide insight into the role of mTOR inhibitors in lung cancer therapy.

Other Novel Approaches

In addition to the evaluation of various molecularly targeted agents, studies are now underway to evaluate novel combinations. This approach involves either the inhibition of multiple steps within a single cell-signaling pathway or coinhibition of two diverse pathways that are critical to the cancer. Multitargeting can be achieved with a single pharmacological agent with a wide spectrum of activity or with a combination of agents that specifically inhibit the relevant pathways. There are several advantages to the use of a single agent that targets multiple pathways, since this allows for better patient compliance and less toxicity when compared to a combination of agents. However, the disadvantage with this approach is that the potency of a single multitargeted agent against each target varies, which might influence the ultimate efficacy of the agent. For instance, vandetanib inhibits both VEGFR and EGFR when given at a high dose (300 mg/day), but the inhibitory effect on EGFR is lower when given at the dose of 100 mg/day [88]. Therefore, at the lower dose it acts predominantly as a VEGFR inhibitor. Although active as a single agent at 300 mg/day, this dose does not appear to offer any advantage over 100 mg/day when used in combination with chemotherapy [89]. Furthermore, the lower dose is better tolerated when given in combination with chemotherapy. Thus, in this instance the multitargeted effect does not contribute to greater efficacy. An example of targeting two pathways with specific inhibitors involves the use of erlotinib and bevacizumab. In a phase II study, this novel combination that inhibits both EGFR and VEGF resulted in a promising median survival of over 12 months in patients with previously treated, advanced NSCLC [90]. This regimen is now being studied in a definitive phase III trial. Thus novel combinations and multitargeted agents may play major roles in the treatment of patients with NSCLC in the near future.

Small Cell Lung Cancer

Small cell lung cancer (SCLC) comprises approximately 15% of the lung cancers diagnosed each year in the United States [2]. The vast majority of patients with this disease have a significant smoking history and it is rarely diagnosed in never-smokers. The common staging system used for SCLC divides patients into either limited-stage or extensive-stage disease. Limited-stage SCLC (LS-SCLC) is defined as unilateral chest involvement and/or the ability to encompass the disease in a "tolerable radiation field." Patients who demonstrate SCLC on both sides of the chest or outside the thorax (brain, bones, liver, adrenal glands, etc.) are classified as having extensive-stage SCLC (ES-SCLC). Approximately 60–70% of patients with SCLC present with extensive-stage disease, which is incurable with currently available treatment options. Untreated, the median survival of patients with ES-SCLC is 6–8 weeks; however, palliative chemotherapy may extend survival to 9–10 months with preservation of quality of life.

Unlike many other malignancies, ES-SCLC has not shared the success of newer treatment approaches, such as chemotherapy dose intensification, maintenance therapy, or molecularly targeted agents. Indeed, the standard of care for patients with ES-SCLC, platinum-based chemotherapy, has remained virtually unchanged over the past 20 years. More effective treatments are urgently needed for this disease that kills over 20,000 patients each year in the United States.

Current Standard of Care

For patients who present with ES-SCLC, the standard treatment typically includes platinum-based chemotherapy utilizing cisplatin or carboplatin in combination with either etoposide or irinotecan. Previously, alkylator-based regimens, such as CAV [cyclophosphamide, doxorubicin (Adriamycin), and vincristine], were used to treat ES-SCLC; however, platinum-based regimens such as cisplatin plus etoposide (PE) were found to have equal efficacy and better tolerability [91]. Similarly, carboplatin is now frequently used instead of cisplatin due to its more favorable toxicity profile, and the combination of carboplatin plus etoposide (CE) has become a favorite regimen among oncologists in the United States. A trial that compared CE to PE demonstrated response rates of 64% vs. 50% and median survival times of 11.8 months vs. 12.5 months for the CE and PE treatment groups, respectively [92]. Overall, the toxicity profile favored CE, including a reduced incidence of severe neutropenia.

Japanese investigators have demonstrated that the combination of cisplatin plus irinotecan (IP) may have superiority over PE in their patient population. A phase III study randomized 154 patients with untreated ES-SCLC to receive cisplatin (60 mg/m^2, day 1) plus irinotecan (60 mg/m^2, days 1,8,15 of a 28-day cycle) or cisplatin (80 mg/m^2, day 1) plus etoposide (100 mg/m^2, days 1–3 of a 21-day cycle) [93]. The response rate (84% vs. 67.5%), median survival (12.8 months vs. 9.4 months; $P=0.002$), and 1-year survival rate (58.4% vs. 37.7%) all favored the IP arm. Side effects were comparable between the two arms with similar rates of myelosuppression but more high-grade diarrhea with IP.

A confirmatory study conducted in the United States failed to demonstrate superiority for the IP regimen. The regimen utilized for this study was slightly different than that in the Japanese study in that the IP was administered as cisplatin 30 mg/m^2 plus irinotecan 65 mg/m^2 on days 1 and 8 of a 21-day cycle. The response rate (48% vs. 43.5%), median survival (9.3 months vs. 10.2 months), and 1-year survival rate (35% vs. 35.2%) for IP and PE, respectively, were nearly identical [94]. Patients receiving PE demonstrated higher rates of febrile neutropenia, whereas IP was associated with higher rates of diarrhea, dehydration, and vomiting. Several explanations were proposed for the different outcomes between these two trials, including differences in the dose and schedule of chemotherapy, possible molecular differences in SCLC between the countries, and differences in the metabolism of irinotecan in each population. Another US trial run by the Southwest Oncology Group (SWOG) utilizing the same doses and schedules of IP and PE as the Japanese study has completed enrollment, but results have not yet been reported. Presently, the platinum–etoposide combination continues to be the standard therapy for patients with ES-SCLC in the United States.

Multidrug Combinations

The Goldie–Coldman mathematical model predicts that the optimal cancer treatment with chemotherapy would entail upfront use of all active agents simultaneously in an attempt to reduce the selection of resistant tumor clones. Therefore, the addition of noncross-resistant agents to platinum plus etoposide-based therapy was considered an appealing strategy to improve efficacy and prolong patient survival. Unfortunately, these multidrug combinations have not demonstrated consistent improvements in survival of patients with ES-SCLC and are fraught with substantial increases in toxicity when compared to platinum-based, two-drug regimens. For example, the triplet combination of cisplatin, etoposide, and paclitaxel (TEP) was compared with standard PE in 133 patients with ES-SCLC [95]. The response rate, median survival, and 1-year survival rate for TEP vs. PE were 50% vs. 48%, 9.5 months vs. 10.5 months ($P = 0.90$), and 38.2% vs. 37.7%, respectively. The treatment-related mortality rate was 13% in the TEP arm and the study was stopped early. Another trial randomized 587 patients to either TEP or PE and, again, the response rate, median survival, and 1-year survival rate were nearly identical: 75% vs. 68%, 10.6 months vs. 9.9 months ($P = 0.17$), and 38% vs. 37%, respectively [96]. The treatment-related death rate was 2.4% with PE and 6.5% with TEP, mostly from neutropenic sepsis. A similar study randomized 614 untreated patients with both LS- and ES-SCLC to carboplatin, etoposide and vincristine or carboplatin, etoposide and paclitaxel [97]. There was no difference in response rate and median survival was 10 months in both arms. Other active agents in SCLC, such as ifosfamide, cyclophosphamide, and epirubicin, have also failed to demonstrate a substantial clinical benefit when added to PE [98]. Thus, two decades of testing various combinations of active chemotherapy agents have failed to substantially improve patient survival beyond that achieved with platinum-based, two-drug therapy. The modest survival gain that is occasionally reported with multidrug regimens is often counterbalanced by an increase in morbidity and mortality.

Alternating Noncross-Resistant Chemotherapy Regimens

Because overlapping toxicities, most notably myelosuppression, prevent the use of multiple agents simultaneously, an alternative approach is to use noncross-resistant regimens in an alternating fashion to expose the cancer to as many effective agents as possible while reducing the toxic events that limit their concurrent use. Given the efficacy of the PE and CAV regimens in ES-SCLC, two large trials compared the alternation of these regimens to PE or CAV alone. A large Japanese study randomized patients with LS- or ES-SCLC to PE, CAV, or alternating PE and CAV [99]. The response rate for PE/CAV was 76% compared with 78% for PE alone and although the median survival appeared to favor PE/CAV (11.8 months vs. 9.9 months; $P = 0.056$), this benefit was not seen in patients with extensive-stage disease. Similarly, a trial in the United States randomized 477 patients with ES-SCLC to one of the same three regimens [91]. The response rates and median survival of patients receiving PE, CAV, and PE/CAV were 60.7%, 50.6%, and 59.4% and 8.6, 8.3, and 8.1 months, respectively. Not surprisingly, patients receiving alternating PE and CAV experienced more myelosuppression than those in the other two arms. For patients who received either PE or CAV alone and then crossed over to receive the other regimen at the time of disease relapse, the response rate was disappointing, ranging from 8% to 28% depending on the response to initial therapy. Forty-one patients initially treated with PE demonstrated a response rate of only 14% for chemosensitive patients and 8% for chemoresistant patients with salvage CAV, with a median survival of 4.3 months for the entire cohort. This raised the question of whether CAV and PE were truly noncross-resistant regimens, since a higher response rate would have been predicted when used as salvage therapy.

Newer agents like topotecan and paclitaxel have demonstrated efficacy against SCLC when used as single agents and have been evaluated in an alternating fashion with PE. One phase II trial of PE alternating with single-agent topotecan (1.5 mg/m^2/day, days 1–5 of a 21-day cycle) in patients with ES-SCLC reported a response rate of 64% and a median survival of 11.5 months [100]. The relatively modest efficacy and the higher degree of myelosuppression resulted in the decision not to develop this regimen further. Another phase II study investigated PE alternating with topotecan (1 mg/m^2/day, days 1–5) plus paclitaxel (200 mg/m^2 on day 5 of a 21-day cycle) with growth factor support [101]. The response rate was 77% with a median survival of 10.5 months and a 1-year survival rate of 37%. The incidence of grade 4 neutropenia was high despite the use of growth factor support. Overall, this approach did not appear to demonstrate an advantage over standard PE therapy. Based on these and other trials, the alternation of noncross-resistant chemotherapy regimens does not offer an improvement in tumor response rate or prolong survival in patients with ES-SCLC when compared to standard therapy with PE.

Dose Intensification

Preclinical models suggest a linear logarithmic relationship between the cytotoxic chemotherapy dose and the degree of tumor cell kill [102]. Chemosensitive malignancies such as germ cell tumors and high-grade lymphoma are curable with higher doses of cytotoxic agents, and given the sensitivity of SCLC to chemotherapy, it was rational to predict a similar outcome. Many trials in patients with ES-SCLC have achieved dose intensification either by increasing the dose of chemotherapy or by shortening the time between courses, thereby increasing the total dose per week of chemotherapy. One early trial utilized cyclophosphamide (50 mg/kg/day, days 1–2), etoposide (400 mg/m^2, days 1–3), and cisplatin (40 mg/m^2, days 1–3) (HDCEP) every 28 days for two cycles followed by four cycles of standard CAV [103]. In 20 patients, the response rate was 90% and the median survival was 9.5 + months. On average, patients were hospitalized for 23 days of each cycle of HDCEP for neutropenia-related complications and 84% of the courses were complicated by neutropenic fever. Despite the high response rate, two treatment-related deaths and a median survival comparable to historical controls rendered this regimen unfavorable in the palliative setting. Similarly, a study evaluating high-dose PE (HDPE) compared with standard-dose PE (SDPE) failed to demonstrate a survival benefit [104]. Over 100 patients were randomized to receive standard-dose or high-dose cisplatin (40 mg/m^2) and etoposide (120 mg/m^2), each given on days 1–5 of a 21-day cycle. Two of the first four patients receiving HDPE died from complications of myelosuppression and the cisplatin and etoposide doses were subsequently reduced to 27 mg/m^2 and 80 mg/m^2, respectively. Still, myelosuppression remained severe for HDPE, and the response rate (86% vs. 83%) and median survival (11.4 months vs. 10.7 months; $P = 0.68$) were comparable between the two arms.

Shortening the duration between treatments also has not shown benefit compared with traditional regimens given at 3-week intervals. A large trial randomized 300 patients with SCLC to receive vincristine (0.5 mg/m^2, day 15), ifosfamide (5 g/m^2, day 1), carboplatin (300 mg/m^2, day 1), and etoposide (120 mg/m^2 intravenously days 1–2 and 240 mg/m^2 orally day 3) (V-ICE) at 28-day or 21-day intervals with or without granulocyte-macrophage colony-stimulating factor (GM-CSF) support [105]. The primary endpoint was to assess whether GM-CSF reduced toxicity from chemotherapy. No reduction in myelosuppression was found with GM-CSF and the response rate of 77% was identical in the 28- and 21-day cycle arms. Although there was a suggestion of a survival benefit with the 21-day regimen, the inclusion of patients with both LS- and ES-SCLC rendered the results uninterpretable for this endpoint.

Another dose intense regimen included cisplatin (25 mg/m^2 weekly), vincristine (1 mg/m^2 every 2 weeks), doxorubicin (40 mg/m^2), and etoposide (80 mg/m^2 every 2 weeks) for a total of 9 weeks of therapy (CODE) and demonstrated a remarkable 2-year survival of almost 30% in a pilot study [106]. The CODE regimen yielded a twofold increase in dose intensity over a 9-week period compared with 18 weeks of alternating CAV with PE. Two large trials evaluated this 9-week regimen of intensive weekly chemotherapy compared with the alternation of CAV and PE administered every 21 days for 18 weeks [107, 108]. Both trials demonstrated an improvement in response rate with CODE over CAV/PE; however, there was no difference in median survival between the study arms. Neutropenia-related complications were much higher with CODE despite growth factor support and one trial demonstrated a treatment-related mortality rate of 8.2% with CODE compared with 0.9% with CAV/PE. The CODE regimen was thus deemed inferior to standard regimens based on greater toxicity and the lack of improvement in patient survival.

Finally, a trial randomized over 200 patients to weekly chemotherapy with the "multiple drug combination" (MDC) of doxorubicin, etoposide, cyclophosphamide, vindesine, vincristine, and methotrexate or to standard therapy of cyclophosphamide, doxorubicin, and etoposide (CDE) [109]. The response rate (69% vs. 62%), median survival (49 weeks vs. 43 weeks; $P = 0.34$), and 2-year survival (8.5% vs. 7.9%) were nearly identical between the two arms. Unfortunately, increasing the dose intensity of active agents in ES-SCLC did not improve upon overall survival and again, severe myelosuppression limited the usefulness of this regimen in palliating patients with ultimately incurable disease.

Autologous Stem Cell Transplantation

Autologous stem cell rescue of the bone marrow has been investigated to allow the administration of high doses of chemotherapy that would otherwise not be possible due to intolerable myelosuppression. Theoretically, this would facilitate the increase of cytotoxic chemotherapy dosage to levels necessary to achieve tumor cell kill equivalent to that achieved in preclinical models. Unfortunately, the majority of trials that evaluated this approach were uncontrolled and had small sample sizes. The first randomized trial assigned patients with

SCLC-ES to either standard chemotherapy (SC) or SC followed by a late-intensification regimen of cyclophosphamide, etoposide, and BCNU with subsequent autologous bone marrow transplantation [110]. No statistical difference in median survival was detected between the treatment arms and there was an 18% toxic death rate with late-intensification chemotherapy. Enrolled patients were relatively young and had a good performance status, adding further concern regarding the application of this approach to routine use. Another study included 69 patients with SCLC, the majority of whom had ES disease, and treated them with four cycles of high-dose ifosfamide, carboplatin, and etoposide followed by stem cell rescue after each cycle [111]. The survival results were modest (median survival, 11 months; 2-year survival rate, 5%) despite a high response rate of 86% in patients with ES-SCLC. Toxicity was considerable with 14% of patients experiencing severe diarrhea, 10% severe mucositis, and a 9% toxic death rate. Finally, a retrospective review of 103 patients with SCLC treated with high-dose chemotherapy followed by autologous stem cell transplant at 22 centers participating in the Autologous Blood and Marrow Transplant Registry suggested that this approach may benefit younger patients and those with earlier stage disease but not older patients or those with extensive-stage disease [112]. The enthusiasm toward this approach has faded over the past several years. Given the lack of survival benefit and high treatment-related mortality, high-dose chemotherapy with stem cell rescue cannot be recommended outside of the clinical trial setting.

Duration of Chemotherapy

Four cycles of combination chemotherapy are considered optimal for treatment of SCLC. Efforts to improve the efficacy of chemotherapy have included increasing the number of cycles and utilizing noncross-resistant chemotherapy for maintenance treatment upon completion of induction therapy.

A randomized trial treated patients with SCLC with a complete response (CR) after six cycles of CDE to either observation or an additional six cycles and demonstrated no benefit with prolonged therapy [113]. Another study randomized almost 700 patients with LS- and ES-SCLC to either 5 or 12 cycles of CDE [114]. The response rate was 75% after five cycles and the number of patients that achieved a CR after the fifth cycle was extremely low. The median survival was 9.3 months in both arms and toxicity in the maintenance arm included severe leukopenia and thrombocytopenia in 79% and 23% of patients, respectively. Toxicity with the maintenance therapy resulted in significant delays in therapy and dose reductions, and only 37% of the patients completed all 12 of the planned cycles. Finally, a large phase III trial with over 600 patients with SCLC found that continuation of CAV improved time to progression but had no impact on overall survival [115].

Utilizing noncross-resistant maintenance therapy after induction chemotherapy also has not demonstrated a substantial survival benefit. A randomized study of over 200 patients compared four standard cycles of PE followed by either observation or 10 cycles of CAV [116]. Median survival was not prolonged with maintenance chemotherapy and only 17% of the patients completed the planned therapy due to toxicity that included profound myelosuppression. More recently, a trial using an intensive induction regimen of cisplatin, ifosfamide, and etoposide (VIP) followed by maintenance oral etoposide for 9 weeks demonstrated an improvement in progression-free survival but no improvement in overall survival compared with the induction-only arm, despite the low toxicity rate of the oral agent [117]. Finally, a phase III study that evaluated standard PE followed by either observation or the addition of four cycles of topotecan failed to demonstrate an improvement in median survival or quality of life [118]. Topotecan is a commonly used agent at the time of relapse after platinum-based therapy and it seemed logical to investigate this agent in the first-line setting. Unfortunately, the median survival (9.3 months vs. 8.9 months; $P = 0.43$), and 1-year survival (28% vs. 25%) were not improved with sequential topotecan administration compared with the standard therapy.

Patients with SCLC are typically older and frequently have tobacco-related comorbidities, making it difficult for them to tolerate prolonged therapy, as many of these trials demonstrate. If induction chemotherapy for ES-SCLC is sufficiently aggressive, maintenance chemotherapy seems to only add further toxicity without improving upon survival. Although a few trials demonstrated an improvement in time to progression with maintenance therapy, the influence of second-line chemotherapy given to patients at the time of relapse after receiving short-course induction therapy likely negates the survival benefit. As newer, less-toxic targeted agents are developed, it is hoped that maintenance treatment with such agents will prolong survival without increasing toxicity, as has been demonstrated with trastuzumab in patients with HER-2-positive breast cancer.

Other Cytotoxic Agents

Over the past few years, a number of new cytotoxic agents have been evaluated in small phase I and II clinical trials in patients with ES-SCLC, mostly in the second-line setting. Thus far, the number of objective responses that have been observed remains modest, but a few agents seem to show promising effectiveness and tolerability. Amrubicin, a fully synthetic anthracycline that inhibits DNA topoisomerase II, is one of the most promising agents. Two phase II studies of amrubicin in patients with recurrent SCLC demonstrated response rates of 37% and 52%, and median survival was approximately 11 months [119, 120]. Interestingly, one study demonstrated a response rate of 50% in 16 patients who were deemed chemoresistant to prior therapy. Trials are ongoing to further evaluate amrubicin, including a randomized phase II trial and a planned phase III trial with topotecan as the control arm.

The alkylating agent VNP40101M has demonstrated response rates of 29% and 5% in patients with chemosensitive disease and chemoresistant disease, respectively [121]. Of note, 3 of 16 patients with brain metastases demonstrated a response in the central nervous system, indicating a potential benefit for patients with central nervous system recurrence. Picoplatin is a platinum analog designed to overcome platinum resistance. A preliminary report from a phase II study indicates potential clinical benefit with a median survival of 6.5 months in chemorefractory patients when single-agent picoplatin was given in the second-line setting [122]. A confirmatory phase III study is currently underway.

Targeted Therapy

The investigation of molecular pathways critical for growth and survival of SCLC is the next logical step toward the discovery of improved therapies. Further understanding of the biology of malignancies has led to "targeted therapy" designed to inhibit the pathways involved in tumorigenesis. Clinical studies in SCLC over the past several years have focused on these targeted agents as single agents and in combination with standard cytotoxic agents.

Antiangiogenic Therapy

SCLC is characterized by overexpression of VEGF, high expression of MMP-3, -11, -14, and high microvessel density, which are all negative prognostic factors [123]. VEGF is overexpressed in up to 80% of SCLCs. Therefore, agents that inhibit angiogenic pathways have been under investigation for the treatment of SCLC. Thalidomide has been shown to repress key angiogenesis genes that lead to downregulation of VEGF and fibroblast growth factor (FGF) secretion [124]. A large phase III study randomized 119 patients with SCLC who responded to two cycles of cisplatin, cyclophosphamide, epirubicin, and etoposide (PCDE) to an additional two cycles of the chemotherapy with or without thalidomide [125]. Patients randomized to receive thalidomide continued the therapy after completion of the four cycles of chemotherapy as maintenance treatment. Thalidomide did not improve the response rate after the fourth cycle of PCDE and although the median and 1-year survival (11.7 months vs. 8.7 months and 49% vs. 30%, respectively) appeared to favor the addition of thalidomide, the difference did not meet statistical significance ($P = 0.16$). Grade ≥ 2 neuropathy was noted in over one-third of the patients treated with thalidomide, which led to dose reductions and low compliance.

Vandetanib is an oral agent that inhibits the VEGF receptor-2, as well as EGFR. A phase II study randomized 107 patients who achieved a CR or a partial response (PR) with more than four cycles of standard chemotherapy to vandetanib or to placebo [126]. Median survival was not improved with vandetanib (10.6 months vs. 11.9 months; $P = 0.90$). Therapy was poorly tolerated with side effects that included prolongation of the QTc interval, hypertension, diarrhea, and rash. Bevacizumab has recently been studied in combination with standard chemotherapeutic agents for the treatment of ES-SCLC. Data from two nonrandomized phase II studies demonstrated modest survival and PFS, although it was unclear if the regimens offered a clear advantage over historical controls with chemotherapy alone [127, 128].

The matrix metalloproteinases (MMP) comprise a family of proteins that, when secreted, digest extracellular matrix and basement membrane, allowing local tumor expansion and facilitating the formation of blood vessels [129]. Over 30 MMPs have been identified and are elevated by IHC in 60–100% of SCLC specimens, making them attractive therapeutic targets. Unfortunately, despite encouraging preclinical data, therapeutic trials have not demonstrated a benefit from MMP inhibitors. For example, a phase III trial of the MMP inhibitor BAY12-9566 in patients with SCLC was closed early due to shorter survival of the patients receiving the study agent when compared to those in the placebo arm. Another similarly designed phase III trial randomized 532 patients who had achieved a CR or a PR with induction chemotherapy to receive the MMP inhibitor marimastat or placebo [130]. Unfortunately, median survival was similar (9.3 months vs. 9.7 months; $P = 0.90$) and significant musculoskeletal toxicity resulted in dose reduction in 50% and discontinuation of the drug in 20% of patients. Although marimastat is one of the most potent inhibitors of MMPs, the inhibition of a few MMPs by this agent is unlikely to impact tumor growth and survival in patients with advanced SCLC.

Other Tyrosine Kinase Inhibitors

The c-kit receptor and its ligand, stem cell factor, appear to confer a survival advantage to SCLC through an autocrine growth pathway. In vitro data suggest that c-kit inhibition may reverse apoptotic inhibition in SCLC [131, 132]. Therefore, imatinib, an inhibitor of c-kit tyrosine kinase, was evaluated as a single agent for the treatment of SCLC. The initial study enrolled an unselected patient group for imatinib therapy and reported no objective responses and no evidence of anticancer activity [133]. Subsequently, another phase II study enrolled only patients whose tumor tissue expressed the c-kit receptor (by IHC) in an attempt to preselect patients who were most likely to benefit. However, this selected patient group also did not seem to benefit from c-kit inhibition with imatinib [134]. Another phase II study evaluating imatinib as maintenance therapy after induction chemotherapy with cisplatin and irinotecan for patients with c-kit-positive ES-SCLC also failed to demonstrate anticancer activity [135]. It is now evident that SCLC does not depend entirely on the c-kit autocrine growth pathway for survival and its inhibition has therefore not translated into clinical benefit. Other multitargeted TKIs such as sorafenib and sunitinib are currently under investigation, but data on their potential efficacy are not yet available.

Bcl-2 Inhibition

A novel approach for the treatment of patients with ES-SCLC targets the apoptotic inhibitor Bcl-2, which is overexpressed in up to 90% of SCLCs and has been implicated in conferring resistance to radiation and chemotherapy [136]. Oblimersen is an oligonucleotide complimentary to Bcl-2 mRNA that activates specific RNase H-mediated mRNA degradation, leading to reduced Bcl-2 protein levels [137]. Based on preclinical models that suggested antitumor activity, clinical trials that studied combinations of oblimersen with chemotherapy were initiated [138]. A pilot study with oblimersen plus paclitaxel in patients with chemorefractory SCLC demonstrated safety of this combination, but no responses were identified [139]. A similarly designed phase I study evaluated oblimersen with carboplatin plus etoposide in chemonaïve patients with ES-SCLC [140]. Sixteen patients received six cycles of chemotherapy with oblimersen and the response rate was 86% with a median survival of 8.6 months. Myelosuppression was the main dose-limiting side effect and no major non-hematologic side effects were identified. However, a randomized study that evaluated the utility of oblimersen when given in combination with chemotherapy failed to demonstrate any additional advantage [141]. Despite the failure of oblimersen in this setting, a number of novel Bcl-2 family inhibitors are currently under development for the treatment of SCLC.

Vaccine Therapy

Vaccine-based therapies have been in the forefront of investigation for the past two decades for the treatment of cancer. Accordingly, vaccine approaches have been investigated for the treatment of patients with SCLC. The *p53* gene is mutated in up to 90% of SCLCs. In addition, *p53* consistently demonstrates a high level of expression, has a long half-life, and is important for tumor survival, making it an appealing therapeutic target [142]. Twenty-nine ES-SCLC patients were treated with platinum-based chemotherapy followed by autologous dendritic cells transduced with wild-type *p53* gene delivered by an adenoviral vector. Although a T-cell-mediated immune response was attained in over half of the subjects, only one patient demonstrated an objective response and the median survival of 11.8 months and 1-year survival rate of 38% did not appear superior to historical controls. The authors postulated that patient-derived antiadenovirus antibodies may have contributed to the lack of clinical benefit. Interestingly, patients with a positive immune response to the vaccine demonstrated a response rate of 75% to subsequent cytotoxic chemotherapy compared with 30% for the patients who did not demonstrate an immune response ($P = 0.08$). This observation could be related to undefined cytotoxic–immunological synergy or simply to patient selection bias. Nevertheless, further studies appear warranted, given the typically low response rate of 5–20% seen with second-line chemotherapy.

A second trial utilized Bec2, an antiidiotypic antibody that mimics the ganglioside antigen GD3, which is overexpressed in about 60% of SCLCs [143]. This large phase III study randomized 515 patients with LS-SCLC to the Bec2/Bacille Calmette-Guerin vaccine or to observation after completing standard therapy [144]. Only one-third of enrolled patients demonstrated a humoral response to the vaccine and no difference in survival between the two arms was detected. Side effects of the vaccine included flu-like symptoms, malaise, and local skin reactions that led to the discontinuation of therapy in some patients. The authors postulated that higher titers of anti-GD3 antibodies may be required to demonstrate a survival benefit and a multivalent vaccine against several targets commonly expressed in SCLC may improve outcome. Similar to other malignancies, however, vaccine therapy has failed to demonstrate a therapeutic benefit in patients with SCLC, although new strategies combining chemotherapy with immunotherapy may warrant further investigation.

Summary

Advanced-stage lung cancer is now a treatable disease with several chemotherapeutic and targeted interventions contributing to qualitative and quantitative improvements in patient outcome. Systemic chemotherapy continues to be the backbone of therapy, although a plateau in efficacy has been noted in multiple therapeutic settings. Novel targeted agents, already under extensive investigation, provide hope for moving the treatment paradigms to the next level. The EGFR and VEGF inhibitors provide proof of principle that molecularly targeted agents can be integrated into existing therapies. In addition to developing newer agents, individualization of therapy based on tumor-specific characteristics remains the ultimate goal since lung cancer is characterized by wide molecular heterogeneity. The utilization of high-throughput genomic technology is being tested for better prognostication and treatment prediction for patients with lung cancer. Although the improvements in therapy have thus far been modest, the plethora of novel agents under investigation provides reason for optimism.

References

1. Jemal A, Siegel R, Ward E, et al. Cancer statistics, 2007. CA Cancer J Clin 2007; 57:43–66.
2. Govindan R, Page N, Morgensztern D, et al. Changing epidemiology of small-cell lung cancer in the United States over the last 30 years: analysis of the surveillance, epidemiologic, and end results database. J Clin Oncol 2006; 24:4539–4544.

3. Ramalingam S, Belani CP. State-of-the-art chemotherapy for advanced non-small cell lung cancer. Semin Oncol 2004; 31:68–74.

4. Albain KS, Crowley JJ, LeBlanc M, et al. Survival determinants in extensive-stage non-small-cell lung cancer: the Southwest Oncology Group experience. J Clin Oncol 1991; 9:1618–1626.

5. Langer C, Li S, Schiller J, et al. Randomized phase II trial of paclitaxel plus carboplatin or gemcitabine plus cisplatin in Eastern Cooperative Oncology Group performance status 2 non-small-cell lung cancer patients: ECOG 1599. J Clin Oncol 2007; 25:418–423.

6. Bunn PA, Jr. Chemotherapy for advanced non-small-cell lung cancer: who, what, when, why? J Clin Oncol 2002; 20:23S–33S.

7. Schiller JH, Harrington D, Belani CP, et al. Comparison of four chemotherapy regimens for advanced non-small-cell lung cancer. N Engl J Med 2002; 346:92–98.

8. Scagliotti G, Parikh P, von Pawel J, et al. Phase III study of pemetrexed plus cisplatin versus gemcitabine plus cisplatin in chemonaive patients with locally advanced or metastatic non-small cell lung cancer. J Thorac Oncol 2007; 2:S306.

9. Wozniak AJ, Crowley JJ, Balcerzak SP, et al. Randomized trial comparing cisplatin with cisplatin plus vinorelbine in the treatment of advanced non-small-cell lung cancer: a Southwest Oncology Group study. J Clin Oncol 1998; 16:2459–2465.

10. Sandler AB, Nemunaitis J, Denham C, et al. Phase III trial of gemcitabine plus cisplatin versus cisplatin alone in patients with locally advanced or metastatic non-small-cell lung cancer. J Clin Oncol 2000; 18:122–130.

11. Gatzemeier U, von Pawel J, Gottfried M, et al. Phase III comparative study of high-dose cisplatin versus a combination of paclitaxel and cisplatin in patients with advanced non-small-cell lung cancer. J Clin Oncol 2000; 18:3390–3399.

12. Rosell R, Gatzemeier U, Betticher DC, et al. Phase III randomised trial comparing paclitaxel/carboplatin with paclitaxel/cisplatin in patients with advanced non-small-cell lung cancer: a cooperative multinational trial. Ann Oncol 2002; 13:1539–1549.

13. Hotta K, Matsuo K, Ueoka H, et al. Meta-analysis of randomized clinical trials comparing Cisplatin to Carboplatin in patients with advanced non-small-cell lung cancer. J Clin Oncol 2004; 22:3852–3859.

14. Kelly K, Crowley J, Bunn PA, Jr. et al. Randomized phase III trial of paclitaxel plus carboplatin versus vinorelbine plus cisplatin in the treatment of patients with advanced non–small-cell lung cancer: a Southwest Oncology Group trial. J Clin Oncol 2001; 19:3210–3218.

15. Fossella F, Pereira JR, Von Pawel J, et al. Randomized, multinational, phase III study of docetaxel plus platinum combinations versus vinorelbine plus cisplatin for advanced non-small-cell lung cancer: the TAX 326 Study Group. J Clin Oncol 2003; 16:3016–3024.

16. Le Chevalier T, Brisgand D, Douillard JY, et al. Randomized study of vinorelbine and cisplatin versus vindesine and cisplatin versus vinorelbine alone in advanced non-small-cell lung cancer: results of a European multicenter trial including 612 patients. J Clin Oncol 1994; 12:360–367.

17. Bonomi P, Kim K, Fairclough D, et al. Comparison of survival and quality of life in advanced non-small-cell lung cancer patients treated with two dose levels of paclitaxel combined with cisplatin versus etoposide with cisplatin: results of an Eastern Cooperative Oncology Group trial. J Clin Oncol 2000; 18:623–631.

18. Smit EF, van Meerbeeck JP, Lianes P, et al. Three-arm randomized study of two cisplatin-based regimens and paclitaxel plus gemcitabine in advanced non-small-cell lung cancer: a phase III trial of the European Organization for Research and Treatment of Cancer Lung Cancer Group–EORTC 08975. J Clin Oncol 2003; 21:3909–3917.

19. Treat J, Belani CP, Edelman M, et al. A randomized phase III trial of gemcitabine in combination with carboplatin or paclitaxel versus paclitaxel plus carboplatin in advanced non-small cell lung cancer: Update of the Alpha Oncology Trial. J Clin Oncol 2005; 23:1096.

20. Alberola V, Camps C, Provencio M, et al. Cisplatin plus gemcitabine versus a cisplatin-based triplet versus nonplatinum sequential doublets in advanced non-small-cell lung cancer: a Spanish Lung Cancer Group phase III randomized trial. J Clin Oncol 2003; 21:3207–3213.
21. Hanna N, Shepherd FA, Fossella FV, et al. Randomized phase III trial of pemetrexed versus docetaxel in patients with non-small-cell lung cancer previously treated with chemotherapy. J Clin Oncol 2004; 22:1589–1597.
22. Schmid M, Malicki D, Nobori T, et al. Homozygous deletions of methylthioadenosine phosphorylase (MTAP) are more frequent than p16INK4A (CDKN2) homozygous deletions in primary non-small cell lung cancers. Oncogene 1998; 17:2669–2675.
23. Schmid M, Sen M, Rosenbach MD, et al. A methylthioadenosine phosphorylase (MTAP) fusion transcript identifies a new gene on chromosome 9p21 that is frequently deleted in cancer. Oncogene 2000; 19:5747–5754.
24. Chattopadhyay S, Zhao R, Tsai E, et al. The effect of a novel transition state inhibitor of methylthioadenosine phosphorylase on pemetrexed activity. Mol Cancer Ther 2006; 5:2549–2555.
25. Rosell R, Taron M, Barnadas A, et al. Nucleotide excision repair pathways involved in Cisplatin resistance in non-small-cell lung cancer. Cancer Control 2003; 10:297–305.
26. Lord RV, Brabender J, Gandara D, et al. Low ERCC1 expression correlates with prolonged survival after cisplatin plus gemcitabine chemotherapy in non-small cell lung cancer. Clin Cancer Res 2002; 8:2286–2291.
27. Cobo M, Isla D, Massuti B, et al. Customizing cisplatin based on quantitative excision repair cross-complementing 1 mRNA expression: a phase III trial in non-small-cell lung cancer. J Clin Oncol 2007; 25:2747–2754.
28. Simon G, Sharma A, Li X, et al. Feasibility and efficacy of molecular analysis-directed individualized therapy in advanced non-small-cell lung cancer. J Clin Oncol 2007; 25:2741–2746.
29. Shepherd FA, Dancey J, Ramlau R, et al. Prospective randomized trial of docetaxel versus best supportive care in patients with non-small-cell lung cancer previously treated with platinum-based chemotherapy. J Clin Oncol 2000; 18:2095–2103.
30. Fossella FV, DeVore R, Kerr RN, et al. Randomized phase III trial of docetaxel versus vinorelbine or ifosfamide in patients with advanced non-small-cell lung cancer previously treated with platinum-containing chemotherapy regimens. The TAX 320 Non-Small Cell Lung Cancer Study Group. J Clin Oncol 2000; 18:2354–2362.
31. Ramlau R, Gervais R, Krzakowski M, et al. Oral topotecan demonstrates clinical activity in relapsed non-small cell lung cancer. Results from an open-label, phase III study comparing oral topotecan to intravenous docetaxel. J Clin Oncol 2005; 23:625.
32. Krzakowski M, Douillard J, Ramlau R, et al. Phase III study of vinflunine versus docetaxel in patients with advanced non-small cell lung cancer previously treated with a platinum-containing regimen. J Clin Oncol 2007; 25:387s.
33. Fukuoka M, Yano S, Giaccone G, et al. Multi-institutional randomized phase II trial of gefitinib for previously treated patients with advanced non-small-cell lung cancer. J Clin Oncol 2003; 21:2237–2246.
34. Kris MG, Natale RB, Herbst RS, et al. Efficacy of gefitinib, an inhibitor of the epidermal growth factor receptor tyrosine kinase, in symptomatic patients with non-small cell lung cancer: a randomized trial. JAMA 2003; 290:2149–2158.
35. Thatcher N, Chang A, Parikh P, et al. Gefitinib plus best supportive care in previously treated patients with refractory advanced non-small-cell lung cancer: results from a randomised, placebo-controlled, multicentre study (Iressa Survival Evaluation in Lung Cancer). Lancet 2005; 366:1527–1537.
36. Perez-Soler R, Chachoua A, Hammond LA, et al. Determinants of tumor response and survival with erlotinib in patients with non–small-cell lung cancer. J Clin Oncol 2004; 22:3238–3247.

37. Shepherd FA, Rodrigues Pereira J, Ciuleanu T, et al. Erlotinib in previously treated non-small-cell lung cancer. N Engl J Med 2005; 353:123–132.
38. Hanna N, Lilenbaum R, Ansari R, et al. Phase II trial of cetuximab in patients with previously treated non-small-cell lung cancer. J Clin Oncol 2006; 24:5253–5258.
39. Sirotnak FM, Zakowski MF, Miller VA, et al. Efficacy of cytotoxic agents against human tumor xenografts is markedly enhanced by coadministration of ZD1839 (Iressa), an inhibitor of EGFR tyrosine kinase. Clin Cancer Res 2000; 6:4885–4892.
40. Herbst RS, Giaccone G, Schiller JH, et al. Gefitinib in combination with paclitaxel and carboplatin in advanced non-small-cell lung cancer: a phase III trial -INTACT 2. J Clin Oncol 2004; 22:785–794.
41. Herbst RS, Prager D, Hermann R, et al. TRIBUTE: a phase III trial of erlotinib hydrochloride (OSI-774) combined with carboplatin and paclitaxel chemotherapy in advanced non-small-cell lung cancer. J Clin Oncol 2005; 23:5892–5899.
42. Rosell R, Daniel C, Ramlau R, et al. Randomized phase II study of cetuximab in combination with cisplatin and vinorelbine vs. CV alone in the first-line treatment of patients with epidermal growth factor receptor (EGFR)-expressing advanced non-small-cell lung cancer. Proc Am Soc Clin Oncol 2004; 23:618.
43. Thienelt CD, Bunn PA, Jr., Hanna N, et al. Multicenter phase I/II study of cetuximab with paclitaxel and carboplatin in untreated patients with stage IV non-small-cell lung cancer. J Clin Oncol 2005; 23:8786–8793.
44. Belani CP, Ramalingam S, Schreeder R, et al. Phase II study of cetuximab in combination with carboplatin and docetaxel for patients with advanced/metastatic non-small cell lung cancer. J Clin Oncol 2007; 25:420s.
45. Crawford J, Swanson P, Prager D, et al. Panitumumab, a fully human antibody, combined with paclitaxel and carboplatin versus paclitaxel and carboplatin alone for first line advanced non-small cell lung cancer: a primary analysis. Eur J Cancer 2005; 3:324.
46. Scartozzi M, Bearzi I, Berardi R, et al. Epidermal growth factor receptor (EGFR) status in primary colorectal tumors does not correlate with EGFR expression in related metastatic sites: implications for treatment with EGFR-targeted monoclonal antibodies. J Clin Oncol 2004; 22:4772–4778.
47. Hirsch FR, Gandara D, McCoy J, et al. Increased EGFR gene copy number detected by FISH is associated with increased sensitivity to gefitinib in patients with bronchioloalveolar carcinoma (S0126). J Clin Oncol 2005; 23:628.
48. Hirsch FR, Varella-Garcia M, McCoy J, et al. Increased epidermal growth factor receptor gene copy number detected by fluorescence in situ hybridization associates with increased sensitivity to gefitinib in patients with bronchioloalveolar carcinoma subtypes: a Southwest Oncology Group study. J Clin Oncol 2005; 23:6838–6845.
49. Hirsch FR, Varella-Garcia M, Bunn PA, Jr., et al. Epidermal growth factor receptor in non-small-cell lung carcinomas: correlation between gene copy number and protein expression and impact on prognosis. J Clin Oncol 2003; 21:3798–3807.
50. Tsao MS, Sakurada A, Cutz JC, et al. Erlotinib in lung cancer – molecular and clinical predictors of outcome. N Engl J Med 2005; 353:133–144.
51. Douillard JY, Kim ES, Hirsch V, et al. Gefitinib versus docetaxel in patients with locally advanced or metastatic non-small cell lung cancer pre-treated with platinum-based chemotherapy: a randomized, open-label phase III study (INTEREST). J Thorac Oncol 2007; 2:S305.
52. Crino L, Zatloukal P, Reck M, et al. Gefitinib versus vinorelbine in chemonaive elderly patients with advanced non-small cell lung cancer (INVITE): a randomized phase II study. J Thorac Oncol 2007; 2:S341.
53. Lynch TJ, Bell DW, Sordella R, et al. Activating mutations in the epidermal growth factor receptor underlying responsiveness of non-small-cell lung cancer to gefitinib. N Engl J Med 2004; 350:2129–2139.

54. Paez JG, Janne PA, Lee JC, et al. EGFR mutations in lung cancer: correlation with clinical response to gefitinib therapy. Science 2004; 304:1497–1500.
55. Paz-Ares L, Sanchez JM, García-Velasco A, et al. A prospective phase II trial of erlotinib in advanced non-small cell lung cancer patients with mutations in the tyrosine kinase domain of the epidermal growth factor receptor (EGFR). J Clin Oncol 2006; 24:369s.
56. Cappuzzo F, Toschi L, Trisolini R, et al. Clinical and biological effects of gefitinib in EGFR FISH positive/phospho-akt positive or never smoker non-small cell lung cancer: Preliminary results of the ONCOBELL trial. J Clin Oncol 2006; 24:369s.
57. Kris MG, Pao W, Zakowski MF, et al. Prospective trial with preoperative gefitinib to correlate lung cancer response with EGFR exon 19 and 21 mutations and to select patients for adjuvant therapy. J Clin Oncol 2006; 24:369s.
58. Mukohara T, Engelman JA, Hanna NH, et al. Differential effects of gefitinib and cetuximab on non-small-cell lung cancers bearing epidermal growth factor receptor mutations. J Natl Cancer Inst 2005; 97:1185–1194.
59. Eberhard DA, Johnson BE, Amler LC, et al. Mutations in the epidermal growth factor receptor and in KRAS are predictive and prognostic indicators in patients with non-small-cell lung cancer treated with chemotherapy alone and in combination with erlotinib. J Clin Oncol 2005; 23:5900–5909.
60. Kobayashi S, Boggon TJ, Dayaram T, et al. EGFR mutation and resistance of non-small-cell lung cancer to gefitinib. N Engl J Med 2005; 352:786–792.
61. Engelman JA, Zejnullahu K, Mitsudomi T, et al. MET amplification leads to gefitinib resistance in lung cancer by activating ERBB3 signaling. Science 2007; 316:1039–1043.
62. Taguchi F, Solomon B, Gregorc V, et al. Mass spectrometry to classify non-small-cell lung cancer patients for clinical outcome after treatment with epidermal growth factor receptor tyrosine kinase inhibitors: a multicohort cross-institutional study. J Natl Cancer Inst 2007; 99:838–846.
63. Ferrara N, Gerber HP, LeCouter J. The biology of VEGF and its receptors. Nat Med 2003; 9:669–676.
64. Ferrara N. Vascular endothelial growth factor as a target for anticancer therapy. Oncologist 2004; 9 Suppl 1:2–10.
65. Hurwitz H, Fehrenbacher L, Novotny W, et al. Bevacizumab plus irinotecan, fluorouracil, and leucovorin for metastatic colorectal cancer. N Engl J Med 2004; 350:2335–2342.
66. Johnson DH, Fehrenbacher L, Novotny WF, et al. Randomized phase II trial comparing bevacizumab plus carboplatin and paclitaxel with carboplatin and paclitaxel alone in previously untreated locally advanced or metastatic non-small-cell lung cancer. J Clin Oncol 2004; 22:2184–2191.
67. Sandler A, Gray R, Perry MC, et al. Paclitaxel–carboplatin alone or with bevacizumab for non-small-cell lung cancer. N Engl J Med 2006; 355:2542–2550.
68. Manegold C, von Pawel J, Zatloukal P, et al. Randomised, double-blind multicentre phase III study of bevacizumab in combination with cisplatin and gemcitabine in chemotherapy-naïve patients with advanced or recurrent non-squamous non-small cell lung cancer: BO17704. J Clin Oncol 2007; 25:388s.
69. Natale RB, Bodkin D, Govindan R, et al. ZD6474 versus gefitinib in patients with advanced NSCLC: Final results from a two-part, double-blind, randomized phase II trial. J Clin Oncol 2006; 24:364s.
70. Socinski MA, Novello S, Sanchez JM, et al. Efficacy and safety of sunitinib in previously treated, advanced non-small cell lung cancer: Preliminary results of a multicenter phase II trial. J Clin Oncol 2006; 24:364s.
71. Gatzemeier U, Blumenschein G, Fosella F, et al. Phase II trial of single-agent sorafenib in patients with advanced non-small cell lung carcinoma. J Clin Oncol 2006; 24:364s.

72. Schiller JH, Flaherty KT, Redlinger M, et al. Sorafenib combined with carboplatin/paclitaxel for advanced non-small cell lung cancer: A phase I subset analysis. J Clin Oncol 2006; 24:412s.

73. Dowlati A, Gray R, Johnson DH, et al. Prospective correlative assessment of biomarkers in E4599 randomized phase II/III trial of carboplatin and paclitaxel ± bevacizumab in advanced non-small cell lung cancer. J Clin Oncol 2006; 24:370s.

74. Schenkein DP. Use of proteasome inhibition in the treatment of lung cancer. Clin Lung Cancer 2004; 6 Suppl 2:S89–S96.

75. Fanucchi MP, Fossella F, Fidias P, et al. Bortezomib + docetaxel in previously treated patients with advanced non-small cell lung cancer: A phase 2 study. J Clin Oncol 2005; 23:629.

76. Davies AM, McCoy J, Lara PN, et al. Bortezomib + gemcitabine /carboplatin results in encouraging survival in advanced non-small cell lung cancer: Results of a phase II Southwest Oncology Group trial (S0339). J Clin Oncol 2006; 24:368s.

77. Lorch JH, Thomas TO, Schmoll HJ. Bortezomib inhibits cell–cell adhesion and cell migration and enhances epidermal growth factor receptor inhibitor-induced cell death in squamous cell cancer. Cancer Res 2007; 67:727–734.

78. Marks PA, Richon VM, Rifkind RA. Histone deacetylase inhibitors: inducers of differentiation or apoptosis of transformed cells. J Natl Cancer Inst 2000; 92:1210–1216.

79. Kelly WK, Richon VM, O'Connor O, et al. Phase I clinical trial of histone deacetylase inhibitor: suberoylanilide hydroxamic acid administered intravenously. Clin Cancer Res 2003; 9:3578–3588.

80. Bali P, Pranpat M, Swaby R, et al. Activity of suberoylanilide hydroxamic Acid against human breast cancer cells with amplification of her-2. Clin Cancer Res 2005; 11:6382–6389.

81. Kim MS, Blake M, Baek JH, et al. Inhibition of histone deacetylase increases cytotoxicity to anticancer drugs targeting DNA. Cancer Res 2003; 63:7291–7300.

82. Ramalingam S, Parise RA, Egorin MJ, et al. Phase I study of vorinostat, a histone deacetylase (HDAC) inhibitor, in combination with carboplatin and paclitaxel for patients with advanced solid malignancies. J Clin Oncol 2006; 24:98s.

83. Witta SE, Gemmill RM, Hirsch FR, et al. Restoring E-cadherin expression increases sensitivity to epidermal growth factor receptor inhibitors in lung cancer cell lines. Cancer Res 2006; 66:944–950.

84. Bjornsti MA, Houghton PJ. The TOR pathway: a target for cancer therapy. Nat Rev Cancer 2004; 4:335–348.

85. Hay N, Sonenberg N. Upstream and downstream of mTOR. Genes Dev 2004; 18:1926–1945.

86. Hudes G, Carducci M, Tomczak P, et al. A phase 3, randomized, 3-arm study of temsirolimus (TEMSR) or interferon-alpha (IFN) or the combination of TEMSR + IFN in the treatment of first-line, poor-risk patients with advanced renal cell carcinoma. J Clin Oncol 2006; 24:2s.

87. Papadimitrakopoulou V, Blumenschein G, Rollins M, et al. A phase I/II study investigating the combination of RAD001 (everolimus) and erlotinib as 2nd /3rd line therapy in patients with advanced non-small cell lung cancer previously treated with chemotherapy. J Clin Oncol 2006; 24:670s.

88. Herbst RS, Heymach JV, O'Reilly MS, et al. Vandetanib (ZD6474): an orally available receptor tyrosine kinase inhibitor that selectively targets pathways critical for tumor growth and angiogenesis. Expert Opin Investig Drugs 2007; 16:239–249.

89. Heymach J, Johnson B, Prager D, et al. A phase II trial of ZD6474 plus docetaxel in patients with previously treated NSCLC: Follow-up results. J Clin Oncol 2006; 24:368s.

90. Herbst RS, O'Neill VJ, Fehrenbacher L, et al. Phase II study of efficacy and safety of bevacizumab in combination with chemotherapy or erlotinib compared with

chemotherapy alone for treatment of recurrent or refractory non small-cell lung cancer. J Clin Oncol 2007; 25:4743–4750.

91. Roth BJ, Johnson DH, Einhorn LH, et al. Randomized study of cyclophosphamide, doxorubicin, and vincristine versus etoposide and cisplatin versus alternation of these two regimens in extensive small-cell lung cancer: a phase III trial of the Southeastern Cancer Study Group. J Clin Oncol 1992; 10:282–291.

92. Skarlos DV, Samantas E, Kosmidis P, et al. Randomized comparison of etoposide–cisplatin vs. etoposide–carboplatin and irradiation in small-cell lung cancer. A Hellenic Cooperative Oncology Group study. Ann Oncol 1994; 5:601–607.

93. Noda K, Nishiwaki Y, Kawahara M, et al. Irinotecan plus cisplatin compared with etoposide plus cisplatin for extensive small-cell lung cancer. N Engl J Med 2002; 346:85–91.

94. Hanna N, Bunn PA, Jr., Langer C, et al. Randomized phase III trial comparing irinotecan/cisplatin with etoposide/cisplatin in patients with previously untreated extensive-stage disease small-cell lung cancer. J Clin Oncol 2006; 24:2038–2043.

95. Mavroudis D, Papadakis E, Veslemes M, et al. A multicenter randomized clinical trial comparing paclitaxel–cisplatin–etoposide versus cisplatin–etoposide as first-line treatment in patients with small-cell lung cancer. Ann Oncol 2001; 12:463–470.

96. Niell HB, Herndon JE, 2nd, Miller AA, et al. Randomized phase III intergroup trial of etoposide and cisplatin with or without paclitaxel and granulocyte colony-stimulating factor in patients with extensive-stage small-cell lung cancer: Cancer and Leukemia Group B Trial 9732. J Clin Oncol 2005; 23:3752–3759.

97. Reck M, von Pawel J, Macha HN, et al. Randomized phase III trial of paclitaxel, etoposide, and carboplatin versus carboplatin, etoposide, and vincristine in patients with small-cell lung cancer. J Natl Cancer Inst 2003; 95:1118–1127.

98. Loehrer PJ, Sr., Ansari R, Gonin R, et al. Cisplatin plus etoposide with and without ifosfamide in extensive small-cell lung cancer: a Hoosier Oncology Group study. J Clin Oncol 1995; 13:2594–2599.

99. Fukuoka M, Furuse K, Saijo N, et al. Randomized trial of cyclophosphamide, doxorubicin, and vincristine versus cisplatin and etoposide versus alternation of these regimens in small-cell lung cancer. J Natl Cancer Inst 1991; 83:855–861.

100. Mavroudis D, Veslemes M, Kouroussis C, et al. Cisplatin–etoposide alternating with topotecan in patients with extensive stage small cell lung cancer. A multicenter phase II study. Lung Cancer 2002; 38:59–63.

101. Jett JR, Hatfield AK, Hillman S, et al. Alternating chemotherapy with etoposide plus cisplatin and topotecan plus paclitaxel in patients with untreated, extensive-stage small cell lung carcinoma: a phase II trial of the North Central Cancer Treatment Group. Cancer 2003; 97:2498–2503.

102. Frei E, 3rd, Canellos GP. Dose: a critical factor in cancer chemotherapy. Am J Med 1980; 69:585–594.

103. Johnson DH, DeLeo MJ, Hande KR, et al. High-dose induction chemotherapy with cyclophosphamide, etoposide, and cisplatin for extensive-stage small-cell lung cancer. J Clin Oncol 1987; 5:703–709.

104. Ihde DC, Mulshine JL, Kramer BS, et al. Prospective randomized comparison of high-dose and standard-dose etoposide and cisplatin chemotherapy in patients with extensive-stage small-cell lung cancer. J Clin Oncol 1994; 12:2022–2034.

105. Steward WP, von Pawel J, Gatzemeier U, et al. Effects of granulocyte-macrophage colony-stimulating factor and dose intensification of V-ICE chemotherapy in small-cell lung cancer: a prospective randomized study of 300 patients. J Clin Oncol 1998; 16:642–650.

106. Murray N, Shah A, Osoba D, et al. Intensive weekly chemotherapy for the treatment of extensive-stage small-cell lung cancer. J Clin Oncol 1991; 9:1632–1638.

107. Furuse K, Fukuoka M, Nishiwaki Y, et al. Phase III study of intensive weekly chemotherapy with recombinant human granulocyte colony-stimulating factor versus

standard chemotherapy in extensive-disease small-cell lung cancer. The Japan Clinical Oncology Group. J Clin Oncol 1998; 16:2126–2132.

108. Murray N, Livingston RB, Shepherd FA, et al. Randomized study of CODE versus alternating CAV/EP for extensive-stage small-cell lung cancer: an Intergroup Study of the National Cancer Institute of Canada Clinical Trials Group and the Southwest Oncology Group. J Clin Oncol 1999; 17:2300–2308.

109. Sculier JP, Paesmans M, Bureau G, et al. Multiple-drug weekly chemotherapy versus standard combination regimen in small-cell lung cancer: a phase III randomized study conducted by the European Lung Cancer Working Party. J Clin Oncol 1993; 11:1858–865.

110. Humblet Y, Symann M, Bosly A, et al. Late intensification chemotherapy with autologous bone marrow transplantation in selected small-cell carcinoma of the lung: a randomized study. J Clin Oncol 1987; 5:1864–1873.

111. Leyvraz S, Perey L, Rosti G, et al. Multiple courses of high-dose ifosfamide, carboplatin, and etoposide with peripheral-blood progenitor cells and filgrastim for small-cell lung cancer: A feasibility study by the European Group for Blood and Marrow Transplantation. J Clin Oncol 1999; 17:3531–3539.

112. Rizzo JD, Elias AD, Stiff PJ, et al. Autologous stem cell transplantation for small cell lung cancer. Biol Blood Marrow Transplant 2002; 8:273–280.

113. Lebeau B, Chastang C, Allard P, et al. Six vs twelve cycles for complete responders to chemotherapy in small cell lung cancer: definitive results of a randomized clinical trial. The "Petites Cellules" Group. Eur Respir J 1992; 5:286–290.

114. Giaccone G, Dalesio O, McVie GJ, et al. Maintenance chemotherapy in small-cell lung cancer: long-term results of a randomized trial. European Organization for Research and Treatment of Cancer Lung Cancer Cooperative Group. J Clin Oncol 1993; 11:1230–1240.

115. Ettinger DS, Finkelstein DM, Abeloff MD, et al. A randomized comparison of standard chemotherapy versus alternating chemotherapy and maintenance versus no maintenance therapy for extensive-stage small-cell lung cancer: a phase III study of the Eastern Cooperative Oncology Group. J Clin Oncol 1990; 8:230–240.

116. Beith JM, Clarke SJ, Woods RL, et al. Long-term follow-up of a randomised trial of combined chemoradiotherapy induction treatment, with and without maintenance chemotherapy in patients with small cell carcinoma of the lung. Eur J Cancer 1996; 32A:438–443.

117. Hanna NH, Sandier AB, Loehrer PJ, Sr., et al. Maintenance daily oral etoposide versus no further therapy following induction chemotherapy with etoposide plus ifosfamide plus cisplatin in extensive small-cell lung cancer: a Hoosier Oncology Group randomized study. Ann Oncol 2002; 13:95–102.

118. Schiller JH, Adak S, Cella D, et al. Topotecan versus observation after cisplatin plus etoposide in extensive-stage small-cell lung cancer: E7593–a phase III trial of the Eastern Cooperative Oncology Group. J Clin Oncol 2001; 19:2114–2122.

119. Onoda S, Masuda N, Seto T, et al. Phase II trial of amrubicin for treatment of refractory or relapsed small-cell lung cancer: Thoracic Oncology Research Group Study 0301. J Clin Oncol 2006; 24:5448–5453.

120. Kudoh S, Yoshimura N, Kimura T. A phase II trial of amrubicin for recurrent or refractory small cell lung cancer. J Clin Oncol 2006; 24:671s.

121. Mekhail T, Gettinger S, Blumenschein G. A phase II trial of VNP40101M in patients with relapsed or refractory small cell lung cancer with or without brain metastases. J Clin Oncol 2007; 25:439s.

122. Bentzion D, Lipatov O, Polyakov I. A phase II study of picoplatin as second line therapy for patients with small cell lung cancer who have resistant or refractory disease or have relapsed within 180 days of completing first-line, platinum-containing chemotherapy. J Clin Oncol 2007; 25:439s.

123. Lucchi M, Mussi A, Fontanini G, et al. Small cell lung carcinoma: the angiogenic phenomenon. Eur J Cardiothorac Surg 2002; 21:1105–1110.

124. D'Amato RJ, Loughnan MS, Flynn E, et al. Thalidomide is an inhibitor of angiogenesis. Proc Natl Acad Sci USA 1994; 91:4082–4085.
125. Pujol JL, Breton JL, Gervais R, et al. Phase III double-blind, placebo-controlled study of thalidomide in extensive-disease small-cell lung cancer after response to chemotherapy: an intergroup study FNCLCC cleo04 IFCT 00-01. J Clin Oncol 2007; 25:3945–3951.
126. Arnold AM, Seymour L, Smylie M, et al. Phase II study of vandetanib or placebo in small-cell lung cancer patients after complete or partial response to induction chemotherapy with or without radiation therapy: National Cancer Institute of Canada Clinical Trials Group Study BR.20. J Clin Oncol 2007; 25:4278–4284.
127. Ready N, Dudek A, Wang X, et al. CALGB 30306: A phase II study of cisplatin, irinotecan and bevacizumab for untreated extensive stage small cell lung cancer. J Clin Oncol 2007; 25:400s.
128. Sandler A, Szwaric S, Dowlati A, et al. A phase II study of cisplatin plus etoposide plus bevacizumab for previously untreated extensive stage small cell lung cancer (E3501): A trial of the Eastern Cooperative Oncology Group. J Clin Oncol 2007; 25:400s.
129. Khokha R, Denhardt DT. Matrix metalloproteinases and tissue inhibitor of metalloproteinases: a review of their role in tumorigenesis and tissue invasion. Invasion Metastasis 1989; 9:391–405.
130. Shepherd FA, Giaccone G, Seymour L, et al. Prospective, randomized, double-blind, placebo-controlled trial of marimastat after response to first-line chemotherapy in patients with small-cell lung cancer: a trial of the National Cancer Institute of Canada-Clinical Trials Group and the European Organization for Research and Treatment of Cancer. J Clin Oncol 2002; 20:4434–4439.
131. Krystal GW, DeBerry CS, Linnekin D, et al. Lck associates with and is activated by Kit in a small cell lung cancer cell line: inhibition of SCF-mediated growth by the Src family kinase inhibitor PP1. Cancer Res 1998; 58:4660–4666.
132. Krystal GW, Carlson P, Litz J. Induction of apoptosis and inhibition of small cell lung cancer growth by the quinoxaline tyrphostins. Cancer Res 1997; 57:2203–2208.
133. Johnson BE, Fischer T, Fischer B, et al. Phase II study of imatinib in patients with small cell lung cancer. Clin Cancer Res 2003; 9:5880–5887.
134. Dy GK, Miller AA, Mandrekar SJ, et al. A phase II trial of imatinib (ST1571) in patients with c-kit expressing relapsed small-cell lung cancer: a CALGB and NCCTG study. Ann Oncol 2005; 16:1811–1816.
135. Schneider BJ, Gadgeel S, Ramnath N, et al. Phase II trial of imatinib maintenance therapy after irinotecan and cisplatin in patients with c-kit positive extensive stage small cell lung cancer. J Clin Oncol 2006; 24:674s.
136. Dole M, Nunez G, Merchant AK, et al. Bcl-2 inhibits chemotherapy-induced apoptosis in neuroblastoma. Cancer Res 1994; 54:3253–3259.
137. Smith MR, Abubakr Y, Mohammad R, et al. Antisense oligodeoxyribonucleotide down-regulation of bcl-2 gene expression inhibits growth of the low-grade non-Hodgkin's lymphoma cell line WSU-FSCCL. Cancer Gene Ther 1995; 2:207–212.
138. Leung S, Miyake H, Zellweger T, et al. Synergistic chemosensitization and inhibition of progression to androgen independence by antisense Bcl-2 oligodeoxynucleotide and paclitaxel in the LNCaP prostate tumor model. Int J Cancer 2001; 91:846–50.
139. Rudin CM, Otterson GA, Mauer AM, et al. A pilot trial of G3139, a bcl-2 antisense oligonucleotide, and paclitaxel in patients with chemorefractory small-cell lung cancer. Ann Oncol 2002; 13:539–455.
140. Rudin CM, Kozloff M, Hoffman PC, et al. Phase I study of G3139, a bcl-2 antisense oligonucleotide, combined with carboplatin and etoposide in patients with small-cell lung cancer. J Clin Oncol 2004; 22:1110–1117.
141. Rudin CM, Salgia R, Wang XF, et al. CALGB 30103: A randomized phase II study of carboplatin and etoposide with or without G3139 in patients with extensive stage small cell lung cancer. J Clin Oncol 2005; 23:662s.

142. D'Amico D, Carbone D, Mitsudomi T, et al. High frequency of somatically acquired p53 mutations in small-cell lung cancer cell lines and tumors. Oncogene 1992; 7:339–46.
143. Brezicka T, Bergman B, Olling S, et al. Reactivity of monoclonal antibodies with ganglioside antigens in human small cell lung cancer tissues. Lung Cancer 2000; 28:29–36.
144. Giaccone G, Debruyne C, Felip E, et al. Phase III study of adjuvant vaccination with Bec2/bacille Calmette-Guerin in responding patients with limited-disease small-cell lung cancer (European Organisation for Research and Treatment of Cancer 08971-08971B; Silva Study). J Clin Oncol 2005; 23:6854–6864.
145. Ohe Y, Ohashi Y, Kubota K, et al. Randomized phase III study of cisplatin plus irinotecan versus carboplatin plus paclitaxel, cisplatin plus gemcitabine, and cisplatin plus vinorelbine for advanced non-small-cell lung cancer: Four-Arm Cooperative Study in Japan. Ann Oncol 2007; 18:317–323.
146. Schiller J, Larson T, Ou S, et al. Efficacy and safety of axitinib (AG-013736) in patients with advanced non-small cell lung cancer: A phase II trial. J Clin Oncol 2007; 25:386s.
147. Gauler T, Besse B, Meric J, et al. Phase II open-label study to investigate efficacy and safety of PTK787/ZK 222584 orally administered once daily or twice daily at 1,250 mg as second-line monotherapy in patients with stage IIIB/IV non-small cell lung cancer. J Clin Oncol 2007; 25:394s.

Site-Directed Therapy for Lung Cancer Metastases

Kevin S. Oh, Baskaran Sundaram, Venkataramu Krishnamurthy, Allan Pickens, Malini Venkatram, Ella A. Kazerooni, Charlie Pan, and James Hayman

Abstract At the time of diagnosis, 40% of patients with non-small cell lung cancer (NSCLC) and nearly 70% of patients with small cell lung cancer (SCLC) have advanced metastatic disease. The prognosis of patients with advanced lung cancer is dismal, with a 5-year overall survival rate of 1–2%. The primary treatment of advanced disease is supportive care and palliative chemotherapy. However, there is a growing body of evidence suggesting that highly selected patients with oligometastatic disease can achieve long-term survival with ablative forms of site-directed therapy, including surgical resection, external beam radiation therapy (EBRT), stereotactic radiosurgery (SRS), stereotactic body radiation therapy (SBRT), and radiofrequency ablation (RFA). This chapter summarizes the experience with site-directed therapy in the management of metastatic lung cancer in the most commonly involved sites: brain, adrenal gland, liver, lung, and bone.

Introduction

Forty percent of patients with non-small cell lung cancer (NSCLC) and nearly 70% with small cell lung cancer (SCLC) have advanced hematogenously metastatic disease at diagnosis. The prognosis for such patients is dismal, with a 5-year overall survival rate of 1–2% [1, 2]. The presence of multiple metastases is indicative of widespread disease which is not curable through the use of currently available therapy. Therefore, the primary goal of therapy is palliation through the use of systemic chemotherapy or molecularly targeted therapy. Local treatment modalities, such as surgery and radiotherapy, are primarily utilized with palliative intent to lessen symptoms at sites of metastatic spread.

In a small subset of patients with oligometastatic NSCLC in which all sites of disease can be treated in a definitive manner, site-directed therapy is sometimes offered with the intention of achieving long-term survival, if not cure. The data

K.S. Oh (✉)
Department of Radiation Oncology, Massachusetts General Hospital, Boston, MA, USA
e-mail: kohz@partners.org

V. Keshamouni et al. (eds.), *Lung Cancer Metastasis*,
DOI 10.1007/978-1-4419-0772-1_16, © Springer Science+Business Media, LLC 2009

supporting the use of definitive site-directed therapy are strongest for patients with a *solitary metastasis*. In highly selected patient populations, definitive site-directed therapy for a solitary metastasis has achieved long-term survival rates of 15–20%. Before offering definitive site-directed therapy, extensive assessment of disease extent must be undertaken using all available modalities, including computed tomography (CT), magnetic resonance imaging (MRI), positron emission tomography (PET), and biopsy of sites of potential metastatic disease, to confirm that the target lesion is truly a solitary metastatic deposit. Frequently, a biopsy is indicated to rule out the possibility of a second primary malignancy. Solitary metastases fall into three distinct clinical scenarios: (1) a synchronous metastasis found at the time of initial cancer diagnosis; (2) a metachronous metastasis arising sometime after the successful treatment of the primary cancer; and (3) a single metastasis in the target organ occurring in the setting of metastatic disease in other organs. Unfortunately, retrospective reports on the utility of site-directed therapy are often confounded by the inclusion of patients in all of these groups despite their clearly different prognoses.

This chapter summarizes the treatment strategies and outcomes of site-directed therapy for patients with advanced lung cancer, focusing primarily on NSCLC occurring in the most common metastatic sites, including the brain, adrenal gland, liver, lung, and bone [3–10]. Patients with extensive-stage SCLC rarely present with solitary sites of metastatic disease, so few reports are available regarding the use of site-directed therapy for this disease. However, patients with extensive-stage SCLC who respond to initial chemotherapy may benefit from prophylactic cranial irradiation (PCI) and definitive thoracic radiation, which will also be discussed.

Brain

NSCLC accounts for 37–56% of all intracranial metastases [11, 12], and brain metastases occur in up to 45% of patients with lung cancer in autopsy series [3–10]. In general, the prognosis for patients with brain metastases is extremely poor. A recursive partitioning analysis of patients with brain metastases from any primary site enrolled in three Radiation Therapy Oncology Group (RTOG) trials reported a median survival of 7.1 months for patients in the most favorable group and only 2.3 months for those in the least favorable group [13]. In this analysis, 61% of patients had primary lung cancer. As evidenced by these dismal statistics, the treatment of brain metastases with local therapeutic modalities is purely palliative in the vast majority of patients.

Multiple Brain Metastases

Approximately 50% of patients with brain metastases from NSCLC have multiple lesions [14]. For patients with multiple brain metastases or poor functional status, corticosteroids and whole brain radiation therapy (WBRT) given with palliative intent are considered the standard of care. For those treated only with corticosteroids, median survival is 1–2 months, while the addition of WBRT improves survival to 3–6 months. The standard fractionation for WBRT in the United States is 30 Gy in 10 fractions delivered by opposed lateral beams, but the optimal schedule remains undefined. In the 1970s, two prospective randomized trials that compared various fractionation schedules in >1,800 patients with brain metastases from multiple primary sites reported no differences in median survival, symptom palliation, or duration of neurologic improvement [15]. In addition, a smaller study suggested that ultra-rapid schedules of 10 Gy in 1 fraction or 6 Gy in 2 fractions may not provide durable responses [16].

Limited Brain Metastases

Several case series have suggested that highly selected patients with solitary or limited intracranial metastases may achieve long-term survival with aggressive surgical resection. Nearly all studies addressing the role of surgery have included a mixture of patients with synchronous and metachronous diseases. Table 1 is a summary of the larger retrospective reports that have examined outcomes after combined resection of the primary tumor and brain metastasis. Overall, this approach has yielded 5-year survival rates of 10–30%. Hankins et al. reported a 5-year survival rate of 45%, but this may be attributable to a large proportion of patients with T1-2 (80%) and node-negative primary lesions (70%) [17]. In several series, the ability to completely resect the primary lung tumor appeared to be a strong, independent prognostic factor on multivariate analysis. Node-positive primary disease has consistently been associated with poor prognosis after brain resection, suggesting that nodal disease reflects the presence of more widespread systemic disease. Therefore, aggressive site-directed treatment of metastatic disease may not be appropriate in such patients.

Several randomized trials have examined the relative contributions of surgical resection, WBRT, and stereotactic radiosurgery (SRS) to the survival, failure pattern, and quality of life of patients with limited brain metastases. Although the most compelling trials included patients with brain metastases from a variety of primary sites, the majority of patients in all of these studies had NSCLC. There are no randomized trials comparing surgical resection to SRS in patients with brain metastases only from NSCLC [18].

In a landmark study, Patchell et al. randomized 48 patients with a single brain metastasis and good performance status to undergo resection followed by WBRT (36 Gy in 3 Gy fractions) or WBRT alone. The use of surgery improved median survival (40 vs. 15 weeks), time to neurologic death, maintenance of performance status, time to recurrence, and intracranial local control [19]. In a

Table 1 Studies of surgical resection for a solitary brain metastasis from NSCLC

Series	Year	N	NSCLC (%)	Solitary (%)	Synchronous/ metachronous (%)	Brain RT (%)	5-year OS (%)	Favorable factors for survival
Mussi [192]	1985	20	100	100	25/75	NR	33.6	
Magilligan [193]	1986	41	90	100	34/66	61	21	MVA: wedge resection
Rossi [194]	1987	40	100	100	85/15	80	12.5	MVA: age <50 years, node-negative disease, better performance status
Torre [195]	1988	21	100	100	100/0	52	NR	UVA: node-negative disease, use of CT for screening
Hankins [17]	1988	19	95	100	68/32	84	45	MVA: complete resection of the primary tumor
Macchiarini [196]	1991	37	100	100	27/73	24	30	UVA: interval >12 months between resection of primary and brain metastasis
Burt [197]	1992	185	100	89	35/65	83	13	MVA: complete resection of the primary tumor
Wronski [198]	1995	231	100	87	37/63	84	12.5	MVA: complete resection of primary tumor, female, age <60 years, supratentorial metastasis, absence of systemic metastases
Saitoh [199]	1999	24	100	100	0/100	42	8.3	MVA: interval >360 days between resection of primary and brain metastasis, lobectomy
Billing [200]	2001	28	100	93	100/0	86	21.4	MVA: node-negative disease
Bonnette [201]	2001	103	100	96	100/0	73	11	MVA: adenocarcinoma

NSCLC = non-small cell lung cancer, RT = radiation therapy, OS = overall survival, NR = not reported, MVA = multivariate analysis, UVA = univariate analysis follow-up study, 95 patients who underwent complete surgical resection were randomized to receive postoperative WBRT (50.4 Gy in 1.8 Gy fractions) or no further treatment after surgery [20]. The addition of WBRT improved intracranial control and rate of neurologic death, but did not impact on median survival or maintenance of performance status. However, most patients in this study who did not receive immediate postoperative WBRT did eventually require WBRT during the course of their disease due to local brain relapse. In both of these studies, patients with radiosensitive histologies, such as SCLC, were excluded.

Analogous trials have been conducted using SRS based on the assumption that it may be a completely ablative and non-invasive substitute for surgery in patients who have unresectable disease or are medically inoperable. An early dose-escalation study of SRS (RTOG 90-05) established the maximal tolerated dose (MTD) based on the size of the metastatic lesion: 24 Gy for tumors <20 mm, 18 Gy for tumors 21–30 mm, and 15 Gy for tumors 31–40 mm [21]. The MTD was not reached in patients with tumors <20 mm. Of note, approximately two-thirds of patients were being treated for recurrent brain metastases after prior WBRT. RTOG 95-08 compared WBRT with or without an SRS boost in 331 patients with 1–3 brain metastases [22]. WBRT was delivered as 37.5 Gy in 15 fractions and SRS doses followed those established by RTOG 90-05. For the subset of patients with a solitary metastasis, WBRT + SRS improved median survival (6.5 vs. 4.9 months, $p = 0.039$), but no significant survival benefit was observed in the overall study population. However, the addition of SRS did improve the 1-year local control (82 vs. 71%, $p = 0.01$), maintenance of performance status, and steroid requirement. A reciprocal study, JROSG 99-1, randomized 132 patients with 1–4 brain metastases to receive SRS with or without WBRT [23]. The addition of WBRT improved intracranial control end-points, including total brain recurrence (47 vs. 76%), distant brain recurrence (42 vs. 64%), local brain recurrence (11 vs. 28%), and need for salvage brain treatment (15 vs. 43%). However, there was no significant overall survival difference, so accrual was terminated early at interim analysis.

In summary, in studies of highly selected patients with good performance status and solitary or limited intracranial metastases, surgical resection has achieved long-term survival rates of 10–30%. Randomized trials support the notion that ablative therapy with either surgical resection or SRS can improve survival and maintain performance status in patients with a solitary brain metastasis. The addition of WBRT after surgical resection or SRS improves intracranial control, but does not significantly impact survival or performance status. For patients with multiple brain metastases, WBRT with palliative intent should remain the mainstay of therapy. The greater the number of brain metastases, the lower the hope that surgical resection or SRS can produce long-term control. The numeric threshold at which surgical resection or SRS should be discounted as a rational treatment option remains controversial.

Prophylactic Cranial Irradiation

Patients with SCLC who achieve a good response after induction chemotherapy remain at high risk for intracranial failure with up to 37% of patients who do not receive prophylactic cranial irradiation (PCI) experiencing brain metastases as an isolated site of first relapse [24]. While patients with gross brain metastases at diagnosis have a dismal prognosis despite treatment, it has been hypothesized that relatively low radiation doses may eradicate occult disease if given prophylactically.

The role of PCI is best defined for patients with limited-stage SCLC, although newer data also support its use in patients with extensive-stage disease. However, there is no evidence that PCI improves survival in patients with NSCLC [25]. The strongest evidence for the use of PCI in patients with SCLC comes from a meta-analysis which included 987 patients with SCLC who achieved a complete response after induction chemotherapy who were enrolled on 7 randomized trials that compared PCI with no PCI [26]. The relative risk of death in the PCI group compared to the control group was 0.84 ($p = 0.01$), which translated into an absolute survival benefit of 5.4% at 3 years. While only 12% of patients in the PCI group had extensive-stage disease, interaction analysis demonstrated that stage of disease did not have a significant effect on the benefit of PCI. More recently, the EORTC conducted a randomized trial comparing PCI with no PCI in 286 patients with extensive-stage SCLC who had *any* response to 4–6 cycles of chemotherapy [27]. Of these patients, 76% had residual thoracic disease and 71% had residual distant disease. PCI significantly decreased the risk of brain metastases (16.8 vs. 41.3%, $p < 0.001$) and improved the 1-year survival rate (27.1 vs. 13.3%, $p = 0.003$). The collective data now appear to support the use of PCI in patients with limited- or extensive-stage SCLC who have achieved a response to initial chemotherapy.

Regarding the optimal fractionation of PCI, the meta-analysis included studies utilizing a wide range of doses and schedules from 8 Gy in a single fraction to 40 Gy in 20 fractions [26]. The schedules with higher total doses led to greater decreases in the risk of brain metastases ($p = 0.02$), but there were no significant differences in survival among the varying regimens.

Adrenal Gland

Autopsy series have reported adrenal metastases in 29–64% of patients with lung cancer [3–10]. However, the incidence of a solitary adrenal metastasis is only 1.6–3.5% [28, 29]. Several small, retrospective series suggest that the resection of a solitary adrenal metastasis due to NSCLC may afford long-term survival in highly selected patients. In an early case series, Twomey et al. reported that two patients with solitary adrenal metastases from large cell lung cancer were alive 6 and 14 years after adrenalectomy and aggressive therapy of the primary lung tumor [30]. This observation encouraged the publication of other small retrospective series over the next two decades [29, 31–35]. Using a MEDLINE search, Abdel-Raheem et al. [36] were able to compile reports on only 18 patients with operable NSCLC who were treated for a metachronous solitary adrenal metastasis from 1965 to 2000. Median survival was 19 months for those who underwent adrenalectomy and chemotherapy (N = 8), 15 months for chemotherapy alone (N = 2), 14 months for adrenalectomy alone (N = 5), and 8 months for palliative radiation alone (N = 2). In 2001, Porte et al. reported a multicenter retrospective study of 43 patients who underwent resection of a solitary adrenal metastasis (32 synchronous, 11 metachronous) [35]. Median survival was 11 months and three patients (7%) survived for over 5 years. Survival was not significantly influenced by histology, stage, adjuvant/neoadjuvant treatment, timing of metastasis (synchronous vs. metachronous), or disease-free interval. The advent of minimally invasive adrenalectomy has led to lower complication rates, less blood loss, and shorter length of stay [37]. Unfortunately, the current data are limited by the small number of highly selected patients that have been reported and the lack of prospective trials. In addition, no consistent clinical or pathologic predictors of survival after adrenalectomy have been identified. Overall, it is not possible to propose a definitive recommendation regarding the potential utility of adrenalectomy for solitary adrenal metastasis in patients with NSCLC.

Liver

The liver is one of the most common sites for metastatic disease [38–41]. The incidence of liver metastases at the time of diagnosis of NSCLC has been reported to be 3.8% [42], but rises to 58% in autopsy series [3–10]. There are few reports of long-term survival after treatment of liver metastasis in patients with NSCLC. Since liver metastases in patients with NSCLC are nearly always a harbinger of widespread systemic disease, the use of definitive site-directed therapy is rarely considered an appropriate management option.

Surgical Resection

Liver metastasectomy has been extensively evaluated in patients with colorectal cancer, with reported 5-year overall survival rates of 25–38% [43–48, 50, 52]. In contrast, only a few case reports are available regarding the resection of liver metastases in patients with NSCLC. In colorectal cancer, isolated liver metastases, without systemic hematogenous spread, are common due to venous drainage of the primary tumor into the portal venous system. However, in NSCLC and most other solid tumors, liver metastases occur in the setting of widespread distant disease due to involvement of the systemic circulation. Therefore, it is not possible to extrapolate the results of metastasectomy or any other definitive site-directed therapy in patients with colorectal cancer to those with other malignancies, including lung cancer. DiCarlo et al. reviewed nine reports of resection of liver metastases in patients with non-colorectal primaries from 1978 to 2003 [53–61]. Only 13 patients in these series had primary lung cancer and survival was reported in only 5 patients (9, 13, 36, >60, and 185 months). A later case study reported one patient with NSCLC who survived 62 months after resection of a liver metastasis [62]. Based on these reports, some would advocate aggressive liver metastasectomy in highly selected patients with NSCLC. However, enthusiasm for this strategy is dampened by the paucity and anecdotal nature of the available data as well as the potential morbidity and mortality that can result from such an invasive approach. Even in colorectal cancer, fewer than 20% of patients with liver-only metastases are eligible for potentially curative resection due to the number or location of lesions [48, 49, 63].

Radiofrequency Ablation

Although surgical resection is considered the gold standard for site-directed therapy for limited liver metastases in patients with colorectal cancer, many patients are medically inoperable or surgically unresectable. In such patients, minimally invasive alternatives, including radiofrequency ablation (RFA), cryoablation, laser or microwave ablation, percutaneous ethanol injection, and transarterial chemoembolization, offer potential options for local disease control. Although initially considered a purely palliative option for patients with liver metastases, thermal ablative procedures, such as RFA, have recently been reported to offer the potential for long-term survival to select groups of patients with colorectal cancer [64, 65]. As with surgical resection, most of the experience with RFA of liver metastases comes from studies in patients with colorectal cancer and gastrointestinal neuroendocrine tumors [64–72]. The published experience with RFA in non-colorectal, non-neuroendocrine liver metastases is very limited [73, 74].

RFA converts radiofrequency waves into heat by utilizing a high-frequency alternating current (100–500 kHz) passed through an uninsulated electrode tip embedded in a tumor. The resulting ionic vibration causes frictional heating of the tissues surrounding the electrode. In general, thermal damage to cells begins at 42°C and the exposure time required for actual cell death decreases exponentially with increasing temperature [75–77]. RFA can be applied via percutaneous, laparoscopic, or open surgical approaches with pros and cons for each of these techniques. The image-guided percutaneous approach is the least invasive and is thus ideal for poor surgical candidates. In general, patients with one to three lesions that are <3.5 cm in diameter and are located in the periphery of the liver can be considered for percutaneous RFA (Fig. 1). Lesions also must not be adjacent to other organs (e.g., bowel, kidney, gallbladder) that can be damaged

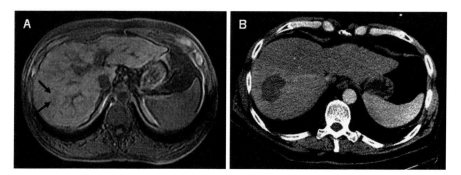

Fig. 1 A 66-year-old man received concurrent chemotherapy and radiation therapy for T1N0 NSCLC. **Panel (a):** Nine months later, MRI (precontrast axial T1 weighted) showed a 2 cm liver tumor (*black arrows*). A biopsy confirmed metastatic NSCLC. **Panel (b):** Contrast-enhanced CT scan performed 1 month after RFA shows that the ablation cavity is larger than the previous tumor, an expected finding after RFA

by the conduction of heat. Laparoscopic RFA has the potential to better define the number and location of liver metastases and the ability to explore the patient for the presence of extrahepatic disease. Laparoscopic RFA should be considered for patients with one or two tumors <4 cm in diameter that are centrally located within the liver [51]. Open surgical RFA is the most invasive approach, but is useful for tumors that are large or situated in difficult locations. An open approach allows temporary occlusion of hepatic vascular inflow, which reduces the heat sink effect during RFA [78–82].

Thus far, RFA has been considered an option primarily for patients who are not candidates for surgical resection. General selection criteria for RFA for liver metastases include unresectable metastases due to technical considerations, poor functional reserve, or patient refusal of surgery; completely treatable by RFA alone or in combination with other site-directed therapies; no evidence of uncontrollable disease at the primary site; and no evidence of extrahepatic metastases. There is no clear consensus regarding limitations on the size and number of lesions that could be treated with RFA, but the size of the tumor remains the major prognostic factor affecting survival [64–66, 83–88]. Successful ablation is possible in >90% of tumors <2.5 cm in size, 70–90% of 2.5–3.5 cm tumors, 50–70% of 3.5–5 cm tumors, and <50% of tumors >5 cm in size. In addition, larger tumors require a higher number of needle repositions to obtain overlapping ablation spheres and longer procedure times, which lead to higher complication rates [89, 90]. Therefore, tumors <3.5 cm are considered ideal, while 5 cm is usually considered the upper limit for RFA. In general, RFA is limited to patients who have five or fewer metastatic lesions from colorectal cancer. However, in NSCLC, it is most reasonable to limit the use of RFA to patients with solitary hepatic lesions.

There is no literature describing the outcome of RFA in patients with liver metastases from lung cancer. Most of the reports on RFA involve patients with liver metastases from colorectal, neuroendocrine, pancreatic, adrenal, or breast cancers [65–74]. In colorectal cancer, RFA for liver metastases results in 1-, 3-, and 5-year survival rates of 90–93, 46–68, and 24–30%, respectively [64, 65, 69, 70]. RFA for liver metastases from neuroendocrine tumors also results in favorable rates for palliation of symptoms and survival [67, 68, 72]. However, due to the aforementioned differences in natural history, these findings cannot be directly applied to patients with metastases from NSCLC.

Stereotactic Body Radiation Therapy

Stereotactic body radiation therapy (SBRT) is highly conformal, hypofractionated radiation applied to extracranial sites. Based on the success of intracranial stereotactic radiosurgery (SRS), initial studies of SBRT in the 1990s reported the safe delivery of ablative doses to tumors in patients who were medically inoperable. The fundamental concepts of SBRT have been nicely reviewed by Timmerman et al. [91]. First, the *radiobiology* of cell survival is uncertain when using radiation therapy at high doses per fraction. The linear-quadratic model has been typically used to describe cell survival with conventionally fractionated radiation therapy (1.8–2 Gy per fraction), but its utility is less clear when high doses per fraction are used [92]. Second, SBRT must be *highly conformal* to deliver high doses to small targets while sparing adjacent critical normal tissue. SBRT planning typically requires multiple static beams (often non-coplanar and non-opposing) or dynamic arcs. Third, reliable *immobilization and stereotactic localization* are required to minimize variations in the delivery of each fraction. Fourth, *motion control* is crucial to monitor and minimize organ motion that occurs during the long treatment times required for SBRT. Abdominal compression, active breathing control (ABC), breath holds, and respiratory gating are common ways of decreasing respiratory motion on either side of the diaphragm. Fiducial markers can be implanted to allow daily target localization.

Blomgren et al. reported the first retrospective experience with SBRT [93]. Soon thereafter, phase I and II trials demonstrated the safety and efficacy of SBRT for liver metastases, with local control rates of 67–93% at 18 months. Although the patients in these trials had a wide variety of primary tumor sites, the majority had colorectal cancer. Herfarth et al. conducted a phase I/II trial of single-dose SBRT in 56 liver metastases with dose escalation from 14 to 26 Gy, but only 4 lesions were of lung origin [94]. SBRT was well tolerated without serious complications. The local control rates were 75% at 6 months, 71% at 12 months, and 67% at 18 months. Wulf et al. reported on multifraction SBRT for 51 hepatic metastases, of which only 3 were of NSCLC origin [95, 96]. Tumors were treated with either "low-dose" (10 Gy × 3 or 7 Gy × 4) or "high-dose" radiation (12–12.5 Gy × 3 or 26 Gy × 1). The local control rate was 92% at 12 months and 66% at 24 months, with better control with high-dose radiation, and overall toxicity was mild. In a phase I study, Schefter et al. evaluated dose-escalated SBRT in 18 patients with 1–3 liver metastases, reaching a dose of 20 Gy × 3 without dose-limiting toxicity [97]. A subsequent analysis of 36 patients, 10 of whom had a primary lung cancer, reported a local control rate of 93% at 18 months and minimal toxicity[98]. Overall, SBRT for liver metastases is well tolerated and provides excellent rates of local control. However, the experience in patients with NSCLC remains limited and it has not been proven that good local control will translate into improved overall survival.

Lung

The incidence of lung metastasis from NSCLC is 24–97% in autopsy series [3–10]. When a patient with NSCLC presents with a suspicious lesion in a separate lobe, all efforts should be undertaken to determine whether or not the lesion is truly solitary. If it is, the possibility that it is a second primary cancer should be considered since patients with NSCLC are at high risk for developing multiple upper aerodigestive cancers. Patients with synchronous lung primaries have a better prognosis than those with clearly metastatic disease. Therefore, in patients with two discrete lung nodules and no apparent lymph node involvement, each tumor should be treated in a definitive manner as if it were a separate primary cancer.

Pulmonary Metastasectomy

Surgical resection remains an important treatment modality for pulmonary metastases from various solid tumors. Pulmonary metastasectomy was first reported by Davis in 1927 [99]. In the early surgical experience, morbidity and mortality were related to loss of lung parenchyma, thus mandating that selected patients had solitary or limited metastases. Current operative techniques have allowed the inclusion of patients with multiple metastases, bilateral disease, and involvement of vital structures.

Patient selection criteria for pulmonary metastasectomy include good risk for surgery, no evidence of uncontrollable disease at the primary site, either absence or good control of extrapulmonary metastases, and potential for complete resection. Selection of patients for pulmonary metastasectomy according to these criteria is associated with the best survival [100]. Indications for resection also may include the need to establish a pathologic diagnosis, to clarify if the lesion is a metastasis or a new primary tumor, or to control symptoms such as hemoptysis or pneumothorax.

Thoracotomy is the most frequently utilized approach for unilateral metastasectomy, primarily because of the ability to bimanually palpate the lung to identify other lesions. Bilateral pulmonary metastases can be resected with sequential thoracotomy, median sternotomy, or clamshell approaches.

Thoracoscopic pulmonary metastasectomy is gaining popularity, but has been criticized for its limited ability to identify other metastases. However, improvements in the resolution of CT have resulted in fewer pulmonary nodules that can be palpated at surgery, but not visualized on preoperative imaging studies. In addition, thoracoscopic instruments and techniques have evolved to allow enhanced visualization and palpation of lung parenchyma. The advantages of thoracoscopic metastasectomy include smaller incisions, less pain, earlier recovery, and fewer postoperative adhesions.

The extent of pulmonary resection is controversial, although survival after pulmonary metastasectomy is clearly dependent on the completeness of resection. Superficial metastases can be excised using staplers, electrocautery, sharp resection with suturing, or laser. More centrally located pulmonary metastases may require a lobectomy or pneumonectomy for complete resection. Some surgeons recommend lobectomy with lymph node dissection because of the possibility of nodal metastases [101]. However, lymph node dissection is generally discouraged due to the low incidence of nodal involvement with pulmonary metastases and the poor survival of patients with nodal metastasis regardless of resection. Pneumonectomy or extended resection is rarely used and should be reserved for special circumstances with acceptable surgical risk and a reasonable chance for long-term survival. Outcomes after pulmonary metastasectomy are dictated by the natural history of the primary malignancy, as evidenced by a wide variation in survival rates [100, 102, 105–114]. Most series report operative mortality of <2% and morbidity of 10% [102–104].

For NSCLC, the most recent American Joint Committee on Cancer (AJCC) staging system distinguishes between intrapulmonary metastases involving the same lobe as the primary ("PM1," staged as T4) and those involving a different lobe ("PM2," staged as M1). Attempts to validate this classification have generated data regarding survival after resection of intrapulmonary metastases from NSCLC. Fukuse et al. reviewed 41 patients who had a postoperative diagnosis of intrapulmonary metastases and reported 3-year survival rates of 49% for PM1 disease (N = 20) and 21% for PM2 disease (N = 21) [115]. In a similar study, Okada et al. reviewed 89 patients who underwent an operation for primary lung cancer and were found to have synchronous ipsilateral intrapulmonary metastases [116]. The 5-year survival rate was 29.6% for PM1 disease (N = 48) and 23.4% for PM2 disease (N = 41). However, in a large-scale analysis of national data collected in Japan in 1994 which included 6,080 patients without intrapulmonary metastases, 317 with PM1 metastases, and 128 with PM2 metastases, Nagai et al. reported 5-year survival rates of 55.1, 26.8, and 22.5%, respectively, with no significant survival differences between patients with PM1 and PM2 disease or PM2 and other M1 diseases [117].

In summary, in highly selected patients, pulmonary metastasectomy can achieve long-term survival with low rates of operative complications. Complete resection is essential, even if multiple resections are required to achieve a favorable outcome. However, most reports of pulmonary metastasectomy have been retrospective and, as such, can be confounded by selection bias and lead-time bias.

Radiofrequency Ablation

While pulmonary metastasectomy remains the site-directed therapy of choice, many patients are not candidates for surgical resection. The pulmonary parenchyma may be ideal for RFA due to its ability to concentrate thermal energy focally within tumor tissue with little energy spreading to the adjacent aerated normal lung parenchyma [118–121]. While many publications have addressed the application of RFA for lung metastases, very few have included a significant number of patients with NSCLC [122–135].

Patient selection criteria for RFA for lung metastases are summarized in Table 2. The majority of patients who undergo RFA are medically inoperable, but have otherwise surgically resectable disease. The best results of RFA have been reported for tumors that are ≤ 3 cm in diameter, although substantial tumor response and local control have been reported in larger tumors [130, 135–139]. Peripheral tumors that are located away from the hilar structures and surrounded by lung parenchyma can be safely and effectively treated with RFA. It is preferred that tumors not be in direct contact with the trachea, esophagus, aorta, or heart, but recent studies have reported that such tumors can be safely and effectively treated [140, 141]. The "heat sink effect" of constant tissue cooling that occurs due to flowing intravascular blood probably protects both small and large pulmonary vasculature from tissue damage, even when they are near the ablation zones [140, 142]. RFA of lung lesions is performed percutaneously under general anesthesia or conscious sedation with CT guidance (Fig. 2). During ablation, ground glass attenuation develops and surrounds the lesion, which is believed to positively correlate with histological tissue necrosis [143–145]. Oversizing the ablation zone by at least 1 cm may be necessary to obtain a tumor-free margin.

The most commonly reported complication of RFA is pneumothorax which occurs in one-third of patients, with a much smaller number requiring a chest

Table 2 Selection criteria for radiofrequency ablation (RFA) of lung metastases

Inclusion criteria
Medically inoperable or technically unresectable
Treatable by RFA alone or with other site-directed therapy
No uncontrollable disease at the primary site
No extrapulmonary metastases
Patient refusal of surgery

Exclusion criteria
Invasion of mediastinal structures
Close proximity to hilar structures or other vital organs
Prior pneumonectomy
Suppurative neoplasm
Active lung or chest wall infection
Contraindication to sedation or anesthesia
Uncontrolled coagulopathy

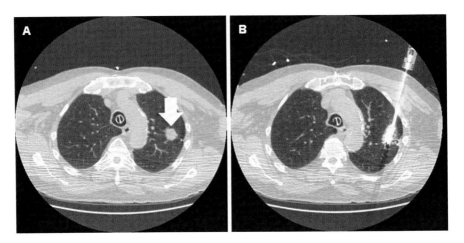

Fig. 2 A 69-year-old man underwent left upper lobe partial resection for lung adenocarcinoma. **Panel (a)**: Three years later, a new left upper lobe lung nodule was noted by CT and was biopsy-proven recurrent adenocarcinoma (*arrow*). Since he was medically inoperable, he underwent RFA. **Panel (b)**: RFA probe in the middle of the nodule along its long axis

tube placement [146–148]. Other reported complications include fever, pulmonary hemorrhage, pleural effusion, hemothorax, pneumonia, and bronchopleural fistula. One study reported minor complications in 65% and major complications in 17% of patients [149].

Few of the pulmonary lesions included in reports on RFA have been metastases from a primary lung cancer. Therefore, data on response, local control, and survival can only be extrapolated from studies that have explored RFA to treat metastatic lung nodules from a variety of primary sites (Table 3). Rates of local control have been reported as high as 80–100%. Simon et al. reported the largest series of RFA for pulmonary metastases (73 nodules including 31 from NSCLC) with 1-, 2-, and 5-year survival rates of 70, 54, and 44%, respectively [130]. Several studies have reported that tumor size <3 cm is associated with improved local control and survival [124, 135, 150].

In summary, radiofrequency ablation is a promising, less invasive, site-directed therapy for lung tumors. At this time, RFA should be reserved for patients who are not candidates for surgical resection. Other common selection criteria include tumors < 3 cm, residual or recurrent disease despite maximal conventional therapy, and disease located away from vital structures. While the rates of response and local control have been favorable, these data have been generated in patients with tumors from a wide variety of primary sites, and any extrapolation to the treatment of intrapulmonary metastasis from NSCLC must be made with caution.

Table 3 Studies of radiofrequency ablation (RFA) for lung metastases

Study	Lesion size (cm)	Metastases: patients (nodules)	NSCLC: patients (nodules)	Follow-up (range) (months)	Response and local control	Survival
Herrere [202]	5.3 (2–16.1)	13	5	6 (1–14)	Response 55%, stable 33%	Death due to progression 38%
Yasui [122]	1.95 ± 1.26	32 (96)	3 (3)	7.1 (1–17)	CR 91%, PR 9%	Death 11% (all extrathoracic)
Akeboshi [136]	2.7 ± 1.3	21 (68)	10	9.2 (5–18)	CR 61%, PR 39%	1 year OS 84% (similar in CR vs. PR)
Kang [203]	NR	27	23	(0.25–0.5)	2 week: FDG-PET negative if <3.5 cm	No deaths
King [129]	NR	19 (44)	0	24 (4.9–30.4)	1 year: CR 36%, PR/ stable 44%	Death 47%
Steinke [128]	4.2	23 (52)	0	14.3 (5.8–27.6)	1 year: CR 43%, PR 13%, stable 10%	1 year OS 78%
VanSonnenberg [204]	4.4*	11	18	(2–26)	90% patients with >90% necrosis	1 year death 13% (all extrathoracic)
Bojarski [145]	3.1 (1–7)	18 (18)	(14)	10.1 (1–30)	1 year: PR 13%, stable 27%	NR
Gadaleta [205]	NR	45	9	18	CR 95%	NR
Ambrogi [135]	2.4	(24)	(40)	23.7	CR 64% (better if <3 cm)	OS 17 months, PFS 13 months <3 cm: OS 20 months, PFS 16 months >3 cm: OS 12 months, PFS 7 months
Thanos [134]	3.8	8 (8)	14	14.3 (5.8–27.6)	Recurrence 5%	Median PFS 29 months OS: 1 year 70%, 2 years 60%, 3 years 45%
Rossi [133]	1.2	16 (21)	15 (15)	11.4 ± 7.7	Recurrence 10%	OS 71%

(Continued)

Table 3 (Continued)

Study	Lesion size (cm)	Metastases: patients (nodules)	NSCLC: patients (nodules)	Follow-up (range) (months)	Response and local control	Survival
Kishi [132]	2.9*	3 (4)	5 (5)	(3–12)	CR 50%	NR
Lagana [131]	NR	7	9	5 (1–12)	CR 90%, recurrence 13%	NR
Hoffman [206]	NR	20 (20)	1	18 (3–36)	Local control 86%	NR
Dbaere [207]	17 ± 9	51 (53)	9	≥12	18 months: incomplete response 12%	18 months: OS 76%, DFS 44%
Simon [130]	NR	(73)	(116)	20.5 (3–74)	NR	OS: 1 year 70%, 2 years 54%, 5 years 44%
Yamakado [126]	19	71 (155)	0	19 (4–42)	Progression 17% (better if <3 cm)	OS: 1 year 84%, 2 years 62%, 3 years 46%; Median OS 31 months
Yan [125]	2.1 ± 1.1	55	0	24 (6–40)	Local PFS: 1 year 74%, 2 years 56%	Median OS 33 months, PFS 15 months OS: 1 year 85%, 2 years 64%, 3 years 46% PFS: 1 year 61%, 2 years 34%

* = calculated by chapter co-author; NSCLC = non-small cell lung cancer; CR = complete response; PR = partial response; OS = overall survival; DFS = disease-free survival; PFS = progression-free survival; FDG-PET = fluorodeoxyglucose-positron emission tomography; NR = not reported

Stereotactic Body Radiation Therapy

SBRT can achieve highly conformal dose distributions in the lung (Fig. 3). The rationale for using SBRT as a minimally invasive ablative therapy in lieu of surgical resection for oligometastases is based on the experience with early-stage NSCLC, in which 3-year local control rates are 80–95%. Timmerman et al. reported a phase I trial of SBRT for medically inoperable patients with cT1-2N0M0 (tumor <7 cm) NSCLC using three fractions with dose escalation starting at 8 Gy per fraction. For lesions >5 cm, the maximal tolerated dose was 72 Gy (24 Gy × 3) [151, 152]. In a subsequent phase II trial using SBRT doses of 60–66 Gy for stage I NSCLC, the 2-year local control rate was 95%, but there was excessive toxicity in patients with central lesions [153]. Other series have reported local control rates ranging from 80 to 95% at 3 years for patients with early-stage NSCLC [154–160].

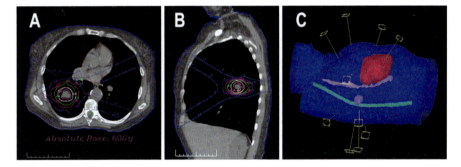

Fig. 3 Dose distribution mapping for SBRT for a solitary lung tumor. **Panel (a):** Axial view. **Panel (b):** Sagittal view. **Panel (c):** Beam arrangement in three dimensions, including non-coplanar beams

For patients with lung metastases, several groups have reported favorable local control rates of 67–98% after treatment with SBRT using either multi-fraction [95, 161–163] or single-fraction regimens [155, 156, 164] (Table 4). However, the collective interpretation of these studies is limited by the inclusion of patients with primary lung lesions and pulmonary metastases from a variety of primary sites with a low proportion of metastases of primary lung origin.

In conclusion, SBRT is safe when patients are appropriately selected for tumor size and location. SBRT provides excellent local control for both primary NSCLC and metastatic lung lesions and can be considered an option for patients who are medically inoperable. However, it is unclear if the high rates of local control will translate into a survival benefit even in highly selected patients. Of note, the currently available data have been generated in patients with tumors from a wide variety of primary sites and any extrapolation to the treatment of metastasis from NSCLC must be made with caution.

Table 4 Studies of stereotactic body radiotherapy (SBRT) for lung metastases

Author	SBRT fractionation	Lung metastases	Metastases from primary lung cancer	Tumor size (range)‡	Median follow-up (months)	Local control rate (%)
Blomgren [208]	21–66 Gy in 1–3 fractions	14	0	Median CTV 48 cc (3–198)	8.2‡	93
Uematsu [209]	32–76 Gy in 5–15 fractions	43	11	Median 2.5 cm (0.8–4.8)	11‡	98
Nakagawa [164]	15–25 Gy × 1*	21	3	Median CTV 7 cc (0.8–126)	10‡	95
Wulf [95]	10 Gy × 3†	11	5	Median CTV 57 cc (5–277)	8‡	76‡
Nagata [161]	12 Gy × 4	9	1	Mean CTV 12.6 cc (0.5–38.6)	18	67
Fritz [155]	30 Gy × 1	31	10	Median CTV 6 cc (2.8–55.8)	22	87
Hara [156]	20–34 Gy × 1	48	11	Mean CTV 5 cc (1–19)	NR	1 year 93 2 years 78‡
Yoon [163]	10–12 Gy × 3–4	53 patients	14 patients	Mean GTV 43.9 cc (4.3–213)	14‡	82‡
Okunieff [162]	2.5–6.5 Gy/ fraction to 50–55 Gy total	125	NR	Median GTV 4.7 cc (0.1–125)	14.9	94

* 8 patients received conventionally fractionated radiation therapy after SBRT
† one target received 7 Gy × 4
‡ including data from primary tumors treated with SBRT
NR = not reported

Thoracic Irradiation in Extensive-Stage SCLC

Despite the fact that most patients with extensive-stage SCLC have a good response to initial chemotherapy, their overall prognosis remains poor with a median survival of 9–12 months. The role of thoracic radiation therapy (TRT) has been well defined in patients with limited-stage disease, but its benefit in extensive-stage patients is less clear. Jeremic et al. conducted a randomized trial in which patients with extensive-stage SCLC who achieved a complete response after initial chemotherapy (N = 109) were then randomized to further chemotherapy alone or concurrent chemotherapy + accelerated hyperfractionated TRT with 54 Gy in 36 fractions delivered twice daily [165]. The inclusion of TRT improved both median survival (17 vs. 11 months) and 5-year survival (9.1

vs. 3.7%, $p = 0.041$) rates. However, several other studies have failed to show a significant survival benefit for TRT in patients with extensive-stage SCLC [166–168].

Bone

Bone metastases are common in patients with NSCLC, with autopsy series documenting rates of 21–41% [3–10]. The median survival for a patient with bone metastasis from NSCLC has been reported as 5–6 months [169]. As such, radiation therapy should generally be given with palliative intent to patients with painful bone metastases, although there are limited case reports of long-term survival after aggressive resection of solitary bone involvement [170]. RTOG 74-02 was the initial large-scale attempt to clarify the optimal conventional fractionation for palliative radiation for symptomatic bone metastases. Patients with solitary bone lesions were randomized to receive 2.7 Gy × 15 or 4 Gy × 5 fractions, while those with multiple lesions were randomized to receive 3 Gy × 10, 3 Gy × 5, 4 Gy × 5, or 5 Gy × 5 fractions. In the initial report, 89% of patients had at least some relief of pain and there were no differences in pain relief between the various fractionation schedules [171]. However, a reanalysis of this data using different end-points and pooling of solitary and multiple lesions found that the high-dose protracted schedules (2.7 Gy × 15 and 3 Gy × 10 fractions) were associated with improved "complete combined relief" (i.e., absence of pain and cessation of narcotic use) [172]. As a result, the standard for conventional fractionation has remained 3 Gy × 10 fractions.

Uncomplicated Bone Metastases

Considering the palliative nature of radiotherapy, numerous attempts have been made to reduce the dose and time required for patients to complete treatment. Multiple randomized trials have shown equivalence between conventional and hypofractionated schedules for uncomplicated bone metastases. These generally excluded patients with prior radiation therapy to the site, impending or true pathologic fracture, compression of the spinal cord or cauda equina, or planned surgery at the involved site.

The Dutch Bone Metastasis Study compared treatment with 8 Gy × 1 fraction to 4 Gy × 6 fractions in 1,171 patients, 25% of whom had primary lung cancer [173]. There were no significant differences in palliative response, analgesic requirement, quality of life, or side effects. However, significantly more retreatments were required in the 8 Gy × 1 fraction group (25 vs. 7%). In a separate analysis of 320 long-term survivors (i.e., alive >1 year), the duration of response and rate of progression were similar in both arms [174]. This suggests that a single 8 Gy fraction can be offered to all patients with a painful bone metastasis, not only those with the worst prognosis. In the United States, RTOG 97-14 randomized nearly 900 patients with 1–3 painful bone metastases to receive 3 Gy × 10 fractions vs. a single 8 Gy fraction and found that there were no significant differences in complete or partial response rates [175]. The re-treatment rate again was significantly higher in the 8 Gy arm (18 vs. 9%, $p < 0.001$), while the 3 Gy × 10 fractions arm produced more frequent grade 2–4 acute toxicity (17 vs. 10%, $p = 0.002$). However, this study was limited to patients with primary breast or prostate cancer. The Bone Pain Trial Working Party randomized 765 patients (12% with primary lung cancer) to receive 8 Gy × 1, 4 Gy × 5, or 3 Gy × 10 fractions and also found no significant differences in survival, time to pain improvement, and durability of palliation [176]. Again, re-treatment was more common in the single-fraction group. More recently, studies from Australia (TROG 96.05) [177] and Norway/Sweden [178] also confirm no significant differences between 8 Gy × 1 fraction and more protracted fractionation schedules.

Complicated Bone Metastases

Because patients with complicated bone metastases were not included in hypo-fractionation trials, they should be treated with conventional fractionated radiation (e.g., 3 Gy × 10 fractions), rather than a single 8 Gy fraction, in coordination with potential surgical intervention. For patients with spinal cord compression, a multidisciplinary approach that includes both radiation oncology and neurosurgery should be pursued. Patchell et al. [179] randomized 101 patients with spinal cord compression to either decompressive surgical resection followed by radiation (3 Gy × 10 fractions) or radiation alone. Eligibility was restricted to patients with a single area of compression, which could span multiple spinal levels, and patients with radiosensitive histologies were excluded. The study was stopped at interim analysis when the surgical arm was found to have dramatically improved likelihood of ambulation after treatment (84 vs. 57%, $p = 0.001$), duration of ambulation (median 122 vs. 13 days, $p = 0.003$), and need for corticosteroids or opioid analgesics. These data provide compelling evidence that surgical decompression should be considered before proceeding with radiation in patients with spinal cord compression at a solitary site. In addition, surgical management should be considered when there is mechanical instability, radioresistant histology, history of prior radiation, no pathologic diagnosis, or compression due to displaced bone.

Stereotactic Body Radiation Therapy

As with other extracranial sites, there is growing interest in the use of SBRT to treat spinal metastases, especially when the patient has progressed through conventionally fractionated therapy. In 1995, Hamilton et al. [180] first described the use of SBRT to treat the spine. Since then, many groups have published on the procedures, safety, and efficacy of spinal SBRT [181–190]. Gerszten et al. reported on 500 patients with spinal metastases treated with SBRT with a mean maximum intratumoral dose of 20 Gy. Long-term pain improvement was achieved in 86% of patients and tumor control was noted in 88–90% of lesions [184]. Most recently, Chang et al. published the results of a phase I/II study of SBRT for spinal metastases in 63 patients [191]. At a median follow-up of 21 months, no neuropathy or myelopathy was observed and the 1-year tumor progression-free survival rate was 84%.

In summary, a single 8 Gy fraction should be considered the standard treatment for uncomplicated bone metastases, as it has been shown to be as effective as, and less burdensome than, more protracted schedules in multiple randomized trials. Since complicated bone metastases were excluded from these trials, we recommend conventionally fractionated radiation schedules in close coordination with the surgical team. SBRT for spinal metastases may be considered for local control and palliative relief for patients undergoing re-treatment and in other situations that preclude standard radiotherapy.

Conclusion

Many patients with NSCLC harbor metastatic disease at diagnosis and their 5-year survival rate is only 1–2%. In many of these patients, site-directed therapy can offer substantial palliation of symptoms and improvement in quality of life. However, a small, select subset of patients with limited metastatic disease may be offered site-directed therapy with the intent of achieving long-term disease control. Although this approach is well documented for patients with oligometastatic disease from other primary cancer sites, the data for definitive site-directed therapy in patients with metastatic lung cancer are very limited outside of the setting of a solitary brain metastasis. In selected subsets of patients with NSCLC and a solitary metastasis, site-directed therapy has been reported to result in long-term survival rates of 15–20%.

Surgical resection remains the gold standard for site-directed therapy, but many patients are medically inoperable due to comorbidities or poor performance status that often accompanies stage IV disease. For such patients, conventional radiotherapy, stereotactic radiosurgery, stereotactic body radiotherapy, and radiofrequency ablation offer less invasive alternatives that still offer high rates of local control. Importantly, due to the paucity of randomized trials, it remains unclear if local control for most sites of oligometastatic disease will translate into improved survival. However, most patients who ultimately succumb after site-directed therapy die from systemic progression, rather than local failure. Therefore, patients selected for site-directed therapy must undergo careful evaluation prior to initiating such therapy, including confirmation of a favorable performance status and a solitary focus of progressive metastatic disease, with otherwise stable systemic disease or an early-stage primary tumor that is amenable to definitive therapy.

References

1. Naruke T, Tsuchiya R, Kondo H, et al. Prognosis and survival after resection for bronchogenic carcinoma based on the 1997 TNM-staging classification: the Japanese experience. Ann Thorac Surg 2001, 71:1759–1764.
2. Mountain CF. Revisions in the International System for Staging Lung Cancer. Chest 1997, 111:1710–1717.
3. Abrams HL, Spiro R, Goldstein N. Metastases in carcinoma: analysis of 1000 autopsied cases. Cancer 1950, 3:74–85.
4. Engelman RM. Bronchiogenic carcinoma: a statistical review of two hundred and thirty-four autopsies. J Thorac Surg 1954, 27:227–237.
5. Guillan RA, Zelman S, Alonso RA. Adenocarcinoma of the lungs: an analysis of 24 cases in men. Am J Clin Pathol 1967, 47:580–584.
6. Koletsky S. Primary carcinoma of the lung: a clinical and pathologic study of one hundred cases. Arch Int Med 1938, 62:636–651.
7. Onuigbo WI. Some pathological data on 2000 adenocarcinomas and squamous cell carcinomas of the lung. Br J Cancer 1963, 17:1–7.
8. Stenbygaard LE, Sørensen JB, Larsen HH, et al. Metastatic pattern in non-resectable non-small cell lung cancer. Acta Oncologica 1999, 38:993–998.
9. Stenbygaard LE, Sørensen JB, Olsen JE. Metastatic pattern at autopsy in non-resectable adenocarcinoma of the lung: a study from a cohort of 259 consecutive patients treated with chemotherapy. Acta Oncologica 1997, 36:301–306.
10. Strauss B, Weller CV. Bronchogenic carcinoma: a statistical analysis of two hundred ninety-six cases with necropsy as to relationships between cell types and age, sex, and metastasis. Arch Pathol 1957, 63:602–611.
11. Jawahar A, Willis BK, Smith DR, et al. Gamma knife radiosurgery for brain metastases: do patients benefit from adjuvant external-beam radiotherapy? An 18-month comparative analysis. Stereotact Funct Neurosurg 2002, 79: 262–271.
12. Varlotto JM, Flickinger JC, Niranjan A, et al. Analysis of tumor control and toxicity in patients who have survived at least one year after radiosurgery for brain metastases. Int J Radiat Oncol Biol Phys 2003, 57:452–464.
13. Gaspar L, Scott C, Rotman M, et al. Recursive partitioning analysis (RPA) of prognostic factors in three Radiation Therapy Oncology Group (RTOG) brain metastases trials. Int J Radiat Oncol Biol Phys 1997, 37:745–751.
14. Nussbaum ES, Djalilian HR, Cho KH, et al. Brain metastases: histology, multiplicity, surgery, and survival. Cancer 1996, 78:1781–1788.
15. Borgelt B, Gelber R, Kramer S, et al. The palliation of brain metastases: final results of the first two studies by the Radiation Therapy Oncology Group. Int J Radiat Oncol Biol Phys 1980, 6:1–9.
16. Borgelt B, Gelber R, Larson M, et al. Ultra-rapid high dose irradiation schedules for the palliation of brain metastases: final results of the first two studies by the Radiation Therapy Oncology Group. Int J Radiat Oncol Biol Phys 1981, 7:1633–1638.
17. Hankins JR, Miller JE, Salcman M, et al. Surgical management of lung cancer with solitary cerebral metastasis. Ann Thorac Surg 1988, 46:24–28.
18. Fuentes R, Bonfill X, Esposito J. Surgery versus radiosurgery for patients with a solitary brain metastasis from non-small cell lung cancer. Cochrane Database Syst Rev 2006, CD004840.

19. Patchell RA, Tibbs PS, Walsh JW, et al. A randomized trial of surgery in the treatment of single metastases to the brain. N Engl J Med 1990, 322:494–500.
20. Patchell RA, Tibbs PA, Regine WF, et al. Postoperative radiotherapy in the treatment of single metastases to the brain: a randomized trial. JAMA 1998, 280:1485–1489.
21. Shaw E, Scott C, Souhami L, et al. Single dose radiosurgical treatment of recurrent previously irradiated primary brain tumors and brain metastases: final report of RTOG protocol 90-05. Int J Radiat Oncol Biol Phys 2000, 47:291–298.
22. Andrews DW, Scott CB, Sperduto PW, et al. Whole brain radiation therapy with or without stereotactic radiosurgery boost for patients with one to three brain metastases: phase III results of the RTOG 9508 randomised trial. Lancet 2004, 363:1665–1672.
23. Aoyama H, Shirato H, Tago M, et al. Stereotactic radiosurgery plus whole-brain radiation therapy vs stereotactic radiosurgery alone for treatment of brain metastases: a randomized controlled trial. JAMA 2006, 295:2483–2491.
24. Arriagada R, Le Chevalier T, Riviere A, et al. Patterns of failure after prophylactic cranial irradiation in small-cell lung cancer: analysis of 505 randomized patients. Ann Oncol 2002, 13:748–754.
25. Lester JF, MacBeth FR, Coles B. Prophylactic cranial irradiation for preventing brain metastases in patients undergoing radical treatment for non-small-cell lung cancer: a Cochrane Review. Int J Radiat Oncol Biol Phys 2005, 63:690–694.
26. Auperin A, Arriagada R, Pignon JP, et al. Prophylactic cranial irradiation for patients with small-cell lung cancer in complete remission. N Engl J Med 1999, 341:476–484.
27. Slotman B, Faivre-Finn C, Kramer G, et al. Prophylactic cranial irradiation in extensive small-cell lung cancer. N Engl J Med 2007, 357:664–672.
28. Ettinghausen SE, Burt ME. Prospective evaluation of unilateral adrenal masses in patients with operable non-small-cell lung cancer. J Clin Oncol 1991, 9:1462–1466.
29. Porte HL, Roumilhac D, Graziana JP, et al. Adrenalectomy for a solitary adrenal metastasis from lung cancer. Ann Thorac Surg 1998, 65:331–335.
30. Twomey P, Montgomery C, Clark O. Successful treatment of adrenal metastases from large-cell carcinoma of the lung. JAMA 1982, 248:581–583.
31. Luketich JD, Burt ME. Does resection of adrenal metastases from non-small cell lung cancer improve survival? Ann Thorac Surg 1996, 62:1614–1616.
32. Luketich JD, Martini N, Ginsberg RJ, et al. Successful treatment of solitary extracranial metastases from non-small cell lung cancer. Ann Thorac Surg 1995, 60:1609–1611.
33. de Perrot M, Licker M, Robert JH, et al. Long-term survival after surgical resections of bronchogenic carcinoma and adrenal metastasis. Ann Thorac Surg 1999, 68:1084–1085.
34. Raviv G, Klein E, Yellin A, et al. Surgical treatment of solitary adrenal metastases from lung carcinoma. J Surg Oncol 1990, 43:123–124.
35. Porte H, Siat J, Guibert B, et al. Resection of adrenal metastases from non-small cell lung cancer: a multicenter study. Ann Thorac Surg 2001, 71:981–985.
36. Abdel-Raheem MM, Potti A, Becker WK, et al. Late adrenal metastasis in operable non-small-cell lung carcinoma. Am J Clin Oncol 2002, 25:81–83.
37. Heniford BT, Arca MJ, Walsh RM, et al. Laparoscopic adrenalectomy for cancer. Semin Surg Oncol 1999, 16:293–306.
38. Baker ME, Pelley R. Hepatic metastases: basic principles and implications for radiologists. Radiology 1995, 197:329–337.
39. Greenlee RT, Murray T, Bolden S, et al. Cancer statistics, 2000. CA Cancer J Clin 2000, 50:7–33.
40. Landis SH, Murray T, Bolden S, et al. Cancer statistics, 1999. CA Cancer J Clin 1999, 49:8–31.
41. Weiss L, Grundmann E, Torhorst J, et al. Haematogenous metastatic patterns in colonic carcinoma: an analysis of 1541 necropsies. J Pathol 1986, 150:195–203.
42. Kagohashi K, Satoh H, Ishikawa H, et al. Liver metastasis at the time of initial diagnosis of lung cancer. Medical Oncol 2003, 20:25–28.

43. Fong Y, Cohen AM, Fortner JG, et al. Liver resection for colorectal metastases. J Clin Oncol 1997, 15:938–946.
44. Gayowski TJ, Iwatsuki S, Madariaga JR, et al. Experience in hepatic resection for metastatic colorectal cancer: analysis of clinical and pathologic risk factors. Surgery 1994, 116:703–710.
45. Nordlinger B, Quilichini MA, Parc R, et al. Hepatic resection for colorectal liver metastases. Influence on survival of preoperative factors and surgery for recurrences in 80 patients. Ann Surg 1987, 205:256–263.
46. Rosen CB, Nagorney DM, Taswell HF, et al. Perioperative blood transfusion and determinants of survival after liver resection for metastatic colorectal carcinoma. Ann Surg 1992, 216:493–504.
47. Singletary SE, Walsh G, Vauthey JN, et al. A role for curative surgery in the treatment of selected patients with metastatic breast cancer. Oncologist 2003, 8:241–251.
48. Hao CY, Ji JF. Surgical treatment of liver metastases of colorectal cancer: Strategies and controversies in 2006. Eur J Surg Oncol 2006, 32:473–483.
49. Lehnert T, Golling M. Indications and outcome of liver metastases resection. Radiologe 2001, 41:40–48.
50. Shumate C. Hepatic resection for colorectal cancer metastases. In: Curley S, ed. Liver Cancer. New York: Springer-Verlag, 1998, 136–149.
51. Siperstein A, Garland A, Engle K, et al. Laparoscopic radiofrequency ablation of primary and metastatic liver tumors: technical considerations. Surg Endoscopy 2000, 14:400–405.
52. Tuttle T. Hepatectomy for noncolorectal metastases. In: Curley S, ed. Liver Cancer. New York: Springer-Verlag, 1998, 201–211.
53. Di Carlo I., Grasso G, Patane D, et al. Liver metastases from lung cancer: is surgical resection justified? Ann Thorac Surg 2003, 76:291–293.
54. Stehlin JS Jr, de Ipolyi PD, Greeff PJ, et al. Treatment of cancer of the liver. Twenty years' experience with infusion and resection in 414 patients. Ann Surg 1988, 208:23–35.
55. Berney T, Mentha G, Roth AD, et al. Results of surgical resection of liver metastases from non-colorectal primaries. Br J Surg 1998, 85:1423–1427.
56. Cobourn CS, Makowka L, Langer B, et al. Examination of patient selection and outcome for hepatic resection for metastatic disease. Surg Gynecol Obstet 1987, 165:239–246.
57. Foster JH. Survival after liver resection for secondary tumors. Am J Surg 1978, 135:389–394.
58. Hamy AP, Paineau JR, Mirallie EC, et al. Hepatic resections for non-colorectal metastases: forty resections in 35 patients. Hepatogastroenterology 2000, 47:1090–1094.
59. Lindell G, Ohlsson B, Saarela A, et al. Liver resection of noncolorectal secondaries. J Surg Oncol 1998, 69:66–70.
60. Schwartz SI. Hepatic resection for noncolorectal nonneuroendocrine metastases. World J Surg 1995, 19:72–75.
61. Tomas-de la Vega JE, Donahue EJ, Doolas A, et al. A ten year experience with hepatic resection. Surg Gynecol Obstet 1984, 159:223–228.
62. Nagashima A, Abe Y, Yamada S, et al. Long-term survival after surgical resection of liver metastasis from lung cancer. Jpn J Thorac Cardiovasc Surg 2004, 52:311–313.
63. Curley SA, Izzo F, Delrio P, et al. Radiofrequency ablation of unresectable primary and metastatic hepatic malignancies: results in 123 patients. Ann Surg 1999, 230:1–8.
64. Gillams AR, Lees WR. Radio-frequency ablation of colorectal liver metastases in 167 patients. Eur Radiol 2004, 14:2261–2267.
65. Solbiati L, Livraghi T, Goldberg SN, et al. Percutaneous radio-frequency ablation of hepatic metastases from colorectal cancer: long-term results in 117 patients. Radiology 2001, 221:159–166.
66. Abdalla EK, Vauthey JN, Ellis LM, et al. Recurrence and outcomes following hepatic resection, radiofrequency ablation, and combined resection/ablation for colorectal liver metastases. Ann Surg 2004, 239:818–825.

67. Berber E, Flesher N, Siperstein AE. Laparoscopic radiofrequency ablation of neuroendocrine liver metastases. World J Surg 2002, 26:985–990.
68. Gillams A, Cassoni A, Conway G, et al. Radiofrequency ablation of neuroendocrine liver metastases: the Middlesex experience. Abdom Imaging 2005, 30:435–441.
69. Jakobs TF, Hoffmann RT, Trumm C, et al. Radiofrequency ablation of colorectal liver metastases: mid-term results in 68 patients. Anticancer Res 2006, 26:671–680.
70. Lencioni R, Crocetti L, Cioni D, et al. Percutaneous radiofrequency ablation of hepatic colorectal metastases: technique, indications, results, and new promises. Invest Radiol 2004, 39:689–697.
71. Pawlik TM, Izzo F, Cohen DS, et al. Combined resection and radiofrequency ablation for advanced hepatic malignancies: results in 172 patients. Ann Surg Oncol 2003, 10:1059–1069.
72. Siperstein AE, Berber E. Cryoablation, percutaneous alcohol injection, and radiofrequency ablation for treatment of neuroendocrine liver metastases. World J Surg 2001, 25:693–696.
73. Abraham J, Fojo T, Wood BJ. Radiofrequency ablation of metastatic lesions in adrenocortical cancer. Ann Intern Med 2000, 133:312–313.
74. Livraghi T, Goldberg SN, Solbiati L, et al. Percutaneous radio-frequency ablation of liver metastases from breast cancer: initial experience in 24 patients. Radiology 2001, 220:145–149.
75. Curley SA. Radiofrequency ablation of malignant liver tumors. Oncologist 2001, 6:14–23.
76. Dickson JA, Calderwood SK. Temperature range and selective sensitivity of tumors to hyperthermia: a critical review. Ann N Y Acad Sci 1980, 335:180–205.
77. Goldberg SN. Radiofrequency tumor ablation: principles and techniques. Eur J Ultrasound 2001, 13:129–147.
78. Aschoff AJ, Merkle EM, Wong V, et al. How does alteration of hepatic blood flow affect liver perfusion and radiofrequency-induced thermal lesion size in rabbit liver? J Magn Reson Imaging 2001, 13:57–63.
79. Chinn SB, Lee FT Jr, Kennedy GD, et al. Effect of vascular occlusion on radiofrequency ablation of the liver: results in a porcine model. AJR Am J Roentgenol 2001, 176:789–795.
80. Curley SA, Izzo F, Ellis LM, et al. Radiofrequency ablation of hepatocellular cancer in 110 patients with cirrhosis. Ann Surg 2000, 232:381–391.
81. Patterson EJ, Scudamore CH, Owen DA, et al. Radiofrequency ablation of porcine liver in vivo: effects of blood flow and treatment time on lesion size. Ann Surg 1998, 227:559–565.
82. Rossi S, Garbagnati F, De Francesco I, et al. Relationship between the shape and size of radiofrequency induced thermal lesions and hepatic vascularization. Tumori 1999, 85:128–132.
83. Aloia TA, Vauthey JN, Loyer EM, et al. Solitary colorectal liver metastasis: resection determines outcome. Arch Surg 2006, 141:460–466.
84. Amersi FF, McElrath-Garza A, Ahmad A, et al. Long-term survival after radiofrequency ablation of complex unresectable liver tumors. Arch Surg 2006, 141:581–587.
85. Berber E, Pelley R, Siperstein AE. Predictors of survival after radiofrequency thermal ablation of colorectal cancer metastases to the liver: a prospective study. J Clin Oncol 2005, 23:1358–1364.
86. van Duijnhoven FH, Jansen MC, Junggeburt JM, et al. Factors influencing the local failure rate of radiofrequency ablation of colorectal liver metastases. Ann Surg Oncol 2006, 13:651–658.
87. de Baere T, Elias D, Dromain C, et al. Radiofrequency ablation of 100 hepatic metastases with a mean follow-up of more than 1 year. AJR Am J Roentgenol 2000, 175:1619–1625.
88. Wood TF, Rose DM, Chung M, et al. Radiofrequency ablation of 231 unresectable hepatic tumors: indications, limitations, and complications. Ann Surg Oncol 2000, 7:593–600.

89. Buscarini E, Savoia A, Brambilla G, Radiofrequency thermal ablation of liver tumors. Eur Radiol 2005, 15:884–894.
90. Goldberg SN, Charboneau JW, Dodd GD 3rd, et al. Image-guided tumor ablation: proposal for standardization of terms and reporting criteria. Radiology 2003, 228:335–345.
91. Timmerman RD, Kavanagh BD, Cho LC, et al. Stereotactic body radiation therapy in multiple organ sites. J Clin Oncol 2007, 25:947–952.
92. Fowler JF. The linear-quadratic formula and progress in fractionated radiotherapy. Br J Radiol 1989, 62:679–694.
93. Blomgren H, Lax I, Naslund I, et al. Stereotactic high dose fraction radiation therapy of extracranial tumors using an accelerator. Clinical experience of the first thirty-one patients. Acta Oncol 1995, 34:861–870.
94. Herfarth KK, Debus J, Lohr F, et al. Stereotactic single-dose radiation therapy of liver tumors: results of a phase I/II trial. J Clin Oncol 2001, 19:164–170.
95. Wulf J, Hadinger U, Oppitz U, et al. Stereotactic radiotherapy of targets in the lung and liver. Strahlenther Onkol 2001, 177:645–655.
96. Wulf J, Guckenberger M, Haedinger U, et al. Stereotactic radiotherapy of primary liver cancer and hepatic metastases. Acta Oncol 2006, 45:838–847.
97. Schefter TE, Kavanagh BD, Timmerman RD, et al. A phase I trial of stereotactic body radiation therapy for liver metastases. Int J Radiat Oncol Biol Phys 2005, 62:1371–1378.
98. Kavanagh BD, Schefter TE, Cardenes HR, et al. Interim analysis of a prospective phase I/II trial of SBRT for liver metastases. Acta Oncol 2006, 45:848–855.
99. Divis G. Einbertrag zur operativen, Behandlung der Lungengeschuuilste. Acta Chir Scand 1927, 62:329.
100. Kondo H, Okumura T, Ohde Y, et al. Surgical treatment for metastatic malignancies. Pulmonary metastasis: indications and outcomes. Int J Clin Oncol 2005, 10:81–85.
101. Pfannschmidt J, Klode J, Muley T, et al. Nodal involvement at the time of pulmonary metastasectomy: experiences in 245 patients. Ann Thorac Surg 2006, 81:448–454.
102. Pastorino U, Buyse M, Friedel G, et al. Long-term results of lung metastasectomy: prognostic analyses based on 5206 cases. The International Registry of Lung Metastases. J Thorac Cardiovasc Surg 1997, 113:37–49.
103. Robert JH, Ambrogi V, Mermillod B, et al. Factors influencing long-term survival after lung metastasectomy. Ann Thorac Surg 1997, 63:777–784.
104. Mason RJ, Nadel JA, eds. Textbook of Respiratory Medicine. 4th edition. Philadelphia: Elsevier Saunders, 2005.
105. Thomford NR, Woolner LB, Clagett OT. The surgical treatment of metastatic tumors in the lungs. J Thorac Cardiovasc Surg 1965, 49:357–363.
106. Ketchedjian A, Daly B, Luketich J, et al. Minimally invasive techniques for managing pulmonary metastases: video-assisted thoracic surgery and radiofrequency ablation. Thorac Surg Clin 2006, 16:157–165.
107. Pastorino U, Buyse M, Friedel G, et al. Long-term results of lung metastasectomy: prognostic analyses bascd on 5206 cases. AATS/WTSA, 1997.
108. McCormack PM, Attiyeh FF. Resected pulmonary metastases from colorectal cancer. Dis Colon Rectum 1979, 22:553–556.
109. Okumura S, Kondo H, Tsuboi M, et al. Pulmonary resection for metastatic colorectal cancer: experiences with 159 patients. J Thorac Cardiovasc Surg 1996, 112:867–874.
110. Saito Y, Omiya H, Kohno K, et al. Pulmonary metastasectomy for 165 patients with colorectal carcinoma: A prognostic assessment. J Thorac Cardiovasc Surg 2002, 124:1007–1013.
111. Cerfolio RJ, Allen MS, Deschamps C, et al. Pulmonary resection of metastatic renal cell carcinoma. Ann Thorac Surg 1994, 57:339–344.
112. Piltz S, Meimarakis G, Wichmann MW, et al. Long-term results after pulmonary resection of renal cell carcinoma metastases. Ann Thorac Surg 2002, 73:1082–1087.

113. Anraku M, Yokoi K, Nakagawa K, et al. Pulmonary metastases from uterine malignancies: results of surgical resection in 133 patients. J Thorac Cardiovasc Surg 2004, 127:1107–1112.
114. Liu D, Labow DM, Dang N, et al. Pulmonary metastasectomy for head and neck cancers. Ann Surg Oncol 1999, 6:572–578.
115. Fukuse T, Hirata T, Tanaka F, et al. Prognosis of ipsilateral intrapulmonary metastases in resected nonsmall cell lung cancer. Eur J Cardiothorac Surg 1997, 12:218–223.
116. Okada M, Tsubota N, Yoshimura M, et al. Evaluation of TMN classification for lung carcinoma with ipsilateral intrapulmonary metastasis. Ann Thorac Surg 1999, 68:326–330.
117. Nagai K, Sohara Y, Tsuchiya R, et al. Prognosis of resected non-small cell lung cancer patients with intrapulmonary metastases. J Thorac Oncol 2007, 2:282–286.
118. Ahrar K, Price RE, Wallace MJ, et al. Percutaneous radiofrequency ablation of lung tumors in a large animal model. J Vasc Interv Radiol 2003, 14:1037–1043.
119. Ahmed M, Liu Z, Afzal KS, et al. Radiofrequency ablation: effect of surrounding tissue composition on coagulation necrosis in a canine tumor model. Radiology 2004, 230:761–767.
120. Miao Y, Ni Y, Bosmans H, et al. Radiofrequency ablation for eradication of pulmonary tumor in rabbits. J Surg Res 2001, 99:265–271.
121. Goldberg SN, Gazelle GS, Compton CC, et al. Radiofrequency tissue ablation in the rabbit lung: efficacy and complications. Acad Radiol 1995, 2:776–784.
122. Yasui K, Kanazawa S, Sano Y, et al. Thoracic tumors treated with CT-guided radiofrequency ablation: initial experience. Radiology 2004, 231:850–857.
123. Yan TD, King J, Ebrahimi A, et al. Hepatectomy and lung radiofrequency ablation for hepatic and subsequent pulmonary metastases from colorectal carcinoma. J Surg Oncol 2007, 96:367–373.
124. Yan TD, King J, Sjarif A, et al. Percutaneous radiofrequency ablation of pulmonary metastases from colorectal carcinoma: prognostic determinants for survival. Ann Surg Oncol 2006, 13:1529–1537.
125. Yan TD, King J, Sjarif A, et al. Treatment failure after percutaneous radiofrequency ablation for nonsurgical candidates with pulmonary metastases from colorectal carcinoma. Ann Surg Oncol 2007, 14:1718–1726.
126. Yamakado K, Hase S, Matsuoka T, et al. Radiofrequency ablation for the treatment of unresectable lung metastases in patients with colorectal cancer: a multicenter study in Japan. J Vasc Interv Radiol 2007, 18:393–398.
127. Vogl TJ, Straub R, Lehnert T, et al. Percutaneous thermoablation of pulmonary metastases. Experience with the application of laser-induced thermotherapy and radiofrequency ablation, and a literature review. Rofo 2004, 176:1658–1666.
128. Steinke K, Glenn D, King J, et al. Percutaneous imaging-guided radiofrequency ablation in patients with colorectal pulmonary metastases: 1-year follow-up. Ann Surg Oncol 2004, 11:207–212.
129. King J, Glenn D, Clark W, et al. Percutaneous radiofrequency ablation of pulmonary metastases in patients with colorectal cancer. Br J Surg 2004, 91:217–223.
130. Simon CJ, Dupuy DE, DiPetrillo TA, et al. Pulmonary radiofrequency ablation: long-term safety and efficacy in 153 patients. Radiology 2007, 243:268–275.
131. Lagana D, Carrafiello G, Mangini M, et al. Radiofrequency ablation of primary and metastatic lung tumors: preliminary experience with a single center device. Surg Endosc 2006, 20:1262–1267.
132. Kishi K, Nakamura H, Kobayashi K, et al. Percutaneous CT-guided radiofrequency ablation of pulmonary malignant tumors: preliminary report. Intern Med 2006, 45:65–72.
133. Rossi S, Dore R, Cascina A, et al. Percutaneous computed tomography-guided radiofrequency thermal ablation of small unresectable lung tumours. Eur Respir J 2006, 27:556–563.

134. Thanos L, Mylona S, Pomoni M, et al. Percutaneous radiofrequency thermal ablation of primary and metastatic lung tumors. Eur J Cardiothorac Surg 2006, 30:797–800.
135. Ambrogi MC, Lucchi M, Dini P, et al. Percutaneous radiofrequency ablation of lung tumours: results in the mid-term. Eur J Cardiothorac Surg 2006, 30:177–183.
136. Akeboshi M, Yamakado K, Nakatsuka A, Percutaneous radiofrequency ablation of lung neoplasms: initial therapeutic response. J Vasc Interv Radiol 2004, 15:463–470.
137. Lee JM, Jin GY, Goldberg SN, et al. Percutaneous radiofrequency ablation for inoperable non-small cell lung cancer and metastases: preliminary report. Radiology 2004, 230:125–134.
138. Hiraki T, Sakurai J, Tsuda T, et al. Risk factors for local progression after percutaneous radiofrequency ablation of lung tumors: evaluation based on a preliminary review of 342 tumors. Cancer 2006, 107:2873–2880.
139. Nguyen CL, Scott WJ, Young NA, et al. Radiofrequency ablation of primary lung cancer: results from an ablate and resect pilot study. Chest 2005, 128:3507–3511.
140. Nomori H, Imazu Y, Watanabe K, et al. Radiofrequency ablation of pulmonary tumors and normal lung tissue in swine and rabbits. Chest 2005, 127:973–977.
141. Iguchi T, Hiraki T, Gobara H, et al. Percutaneous radiofrequency ablation of lung tumors close to the heart or aorta: evaluation of safety and effectiveness. J Vasc Interv Radiol 2007, 18:733–740.
142. Steinke K, Haghighi KS, Wulf S, et al. Effect of vessel diameter on the creation of ovine lung radiofrequency lesions in vivo: preliminary results. J Surg Res 2005, 124:85–91.
143. Yamamoto A, Nakamura K, Matsuoka T, et al. Radiofrequency ablation in a porcine lung model: correlation between CT and histopathologic findings. AJR Am J Roentgenol 2005, 185:1299–1306.
144. Tominaga J, Miyachi H, Takase K, et al. Time-related changes in computed tomographic appearance and pathologic findings after radiofrequency ablation of the rabbit lung: preliminary experimental study. J Vasc Interv Radiol 2005, 16:1719–1726.
145. Bojarski JD, Dupuy DE, Mayo-Smith WW. CT imaging findings of pulmonary neoplasms after treatment with radiofrequency ablation: results in 32 tumors. AJR Am J Roentgenol 2005, 185:466–471.
146. Gillams AR, Lees WR. Analysis of the factors associated with radiofrequency ablation-induced pneumothorax. Clin Radiol 2007, 62:639–644.
147. Hiraki T, Tajiri N, Mimura H, et al. Pneumothorax, pleural effusion, and chest tube placement after radiofrequency ablation of lung tumors: incidence and risk factors. Radiology 2006, 241:275–283.
148. Yamagami T, Kato T, Hirota T, et al. Pneumothorax as a complication of percutaneous radiofrequency ablation for lung neoplasms. J Vasc Interv Radiol 2006, 17:1625–1629.
149. Sano Y, Kanazawa S, Gobara H, et al. Feasibility of percutaneous radiofrequency ablation for intrathoracic malignancies: a large single-center experience. Cancer 2007, 109:1397–1405.
150. Ng K, Yan TD, Zhu JC, et al. Percutaneous radiofrequency ablation of lung tumours: prognostic risk factors for local progression. ANZ J Surg 2007, 77:A89.
151. Timmerman R, Papiez L, McGarry R, et al. Extracranial stereotactic radioablation: results of a phase I study in medically inoperable stage I non-small cell lung cancer. Chest 2003, 124:1946–1955.
152. McGarry RC, Papiez L, Williams M, et al. Stereotactic body radiation therapy of early-stage non-small-cell lung carcinoma: phase I study. Int J Radiat Oncol Biol Phys 2005, 63:1010–1015.
153. Timmerman R, McGarry R, Yiannoutsos C, et al. Excessive toxicity when treating central tumors in a phase II study of stereotactic body radiation therapy for medically inoperable early-stage lung cancer. J Clin Oncol 2006, 24:4833–4839.
154. Baumann P, Nyman J, Lax I, et al. Factors important for efficacy of stereotactic body radiotherapy of medically inoperable stage I lung cancer. A retrospective analysis of patients treated in the Nordic countries. Acta Oncol 2006 45:787–795.

155. Fritz P, Kraus HJ, Muhlnickel W, et al. Stereotactic, single-dose irradiation of stage I non-small cell lung cancer and lung metastases. Radiat Oncol 2006, 1:30.
156. Hara R, Itami J, Kondo T, et al. Clinical outcomes of single-fraction stereotactic radiation therapy of lung tumors. Cancer 2006, 106:1347–1352.
157. Nagata Y, Takayama K, Matsuo Y, et al. Clinical outcomes of a phase I/II study of 48 Gy of stereotactic body radiotherapy in 4 fractions for primary lung cancer using a stereotactic body frame. Int J Radiat Oncol Biol Phys 2005, 63:1427–1431.
158. Nyman J, Johansson KA, Hulten U. Stereotactic hypofractionated radiotherapy for stage I non-small cell lung cancer–mature results for medically inoperable patients. Lung Cancer 2006, 51:97–103.
159. Xia T, Li H, Sun Q, et al. Promising clinical outcome of stereotactic body radiation therapy for patients with inoperable Stage I/II non-small-cell lung cancer. Int J Radiat Oncol Biol Phys 2006, 66:117–125.
160. Zimmermann FB, Geinitz H, Schill S, et al. Stereotactic hypofractionated radiation therapy for stage I non-small cell lung cancer. Lung Cancer 2005, 48:107–114.
161. Nagata Y, Negoro Y, Aoki T, et al. Clinical outcomes of 3D conformal hypofractionated single high-dose radiotherapy for one or two lung tumors using a stereotactic body frame. Int J Radiat Oncol Biol Phys 2002, 52:1041–1046.
162. Okunieff P, Petersen AL, Philip A, et al. Stereotactic body radiation therapy for lung metastases. Acta Oncol 2006, 45:808–817.
163. Yoon SM, Choi EK, Lee SW, et al. Clinical results of stereotactic body frame based fractionated radiation therapy for primary or metastatic thoracic tumors. Acta Oncologica 2006, 45:1108–1114.
164. Nakagawa K, Aoki Y, Tago M, et al. Megavoltage CT-assisted stereotactic radiosurgery for thoracic tumors: original research in the treatment of thoracic neoplasms. Int J Radiat Oncol Biol Phys 2000, 48:449–457.
165. Jeremic B, Shibamoto Y, Nikolic N, et al. Role of radiation therapy in the combined-modality treatment of patients with extensive disease small-cell lung cancer: A randomized study. J Clin Oncol 1999, 17:2092–2099.
166. Brincker H, Hindberg J, Hansen PV. Cyclic alternating polychemotherapy with or without upper and lower half-body irradiation in small cell anaplastic lung cancer. A randomized study. Eur J Cancer Clin Oncol 1987, 23:205–211.
167. Lebeau B, Chastang C, Brechot JM, et al. A randomized trial of delayed thoracic radiotherapy in complete responder patients with small-cell lung cancer. Chest 1993, 104:726–733.
168. Nou E, Brodin O, Bergh J. A randomized study of radiation treatment in small cell bronchial carcinoma treated with two types of four-drug chemotherapy regimens. Cancer 1988, 62:1079–1090.
169. Stanley KE. Prognostic factors for survival in patients with inoperable lung cancer. J Natl Cancer Inst 1980, 65:25–32.
170. Hirano Y, Oda M, Tsunezuka Y, et al. Long-term survival cases of lung cancer presented as solitary bone metastasis. Ann Thorac Cardiovasc Surg 2005, 11:401–404.
171. Tong D, Gillick L, Hendrickson FR. The palliation of symptomatic osseous metastases: final results of the study by the Radiation Therapy Oncology Group. Cancer 1982, 50:893–899.
172. Blitzer PH. Reanalysis of the RTOG study of the palliation of symptomatic osseous metastasis. Cancer 1985, 55:1468–1472.
173. Steenland E, Leer JW, van Houwelingen H, et al. The effect of a single fraction compared to multiple fractions on painful bone metastases: a global analysis of the Dutch Bone Metastasis Study. Radiother Oncol 1999, 52:101–109.
174. van der Linden YM, Steenland E, van Houwelingen HC, et al. Patients with a favourable prognosis are equally palliated with single and multiple fraction radiotherapy: results on survival in the Dutch Bone Metastasis Study. Radiother Oncol 2006, 78:245–253.

175. Hartsell WF, Scott CB, Bruner DW, et al. Randomized trial of short- versus long-course radiotherapy for palliation of painful bone metastases. J Natl Cancer Inst 2005, 97:798–804.

176. Bone Pain Trial Working Party. 8 Gy single fraction radiotherapy for the treatment of metastatic skeletal pain: randomised comparison with a multifraction schedule over 12 months of patient follow-up. Radiother Oncol 1999, 52:111–121.

177. Roos DE, Turner SL, O'Brien PC, et al. Randomized trial of 8 Gy in 1 versus 20 Gy in 5 fractions of radiotherapy for neuropathic pain due to bone metastases (Trans-Tasman Radiation Oncology Group, TROG 96.05). Radiother Oncol 2005, 75:54–63.

178. Kaasa S, Brenne E, Lund JA, et al. Prospective randomised multicenter trial on single fraction radiotherapy (8 Gy x 1) versus multiple fractions (3 Gy x 10) in the treatment of painful bone metastases. Radiother Oncol 2006, 79:278–284.

179. Patchell RA, Tibbs PA, Regine WF, et al. Direct decompressive surgical resection in the treatment of spinal cord compression caused by metastatic cancer: a randomised trial. Lancet 2005, 366:643–648.

180. Hamilton AJ, Lulu BA, Fosmire H, et al. Preliminary clinical experience with linear accelerator-based spinal stereotactic radiosurgery. Neurosurg 1995, 36:311–319.

181. Benzil DL, Saboori M, Mogilner AY, et al. Safety and efficacy of stereotactic radiosurgery for tumors of the spine. J Neurosurg 2004, 101: 413–418.

182. Bilsky MH, Yamada Y, Yenice KM, et al. Intensity-modulated stereotactic radiotherapy of paraspinal tumors: a preliminary report. Neurosurg 2004, 54:823–830.

183. De Salles AA, Pedroso AG, Medin P, et al. Spinal lesions treated with Novalis shaped beam intensity-modulated radiosurgery and stereotactic radiotherapy. J Neurosurg 2004, 101:435–440.

184. Gerszten PC, Welch WC. Cyberknife radiosurgery for metastatic spine tumors. Neurosurg Clin N Am 2004, 15:491–501.

185. Medin PM, Solberg TD, De Salles AA, et al. Investigations of a minimally invasive method for treatment of spinal malignancies with LINAC stereotactic radiation therapy: accuracy and animal studies. Int J Radiat Oncol Biol Phys 2002, 52:1111–1122.

186. Milker-Zabel S, Zabel A, Thilmann C, et al. Clinical results of retreatment of vertebral bone metastases by stereotactic conformal radiotherapy and intensity-modulated radiotherapy. Int J Radiat Oncol Biol Phys 2003, 55:162–167.

187. Ryu S, Yin FF, Rock J, et al. Image-guided and intensity-modulated radiosurgery for patients with spinal metastasis. Cancer 2003, 97:2013–2018.

188. Ryu S, Rock J, Rosenblum M, et al. Patterns of failure after single-dose radiosurgery for spinal metastasis. J Neurosurg 2004, 101:402–405.

189. Ryu SI, Chang SD, Kim DH, et al. Image-guided hypo-fractionated stereotactic radiosurgery to spinal lesions. Neurosurg 2001, 49:838–846.

190. Yin FF, Ryu S, Ajlouni M, et al. Image-guided procedures for intensity-modulated spinal radiosurgery. Technical note. J Neurosurg 2004, 101:419–424.

191. Chang EL, Shiu AS, Mendel E, et al. Phase I/II study of stereotactic body radiotherapy for spinal metastasis and its pattern of failure. Spine 2007, 7:151–160.

192. Mussi A, Janni A, Pistolesi M, et al. Surgical treatment of primary lung cancer and solitary brain metastasis. Thorax 1985, 40:191–193.

193. Magilligan DJ Jr, Duvernoy C, Malik G, et al. Surgical approach to lung cancer with solitary cerebral metastasis: twenty-five years' experience. Ann Thorac Surg 1986, 42:360–364.

194. Rossi NP, Zavala DC, VanGilder JC. A combined surgical approach to non-oat-cell pulmonary carcinoma with single cerebral metastasis. Respiration 1987, 51:170–178.

195. Torre M, Quaini E, Chiesa G, et al. Synchronous brain metastasis from lung cancer. Result of surgical treatment in combined resection. J Thorac Cardiovasc Surg 1988, 95:994–997.

196. Macchiarini P, Buonaguidi R, Hardin M, et al. Results and prognostic factors of surgery in the management of non-small cell lung cancer with solitary brain metastasis. Cancer 1991, 68:300–304.

197. Burt M, Wronski M, Arbit E, et al. Resection of brain metastases from non-small-cell lung carcinoma. Results of therapy. Memorial Sloan-Kettering Cancer Center thoracic surgical staff. J Thorac Cardiovasc Surg 1992, 103:399–410.
198. Wronski M, Arbit E, Burt M, et al. Survival after surgical treatment of brain metastases from lung cancer: a follow-up study of 231 patients treated between 1976 and 1991. J Neurosurg 1995, 83:605–616.
199. Saitoh Y, Fujisawa T, Shiba M, et al. Prognostic factors in surgical treatment of solitary brain metastasis after resection of non-small-cell lung cancer. Lung Cancer 1999, 24:99–106.
200. Billing PS, Miller DL, Allen MS, et al. Surgical treatment of primary lung cancer with synchronous brain metastases. J Thorac Cardiovasc Surg 2001, 122:548–553.
201. Bonnette P, Puyo P, Gabriel C, et al. Surgical management of non-small cell lung cancer with synchronous brain metastases. Chest 2001, 119:1469–1475.
202. Herrera LJ, Fernando HC, Perry Y, et al. Radiofrequency ablation of pulmonary malignant tumors in nonsurgical candidates. J Thorac Cardiovasc Surg 2003, 125:929–937.
203. Kang S, Luo R, Liao W, et al. Single group study to evaluate the feasibility and complications of radiofrequency ablation and usefulness of post treatment position emission tomography in lung tumours. World J Surg Oncol 2004, 2:30.
204. VanSonnenberg E, Shankar S, Morrison PR, et al. Radiofrequency ablation of thoracic lesions: part 2, initial clinical experience: technical and multidisciplinary considerations in 30 patients. AJR Am J Roentgenol 2005, 184:381–390.
205. Gadaleta C, Catino A, Mattioli V. Radiofrequency thermal ablation in the treatment of lung malignancies. In Vivo 2006, 20:765–767.
206. Hoffmann RT, Jakobs TF, Lubienski A, et al. Percutaneous radiofrequency ablation of pulmonary tumors: Is there a difference between treatment under general anaesthesia and under conscious sedation? Eur J Radiol 2006, 59:168–174.
207. de Baere T, Palussiere J, Auperin A, et al. Midterm local efficacy and survival after radiofrequency ablation of lung tumors with minimum follow-up of 1 year: prospective evaluation. Radiology 2006, 240:587–596.
208. Blomgren H, Lax I, Göranson H, et al. Radiosurgery for tumors in the body: clinical experience using a new method. J Radiosurg 1998, 1:63–74.
209. Uematsu M, Shioda A, Tahara K, et al. Focal, high dose, and fractionated modified stereotactic radiation therapy for lung carcinoma patients: a preliminary experience. Cancer 1998, 82:1062–1070.

Systems Approach for Understanding Metastasis

Peter J. Woolf, Angel Alvarez, and Venkateshwar G. Keshamouni

Abstract A systems approach to analysis is based on the belief that the component parts of a system will act differently when isolated from its environment or other parts of the system. In other words, the whole is greater than the sum of its parts due to the relationship and the interaction between the parts. In biology, the goal of a systems approach is to understand the operation of complex biological systems by providing the missing link between molecules and physiology. Currently systems biology encompasses many different approaches with an ultimate aim of developing predictive models for complex human diseases including cancer. This chapter will highlight some of the tools and efforts of systems biology that are applied to cancer and will discuss how these efforts can be further extended to the much needed understanding and targeting of lung tumor metastasis.

Introduction

The traditional reductionist approach of studying the functions of individual genes one or a few at a time has been extremely fruitful in cancer biology in identifying oncogenes, tumor suppressors, and key molecular pathways regulated by them. This approach has led to the development of a conceptual framework, defined by six hallmarks, that govern cellular transformation and tumor development [1]. Despite considerable success of the reductionist approach, many fundamental questions in tumor biology remain unanswered, particularly how a tumor cell acquires the ability to metastasize and colonize a distant site is probably the most puzzling questions of cancer biology. Therefore, understanding the molecular mechanisms involved is an essential step in developing therapeutics against tumor metastasis, which is responsible for more than 90% of cancer-related mortality.

P.J. Woolf (✉)
Department of Chemical Engineering and Biomedical Engineering, University of Michigan, Ann Arbor, MI 48109, USA
e-mail: pwoolf@umich.edu

V. Keshamouni et al. (eds.), *Lung Cancer Metastasis*,
DOI 10.1007/978-1-4419-0772-1_17, © Springer Science+Business Media, LLC 2009

Development of various "omic" technologies has led to the identification and quantitation of large lists of genes, proteins, miRNAs, and metabolites that are modulated during cellular transformation, tumor growth, and metastasis. However, this has not led to the proportionate increase in understanding of the underlying mechanisms. It is now well recognized that many of these molecules and the linear signaling pathways derived from them do not function in isolation but interact with other pathways and molecules forming robust functional modules [2]. Identifying such modules in the complex biological processes including tumor metastasis and understanding their behavior and function require a new holistic approach of systems biology. In other words, systems biology is a rational continuation of successful experimental biology initiated by the molecular biosciences [3, 4].

The systems approach is based on the belief that the whole is greater than the sum of its parts, due to the relationship and the interaction between the parts. The goal of systems biology is to understand the operation of complex biological systems from various hierarchical levels of pathways and networks that make up a complex biological system and to decipher how molecules of these

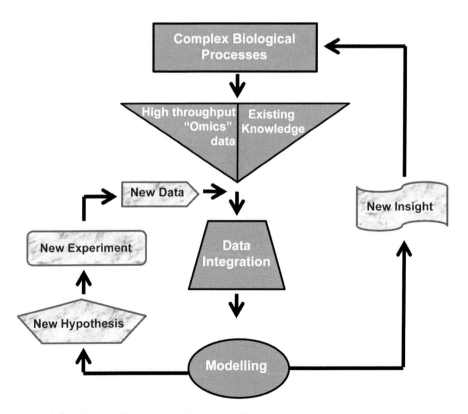

Fig. 1 A flowchart depicting a typical systems biology approach

pathways and networks jointly bring about cell behavior by cooperating in mechanisms [3, 4]. To achieve such a global view of tumor metastasis it is important to take an approach that systematically integrates various "omic" data sets and combines with the existing knowledge, thus accounting for both known and unknown while inferring new mechanistic insights (Fig. 1). Providing a systems level view of metastasis, we can also identify leverage points in the signaling and regulatory networks that represent promising drug targets against metastatic disease [5]. Such an effort involves sophisticated computational strategies and mathematical modeling [6].

Existing cellular and animal models even though provided major insights are not truly predictive of what will happen in vivo in human tumors [7]. This is mainly due to lack of a thorough understanding of how a particular pathway affects a given cellular phenotype and therefore not permitting us to make quantitative predictions about how specific changes to a pathway will influence cellular phenotype. Systems biology promises to bridge this gap by computing mechanistic and dynamic simulations of cancer cells. With these models, we would be able to conduct in silico experiments that could address complicated mechanistic questions [7]. In this chapter, we will describe the data sources and tools used in systems biology, provide examples of how these tools are applied for better understanding of cancer biology, and discuss their potential application in gaining mechanistic insights into the process of metastasis. The goal is to provide a qualitative overview of the methods used without getting lost in the details of the modeling tools.

Data Sources for Systems Biology

Systems biology scale data for cancer research can be divided into two broad categories: observational and relational data. Broadly speaking, observational data describe "what is happening," while relational data describe "what could happen." Examples of observational data include gene expression profiles, measurements of protein concentration, metabolomic measurements, and imaging. All of these measurements provide information about the current state of the cell. In contrast, relational data such as protein–protein interaction maps, pathway networks, transcription networks, and metabolic networks provide relational data about the cell. Sometimes observational and relational data can be similar, for example, an immunoassay on a cell may indicate that in a particular cell, proteins A and B are in a complex, while a protein-binding network suggests that two proteins can form a complex. As this case illustrates, nearly all relational data are derived from observational data.

Why do we bother to distinguish between observational and relational data in systems biology? The central reason is that relational data are generally richer and more widely available, but are not able to predict observational data. In the context of developing cancer therapies, knowing the relational structure or topology of a signaling pathway is only marginally useful without the associated observational data that would allow one to identify key regulators. In a modeling context, relational data provide a model structure, while observational data provide the parameters that make the model quantitative.

A key goal of systems biology in cancer research is developing techniques to merge observational and relational data to make mechanistically sound predictions. Developing these tools, however, is hampered by a number of problems. First, the data sources are sparse. With the possible exception of gene expression profiling, no current observational assay captures the full set of species that govern cellular behavior. Worse, most observational data are sampled infrequently from a small number of experiments. The situation is similar for relational data. Although we have significant repositories of protein–protein–binding data (e.g., BIND [www.bind.ca], MIMI [mimi.ncibi.org]) and pathway maps (e.g., KEGG [http://www.genome.jp/kegg/]), these sources of relational data represent only a fraction of the suspected interactions. A second challenge is the noisiness of the data. Biological assays are notoriously error prone and sample-to-sample variation is high. Ideally we could circumvent this noise by taking more samples, but as noted above large data sets are the exception rather than the rule.

Modeling Tools for Systems Biology

The first step in creating a systems level model for a complex process such as tumorigenesis is to qualitatively define what kind of model is desired. Each class of model varies in its ease of creation, detail of its approximation to reality, and generalizability. The models used in systems biology can be broadly distinguished along the following lines:

Deterministic vs. Stochastic: Deterministic models make predictions that do not change if run many times from the same starting position, while stochastic models assume some level of intrinsic noise and as such will give variable outcomes if run repeatedly. In general, stochastic models are more realistic; however, when analyzing large numbers of elements, such as the number of sodium ions in a cell, deterministic and stochastic models tend to converge.

Linear vs. Nonlinear: Linear models assume that variables change in proportion to each other, while nonlinear models can allow more complex behaviors such as switches, saturating responses, and biphasic profiles, for example.

Static vs. Dynamic: Static models describe relationships between variables measured at the same time, while dynamic models describe relationships between variables measured across time. As an example, models that associate biomarkers with tumor type are static, while models that describe tumor growth through time are dynamic.

Discrete vs. Continuous: Discrete models describe the entities in a variable as non-divisible bodies, while continuous models describe the variables as quantities that can continuously vary. As an example, a tumor model that describes the population dynamics of a tumor stem cell would allow the stem cell number to only take integer values $(0,1,2,\ldots)$, thereby not allowing one to have 2.654 stem cells. In contrast, a model of a signaling pathway in a cancer stem cell may describe the concentration of a signaling protein such as MAPK as a continuous value, such as 3.545. Although we know that molecular entities are discrete, continuous models are able to provide a good description of their behavior when the molecules are at sufficiently high concentration (>1000/cell).

Spatial vs. Non-spatial: Spatial models account for the positions and shapes of the system, while non-spatial models assume that everything in the system has equal access to everything else. Some problems such as tumor morphogenesis, tumor vascularization, and metastatic invasion are inherently spatial, while other domains such as signal transduction and gene regulatory cascades are often modeled as non-spatial. Although spatial models are intrinsically more accurate (everything has a three-dimensional position), spatial models are significantly more computationally demanding and in general require a deeper understanding of the biophysical properties of the environment to accurately model.

In the following sections, we will discuss four of the most commonly used systems biology modeling tools and provide examples of how they have been used to illuminate aspects of cancer biology and clinical treatment. Broadly, the first two methods focus on differential equation-based models, while the last two methods focus on Bayesian techniques. Other methods such as classical statistical methods ([8, 2] + many others) and Boolean models such as are described in [3] and [9] are also used but will not be discussed in this chapter.

Ordinary Differential Equations (Deterministic, Linear or Nonlinear, Dynamic, Continuous)

One of the most common model types used in systems biology consists of ordinary differential equations. These calculus-based models describe how each variable changes with time due to changes in inputs (flows into or production) and outputs (flows out, degradation, and reactions). Because these models are cast in the language of differential equations, they can be analyzed using a large body of theory and computational tools already developed for use in other fields.

As an example, recent work by Hornberg et al. [10] produced a mechanistically realistic model of the epidermal growth factor-induced mitogen-activated protein kinase network. The work was motivated by the desire to determine which signaling elements in this pathway are responsible for cell growth in oncogenesis. The underlying model consisted of 148 reactions between 103 different signaling species. In analyzing this model, the authors found that the signal transduction pathways that mediate oncogenesis are integrated in a non-random way and show particular sensitivity to well-known oncogenes such as Raf. Models such as these have the advantage that they are sufficiently mechanistically realistic that they can accurately predict the impact of gene mutations and changes in gene expression.

Although there are many examples of differential equation models available, this modeling approach suffers from two limitations. First, construction of these models is generally done by hand based on expert knowledge. Hand construction of these models intrinsically limits their size and makes their update challenging as it requires people who are intimately familiar with the model to maintain the model. Second, differential equation models have many parameters that are difficult to determine from experimental data. In the future, more higher quality data will help alleviate problems with these parameters, but subtler problems such as model equivalence and inherently non-decomposable parameter sets will still pose challenges.

Stochastic Differential Equations (Stochastic, Nonlinear, Dynamic, Continuous)

Stochastic differential equations are similar to ordinary differential equation models described above, except that these models allow us to model uncertainty in each variable. While these models are more complex to state, they more accurately reflect uncertainty about the underlying process.

An example of a stochastic model is the Dayananda model for prostate-specific antigen (PSA) change following radiotherapy [11]. Using such a model, one can simulate the time trajectory of PSA to test the effect of different therapeutic options. Unfortunately, due to the complexity of stochastic differential equation models, they are rarely used to model a large number of variables at this time.

Bayesian Networks (Stochastic, Nonlinear, Static, Discrete)

Three features of Bayesian networks (BNs) make them well suited for modeling complex diseases such as tumor metastasis: (1) BNs make quantitative predictions; (2) BNs are human interpreand (3) BNs are robust to noise and nonlinear inputs used for cancer diagnosis and mechanism inference. Once a Bayesian network model is made, it is possible to make quantitative predictions about the outcome of each variable. These predictions can be applied to both discrete variables (e.g., alive or dead) and continuous variables (e.g., gene expression data or clinical measures). Using either approximate or exact inference algorithms, we can fill in missing data or make temporal predictions about how a patient will respond to a particular treatment. The quantitative predictions produced by a Bayesian network have the added advantage that they automatically provide error estimates on the predictions in the form of probability distributions and are directly comparable to experimental data.

A second attractive feature of Bayesian networks is that the resulting graph structures are in an intuitive, graphical form. Graph visualization tools such as Cytoscape [12] or GraphViz [13] allow users to display a Bayesian network or compilation of multiple Bayesian networks in a way that is similar to the biochemical reaction diagrams and therefore familiar to biologists and clinicians. The ability to intuitively communicate the results of a model to researchers, clinicians, and patients is important as it allows all of the stakeholders to participate in any decision made based on the information.

A third feature of Bayesian networks is their robustness to noise and nonlinear inputs. Clinical data often contain significant noise or uncertainty. This noise makes analysis difficult for both the human mind and a wide variety of modeling approaches. However, because Bayesian networks are fundamentally probabilistic, they are well suited to handle noise and sometimes contradictory data in a rational and systematic way. This probabilistic feature also generates models that are relatively agnostic to the complexity of the relationships predicted. For example, a Bayesian network can model linear, nonlinear, or more complicated multi-state relationships equally well. The reason for this flexibility is that the approach does not assume an underlying analytical function to interrelate the data.

In a research context, a Bayesian analysis has an advantage that it is a compact, porand interactive method of communicating a complex set of relationships between variables based on both experimental data and opinion. Such networks can be scrutinized and interpreted in a consistent way.

In both clinical and research contexts in cancer research, Bayesian networks have been used to assist in two areas of (1) biomarker prediction and (2) disease mechanism inference. Below we will discuss each of these areas in turn with examples of how they have been used in understanding the systems biology of oncogenesis.

Bayesian Network Cancer Diagnosis Classifiers

Static Bayesian network engines for disease diagnosis have a long history of fruitful application to medicine [9–11]. As an example, recent work in the area of breast cancer diagnosis from mammograms [14] merges information from literature and expert knowledge. In this work, the authors hand create a Bayesian network to identify individualized risk factors from the appearance of microcalcifications in mammography (BI-RADS – Breast Imaging Reporting and Data System) to retrospectively evaluate whether a Bayesian network can infer patient's probability of breast cancer. Using this approach, the authors find that the automated Bayesian diagnosis is as accurate as a human mammographer trained in the area. In another breast cancer study, Cruz-Ramirez et al. [15] use a Bayesian network learning approach to identify which histological features from a breast biopsy are most predictive of clinical

Fig. 2 A Bayesian network representing a joint probability distribution of 11 variables associated with the prognosis in breast cancer. Figure modified from the work of Cruz-Ramirez et al. [15]. In this figure, the outcome node has only two values: benign or malignant breast cancer. Age was set to have one of three possible values based on patients' age segregation. The remaining variables are binned based on expert classification as absent or present

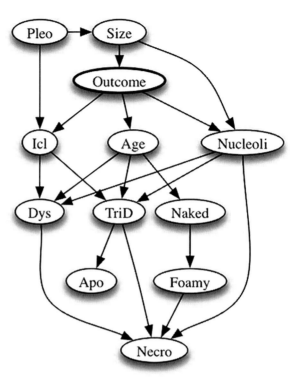

outcome. The Bayesian networks the authors produce, such as is shown in Fig. 2, provide a useful tool to represent these relationships in a compact and easily interpreted way. The authors also used a Bayesian network approach to evaluate the consistency in prognosis made by experts using data sampled from the network.

An important characteristic that makes Bayesian networks attractive to cancer biology researchers is the network's ability to use expert opinion and literature knowledge to impose constraints to the graph learning process. This intelligent constraint ensures that known, important relationships are accounted for in learning the final model. As an example of the role of prior information, Antal et al. [16] showed that Bayesian networks generated with no prior knowledge provide an accurate representation of what is expected based on textual and expert prior information. During their analysis they showed the good performance of Bayesian networks in the classification of ovarian tumors using only clinical data for the network generation. Also, they observed that this performance improved significantly when text and expert knowledge is provided as prior. Utilizing a similar approach of integrating histopathological data, gene and protein expression signatures (comparing primary vs. corresponding metastatic tumor) with existing knowledge of pathways, genes implicated in the process of metastasis, and other clinical parameters, in future, one can probably be able to predict whether a particular primary tumor leads to the metastatic spread of the disease.

Bayesian Networks for Cancer Mechanism Inference

A second application of Bayesian networks in cancer research is to integrate large data sets together to identify molecular mechanisms for disease. Data resources such as gene expression arrays, high throughput proteomic measurements, and pathology imaging databases represent rich sources for information to identify the causes and mechanisms of complex diseases such as cancer. However, merging these data resources is challenging due to the noise, sparsity, and ambiguity of the data. Fortunately, Bayesian networks are able to overcome many of these problems of data integration to yield a more complete view of these data. Excellent overviews describing the use of Bayesian networks in this data integration problem can be found elsewhere [15–17].

One common problem is the integration of multiple kinds of data to yield a predictive model. As an example, Sachs et al. [18] used a Bayesian network approach to integrate multiple data types describing T-cell signaling to create a predictive model. The data included proteomic measurements on single cells under a wide range of known pharmacological interventions. By merging both the proteomic measurements and the knowledge of the targets of the interventions, the authors were able to construct a Bayesian model that recapitulates much of the known signaling pathway from data alone. Subsequent analysis of this same data found that Bayesian networks consistently outperformed competing method such as relevance networks and graphical Gaussian models in terms of model accuracy [17]. A second example of data integration is the work by Woolf et al. [20] on integrating protein phosphorylation data and stem cell differentiation states to produce a mechanistically relevant model of ES cell regulation. Similarly, work by Sachs et al. [18] has demonstrated that Bayesian models of proteomic data can faithfully reproduce aspects of ERK and FAK signaling. Such models can be easily extended to other signaling pathways and processes that are critical for tumor metastasis such as TGF-b-induced epithelial–mesenchymal transitions (EMT). During EMT, epithelial tumor cells undergo a phenotypic switch into a fibroblast-like morphology and lose their epithelial markers in order to acquire migratory and invasive abilities essential for metastasis (see Chapter 4). The cell culture models of EMT serve as in vitro correlates for the multistep, complex process of metastasis. Efforts are underway in our laboratories making quantitative measurements of gene, protein, miRNA, and metabolite expression and to integrate these data sets using Bayesian modeling tools. Our preliminary analysis of gene and protein expression during EMT identified post-transcriptional regulation of actin and cofilin expression, which play a critical role in actin-cytoskeletal remodeling during EMT [19].

Another area of interest for data integration in cancer research is the effect of drugs or metabolites on cellular behavior. For example, in 2005, Chang et al. [20] used a Bayesian network approach to integrate gene expression data and drug perturbations to identify biologically relevant drug signaling pathways and targets. Their work focused on gene expression changes in the NCI60 set of cell lines in response to a series of commonly used cancer drugs. Similarly, in 2003, Conti et al. [21] used a Bayesian network approach to relate a phenotypic outcome of colorectal polyps to diet, metabolite measurements, and lifestyle. These works demonstrate that Bayesian networks are able to bridge the gap between these different kinds of data to yield biologically meaningful results.

Dynamic Bayesian Networks (Stochastic, Nonlinear, Dynamic, Discrete)

Beyond analyzing static relationships between variables, Bayesian networks can also identify temporal patterns in clinical and molecular data. When used in this way, these networks are called dynamic Bayesian networks (DBNs) [24, 25]. DBNs represent a powerful method for analyzing noisy temporal data as occurs in human disease states and represent a possible solution to the shortfalls associated with the oversimplification of disease models that is often employed when analyzing time-varying data. In contrast to static Bayesian networks, a DBN engine captures time-varying clinical parameters and predicts a time course of both disease progression and the impact of clinical interventions. In addition, DBNs also allow for cyclic feedback between variables, allowing investigators to interpret identified connections between nodes as temporal causation. DBNs have been applied to bioinformatic analysis of gene expression data [26–28] and temporal neural signaling [22] and have generated insights that could not be obtained from static Bayesian analysis. DBN modeling was also recently used to understand visual field deterioration [23] and to integrate multi-patient clinical data [24].

Conclusions

Developing a systems level understanding of cancer will require a mixture of plentiful quantitative data and sophisticated computational approaches to synthesize those data. Current efforts to create these systems level models using differential equations or Bayesian networks represent a promising but still small step toward developing a complete understanding of the molecular events that cause a healthy cell to become a tumor and how a tumor cell acquires the ability to metastasize.

In the future, we may well find that we are able to accurately predict the impact of various treatments, but still not have a satisfying *understanding* of the mechanism that caused that response. We already see some of this lack of coherent understanding when examining the literature on major signaling pathways such as MAPK or EGF – much is known but with each discovery we find that these pathways are connected in more and more complex ways. If this future is true, then we will become increasingly reliant on the computational models that are able to integrate these numerous connections between pathways to guide future therapies and patient classification.

References

1. Hanahan, D. and R.A. Weinberg. The hallmarks of cancer. Cell *100*: 57–70, 2000.
2. Ge, H., A.J. Walhout, and M. Vidal. Integrating 'omic' information: a bridge between genomics and systems biology. Trends Genet *19*: 551–60, 2003.
3. Bruggeman, F.J., J.J. Hornberg, F.C. Boogerd, and H.V. Westerhoff. Introduction to systems biology. Exs *97*: 1–19, 2007.
4. Bruggeman, F.J. and H.V. Westerhoff. The nature of systems biology. Trends Microbiol *15*: 45–50, 2007.
5. Butcher, E.C., E.L. Berg, and E.J. Kunkel. Systems biology in drug discovery. Nat Biotechnol *22*: 1253–9, 2004.
6. Kitano, H. Computational systems biology. Nature *420*: 206–10, 2002.
7. Khalil, I.G. and C. Hill. Systems biology for cancer. Curr Opin Oncol *17*: 44–8, 2005.
8. Zhu, Y., H. Li, D.J. Miller, Z. Wang, J. Xuan, R. Clarke, E.P. Hoffman, and Y. Wang. caBIG VISDA: modeling, visualization, and discovery for cluster analysis of genomic data. BMC Bioinformatics *9*: 383, 2008.
9. Zhang, R., M.V. Shah, J. Yang, S.B. Nyland, X. Liu, J.K. Yun, R. Albert, and T.P. Loughran, Jr. Network model of survival signaling in large granular lymphocyte leukemia. Proc Natl Acad Sci USA *105*: 16308–13, 2008.
10. Hornberg, J.J., B. Binder, F.J. Bruggeman, B. Schoeberl, R. Heinrich, and H.V. Westerhoff. Control of MAPK signalling: from complexity to what really matters. Oncogene *24*: 5533–42, 2005.
11. Dayananda, P.W., J.T. Kemper, and M.M. Shvartsman. A stochastic model for prostate-specific antigen levels. Math Biosci *190*: 113–26, 2004.
12. Shannon, P., A. Markiel, O. Ozier, N.S. Baliga, J.T. Wang, D. Ramage, N. Amin, B. Schwikowski, and T. Ideker. Cytoscape: a software environment for integrated models of biomolecular interaction networks. Genome Res *13*: 2498–504, 2003.
13. Gansner, E.R. and S.C. North. An open graph visualization system and its applications to software engineering. Software Practice and Experience *30*: 1203–33, 2000.
14. Burnside, E.S., D.L. Rubin, J.P. Fine, R.D. Shachter, G.A. Sisney, and W.K. Leung. Bayesian network to predict breast cancer risk of mammographic microcalcifications and reduce number of benign biopsy results: initial experience. Radiology *240*: 666–73, 2006.
15. Cruz-Ramirez, N., H.G. Acosta-Mesa, H. Carrillo-Calvet, L.A. Nava-Fernandez, and R.E. Barrientos-Martinez. Diagnosis of breast cancer using Bayesian networks: a case study. Comput Biol Med *37*: 1553–64, 2007.
16. Antal, P., G. Fannes, D. Timmerman, Y. Moreau, and B. De Moor. Using literature and data to learn Bayesian networks as clinical models of ovarian tumors. Artif Intell Med *30*: 257–81, 2004.
17. Werhli, A.V., M. Grzegorczyk, and D. Husmeier. Comparative evaluation of reverse engineering gene regulatory networks with relevance networks, graphical Gaussian models and Bayesian networks. Bioinformatics *22*: 2523–31, 2006.

18. Driscoll, T. and R. Mitchell. Fatal work injuries in New South Wales. N S W Public Health Bull *13*: 95–9, 2002.
19. Keshamouni, V.G., P. Jagtap, G. Michailidis, J.R. Strahler, R. Kuick, A.K. Reka, P. Papoulias, R. Krishnapuram, A. Srirangam, T.J. Standiford, P.C. Andrews, and G.S. Omenn. Temporal quantitative proteomics by iTRAQ 2D-LC-MS/MS and corresponding mRNA expression analysis identify post-transcriptional modulation of actin-cytoskeleton regulators during TGF-beta-Induced epithelial-mesenchymal transition. J Proteome Res *8*: 35–47, 2009.
20. Chang, J.H., K.B. Hwang, S.J. Oh, and B.T. Zhang. Bayesian network learning with feature abstraction for gene-drug dependency analysis. J Bioinform Comput Biol *3*: 61–77, 2005.
21. Conti, D.V., V. Cortessis, J. Molitor, and D.C. Thomas. Bayesian modeling of complex metabolic pathways. Hum Hered *56*: 83–93, 2003.
22. Smith, V.A., J. Yu, T.V. Smulders, A.J. Hartemink, and E.D. Jarvis. Computational inference of neural information flow networks. PLoS Comput Biol 2: e161, 2006.
23. Tucker, A., V. Vinciotti, X. Liu, and D. Garway-Heath. A spatio-temporal Bayesian network classifier for understanding visual field deterioration. Artif Intell Med *34*: 163–77, 2005.
24. Xiang, Z., R.M. Minter, X. Bi, P.J. Woolf, and Y. He. miniTUBA: medical inference by network integration of temporal data using Bayesian analysis. Bioinformatics *23*: 2423–32, 2007.
25. Dojer, N., A. Gambin, A. Mizera, B. Wilczynski, and J. Tiuryn. Applying dynamic Bayesian networks to perturbed gene expression data. BMC Bioinformatics 7: 249, 2006.
26. Li P., C. Zhang, E.J. Perkins, P. Gong, and Y. Deng. Comparison of probabilistic Boolean network and dynamic Bayesian network approaches for inferring gene regulatory networks. BMC Bioinformatics, *8* Suppl 7: S13, 2007.
27. Kim, S., S. Imoto, and S. Miyano. Dynamic Bayesian network and nonparametric regression for nonlinear modeling of gene networks from time series gene expression data. Biosystems, *75*(1-3): 57–65, 2004.
28. Kim, S.Y., Imoto, and S. Miyano. Inferring gene networks from time series microarray data using dynamic Bayesian networks. Brief Bioinform, *4*(3): 228–235, 2003.

Subject Index

A

AAH, *see* Atypical adenomatous hyperplasia

Abcg2-knockout mice, 51

Acquired immune system, 218

Actin-binding proteins, 101–102

Activated fibroblasts, 194, 201, 204

Active breathing control (ABC), 360

Acute myeloblastic leukemia, 32

Acute myeloid leukemia, 49

Acylphosphatase, 301

Adenocarcinomas (ACs), 6
- COX-2 expression in, 118–119
- CXCL10 production and, 160
- HABP2 and CRYM expression in, 206
- incidence of, 318
- lung A549, 77–78
- models of, 246, 256
- MTAP deletions in, 320
- myofibroblasts of, 198, 205
- phase-contrast and immunofluorescence microscopy of human lung, 73
- precursor lesions of, 8
- subtype, 7

Adenosine triphosphate-binding cassette, transporters family, 51

Adherens junctions, 98, 137

Adjuvant therapy, 42, 259, 260, 319, 321

Adrenal metastases, 356–357

Aging-associated changes, in gene expression, 200

AJ, *see* Adherens junctions

Akt kinase activity, 275

Albumin, 300, 301

Alkylating agent VNP40101M, 338

Alpha-1 anti-trypsin (AAT), 305

A549 lung adenocarcinoma cells
- culture, 97
- EMT process in, 77–78, 102
- tumor vascularity, 161

Alveolar macrophages (AMs), 118, 218, 230, 302

AML, *see* Acute myeloblastic leukemia

Amoeboid cells, 36

Amoeboid motility, 33

Amphiregulin, 198, 201

Amrubicin, 337, 338

Angiogenesis, 194, 200, 204, 224–225, 291
- angiogenic signal and, 137
- cell–matrix interaction importance in, 138
- factors regulating, 139
  - angiogenic and angiostatic mediators, 140
  - angiopoietin/TIE receptor–ligand system, 143–144
  - angiostatin, 142–143
  - CXC chemokines, 144
  - endostatin, 143
  - FGF, 141
  - FGF receptors, 141
  - VEGF, 141–142
  - VEGF receptors, 142
- inhibition in lung cancer metastasis, 144–146
- inhibition of, 136
- sequence of events in, 136
  - angiogenic signal, 137
  - cell migration, 137–138
  - cell proliferation, 138
  - ECPs, 139
  - endothelial detachment, 137
  - proteolysis, 137
  - tube formation, 138
  - vessel maturation, 138–139

Angiogenesis inhibitors, 38, 39

Angiogenic and angiostatic mediators, 140

Angiogenic chemokines, 155–158

Angiogenic ELR-containing chemokine ligands, 156

V. Keshamouni et al. (eds.), *Lung Cancer Metastasis*,
DOI 10.1007/978-1-4419-0772-1, © Springer Science+Business Media, LLC 2009